AEHLERT'S

EMT

BASIC

STUDY GUIDE

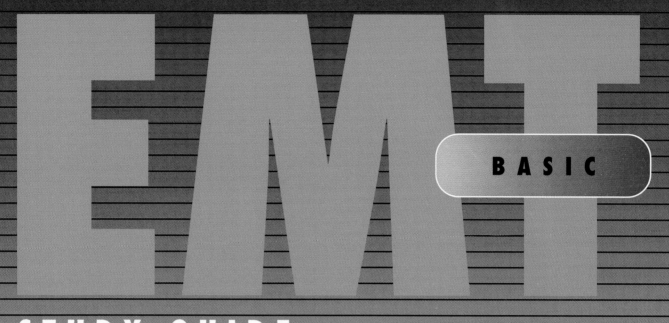

AEHLERT'S EMT BASIC STUDY GUIDE

BARBARA AEHLERT, RN

Southwest EMS Education
Glendale, Arizona

Questions and Answers by

GARRET OLSON, CEP

Mesa, Arizona

Photography by

Vincent Knaus

Chief Pat Bailey

and Greg Ruiz, CEP

Illustrations by

Kimberly M. Battista

and Graham T. Johnson

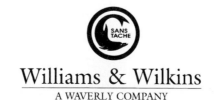

Williams & Wilkins
A WAVERLY COMPANY

BALTIMORE • PHILADELPHIA • LONDON • PARIS • BANGKOK
BUENOS AIRES • HONG KONG • MUNICH • SYDNEY • TOKYO • WROCLAW

Editor: Elizabeth A. Nieginski
Manager, Development Editing: Julie Scardiglia
Managing Editor: Darrin Kiessling
Marketing Manager: Christine Kushner
Development Editor: Kathleen Hunter Seogna, Rosanne Hallowell
Production Coordinator: Danielle Hagan
Text/Cover Designer: Karen S. Klinedinst
Typesetter: Maryland Composition Co., Inc.
Printer/Binder: Transcontinental

© 1998 Williams & Wilkins

351 West Camden Street
Baltimore, Maryland 21201-2436 USA

Rose Tree Corporate Center
1400 North Providence Road (Berne logo)
Building II, Suite 5025
Media, Pennsylvania 19063-2043 USA

Accurate indications, adverse reactions and dosage schedules for drugs are provided in this book, but it is possible that they may change. The reader is urged to review the package information data of the manufacturers of the medications mentioned.

Printed in Canada

First Edition,
Library of Congress Cataloging-in-Publication Data

Aehlert, Barbara.
   [EMT-basic study guide]
   Aehlert's EMT-basic study guide / Barbara Aehlert; questions and answers by Garret Olson; photography by Vincent Knaus, Chief Pat Bailey, and Greg Ruiz; illustrations by Kimberly M. Battista and Graham T. Johnson. — 1st ed.
      p.   cm.
   Includes index.
   ISBN 0–683–30217–5
   1. Emergency medicine—Outlines, syllabi, etc.   2. Emergency medical technicians—Outlines, syllabi, etc.   I. Title.
RC86.92.A35   1998
616.02′5′076—dc21   97–38043
                                                                   CIP

The publishers have made every effort to trace the copyright holders for borrowed material. If they have inadvertently overlooked any, they will be pleased to make the necessary arrangements at the first opportunity.

To purchase additional copies of this book, call our customer service department at **(800) 638-0672** or fax orders to **(800) 447-8438**. For other book services, including chapter reprints and large quantity sales, ask for the Special Sales department.

Canadian customers should call **(800) 665-1148**, or fax **(800) 665-0103**. For all other calls originating outside of the United States, please call **(410) 528-4223** or fax us at **(410) 528-8550**.

Visit Williams & Wilkins on the Internet: http://www.wwilkins.com or contact our customer service department at **custserv@wwilkins.com**. Williams & Wilkins customer service representatives are available from 8:30 am to 6:00 pm, EST, Monday through Friday, for telephone access.

98 99 00 01 02
1 2 3 4 5 6 7 8 9 10

For my mother,

Ronella Su Grisham

CONTENTS

ONE   PREPARATORY INFORMATION

FOUR MEDICAL, BEHAVIORAL, AND OBSTETRIC AND GYNECOLOGICAL EMERGENCIES

FIVE   TRAUMA

SIX   INFANTS AND CHILDREN

SEVEN   OPERATIONS

EIGHT   ADVANCED AIRWAY (ELECTIVE)

FOREWORD

by Ed Kalinowski

As the science of prehospital medical care continues to improve, the knowledge base for Emergency Medical Technician-Basics continues to grow. To absorb the critical information necessary in this demanding career, EMT-Basics need resources that are concise, yet comprehensive and up-to-date. *Aehlert's EMT-Basic Study Guide* is such a resource. Written in a style that provides the learner with quality knowledge in an easy-to-understand format, this guide allows learners to quickly access critical information and to understand the nuances of their profession. It provides both the core material EMT-Basics need to know as well as the enrichment material many instructors consider vital.

Barbara Aehlert truly understands prehospital emergency care. Her combined experience as both a provider and instructor in a number of prehospital arenas, her tenure as a director of emergency medical services, and her background in writing other popular books and instructional materials for prehospital providers and emergency care personnel, including EMT-Basics, is reflected in the depth, comprehensiveness, and user-friendly features of this study guide. Aehlert's ability to clearly communicate the body of knowledge essential for the EMT-Basic student demonstrates that she has her finger on the pulse of prehospital emergency medicine.

Edward J. Kalinowski, BSN, MEd, DrPH
Associate Professor, Kapiolani Community College
University of Hawaii
Honolulu, Hawaii

ABOUT THIS BOOK

Aehlert's EMT-Basic Study Guide, written in an easy-to-understand format, was created to provide the EMT-Basic with the essential information contained in the revised 1994 EMT-Basic National Standard Curriculum. It was also written to assist the EMT-Basic student in preparing for local, state, and national examinations.

The EMT-Basic student will find this text a useful reference throughout his or her education program. Certified EMT-Basics will also find this text a helpful tool in preparation for recertification or refresher training.

Each chapter opens with a list of objectives, followed by a brief "Motivation for Learning" section. This "Motivation for Learning" summarizes the importance of mastering the chapter content and explains how the EMT-Basic will use the material in daily practice. Each chapter is presented in outline format for quick reference and includes a self-test with an accompanying rationale for each answer. A comprehensive post-test is provided in Appendix B for further self-evaluation. Numerous photographs and line drawings enhance the information presented in the chapters.

As all EMT-Basics must take the certification examination and are recertified periodically, test-taking is an integral part of being an EMT-B. Therefore, this text includes a "Test-Taking Preparation" section, Appendix A. Written by Garret Olson, CEP, this appendix helps students create a game plan to assist them in preparing for the certification exam. Included in the appendix are a sample study schedule, test-taking strategies, and a preparation checklist.

Since publication of the EMT-Basic curriculum, the American Heart Association (AHA) guidelines have been updated in the 1994 Edition of the *Textbook of Advanced Cardiac Life Support*. Current information regarding use of the automated external defibrillator (AED) is reflected throughout this text.

It is our sincere hope that the reader will find *Aehlert's EMT-Basic Study Guide* a useful aid and reference. Your comments are welcome and will be used to determine material for future editions of this book.

AN IMPORTANT NOTE ABOUT ENRICHMENT MATERIAL

All cognitive objectives of the EMT-Basic National Standard Curriculum are covered in this text. Material not included in the new curriculum but deemed essential by the author—and other instructors nationwide—is also included (e.g., stroke, heart attack, chest, and abdominal injuries). Objectives that cover this supplemental material are marked with an icon (✳) and highlighted in blue to distinguish them from the curriculum objectives. In the text, sections that cover this material are clearly labeled "Enrichment."

ACKNOWLEDGMENTS

AUTHOR ACKNOWLEDGMENTS

Barbara Aehlert, RN

Many people were involved in the development and production of this text. I offer my sincere thanks to:

- Garret Olson for writing the material on test-taking tips and assuming the monumental task of writing the questions, answers, and rationales that appear in this text. I appreciate your long hours and willingness to keep pace with me as we worked together to meet our deadlines. Additional thanks for your assistance in coordinating the personnel and equipment for the photo shoot with the Mesa Fire Department.

- The City of Mesa Fire Department for generously providing the use of their personnel, vehicles, equipment, and facilities for many photographs in this text. A special thanks to Chief John Oliver; Chief Dennis Compton; Chief Gary Bradbury; Chief Rod Lilly; Captain Alex Fintner, Public Information Officer; Captain Joe Garcia; Keith Pyers, CEP; and Randy Schumacher, CEP.

- The City of Glendale Fire Department for providing personnel, vehicles, and equipment for photographs in this text. A special thanks to Chief Brooke Edwards; Chief Mike White, Ed Tirone, CEP; Captain Crystal Sorenson, CEP; and the crews of Engines 150 and 151.

- The City of Tempe Fire Department for graciously allowing the use of many of the scene photographs in this text, including one used for the cover. A special thanks to Chief Pat Bailey and Greg Ruiz, CEP, the photographers.

- Williams and Wilkins for providing an outstanding staff with which to work.

- Julie Scardiglia for her friendship, humor, and words of encouragement when they were needed most.

- Elizabeth Nieginski for her belief in the merit of this project.

- Kathleen Scogna for her tireless work on the manuscript.

- Vincent Knaus for his exceptional skills as a photographer. A special thanks for the cover photograph featuring the Mesa Fire Department.

- Kimberly Battista for her gift as a medical illustrator.

- The manuscript reviewers: Captain Jim Hansen; MaryAlice Witzel, RN; Ed Kalinowski; Tim McQuade; Shirley Hosler, RN; and Captain Mark Burdick. Your comments and suggestions were essential in the development of this text.

- A very special thanks to Ed Kalinowski, Hawaii EMS Training Coordinator. You have been consistently diligent and thorough in your reviews of my material, and your suggestions have greatly improved it. Also, my sincere thanks for agreeing to write the Foreword for this text.

- Andrea and Sherri Aehlert; Garret, Sue, and Mitchell Olson; Elizabeth Niegirski; and Julie Scardiglia for volunteering as patient models.

- My husband, Dean, whose love, patience, and understanding make it all possible.

CONTRIBUTING AUTHOR ACKNOWLEDGMENTS

Garret Olson, CEP

To my wife, Susan, and son, Mitchell, thank you for your love, support, and patience. You give meaning to all I do.

Thank you, Chief Gary Olson (a.k.a. Dad), for your work ethic, which will always be my measuring stick. Thank you, Mom, for being cooler than June Cleaver.

Thanks to the Mesa Fire Department and Mesa Community College for the countless opportunities to interact with and affect the EMS community and its "customers."

Special thanks to Julie Scardiglia, Kathleen Scogna, and Vincent Knaus for making this book such a great experience.

And finally: Michael Jordan plays basketball. Mozart wrote music. Barbara Aehlert teaches EMS. If you know Barb, the parallels are obvious. Barb, personally and professionally, you are one of my most valued acquaintances. Thank you for including me on this project.

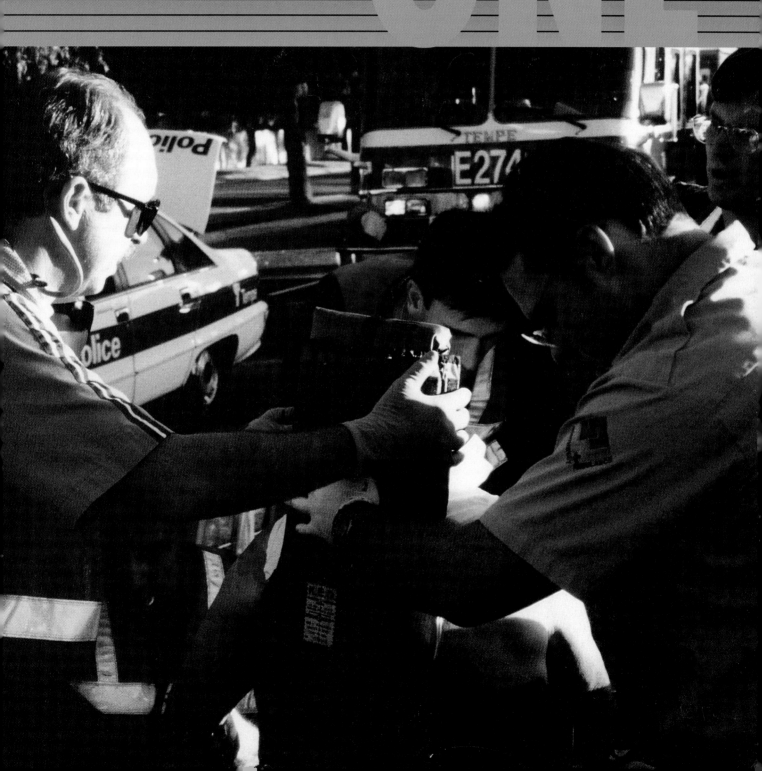

1 INTRODUCTION TO EMERGENCY CARE

OBJECTIVES

*1-1 Describe the development of Emergency Medical Services (EMS) in the United States.

*1-2 List and describe the 10 essential components of an EMS system as identified by the National Highway Traffic Safety Administration's Technical Assistance Program.

*1-3 Describe the four nationally recognized levels of prehospital care providers.

1-4 Differentiate the roles and responsibilities of the EMT-Basic from other prehospital care providers.

1-5 Define the terms "health care system" and "EMS system."

*1-6 Identify the five stages of EMS system response.

1-7 Describe the EMT-Basic's roles and responsibilities in maintaining personal safety.

1-8 Discuss the roles and responsibilities of the EMT-Basic in maintaining the safety of the crew, patient, and bystanders.

*1-9 Describe the professional attributes desirable in an EMT-Basic.

*1-10 Describe the benefits of continuing education.

*1-11 Describe the methods by which continuing education may be obtained.

1-12 Define quality improvement and discuss the EMT-Basic's role in this process.

1-13 Define medical direction and discuss the EMT-Basic's role in this process.

*1-14 Given a scenario, differentiate between on-line medical direction and off-line medical direction.

MOTIVATION FOR LEARNING

EMS has developed from the days when the local funeral home and other services served as the ambulance provider into a complex, sophisticated system. Today, EMT-Basics work side by side with other health care professionals to help deliver professional prehospital emergency medical care.

OVERVIEW OF EMERGENCY MEDICAL SERVICES (EMS)

THE NHTSA TECHNICAL ASSISTANCE PROGRAM

In 1988, the **National Highway Traffic Safety Administration (NHTSA)** established an assessment program (called the Technical Assistance Program) that identified 10 essential components of an EMS system *(Figure 1-1)*.

EMS SYSTEM—NHTSA COMPONENTS

1. **Regulation and policy.** To provide a quality, effective system of emergency medical care for adults and children, each EMS system must have in place legislation that provides for a lead EMS agency, as well as a funding mechanism, regulations, and operational policies and procedures.
2. **Resource management.** Adult and pediatric victims of medical or traumatic emergencies must have equal access to basic emergency care. Basic emergency care includes the triage and transport of all victims by appropriately certified personnel in a licensed and equipped ambulance to a facility that is appropriately equipped and staffed and ready to administer to the needs of the patient.
3. **Human resources and training**
   a. At a minimum, all transporting prehospital personnel should be trained to the EMT-Basic level.
   b. In an effective EMS system, training programs are routinely monitored, instructors meet certain requirements, and the curriculum is standardized throughout the state.
4. **Transportation**
   a. Most patients can be effectively transported in a ground ambulance staffed by qualified emergency medical personnel.
   b. Other patients with more serious injuries or illnesses may require rapid transportation by rotor craft or fixed-wing air medical services.
   c. Routine, standardized methods for inspection and licensing of all emergency medical transport services are essential to maintain a constant state of readiness throughout the state.
5. **Facilities.** Seriously ill or injured patients must be delivered in a timely manner to the closest appropriate facility.
6. **Communications.** Beginning with the universal system access number (9-1-1), the communications network should provide the following to ensure adequate EMS system response and coordination:
   a. Prioritized dispatch
   b. Dispatch-to-ambulance communication
   c. Ambulance-to-ambulance communication
   d. Ambulance-to-hospital communication
   e. Hospital-to-hospital communication
7. **Public information and education**
   a. Efforts must serve to enhance the public's role in the EMS system, its ability to access the system, and the prevention of injuries.
   b. In many areas, EMS personnel provide system access information and present injury prevention programs that lead to better use of EMS resources and improved patient outcomes.
8. **Medical direction**
   a. EMS is a medical care system that includes medical practice delegated by physicians to nonphysician providers.
   b. It is the physician's obligation to be involved in all aspects of the patient care system.
   c. Specific areas of physician involvement include:

      (1)   Planning and protocols
      (2)   On-line medical direction and consultation
      (3)   Audit and evaluation of patient care

9. **Trauma systems.** States must develop a system of specialized care for the triage and transfer of trauma patients including designated trauma centers.

10. **Evaluation**
    a. Each EMS system must be responsible for evaluating the effectiveness of services provided to adult and pediatric victims of medical or trauma-related emergencies.
    b. An effective EMS system evaluates itself against preestablished standards and objectives in order to improve services, particularly direct patient care.
    c. These requirements are part of an ongoing **quality improvement** system to review system performance.
    d. The evaluation process should be educational and ongoing.

IMPORTANT ELEMENTS OF THE EMS SYSTEM

ACCESSING THE EMS SYSTEM

1. **9-1-1**
    a. 9-1-1 is also called the universal access number.
    b. 9-1-1 calls come into a single location called the **public service answering point (PSAP).**
    c. Enhanced 9-1-1 provides additional information to the dispatcher, including the caller's street or billing address and phone number.

2. **Non–9-1-1**
    a. The caller dials a seven-digit number to access EMS.
    b. Separate numbers for police, fire, ambulance, and other services still exist in some communities in the United States.

1797 During the Napoleonic Wars, Baron Dominique Jean Larrey, a French surgeon general, invents a system of service to the injured. Light carriages transport casualties from the field to aid stations, and the medical crews operating the carriages are trained to control hemorrhage and splint fractures.

1915 The first known air medical transport is used during the retreat of the Serbian army from Albania.

Mid-1940s Rural communities begin volunteer fire protection and first-aid services.

1960 Cardiopulmonary resuscitation (CPR) is shown to be useful.

1962 Michigan Instruments introduces "The Thumper."

1800 —— 1900 —— 1940 ——————— 1960 ——

1860s The United States Army is believed to have used the first ambulance service in the United States in 1865.

The first civilian ambulance services in the United States begin as hospital-based services in Cincinnati and New York City.

1950s Mobile Army Surgical Hospital (MASH) units use helicopters for evacuation in the Korean War; the rapid evacuation of patients increases survival.

1958 Dr. Peter Safar demonstrates the benefits of mouth-to-mouth ventilation.

1960 Laerdal introduces Resusci-Anne.

Ambu introduces the bag-valve-mask resuscitator.

1965 PhysioControl introduces the *LifePak 33* defibrillator/monitor.

Fig. 1-1. EMS time line.

LEVELS OF TRAINING

1. A **first responder** is the first person with emergency care training who arrives at the scene (e.g., schoolteacher, law enforcement personnel, lifeguard).
   a. A first responder uses a minimal amount of equipment to perform the initial patient assessment and intervention.
   b. A first responder is also trained to assist other EMS providers.
2. An **emergency medical technician (EMT)** is a member of the emergency medical services team who provides prehospital emergency care.
   a. An **EMT-Basic** has taken a minimum 110-hour course as required by the United States Department of Transportation (DOT).
   b. An **EMT-Intermediate** has additional training in skills such as patient assessment, intravenous therapy, advanced airway procedures, defibrillation, and administration of some medications.
   c. An **EMT-Paramedic** has additional training in skills such as patient assessment, intravenous therapy, invasive airway procedures, electrocardiogram (ECG) interpretation, manual defibrillation, and administration of additional medications.

HEALTH CARE SYSTEM (or Health Care Delivery System)

The **health care system** is a network of people, facilities, and equipment designed to provide for the general health care needs of the population.
1. This system may exist at local, regional, or national levels.
2. It consists of specialty facilities such as:
   a. Trauma centers
   b. Burn centers
   c. Children's hospitals
   d. Poison centers
   e. Neurological centers

THE EMS SYSTEM

The EMS system is network of emergency medical personnel, supplies, and equipment designed to function in a coordinated manner.

1966 Modern EMS begins with the publication of *Accidental Death and Disability, The Neglected Disease of Modern Society* by The National Academy of Sciences-National Research Council (NAS/NRC). Called the "White Paper," this study exposes the inadequacies of prehospital services in continuity of training of emergency responders (ambulance attendants, police and fire personnel), medical direction, vehicle transport, local government support of emergency medical services, and citizen knowledge of first aid. It calls for increased government support of prehospital services and suggests guidelines for EMS system development, prehospital personnel training, and upgrading of transport vehicles and their equipment.

1968 9-1-1 is designated as the universal emergency telephone number.

9-1-1

1970 The National Registry of Emergency Medical Technicians (NREMT) is founded.

1971 *"Emergency!"* television program airs with paramedics Johnny Gage and Roy Desoto.

— **1965** —————————————————————— **1970** —

1966 The Highway Safety Act of 1966 charges the Department of Transportation (DOT) National Highway Traffic Safety Administration (NHTSA) with improving EMS, including helping states develop EMS programs. The Act provides funding for development of highway safety programs in order to reduce number of highway-related deaths. It also provides funding for a course curriculum to train Emergency Medical Technician-Ambulance and directs states to develop EMS programs or risk losing part of their federal highway funding.

1967 George Hurst invents the "Jaws of Life."

1968 The American College of Emergency Physicians (ACEP) is founded.

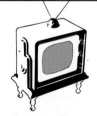

1969 The first nationally recognized EMT-Ambulance curriculum is published.

1. The EMS system is part of the health care system and may exist at local, regional, state, or national levels.
2. The stages of EMS system response include:
   a. Citizen access
   b. Prehospital (**out-of-hospital**), including first responders, EMT-Basics, advanced life-support personnel, and equipment
   c. Hospital emergency department
   d. Critical care
   e. Long-term care and rehabilitation

ROLES AND RESPONSIBILITIES OF THE EMT-BASIC

1. **Personal safety and safety of crew, patient, and bystanders**
   a. The EMT-Basic's most important priority is personal safety.
   b. After receiving a call from the dispatcher, the EMT-Basic drives the emergency vehicle to the given address or location using the most expeditious route, depending on traffic and weather. The EMT-Basic also observes traffic ordinances and regulations concerning emergency vehicle operation.
   c. On arrival at the scene, the EMT-Basic parks the emergency vehicle in a safe location to avoid additional injury.
   d. The EMT-Basic then "sizes up" the scene before beginning patient care to determine:
      (1) Scene safety (Is the scene safe to enter?)
      (2) Mechanism of injury or nature of illness
      (3) Total number of patients
      (4) Need for additional help
   e. In the absence of law enforcement, the EMT-Basic creates a safe traffic environment for protection of the injured and those assisting in the care of injured patients. Creation of a safe traffic environment may include:
      (1) Placement of road flares
      (2) Removal of debris
      (3) Redirection of traffic
2. **Patient assessment and emergency care**
   a. In general, patient assessment and emergency care involve the following:
      (1) Determination of the nature and extent of illness or injury
      (2) Establishment of priorities for required emergency care

1972 The Department of Labor officially recognizes the EMT-Ambulance as an occupational specialty.

1973 The Emergency Medical Services System (EMSS) Act provides federal guidelines and funding for the development of regional EMS systems and identifies 15 essential components of an EMS system.

1974 Glenn Hare patents the cervical collar.

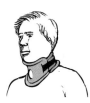

1976 Dr. Burt Kaplan and David Clark Company patent military anti-shock trousers (MAST).

1981 Rick Kendrick invents the Kendrick Extrication Device (KED).

─ **1970** ──────────────── **1975** ──────────────── **1980** ────────

1972 Demonstration projects are begun in some states to develop model regional EMS systems.

1975 The National Association of Emergency Medical Technicians (NAEMT) is founded.

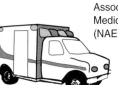

1981 The Omnibus Budget Reconciliation Act consolidates EMS funding into state preventive health and health services block grants and eliminates funding under the EMSS Act.

    (3) Rendering of emergency medical care to adult, infant, and child medical and trauma patients based on assessment findings

  b. Specific responsibilities of the EMT-Basic in patient assessment and emergency care include:

    (1) Opening and maintaining an airway

    (2) Ventilating patients

    (3) Cardiopulmonary resuscitation (CPR), including use of automated external defibrillators (AEDs)

    (4) Controlling hemorrhage; management of shock (hypoperfusion); bandaging wounds; and immobilization of painful, swollen, deformed extremities

    (5) Assisting in childbirth

    (6) Management of respiratory, cardiac, diabetic, allergic, behavioral, and environmental emergencies and suspected poisonings

    (7) Searching for a medical identification emblem to help determine the type of emergency care needed

    (8) Assisting patients with prescribed medications, including sublingual nitroglycerin, epinephrine auto-injectors, and hand-held aerosol inhalers

    (9) Administration of oxygen, oral glucose, and activated charcoal when indicated

3. Lifting and moving patients

  a. Responsibilities of the EMT-Basic in lifting and moving patients include:

    (1) Lifting the stretcher, placing it in the ambulance, and ensuring that the patient and stretcher are secured

    (2) Assisting in lifting and carrying the patient out of the ambulance and into receiving facility

  b. Lifting and moving patients requires knowledge of body mechanics, lifting and carrying techniques, principles of moving patients, and familiarity with equipment.

4. Transport and transfer of care. The EMT-Basic's responsibilities in transport and transfer of care include:

  a. Determining the most appropriate facility to which the patient will be transported, unless otherwise indicated by medical direction. This responsibility requires knowledge of the patient's condition and the extent of injuries as well as the relative locations and staffing of emergency hospital facilities.

  b. Identifying assessment findings that may require communication with medical direction

1984 The EMS for Children (EMS-C) Program provides funds for enhancing the EMS system to better serve pediatric patients.

1988 National Highway Traffic Safety Administration (NHTSA) begins a statewide EMS system Technical Assistance Program and identifies 10 essential components of an EMS system.

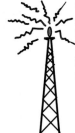

1993 The Federal Communications Commission approves Emergency Medical Radio Services, providing 10 duplex 470 megahertz channels for exclusive emergency medical radio services use.

1986 Life Support Products develops the Automatic Transport Ventilator (ATV).

1994 The DOT EMT-Basic curriculum is revised.

─1984 ─────────────── 1988 ─────────────── 1992 ─────────────── 1996─

1985 The National Research Council publishes *Injury in America: A Continuing Public Health Problem.* This report describes a lack of progress in addressing the problem of accidental death and disability.

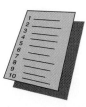

1990 The Trauma Care Systems and Development Act encourages development of trauma systems and provides funding to states for trauma systems planning, implementation, and evaluation.

1995 Congress does not reauthorize funding of the Trauma Care Systems and Development Act.

    c. Reporting verbally and in writing observations and emergency medical care of the patient at the emergency scene and en route to the receiving facility

    d. Providing assistance to the receiving facility staff upon request

5. Record keeping and data collection

    a. Record keeping is an important aspect of prehospital care.

    b. The **prehospital care report** (PCR) information is used by health care providers to note changes in patient condition; these changes are important to health care personnel assuming care of the patient.

    c. PCR information is also essential in quality assessment of emergency medical care.

6. Patient advocacy. The EMT-Basic is responsible for protecting the patient's rights, privacy, and dignity.

PROFESSIONAL ATTRIBUTES OF THE EMT-BASIC

1. Appearance and characteristics of the EMT-Basic include:

    a. Neat, clean, positive image

    b. Self-confidence, emotional stability, good judgement, tolerance for high stress, and a pleasant personality

2. Knowledge and skills. The EMT-Basic must maintain up-to-date knowledge and skills through **continuing education** and refresher courses.

    a. Continuing education and refresher courses are beneficial for the following reasons:

        (1) They help the EMT-Basic retain skills and knowledge learned during initial training.

        (2) They provide information about advances in medicine, skills, and equipment.

        (3) They educate the EMT-Basic about changes in local protocols and national guidelines.

    b. Continuing education may occur in different forms:

        (1) Skill labs

        (2) Lectures and workshops

        (3) Conferences and seminars

        (4) Case reviews and/or quality improvement reviews

        (5) Reading professional journals

        (6) Reviewing videotapes and/or audiotapes

3. Physical demands. The EMT-Basic must be able to meet the following physical demands:

    a. Lift, carry, and balance (at times) patients in excess of 125 pounds (250 pounds with assistance)

    b. Work long hours that may include 24-hour continuous shifts

    c. Drive the ambulance in a safe manner

    d. Accurately discern street names through map reading and correctly distinguish house numbers or business locations

    e. Use the telephone for transmitting and responding to a physician's advice

    f. Give concise and accurate verbal descriptions of a patient's condition to health care professionals

    g. Accurately summarize all data in the form of a written report

4. Temperament. The EMT-Basic must be able to adapt to the following situations:

    a. Dealing with people beyond giving and receiving instructions

    b. Performing under stress when confronted with emergency, critical, unusual, or dangerous situations; or in situations in which working speed and sustained attention are "make-or-break" aspects of the job

    c. Performing a variety of duties; able to change tasks without loss of efficiency or composure

QUALITY IMPROVEMENT

1. **Definition. Quality improvement** is a system of internal and external reviews and audits of all aspects of an EMS system to identify those aspects needing improvement to assure that the public receives the highest quality of prehospital care.
2. The EMT-Basic plays a variety of roles in quality improvement, including:
   a. Documentation
   b. Running reviews and audits
   c. Gathering feedback from patients and hospital staff
   d. Conducting preventive maintenance on vehicles and equipment
   e. Continuing education
   f. Skill maintenance

MEDICAL DIRECTION

1. **Definition. Medical direction** is provided by the physician responsible for management, supervision, and guidance of all aspects of an EMS system to ensure its quality of care. Every ambulance service and rescue squad must have physician medical direction.
2. **Types of medical direction**
   a. On-line medical direction (also called direct medical direction) is medical supervision of EMS personnel by a physician or physician designee by means of a radio, telephone, or the presence of the physician or designee on the scene.
   b. Off-line medical direction (also called indirect medical direction) is medical direction of prehospital personnel through use of protocols, standing orders, training programs, case review, and quality improvement review.
3. **Relationship of the EMT-Basic to medical direction**
   a. The EMT-Basic is the designated agent of physician medical director.
   b. The care rendered by an EMT-Basic is considered an extension of the medical director's authority (although this relationship varies by state law).

REVIEW QUESTIONS

Directions: Each of the numbered items or incomplete statements in this section is followed by answers or by completions of the statement. Select the ONE lettered answer or completion that is BEST in each case.

1. According to the Highway Safety Act of 1966, which of the following is a federal agency responsible for improving and coordinating Emergency Medical Services (EMS)?

   (A)   Department of Transportation (DOT)
   (B)   Occupational Health and Safety Act (OSHA)
   (C)   American College of Emergency Physicians (ACEP)
   (D)   National Registry of Emergency Medical Technicians (NREMT)

2. In 1966, a critique of prehospital medical services was published. This paper, often referred to as the "White Paper," exposed the inadequacies of prehospital care providers, medical direction, transport systems, local government support, and citizen knowledge. What is the formal title of this paper that sparked the beginning of modern EMS?

   (A) *Emergency!*
   (B) *Injury in America: A Continuing Public Health Problem*
   (C) *Death in Streets of America: Our Failings in Prehospital Care*
   (D) *Accidental Death and Disability: The Neglected Disease of Modern Society*

3. The term "enhanced 9-1-1" refers to the capability of the 9-1-1 system to

   (A) locate and dispatch the closest appropriate unit
   (B) prioritize and triage medical calls-for-assistance
   (C) provide the dispatcher with the caller's address and phone number
   (D) dispatch health care providers without the assistance of a dispatcher

4. Nationally, there are four recognized levels of training for prehospital emergency care providers. Which of the following correctly identifies the level of training for the provider who has successfully completed a 110-hour (minimum) course?

   (A) First responder
   (B) EMT-Basic
   (C) EMT-Intermediate
   (D) EMT-Paramedic

5. According to the role and responsibilities of the EMT-Basic, which of the following is the EMT-Basic's most important priority?

   (A) Appearance
   (B) Patient safety
   (C) Personal safety
   (D) Patient assessment

6. EMT-Basics, like all health care providers, must be advocates for their patients. Patient advocacy means assuring

   (A) the patient's rights, privacy, and dignity
   (B) all injured patients receive medical treatment despite their wishes
   (C) the patient's friends and coworkers understand the patient's medical condition
   (D) all patients are transported to the "best" medical facility, despite insurance company contracts and agreements

7. When interacting with other health care professionals and patients, EMT-Basics must possess the proper temperament. Which of the following traits is most critical to the EMT-Basic?

   (A) Adaptability
   (B) Friendliness
   (C) Fast driving skills
   (D) Precise diagnostic skills

8. Medical direction is a key component of any EMS system. It is a broad term for a system that every ambulance service and rescue squad must have. Medical direction is best defined as:

   (A) knowing the location and routes to various hospitals
   (B) a physician responsible for management, supervision, and guidance for the EMS system

(C) medical supervision of EMS personnel by a physician or a physician designee via radio, telephone, or direct contact

(D) the use of protocols, standing orders, and quality improvement review to guide the actions of EMT-Basic's in the absence of direct medical control

Directions: Each of the numbered items or incomplete statements in this section is negatively phrased, as indicated by a capitalized word such as NOT, LEAST, or EXCEPT. Select the ONE lettered answer or completion that is BEST in each case.

9. According to the program set forth by the National Highway Traffic Safety Administration (NHTSA) in 1988, which of the following is NOT one of the ten essential components of an EMS system?

(A) Medical direction
(B) Regulation and policy
(C) Human resources and training
(D) Full-time prehospital care providers

10. One of the roles and responsibilities of the EMT-Basic is scene "size-up." Which of the following is NOT a component of scene size-up?

(A) Scene safety
(B) Sorting the patients by seriousness of injury
(C) Identifying the mechanism of injury or nature of illness
(D) Identifying the total number of patients and calling for additional help as necessary

ANSWERS AND RATIONALES

1-A. The DOT is the agency responsible for EMS on a national level. OSHA is responsible for safety in the workplace. ACEP, founded in 1968, is an advisory board composed of physicians. NREMT, founded in 1970, is the agency that provides certification on a national level.

2-D. Published by the National Academy of Sciences National Research Council (NAS/NRC), *Accidental Death and Disability: The Neglected Disease of Modern Society* served as a wake-up call to America about the poor state of prehospital services. This paper was a catalyst for the development of our modern EMS system. *Emergency!* was a television program that aired in the early 1970's and depicted the lives of firefighter-paramedics in southern California. Published by the NAS/NRC in 1985, *Injury in America: A Continuing Public Health Problem*, described deficiencies in our "modern" EMS system.

3-C. The "enhanced 9-1-1" system gives the dispatch agency information about the caller's location and call-back telephone number. The dispatcher, however, should confirm this information with the caller. Communication systems capable of locating and dispatching the geographically closest rescue/ambulance unit use technology called Automatic Vehicle Locator (AVL). In AVL, global positioning satellites pinpoint the location of rescue units to within several meters. The ability to prioritize and triage a medical call-for-assistance is the job of the emergency medical dispatcher. Emergency medical dispatchers provide a vital link between the caller and rescue crews. Often, they give life-saving prearrival instructions to the caller (e.g., CPR techniques).

4-B. The EMT-Basic must complete a minimum 110-hour initial training program. The EMT-Intermediate has additional responsibilities beyond those of the EMT-Basic including intravenous therapy, advanced airway procedures, and administration of some medications. The EMT-Paramedic is the highest level of EMT certification and may perform such skills as ECG interpretation, manual defibrillation, invasive airway procedures, and administration of additional medications. A first responder is the first person with limited first-aid training who arrives at the scene. First responders include lifeguards, police officers, and teachers.

5-C. A neat appearance, regard for patient safety, and strong patient assessment skills are highly desirable in an EMT-Basic. However, the first priority of the EMT is his or her own safety. EMT-Basics who sustain injury or contamination due to poor safety practices hinder the overall EMS operation: becoming injured or contaminated depletes the resources available to treat the initial patient(s).

6-A. Patient advocacy refers to protecting the patient's rights, privacy, and dignity. EMT-Basics must be professional when dealing with patients. While it is advisable that all injured patients receive some form of medical treatment, patients have the right to refuse treatment (see Chapter 3). Making sure that the patient's friends and coworkers understand the patient's medical condition can be an infringement of the patient's privacy. "Generic" patient information is best (i.e., "We are doing all we can for your friend," or "Your friend seems to be responding appropriately"). When transporting a patient to a hospital, the EMT-Basic must assure that the patient is transported to the "correct" facility. Factors such as the patient's insurance carrier, patient condition, distance, and patient preference must be taken into account. When in doubt about a patient's destination, contact medical direction for assistance.

7-A. EMT-Basics must be able to adapt to dealing with a diverse population, performing under stress, and performing a variety of duties. EMT-Basics are not physicians and should not diagnose injuries or diseases. Safe and prudent driving is desired; fast driving can be hazardous. Insensitivity is not acceptable in any health care provider.

8-B. A medical director is a physician responsible for the management, supervision, and guidance of all aspects of an EMS system to assure its quality of care. Responses C and D describe the two types of medical direction, on-line medical direction and off-line medical direction, respectively.

9-D. The ten essential components of an EMS system are: (1) regulations and policy; (2) resource management; (3) human resources and training; (4) transportation; (5) facilities; (6) communications; (7) public information and education; (8) medical direction; (9) trauma systems; and (10) evaluation. Many EMS systems are administered on a volunteer basis; therefore, full-time prehospital care providers are not one of the components of an EMS system.

10-B. Scene size-up is a rapid initial assessment of the safety of the scene, mechanism of injury or nature of the illness, total number of patients, and the additional resources that will be necessary to provide appropriate care. Sorting patients by seriousness of injury is referred to as "triage." Triage involves a rapid initial assessment of each patient. In multiple-patient incidents, triage should begin as soon as possible after the scene size-up.

BIBLIOGRAPHY

Arterburn RT: EMS Evolution. *Emergency* 26 (10):56–61, 1994.

Barber, JM: *Emergency Patient Care for the EMT-A.* Reston, VA, Reston Publishing Company, 1981.

Crosby LA, Lewallen DG (eds): *Emergency Care and Transportation of the Sick and Injured*, 6th ed. Rosemont, IL, American Academy of Orthopaedic Surgeons, 1995.

Grant HD, Murray RH Jr, Bergeron JD: *Emergency Care*, 7th ed. Englewood Cliffs, NJ, Prentice-Hall, 1995.

Hafen BQ, Karren KJ, Mistovich JJ: *Prehospital Emergency Care*, 5th ed. Upper Saddle River, NJ, Prentice-Hall, 1996.

McSwain NE, White RD, Paturas JL, et al (eds): *The Basic EMT: Comprehensive Prehospital Patient Care*. St. Louis, Mosby-Year Book, 1996.

Stoy WA: *Mosby's EMT-Basic Textbook*. St. Louis, Mosby-Year Book, 1996.

United States Department of Transportation, National Highway Traffic Safety Administration. *Emergency Medical Technician: Basic. National Standard Curriculum*, 1994.

OBJECTIVES

*2-1   Describe the stages of the grieving process.

2-2   List the possible emotional reactions the EMT-Basic may experience when faced with trauma, illness, death, and dying.

2-3   Discuss the possible reactions a family member may exhibit when confronted with death and dying.

2-4   Describe the steps in the EMT-Basic's approach to the family confronted with death and dying.

*2-5   Identify common causes of stress in EMS.

2-6   Identify the physical, behavioral, mental, and emotional warning signs of critical incident stress.

2-7   State possible steps that the EMT-Basic may take to help reduce or alleviate stress.

2-8   State the possible reactions that family members of the EMT-Basic may exhibit as a result of their outside involvement in EMS.

● MOTIVATION FOR LEARNING ●

EMT-Basics encounter many stressful situations when providing emergency medical care to patients, including death and terminal illness, major traumatic situations, and child abuse. EMT-Basics interact with angry, frightened, violent, and seriously injured and ill patients and family members. Therefore, EMT-Basics must learn how to assist the patient, the patient's family, their own families, and other EMT-Basics in dealing with stress. The EMT-Basic must practice personal safety precautions in all scene situations. To reduce the risk of communicable disease, the EMT-Basic should treat all patients as potentially infectious, always use appropriate personal protective equipment when providing medical care, and wash his or her hands after every patient contact.

*2-9   Define the terms critical incident, critical incident stress debriefing, and defusing.

*2-10   Describe the components of critical incident stress management (CISM).

*2-11   Explain the need to determine scene safety.

*2-12   Define the terms bacteria, body substance isolation (BSI), carrier, communicable disease, exposure, host, infection, infectious disease, microorganism, Occupational Safety and Health Administration (OSHA), parasite, pathogen, universal precautions, and virus.

*2-13   Identify the body's normal defenses against infection.

*2-14   List four methods of disease transmission.

*2-15   List four classifications of communicable diseases.

*2-16   Give an example of engineering and work practices.

*2-17   Identify the single most important method of preventing the spread of infection.

*2-18   Describe when hand washing should be performed.

*2-19   Describe proper hand-washing procedure.

2-20   Describe the steps to take for personal protection from airborne and blood-borne pathogens.

*2-21   Describe the procedure for proper documentation and management of an exposure incident.

2-22   Given a scenario, identify the personal protective equipment (PPE) necessary for each of the following situations:
   -Hazardous materials exposure
   -Rescue operations
   -Violent scenes
   -Crime scenes
   -Exposure to bloodborne pathogens
   -Exposure to airborne pathogens

EMOTIONAL ASPECTS OF EMERGENCY CARE

DEATH AND DYING

1. **Stages of death and dying**
   a. **Denial ("Not me")**
      (1)   **Denial** is a defense mechanism and is characterized by an inability or refusal to believe the reality of the event.
      (2)   Denial creates a buffer against the shock of dying and dealing with the illness or injury.
   b. **Anger ("Why me?")**
      (1)   Patient's **anger** is related to his or her inability to control the situation; the anger is displaced and projected onto anything and everything.
      (2)   Anger is characterized by abusive language and criticism of anyone who offers help.
      (3)   When confronted with an angry patient, the EMT-Basic should not take anger or insults personally and should be tolerant and empathetic. The EMT-Basic should not become defensive and should use good listening and communication skills.
   c. **Bargaining ("OK, but first let me . . . ")**
      (1)   The patient attempts to enter into an "agreement" that he or she hopes

may postpone or change the inevitable. The patient may bargain with themselves, his or her family, God, or medical professionals. **Bargaining** reflects the patient's need for time to accept the situation.

    (2) Bargaining is characterized by statements such as, "If I could live to . . . "

d. Depression ("OK, but I haven't . . .")

    (1) **Depression** is a reaction to anticipated death.

    (2) A depressed patient is sad and feels a great sense of loss.

e. Acceptance ("OK, I am not afraid")

    (1) The patient realizes his or her fate and understands that death is certain. **Acceptance** does not mean that the patient is happy about dying; rather, the patient believes that he or she has done all that is possible in preparation to die.

    (2) Family members may require more support during this stage than the patient.

2. Dealing with the dying patient, family members, and bystanders

  a. Patient needs include:

    (1) Dignity

    (2) Respect

    (3) Sharing

    (4) Communication

    (5) Privacy

    (6) Control

  b. Family members may express rage, anger, and despair.

  c. When dealing with death and dying, the EMT-Basic should do the following:

    (1) Listen empathetically

    (2) Do not falsely reassure

    (3) Use a gentle tone of voice

    (4) Let the patient know everything that can be done to help will be done

    (5) Use a reassuring touch, if appropriate

    (6) Comfort the family

STRESSFUL SITUATIONS

1. Common causes of stress in EMS. The EMT-Basic will experience personal stress and will encounter patients and bystanders in severe stress.

  a. Environmental stressors include:

    (1) Lights, siren, alarm noise

    (2) Long hours and shifts

    (3) Absence of challenge between calls

    (4) Weather conditions and temperature extremes

    (5) Confined work spaces

    (6) Emergency driving and rapid scene response

    (7) Demanding physical labor

    (8) Multiple role responsibilities

    (9) Dangerous situations

  b. Psychosocial stressors include:

    (1) Family relationships

    (2) Conflicts with supervisors or coworkers

    (3) Agitated, combative, or abusive patients

    (4) Dealing with critically ill and injured or dying patients

    (5) Patients under the influence of drugs or alcohol

    (6) Incompatibility with partner

  c. Personal stressors include:

    (1) Life-and-death decision making

    (2) Personal expectations

    (3) Feelings of guilt and anxiety

    (4) Dealing with death and dying

2. **High-stress situations** include the following:
   a. Mass casualty incidents
   b. Infant and child trauma
   c. Amputations
   d. Infant, child, elder, or spousal abuse
   e. Death or injury of a coworker or other public safety personnel
   f. Death of a child
   g. Emergency response to illness or injury of a friend or family member

STRESS MANAGEMENT

The EMT-Basic can take steps to reduce and alleviate stress.
1. Recognize the warning signs of critical incident stress.
   a. **Physical signs of stress** *(Figure 2-1)* include:
      (1) Chest pain or tightness, palpitations
      (2) Exhaustion, fatigue
      (3) Difficult or rapid breathing
      (4) Nausea, vomiting
      (5) Dry mouth
      (6) Tremors of the lips or hands

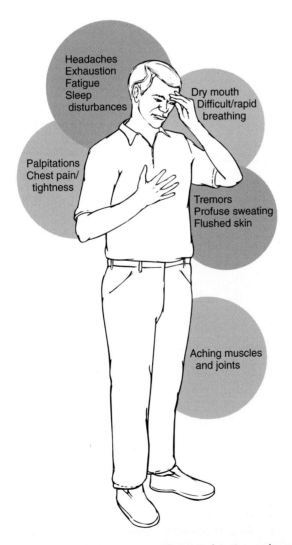

Fig. 2-1. Physical signs of stress include chest pain or tightness, palpitations, exhaustion, fatigue, difficult or rapid breathing, nausea, vomiting, dry mouth, tremors of the lips or hands, profuse sweating, flushed skin, sleep disturbances, aching muscles and joints, and headaches.

       (7) Profuse sweating, flushed skin
       (8) Sleep disturbances
       (9) Aching muscles and joints
     (10) Headaches

  b. Behavioral signs of stress include:
     (1) Crying spells
     (2) Hyperactivity or underactivity
     (3) Withdrawal or a desire to be isolated from others
     (4) Changes in eating habits
     (5) Increased substance use or abuse, including smoking, alcohol consumption, medications, and illegal substances
     (6) Excessive humor or silence
     (7) Violence

  c. Mental (cognitive) signs of stress include:
     (1) Inability to make decisions
     (2) Disorientation or decreased level of awareness
     (3) Memory problems or inability to concentrate
     (4) Lowered attention span
     (5) Disruption in logical thinking

  d. Emotional signs of stress include:
     (1) Panic reactions
     (2) Denial
     (3) Fear
     (4) Guilt
     (5) Anger
     (6) Feelings of hopelessness, abandonment, and numbness
     (7) General loss of control
     (8) Depression

2. Make **lifestyle changes.**
  a. Modify diet.
     (1) Reduce sugar, caffeine, and alcohol intake.
     (2) Avoid fatty foods.
     (3) Increase carbohydrate intake.
  b. Exercise. Exercise is beneficial for the following reasons:
     (1) It provides a physical release for stress
     (2) It prepares the EMT-Basic to handle the physical demands of the job
  c. Learn to relax by practicing relaxation techniques such as meditation, visual imagery, and controlled breathing exercises.
  d. Learn to manage time efficiently and develop a time-management plan.
     (1) Develop an awareness of how one's time is spent.
     (2) Determine long-term goals.
     (3) Establish priorities to allow time for physical activities, mental enrichment, social interactions, and spiritual well-being.
     (4) Implement plan.
  e. Change work schedule.
     (1) Request work shifts that allow more time to relax with family and friends.
     (2) Request a rotation of duty assignment to a less busy area.
  f. Seek professional help.

RESPONSE OF FAMILY AND FRIENDS OF THE EMT-BASIC

Because the job of an EMT-Basic can be stressful, family and friends may respond to this stress. Typical responses include:

1. Lack of understanding of prehospital care
2. Fear of separation or being ignored
3. Frustration caused by the "on-call" nature of the job and the inability to plan activities
4. Frustration caused by wanting to share

CRITICAL INCIDENT STRESS MANAGEMENT (CISM)

1. **Definitions**
   a. A **critical incident** is a situation that causes a prehospital care provider to experience unusually strong emotions and may interfere with the provider's ability to function immediately or later.
   b. A **critical incident stress debriefing (CISD)** is a group meeting led by a mental health professional and peer support personnel to allow rescuers to share thoughts, emotions, and other reactions to a critical event.
   c. A **defusing** is a shorter, less structured version of a debriefing for rescuers held immediately after a critical event.

2. **Overview**
   a. A comprehensive CISM program includes the following:
      (1) Preincident stress education
      (2) On-scene peer support
      (3) One-on-one support
      (4) Disaster support services
      (5) Defusings
      (6) CISD
      (7) Follow-up services
      (8) Spouse and family support
      (9) Community outreach programs
      (10) Other health and welfare programs such as wellness programs
   b. CISM can successfully reduce or alleviate stress because:
      (1) Feelings are ventilated quickly
      (2) The debriefing or defusing environment is nonthreatening

3. **Critical Incident Stress Debriefing (CISD)**
   a. The goals of CISD include:
      (1) Reducing the impact of a critical event
      (2) Accelerating the normal recovery process after experiencing a critical incident
      (3) Preventing development of post-traumatic stress disorder
   b. Benefits of CISD include:
      (1) Allows emergency workers to share feelings and emotions and provides emotional reassurance
      (2) Educates emergency workers about stress reduction and coping techniques
   c. **The CISD process**
      (1) Ideally, a CISD should be held within 24 to 72 hours of a critical incident.
      (2) CISDs are led by a mental health professional and several peer counselors.
      (3) Usually, all emergency workers involved in the incident participate in a CISD.
      (4) Sessions are nonthreatening and confidential.

4. **Defusing**
   a. The goal of a defusing is to stabilize emergency workers so that they can return to service or, if they are at the end of their shift, return home without unusual stress.
   b. Benefits of defusing include:
      (1) Allows emergency workers to share feelings and emotions and provides emotional reassurance
      (2) Educates emergency workers about stress reduction and immediate management techniques
   c. **The defusing process**
      (1) A defusing is a shorter and less structured version of a debriefing.
      (2) It concentrates on the most seriously affected workers.
      (3) A defusing is held within 1 to 4 hours of a critical event.
      (4) Sessions last about 30 to 45 minutes.

(5) Defusings are often led by peer counselors but may be led by a mental health professional.

(6) A defusing may eliminate the need for a formal debriefing.

SCENE SAFETY

RESPONSIBILITIES OF THE EMT-BASIC

The EMT-Basic is responsible for ensuring his or her own safety as well as the safety of the crew, patient, and bystanders.

DISEASE PREVENTION

Part of this responsibility includes taking precautions to prevent the spread of diseases.

DISEASE PREVENTION

TERMINOLOGY

1. **Bacteria** are one-celled organisms that can live outside the human body and do not depend on other organisms to live and grow.
2. **Body Substance Isolation (BSI)** refers to self-protection against *all* body fluids and substances (blood, urine, semen, feces, vaginal secretions, tears, saliva, cerebrospinal fluid, etc.).
3. A **carrier** is a person or animal that shows no signs or symptoms of illness but has pathogens in or on its body that can be transferred to others.
4. A **communicable (contagious) disease** is a disease that can be spread from one person or animal to another, either directly or indirectly.
5. **Exposure** is contact with infected blood, body fluids, tissues, or airborne droplets, either directly or indirectly.
6. A **host** is a plant, person, or animal capable of harboring and providing nourishment for another organism (the parasite).
7. An **infection** is the invasion and growth of microorganisms in a host, with or without detectable signs of illness.
8. An **infectious disease** is a communicable disease caused by microorganisms such as bacteria.
9. A **microorganism** is an organism too small to be seen with the unaided eye; bacteria, some fungi, and protozoa are microorganisms.
10. **Department of Labor, Occupational Safety and Health Administration (OSHA)** is a branch of the federal government responsible for safety in the workplace.
11. A **parasite** is a plant or animal that lives on or within and obtains nourishment from another living organism.
12. A **pathogen** is a microorganism capable of producing disease.
13. **Universal precautions** refers to self-protection against diseases transmitted via blood.
14. A **virus** is a type of infectious agent that depends on other organisms to live and grow.

DEFENSES AGAINST DISEASE

1. **First-line defenses**
   a. Every body surface that is exposed to the environment is involved in the body's first line of defense against disease.
   b. This defensive barrier includes the skin and mucous membranes of the digestive, respiratory, and genitourinary tracts.
   c. As long as the skin and mucous membranes are intact, most pathogens cannot enter the body.

2. **Second-line defenses**
   a. When the body's first line of defense is broken, the body's second line of defense is activated.
   b. The body's second line of defense is an inflammatory response. In this response, white blood cells (leukocytes) attempt to prevent further invasion by walling off, destroying, or neutralizing the invading microorganism.
3. **Third-line defenses**
   a. The body's third line of defense is the immune system.
   b. The immune system is activated by the presence of "foreign" proteins, called antigens, that are found on the surface of many microorganisms, such as bacteria. The immune system responds to these antigens by attempting to suppress or kill the invading microorganisms.

METHODS OF DISEASE TRANSMISSION *(FIGURE 2-2)*

1. **Contact**
   a. Contact is **direct** when the pathogen is physically transferred between an infected person and a susceptible host, e.g., sexual contact with an infected person or contact with excretions from an open sore or ulcer.

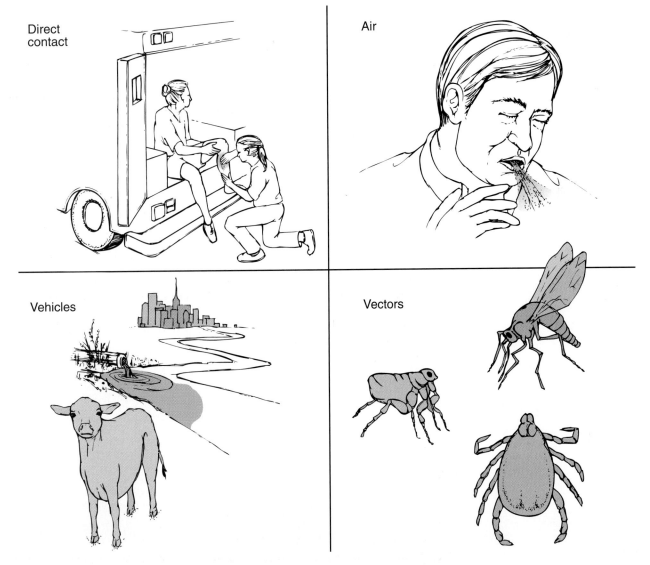

Direct contact   Air

Vehicles   Vectors

Fig. 2-2. Methods of communicable disease transmission.

b. Contact is **indirect** when a susceptible host comes in contact with contaminated substances or inanimate objects, e.g., intravenous tubing, needles, toys, eating utensils and glasses, towels, sheets, and wound dressings.

2. **Air.** Pathogens can be transmitted in droplets or residue of evaporated droplets that remain suspended in the air through coughing, talking, and sneezing.

3. **Vehicles**
   a. A vehicle is an inanimate object by which or upon which a pathogen is transmitted from an infected person to a susceptible host.
   b. Vehicles include:
      (1) Liquids, e.g., water, drugs, blood
      (2) Food, e.g., improperly handled or stored food and fresh fruits and vegetables

4. **Vectors**
   a. A vector is an insect that can transmit a pathogen to humans or other animals that it bites or stings.
   b. Vectors include mosquitoes, fleas, ticks, and lice.

5. **Other methods.** Some animals, such as cows and pigs, harbor pathogens that can be transmitted to humans. Pathogens can be transmitted through eating contaminated animal products or through direct contact with the urine or feces of a contaminated animal.

CLASSIFICATION OF COMMUNICABLE DISEASES

1. Airborne diseases are spread by droplets produced by coughing or sneezing. Examples include:
   a. Tuberculosis
   b. Measles
   c. Meningitis
   d. Rubella
   e. Chickenpox (varicella)

2. Bloodborne diseases are spread by contact with blood or body fluids of an infected person. Examples include:
   a. Hepatitis B virus (HBV)
   b. Hepatitis C
   c. Human immunodeficiency virus (HIV)
   d. Syphilis

3. Foodborne diseases are spread by improper handling of food or by poor personal hygiene. Examples include:
   a. Salmonella (food poisoning)
   b. Hepatitis A

4. Sexually transmitted diseases are spread by either blood or sexual contact. Examples include:
   a. Chlamydia
   b. Gonorrhea
   c. HIV

BODY SUBSTANCE ISOLATION (BSI) STANDARDS AND REGULATIONS

1. The **Centers for Disease Control (CDC)** has developed standards to reduce the risk of infection. These standards have been adopted by OSHA and apply to all emergency workers.

2. Federal standards and regulations attempt to reduce or eliminate the likelihood of disease transmission by using engineering and work practice controls.

ENGINEERING AND WORK PRACTICE CONTROLS

1. Maintain good personal health and hygiene habits, including:
   a. General cleanliness

b. Hand washing
   (1) Hand washing is the single most important method of preventing the spread of disease.
   (2) It should be performed:
      (a) Before and after contact with a patient
      (b) Before performing a procedure
      (c) After glove removal
      (d) Between patients
   (3) Procedure:
      (a) Remove gloves and jewelry
      (b) Use soap and water
      (c) Vigorously rub hands together to work up a lather; washing should also include exposed forearms
      (d) Rinse hands and use a paper towel to dry them
      (e) Use a paper towel to turn off the faucet
   (4) Wearing gloves does NOT eliminate the need for hand washing after each patient contact.
   (5) A waterless hand-cleansing solution can be used initially on the scene; follow with a complete hand washing with soap and water after completing patient care activities.
2. Maintain immunizations and screenings, including:
   a. Tetanus prevention (booster every 10 years)
   b. Hepatitis B vaccine
   c. Influenza vaccine (yearly)
   d. MMR (measles, mumps, and rubella) vaccine (if needed)
   e. Periodic tuberculosis screening
3. Properly clean, disinfect, and dispose of used materials and equipment.
   a. Contaminated materials should be placed in appropriately labeled leakproof containers or bags.
   b. Contaminated materials should be disposed of properly with other contaminated materials.

PERSONAL PROTECTIVE EQUIPMENT (PPE)

1. **Overview**
   a. PPE provides a barrier between the emergency worker and infectious material.
   b. It must be worn when an exposure to blood or other potentially infectious material can be reasonably anticipated.
   c. PPE includes eye protection, protective gloves, gowns, and masks.
2. **Eye protection**
   a. Eye protection is not required for routine patient care but should be worn when splashing of body fluids into the face or eyes of the emergency worker is likely (e.g., childbirth; arterial bleeding).
   b. If prescription eyeglasses are worn, removable side shields can be applied to them.
   c. Goggles are NOT required.
3. **Protective gloves**
   a. Disposable vinyl or latex gloves should be used for contact with blood or bloody body fluids.
   b. They should be changed between contact with different patients.
   c. Vinyl or latex gloves should never be reused.
   d. Utility gloves are needed for cleaning vehicles and equipment.
4. **Gowns**
   a. Gowns should be used in situations in which large amounts of blood or body fluids are anticipated (e.g., during childbirth, major trauma).
   b. Disposable gowns should be used whenever possible
   c. After patient care activities are complete, the EMT-Basic should appropriately

discard the gown and, if possible, change uniform.

    d. In some situations, use of a gown may pose a risk to the emergency worker.

        (1) They may be hazardous during firefighting or extrication procedures.

        (2) The EMT-Basic should check departmental or agency policy concerning gown use.

5. Masks

    a. Surgical-type face masks should be worn by emergency workers to protect against possible blood or other body fluid splatter and/or in situations in which an airborne disease is suspected.

    b. Patients with a known or suspected airborne disease should wear a disposable surgical-type mask.

    c. For patients with known or suspected tuberculosis:

        (1) A **High-Efficiency Particulate Air (HEPA)** respirator should be worn by emergency workers.

        (2) A disposable surgical-type mask should be worn by the patient.

DOCUMENTING AND MANAGING AN EXPOSURE

1. Immediately wash the area of contact thoroughly.

2. Document the situation in which the exposure occurred.

3. Describe the actions taken to reduce the chances of infection.

    a. Inform your designated infection control officer, physician, or other designated individual according to policy.

    b. Know your agency's policy regarding when and how soon to have medical follow-up after an exposure incident.

4. Comply with all required reporting responsibilities and time frames.

5. Cooperate with the investigation of the incident.

6. If applicable, obtain proper immunization boosters.

7. Complete medical follow-up.

INJURY PREVENTION

HAZARDOUS MATERIALS SCENE

1. Identify possible hazards.

    a. Use binoculars to identify hazards before approaching the scene.

    b. Look for signs or placards that provide information about the contents.

    c. If necessary, refer to *Hazardous Materials: The Emergency Response Guidebook*, published by the United States Department of Transportation.

        (1) This book contains reference information about hazardous materials and their identification numbers.

        (2) It should be readily accessible.

    d. Hazardous materials incidents should be controlled by special "HazMat" teams.

    e. Provide emergency care only after the scene is safe and the patient is decontaminated.

2. Protective clothing for a hazardous material scene includes:

    a. Hazardous material suits

    b. Self-Contained Breathing Apparatus (SCBA)

RESCUE SCENE

1. Identify and reduce potential life threats.

    a. Potential life threats include electricity, fire, explosion, and hazardous materials.

    b. Request rescue teams for extensive or heavy rescue.

    c. Observe safe rescue practices.

    d. Use protective gear.

2. Protective clothing for a **rescue** scene includes:
  a. Turnout gear
  b. Puncture-proof gloves
   (1) Wearing disposable medical gloves under structural firefighting gloves is controversial. It is recommended in situations in which sharp objects may puncture medical gloves, such as vehicle extrication.
   (2) However, it may be hazardous for structural firefighting activities. Check departmental or agency protocol.
3. Helmet with ear protection and a chin strap
4. Eye protection (safety glasses or goggles)
5. Boots with steel toes and insoles

VIOLENT SCENE

1. The scene should always be controlled by law enforcement before the EMT-Basic provides patient care. At a violent scene, it may be necessary to control the perpetrator of the crime, bystanders, and family members.
2. Do not disturb the scene unless absolutely necessary for medical care.
3. Preserve the evidence needed for investigation and prosecution.

REVIEW QUESTIONS

Directions: Each of the numbered items or incomplete statements in this section is followed by answers or by completions of the statement. Select the ONE lettered answer or completion that is BEST in each case.

1. When dealing with the family members of a dying patient, the EMT-Basic can expect to deal with a variety of reactions. Typically, these reactions will include

   (A) anger, rage, and despair
   (B) headache and unconsciousness
   (C) chest pain and difficulty breathing
   (D) abdominal pain and rectal bleeding

2. Certain lifestyle changes may assist prehospital personnel in coping with the stress of their profession. One example of a recommended change is

   (A) decreasing carbohydrate intake
   (B) substituting saturated fats for unsaturated fats
   (C) balancing work with recreation, family and health
   (D) increasing caffeine intake to compensate for low energy levels

3. Recognizing the early warning signs of excess stress is important. Physical signs of stress may include

   (A) chest pain
   (B) exhaustion and fatigue
   (C) difficult or rapid breathing
   (D) all of the above

4. What are the goals of Critical Incident Stress Debriefing (CISD)?

  (A) Identify mistakes made during the incident and create an action plan to avoid future mistakes
  (B) Reduce the impact the incident has on prehospital care providers, to accelerate the recovery process, and to help prevent post-traumatic stress disorder
  (C) Identify the health care providers most affected by the incident and refer those individuals to a behavioral health facility
  (D) Allow the media an opportunity to interview prehospital personnel to increase public education and awareness

5. Body Substance Isolation (BSI) refers to

  (A) avoiding interaction with possibly contagious patients
  (B) proper documentation of all exposures to contagious patients
  (C) self-protection methods against all body fluids and substances
  (D) all of the above

6. What are the body's three lines of defense against disease?

  (A) Protective gloves, eye protection, and gown
  (B) The dermis, epidermis, and subcutaneous fat layer
  (C) The respiratory, lymphatic, and circulatory systems
  (D) The skin and mucous membranes, inflammation, and the immune system

7. Which of the following statements about hand washing is FALSE?

  (A) Remove jewelry before washing
  (B) Wearing gloves eliminates the need for hand washing
  (C) Hands must be vigorously rubbed together during hand washing
  (D) Waterless washing solutions act as a good temporary measure until soap and water are available

8. When responding to a known hazardous materials incident

  (A) immediate stabilization of chemicals is the first priority
  (B) make attempts to identify hazards before entering the scene
  (C) approaching from downwind assists in chemical identification
  (D) full body substance isolation (protective gloves, eye wear, mask, and gown) will provide adequate protection

Directions: Each of the numbered questions or incomplete statements in this section refers to a scenario that precedes them. The numbered questions or incomplete statements are followed by answers or by completions of the statement. Select the answer or completion of the statement that is BEST in each case.

You and your partner are called to the scene of a car versus bicycle collision. Upon arrival, you find an 8-year-old female patient lying in the street bleeding heavily from a severe head injury. She is extremely combative and screaming.

Questions 9–12

9. Which of the following would be the appropriate level of personal protective equipment (PPE) in this situation?

  (A) Protective gloves only
  (B) Protective gloves and eye protection

    (C)   Protective gloves, gown, and mask
    (D)   Protective gloves, eye protection, gown, and mask

10. While stabilizing the patient in preparation for transport, the patient's father arrives at the scene. He approaches you and asks about his daughter's condition. Your most appropriate response would be to

    (A)   instruct the father to ask a bystander what happened
    (B)   inform the father that everything is going to be just fine
    (C)   not reveal anything about the patient's condition for legal reasons
    (D)   briefly tell the father about the injuries and your treatment plan

11. After transporting the patient to an appropriate facility, you begin to decontaminate the ambulance. You find a blood-soaked sock that had been removed from the patient. You should

    (A)   give the sock to the patient's father
    (B)   throw the sock in a nearby trash can
    (C)   place the sock on the patient's hospital bed
    (D)   place the sock in a leakproof container with other contaminated material

12. While returning to quarters, you notice your partner seems upset. He is unusually quiet, does not eat dinner that evening, and cannot sleep. He may benefit from

    (A)   tranquilizers
    (B)   requesting to work extra shifts
    (C)   returning to his normal routine
    (D)   contacting a CISM team member

Between calls, your ambulance crew goes to the emergency department to retrieve a backboard that was used earlier on an assault patient. You run to the storage area, grab the backboard with your bare hands, and return to the ambulance. When you return to the ambulance, you notice your hands are covered with blood.

Questions 13–15

13. As a result of this exposure, you may be susceptible to which of the following communicable diseases?

    (A)   Salmonella and chlamydia
    (B)   Tuberculosis (TB) and meningitis
    (C)   Hepatitis B virus (HBV) and human immunodeficiency virus (HIV)
    (D)   All of the above

14. Your first step toward decontamination should be to

    (A)   get a complete physical examination
    (B)   wash your hands with soap and water
    (C)   complete exposure documentation forms
    (D)   contact your agency's Infection Control Officer

15. This exposure is an example of which method of communicable disease transmission?

    (A)   Air
    (B)   Vector
    (C)   Vehicle
    (D)   Contact

1-A. Anger, rage, and despair are common responses family members may experience when faced with the death of a loved one. Family members experiencing chest pain, difficulty breathing, abdominal pain, rectal bleeding, headaches and/or unconsciousness should be evaluated, treated, and transported if appropriate.

2-C. Recommended lifestyle changes to assist coping abilities include balancing work, recreation, family, and health; modifying diet (avoiding fatty foods, increasing carbohydrates); exercising; learning to relax; and changing work schedules.

3-D. In addition to the signs listed, other physical signs of stress include nausea, vomiting, tremors, sweating, sleep disturbances, aching muscles and joints, and headaches.

4-B. Critical Incident Stress Debriefing (CISD) is aimed at helping prehospital care providers in coping with particularly stressful incidents. Debriefings should ideally be held within 24 to 72 hours of a critical incident. Debriefings are led by a mental health professional and several peer counselors and usually involve all emergency workers involved in the incident. Debriefing sessions are nonthreatening and confidential and provide emotional reassurance and education about stress reduction education and coping techniques.

5-C. Body substance isolation (BSI) precautions are the protective measures all health care providers must take to decrease the chances of disease transmission. Avoiding diseased patients is not an option for prehospital health care providers. While proper documentation is important, documentation comes only after an exposure. BSI is aimed at prevention.

6-D. The body's lines of defense are the skin and mucous membranes, inflammation, and the immune system. Protective gloves, eye wear, and gowns are body substance isolation precaution measures. The dermis, epidermis, and subcutaneous fat are the three layers of skin. The respiratory, lymphatic, and circulatory systems are body systems that may be affected by disease.

7-B. Wearing gloves does NOT eliminate the need for hand washing. The effectiveness of hand washing is maximized when jewelry is removed, soap and water are used, and the hands are vigorously rubbed together. Waterless hand-cleaning solutions are good for an initial cleaning on scene but must be followed by proper washing.

8-B. Identifying the materials involved before entering the scene will assist personnel in determining the level of protective equipment necessary, the resources needed to stabilize the scene, the type of patient reactions to expect, and special concerns such as evacuation needs. Stabilization of hazardous materials incidents is the responsibility of specially trained and equipped technicians. Body substance isolation may be fatally inadequate in many hazardous materials scenes. Responders should always attempt to approach the scene from upwind.

9-D. The patient's heavy bleeding combined with her combativeness call for the highest level of personal protective measures. The risk of blood becoming airborne and coming in contact with health care providers is high. In this scenario, you also want to limit the exposure hazard of any bystanders that stopped to help the patient. A reflective ("traffic") vest should be worn for additional safety of the EMT-Basics.

10-D. Remember to be respectful and honest when interacting with family members. As healthcare providers, EMT-Basics must assume responsibility for communicating with family members in the prehospital setting.

11-D. The sock is one of the patient's personal effects; however, covered with blood, the sock must be considered contaminated and secured appropriately.

12-D. A Critical Incident Stress Management (CISM) team member may help accelerate the normal recovery process and lessen the impact of this incident. Tranquilizers would only mask the difficulty your partner is having. Working extra shifts or returning to a normal routine are not attempts to cope with this acute problem and may have a detrimental effect on the recovery process.

13-C. Hepatitis B virus (HBV) and human immunodeficiency virus (HIV) are bloodborne diseases. Tuberculosis (TB) and meningitis are airborne diseases. Salmonella is foodborne and chlamydia is a sexually transmitted disease.

14-B. Hand washing is the single most important method of preventing the spread of infection and must be done immediately. Documentation, notification, and evaluation should be performed in accordance with agency guidelines, but should be done after washing the hands.

15-D. Physical transfer, either direct or indirect, is classified as a contact transmission. Vector transmission occurs when the host is infected via an insect. Vehicle transmission is infection by contaminated items such as food or water. Air transmission occurs when the disease is atomized and transmitted via droplets or droplet residue suspended in the air.

BIBLIOGRAPHY

Anderson KN, Anderson LE, Glanze WD (eds): *Mosby's Medical, Nursing, & Allied Health Dictionary*, 4th ed. St. Louis, Mosby-Year Book, 1994.

Crosby LA, Lewallen DG (eds): *Emergency Care and Transportation of the Sick and Injured*, 6th ed. Rosemont, IL, American Academy of Orthopaedic Surgeons, 1995.

Grant HD, Murray RH Jr, Bergeron JD: *Emergency Care*, 7th ed. Englewood Cliffs, NJ, Prentice-Hall, 1995.

Hafen BQ, Karren KJ, Mistovich JJ: *Prehospital Emergency Care*, 5th ed. Upper Saddle River, NJ, Prentice-Hall, 1996.

Kozier B, Erb G, Blais K, et al: *Fundamentals of Nursing: Concepts, Process, and Practice*, 5th ed. Redwood City, CA, Addison-Wesley, 1995.

McSwain NE, White RD, Paturas JL, et al (eds): *The Basic EMT: Comprehensive Prehospital Patient Care*. St. Louis, Mosby-Year Book, 1996.

Mitchell JT: *Emergency Services Stress: Guidelines for Preserving the Health and Careers of Emergency Services Personnel*. Englewood Cliffs, NJ, Prentice-Hall, 1990.

O'Toole M (ed): *Miller-Keane Encyclopedia and Dictionary of Medicine, Nursing, and Allied Health*. Philadelphia, WB Saunders, 1992.

Potter PA, Perry AG: *Fundamentals of Nursing: Concepts, Process, and Practice*, 3rd ed. St. Louis, Mosby-Year Book, 1993.

Ramos JA, Sharma M: *Practical Stress Management: A Comprehensive Workbook for Managing Change and Promoting Health*. Boston, Allyn and Bacon, 1995.

Stoy WA: *Mosby's EMT-Basic Textbook*. St. Louis, Mosby-Year Book, 1996.

United States Department of Transportation, National Highway Traffic Safety Administration. *Emergency Medical Technician: Basic. National Standard Curriculum*, 1994.

Yvorra JG (ed): *Mosby's Emergency Dictionary Quick Reference for Emergency Responders*. St. Louis, Mosby-Year Book, 1989.

3 MEDICAL–LEGAL AND ETHICAL ISSUES

MOTIVATION FOR LEARNING

Every day, the EMT-Basic faces many medical, legal, and ethical questions. The EMT-Basic must learn how to make correct decisions when medical–legal and ethical questions arise.

3-10   Differentiate between expressed and implied consent.

3-11   Explain the role of consent of minors in providing care.

3-12   Identify the steps to take if a patient refuses care.

3-13   Discuss the issues of abandonment, false imprisonment, assault, and battery and their implications to the EMT-Basic.

3-14   Explain the purpose of advance directives and how the EMT-Basic should care for a patient who has an advance directive.

3-15   Discuss the responsibilities of the EMT-Basic relative to resuscitation efforts for patients who are potential organ donors.

3-16   Describe the actions an EMT-Basic should take to preserve evidence at a crime scene.

3-17   List the specific types of situations an EMT-Basic is required to report in most states.

LEGAL DUTIES AND ETHICAL RESPONSIBILITIES

LEGAL DUTIES

The EMT-Basic has legal duties to the patient, medical director, and public that are set by statutes and regulations and are also based on generally accepted standards.

ETHICAL RESPONSIBILITIES

1. **Definition—Ethics. Ethics** are principles that identify conduct deemed morally desirable, i.e., what a person *ought* to do.
2. **Responsibilities of the EMT-Basic.** The EMT-Basic has a responsibility to make the physical and emotional needs of the patient a priority by:
   a. Responding to the physical and emotional needs of every patient with respect
   b. Maintaining mastery of skills
   c. Participating in continuing education and refresher programs
   d. Critically reviewing performance and seeking improvement
   e. Reporting honestly and accurately and respecting confidentiality
   f. Working cooperatively and with respect for other emergency professionals

THE LEGAL SYSTEM

TYPES OF LAW

1. **Civil (tort) law**
   a. **Civil law** is a branch of law that deals with torts (civil wrongs) committed by one individual against another. Examples include divorce and breach of contract.
   b. Court provides a remedy in the form of an action for damages.
2. **Criminal law**
   a. **Criminal law** is the area of law in which the federal, state, or local government prosecutes individuals on behalf of society for violating laws designed to safeguard society.
   b. Criminal laws are punishable by fine, imprisonment, or both.
3. **Common law**
   a. **Common law** is "case" or "judge-made" law.
   b. Common laws are derived from society's acceptance of customs or norms over time.

THE LAW AND THE EMT-BASIC

1. **Scope of practice**
   a. **Definition. Scope of practice** is the duties and skills an EMT-Basic is legally allowed and expected to perform when necessary.
   b. State laws and regulations often use the United States Department of Transportation EMT-Basic National Standard Curriculum to define the EMT-Basic's scope of practice.
   c. Medical direction and/or the local, regional, or state emergency medical services (EMS) community may broaden or limit the EMT-Basic's scope of practice through the use of standing orders and protocols.
2. **Medical direction**
   a. The EMT-Basic's ability to function is contingent on medical direction.
   b. Specific procedures require permission from medical direction before they can be performed by the EMT-Basic. These procedures are:
      (1) Advanced airway procedures
      (2) Assisting a patient with medications
   c. Medical direction may be off-line or on-line, depending on state and local requirements.
      (1) Telephone and/or radio communication are on-line medical direction.
      (2) Approved standing orders and protocols are off-line medical direction.
3. **Medical Practice Act**
   a. A **medical practice act** is legislation that governs the practice of medicine; this act varies from state to state.
   b. It may prescribe how and to what extent a physician may delegate authority to an EMT-Basic to render emergency medical care.
4. Legal responsibilities of the EMT-Basic are as follows:
   a. Act in a reasonable and prudent manner
   b. Provide a level of care and transportation consistent with education and training
5. **Negligence**
   a. **Definition. Negligence** is a deviation from the accepted standard of care, resulting in further injury to the patient.
   b. Negligence can result in legal accountability and liability.
   c. Negligence occurs when the following conditions are met:
      (1) There was a duty to act.
      (2) This duty was breached.
      (3) Injury and/or damages (physical or psychological) were inflicted.
      (4) The actions of the EMT-Basic caused the injury and/or damage (proximate cause).
   d. **Duty to act**
      (1) The duty to act may be a formal contractual or an implied duty.
         (a) **Implied duty:**
            (i) Occurs, for example, when a patient calls for an ambulance and the dispatcher confirms that an ambulance will be sent
            (ii) May be undertaken voluntarily by beginning to care for a patient
         (b) **Formal duty** occurs when, for example, an ambulance service has a written contract with a municipality, with specific clauses specifying when service must be provided or may be refused.
      (2) The legal duty to act may not exist.
         (a) In some states, while off duty or if driving an emergency vehicle outside the company's service area, the EMT-Basic has no legal duty to act if he or she observes or comes upon an accident.
         (b) Although a legal duty to act may not exist, a moral or ethical duty to act may exist.
         (c) EMT-Basics must know their specific state regulations regarding duty to act.

    (3) **Duties of the EMT-Basic** include:
        (a) Duty to respond and render care
        (b) Duty to obey laws and regulations
        (c) Duty to operate an emergency vehicle reasonably and with due regard for the safety of others
        (d) Duty to provide care and transportation to the expected standard
        (e) Duty to provide care and transportation consistent with the scope of practice and local medical protocols
        (f) Duty to continue care and transportation through to its appropriate conclusion

e. Breach of duty
    (1) **Standard of care**
        (a) **Definition. Standard of care** is exercising the degree of care, skill, and judgement that would be expected under similar circumstances by a similarly trained, reasonable EMT-Basic.
        (b) Standard of care is established by court testimony and reference to published codes, standards, criteria, and guidelines applicable to the situation.
    (2) Breach of duty may occur by:
        (a) **Malfeasance,** or performing a wrongful or unlawful act. For example, before abortion was legalized, performing one was an act of malfeasance.
        (b) **Misfeasance,** or performing a legal act in a harmful or injurious way. For example, performing cardiopulmonary resuscitation (CPR) in such a manner that the patient's chest is crushed may constitute an act of misfeasance.
        (c) **Nonfeasance,** or failure to perform a required act or duty

f. Damages occur if the patient is injured, either physically or psychologically, by the breach of duty.

g. Proximate cause is established (usually by expert testimony) when:
    (1) The action or inaction of the EMT-Basic was the cause of, or contributed to, the patient's injury
    (2) The EMT-Basic could reasonably foresee that his or her action or inaction would result in the damage

h. The EMT-Basic can protect himself or herself against negligence claims by:
    (1) Maintaining a professional attitude and conduct
    (2) Taking appropriate education and training and continuing education courses
    (3) Receiving appropriate medical direction (on- and off-line)
    (4) Giving a consistently high standard of care
    (5) Performing accurate, thorough documentation

THE EMT-BASIC–PATIENT RELATIONSHIP

CONFIDENTIALITY

1. Confidential information includes:
    a. Patient history
    b. Assessment findings
    c. Treatment rendered
2. **Release of information**
    a. Release of information requires a written release form signed by the patient or legal guardian. The EMT-Basic should not release information on request, either written or verbal, unless legal guardianship has been established.
    b. Permission is not required for release of certain information, including:

      (1) To other health care providers with a need to know to continue or provide care

      (2) When required by law, i.e., if state law requires reporting incidents such as sexual assault, abuse, or gunshot wounds

      (3) When required for third party billing forms

      (4) In response to a proper subpoena

   c. Releasing patient information without proper permission may lead to charges of libel or slander.

      (1) **Libel** is injuring a person's character, name, or reputation by false and malicious writings.

      (2) **Slander** is injuring a person's character, name, or reputation by false and malicious spoken words.

CONSENT

Conscious, competent patients have the right to decide what medical care and transportation to accept.

  1. Expressed consent

   a. Expressed consent may be given:

      (1) Verbally

      (2) By written communication

      (3) Nonverbally, i.e., expressed by action or allowing care to be rendered

   b. Patient must be of legal age and able to make a rational decision

   c. Patient must be informed of the steps of the procedures and all related risks, including:

      (1) The nature of the illness or injury

      (2) The recommended treatment

      (3) The risks and dangers of treatment

      (4) Alternative treatments and their risks

      (5) Dangers of refusing treatment (including transport)

   d. Expressed consent must be obtained from every conscious, mentally competent adult before rendering treatment.

   e. A conscious, competent adult can revoke consent at any time during care and transport.

   f. Failure to obtain a patient's consent can result in a claim of battery.

  2. Implied consent

   a. Definition. Implied consent is consent assumed from a patient requiring emergency intervention who is mentally, physically, or emotionally unable to provide expressed consent.

      (1) Implied consent is based on the assumption that the patient would consent to lifesaving interventions if he or she were able to do so.

      (2) Implied consent is sometimes called the **emergency doctrine.**

   b. It is effective only until patient no longer requires emergency care or regains competence to make decisions.

  3. Minors

   a. Consent for treatment of minors must be obtained from the parent or legal guardian.

   b. When life-threatening situations exist and the parent or legal guardian is not available for consent, emergency treatment should be rendered based on implied consent.

   c. Emancipated minors

      (1) In most states, a person is a minor until age 18, unless emancipated.

      (2) In general, the courts deem an emancipated minor to be one who:

         (a) Is married

         (b) Is a parent

         (c) Is economically independent (living independently and is self-supporting)

        (d) Maintains a separate home

        (e) Is in the armed forces

    (3) Nonemancipated minors are not able to give or withhold consent.

d. Mentally incompetent adults

    (1) If the mentally incompetent adult has a legal guardian, consent may be given or withheld by the guardian.

    (2) If no one legally able to give consent can be contacted, emergency treatment should be rendered based on implied consent.

e. Prisoners or arrestees

    (1) Court or police who have custody may authorize emergency treatment.

    (2) Such emergency care is usually limited to care needed to save life or limb.

REFUSAL OF CARE

1. A mentally competent adult has the right to refuse treatment.

    a. The patient may withdraw consent for treatment at any time.

    b. An example of refusal of care is an unconscious patient who regains consciousness and refuses transport to the hospital.

2. When confronted with a patient who refuses care, the EMT-Basic should do the following:

    a. Ensure that the patient can make a rational, informed decision, e.g., he or she is not under the influence of alcohol or other drugs or is affected by the illness or injury

    b. Inform the patient why he or she should receive care and what may happen to him or her if this care is not given; use specific and nontechnical words when talking to the patient

    c. Make multiple attempts to convince the patient to accept care

    d. Consult medical direction. The EMT-Basic should never make an independent decision not to transport a patient.

    e. Request that the patient and a disinterested witness (e.g., not a family member or friend of the patient) sign a "release from liability" form

    f. Advise the patient that he or she may call again for help if needed

    g. Attempt to get family or friends to stay with the patient

    h. Thoroughly document assessment findings and emergency medical care given on the prehospital care report

    i. When in doubt, the best decision is to provide care.

LEGAL COMPLICATIONS RELATED TO CONSENT

1. Abandonment

    a. Definition. Abandonment is termination of care without reasonable notice or turning the patient over to less-qualified personnel when the patient still needs and desires continuing attention.

    b. Abandonment can occur in the field or when a patient is delivered to the emergency department.

2. False imprisonment

    a. Definition. False imprisonment is intentional and unjustifiable detention.

    b. False imprisonment may be charged by a patient who is transported without consent or who is restrained without proper cause or authority.

    c. It can be a civil or criminal violation.

3. Assault

    a. Definition. Assault is threatening, attempting, or causing fear of offensive physical contact with a patient or other individual.

    b. Assault may be a civil or criminal violation.

4. Battery

    a. Definition. Battery is unlawful touching of another person without consent.

    b. Battery may be a civil or criminal violation.

ADVANCE DIRECTIVES

1. **Definition.** An **advance directive** is a written document that specifies a person's health care wishes when he or she becomes unable to make decisions for himself or herself.
2. Types of advance directives include:
   a. Living will
   b. **Durable power of attorney for health care,** which is a written document that identifies a legal guardian to make decisions for a patient when the patient can no longer make such decisions.
   c. Do not resuscitate (DNR) orders
3. **Legal considerations**
   a. A patient has the right to refuse resuscitative efforts.
   b. In general, an advance directive requires a written order from a physician.
   c. Medical direction must establish and implement policies for dealing with advance directives.
   d. When in doubt or when written orders are not present, the EMT-Basic should begin resuscitation efforts.

SPECIAL SITUATIONS

ORGAN DONORS AND HARVESTING

1. Organ donorship requires a signed legal permission document, such as:
   a. Separate donor card
   b. Intent to be a donor on the reverse of patient's driver's license
2. A potential organ donor should not be treated differently from any other patient requesting treatment.
3. EMT-Basic's role in organ harvesting includes:
   a. Identifying the patient as a potential donor
   b. Establishing communication with medical direction
   c. Providing emergency care that will help maintain viable organs

MEDICAL IDENTIFICATION INSIGNIA

1. Medical identification insignia may be a bracelet, necklace, or card.
2. These insignia indicate that the patient has a serious medical condition, such as allergies, diabetes, or epilepsy.

CRIME SCENES

1. Dispatch should notify law-enforcement personnel about the presence of a potential crime scene.
2. Responsibilities of the EMT-Basic at a crime scene include:
   a. Protecting self and other EMS personnel
   b. Caring for the patient(s) as necessary
   c. Notifying law enforcement if not already involved
   d. Observing and documenting any items moved or anything unusual at the scene
   e. Protecting potential evidence by:
      (1) Leaving holes in clothing from bullet or stab wounds intact, if possible
      (2) Not disturbing any item at the scene unless emergency care requires it

SPECIAL REPORTING SITUATIONS

COMMON TYPES OF SPECIAL REPORTING SITUATIONS

Commonly required reporting situations are established by state legislation and may vary from state to state but often include:

1. Child abuse or neglect
2. Elder abuse
3. Spousal abuse
4. Sexual assault
5. Gunshot and stab wounds
6. Animal bites
7. Suspected infectious disease exposure

OTHER REPORTING SITUATIONS

Other situations the EMT-Basic may be required to report include:
1. Use of patient restraints to treat or transport a patient against his or her will
2. Attempted suicide
3. Situations in which a patient appears to be mentally incompetent or intoxicated

REVIEW QUESTIONS

Directions: Each of the numbered items or incomplete statements in this section is followed by answers or by completions of the statement. Select the ONE lettered answer or completion that is BEST in each case.

1. The EMT-Basic's scope of practice is best defined as

    (A) any measure necessary to save a life
    (B) the legal duties and skills performed when necessary
    (C) performing skills listed in nationally published EMS journals
    (D) any measure authorized by a physician at the scene of an accident

2. You are dispatched for a "man down, unknown medical problem." Upon arrival, you find a 43-year-old man sleeping next to a trash can. He smells strongly of alcohol and responds to loud verbal stimuli by moaning unintelligibly. While documenting this incident, you include the following statement in your narrative, "the patient is a filthy alcoholic." In written form, this statement is

    (A) libelous
    (B) slanderous
    (C) appropriate
    (D) required for accurate documentation

3. You are called to a long-term care facility for an 89-year-old female patient found not breathing and pulseless. Cardiopulmonary resuscitation (CPR) has not been initiated. The health care provider on the scene states the patient is a "no code." She states she knows the patient has "DNR" papers but the staff has not been able to locate them. Without these papers, your best course of action will be to

    (A) call the coroner
    (B) begin treating the patient
    (C) transport the patient without beginning treatment
    (D) allow the facility staff as much time as necessary to locate the necessary documents

4. You are dispatched to a local elementary school for an 8-year-old male patient with an injured arm. You find the patient in the nurse's office complaining of severe right wrist pain. The child tells you he fell off the monkey bars at the school. While

examining the child, you note he is covered with bruises in various stages of healing. The child states, "My Dad hits me when he drinks." You should

(A) call both parents to the school for questioning
(B) call the father to the school to question him about possible abuse
(C) treat the child's injury and ask the school nurse to keep her eye on the child
(D) treat the child's injured arm, document your findings and the child's statement, and inform the physician at the receiving facility of the situation

Directions: Each of the numbered questions or incomplete statements in this section refers to a scenario that precedes them. The numbered questions or incomplete statements are followed by answers or by completions of the statement. Select the answer or completion of the statement that is BEST in each case.

You are dispatched to the scene of a motor vehicle collision. Upon arrival, you observe that a cement-mixer truck has rear-ended a subcompact car. The only person in the car, a 74-year-old woman, was not wearing her seat belt during impact and is complaining of severe abdominal pain. You and your partner quickly remove the patient from the vehicle and package her for transport to the closest appropriate medical facility. Despite your efforts, the patient suffers a cardiopulmonary arrest en route to the hospital and is subsequently pronounced dead in the emergency department.

Questions 5–9

5. If a family member of the deceased decides to sue you, the case would be tried according to

(A) criminal law
(B) common law
(C) civil (tort) law
(D) all of the above

6. If it were determined that you failed to provide appropriate treatment during your care of this patient, you may be prosecuted by the federal, state, or local government. This case would be tried according to

(A) criminal law
(B) common law
(C) civil (tort) law
(D) all of the above

7. During the court proceeding, the prosecutor charges you with negligence. The prosecutor must prove four facts to prove negligence. The first fact is that you had a formal or implied obligation to render assistance. The term used for this obligation is

(A) licensure
(B) duty to act
(C) certification
(D) advance directive

8. The second component of negligence concerns your failure to meet the obligation to render assistance. This is called

(A) consent
(B) abandonment

(C)   breach of duty
(D)   standard of care

9. The prosecutor successfully illustrates your obligation to render assistance and your failure to meet said obligation. The final components of negligence are injury or damages were inflicted and

(A)   your action or inaction was the cause
(B)   you willfully caused the injury or damage
(C)   the patient lost money because of the injury or damage
(D)   a person of higher certification or licensure could have prevented the injury or damage

Your rescue crew is called to the scene of a 32-year-old man who was hit in the head by a softball. Upon arrival you find your patient semiconscious on the pitcher's mound at a local park. He is bleeding from a laceration at the left orbit. He does not respond to verbal stimuli (questioning) and has a purposeful response to painful stimuli (i.e., he moves away when you pinch his hand).

Questions 10–15

10. After sizing up the scene and taking body substance isolation precautions, you approach the patient and begin treatment. You are treating this patient based on

(A)   your civic duty
(B)   implied consent
(C)   expressed consent
(D)   common law doctrine

11. While being packaged for transport to a local emergency department, the patient regains consciousness and can answer all of your questions appropriately. You ask the patient if he would like you to continue medical treatment. This form of consent is called

(A)   minor consent
(B)   implied consent
(C)   expressed consent
(D)   common law doctrine

12. If you did not request permission to treat this patient, touching him may be considered

(A)   assault
(B)   battery
(C)   negligence
(D)   abandonment

13. The patient states he does not want you to treat him. Which of the following statements regarding this patient's refusal of care is correct?

(A)   The patient cannot refuse treatment because you have already begun care
(B)   The patient cannot refuse treatment because he was previously unconscious
(C)   The patient can refuse treatment only if law-enforcement personnel are present at the scene
(D)   The patient can refuse treatment if he is mentally competent and his refusal is expressed and informed

14. Assuming this patient meets the criteria to refuse treatment, you might be charged with which of the following if you insist on transporting him against his will?

   (A)   Negligence
   (B)   Abandonment
   (C)   Breach of duty
   (D)   False imprisonment

15. After explaining the possible consequences of refusing treatment, the patient agrees to be treated and transported. When you arrive at the hospital, you find the emergency department is extremely busy and are unable to locate a nurse or physician to assume care of your patient. The unit clerk instructs you to leave the patient by the trauma room and she will make sure the next available nurse assumes care of the patient. This option

   (A)   is not acceptable and would constitute abandonment
   (B)   is acceptable only if the patient is in critical condition
   (C)   is acceptable since the patient is already in the emergency department
   (D)   is acceptable since the unit clerk is employed by the hospital and knows CPR

ANSWERS AND RATIONALES

1-B.   Scope of practice refers to the skills and techniques the EMT-Basic is trained, certified, and authorized to perform based on coordination with the medical director. Parameters must be set so these skills are performed at the appropriate time. For example, EMT-Basics should be trained and competent in assisting ventilations with a bag-valve-mask device; however, not all patients require ventilatory assistance.

2-A.   Your interpretation of this patient's lifestyle is not pertinent to your documentation. Your documentation should be purely factual. While it is a fact that you noted the patient's breath smelled of an alcohol-like substance, your conclusion that the smell was alcohol may be premature and incorrect. Document facts and objective findings, not conclusions. Written comments such as "the patient is a filthy alcoholic" may injure a person's character, name, or reputation and are considered libelous. If expressed verbally, these comments would be considered slanderous.

3-B.   When an advance directive is not at hand (or looks suspicious or incomplete), the best decision is to provide care until you can contact medical direction for instructions. Some states require that you have in hand the original directive, not a copy. Consult medical direction to determine local protocols regarding advance directives.

4-D.   Unless you are trained and responsible for law enforcement (in addition to your responsibilities as an EMT-Basic), your involvement in this situation should be limited to treating the patient and ensuring that the proper authorities have been notified. Consult medical direction to determine who are considered the "proper authorities" in your area. Other situations that may require special notification procedures include spousal abuse, elder abuse, sexual assault, gunshot and stab wounds, animal bites, and suspected infectious disease exposure.

5-C.   Civil (tort) law concerns issues of potential wrongdoing between individuals. Criminal law deals with violations of law to be prosecuted by federal, state, or local government. Criminal law violations may include incarceration, fines, or both. Common law is based on a "judge-made" law to enforce societal customs or norms.

6-A.   Laws enforced by the federal, state, or local government are decided according to criminal law. Criminal laws are punishable by fines, imprisonment, or both.

7-B. Duty to act is the term given to one's obligation to render assistance. This duty may be (1) implied in which you verbalize an intent to help or volunteer assistance or (2) may be a formal duty in which you have a contractual agreement to render assistance when needed. The legality of one's duty to act while "off-duty" varies from state to state.

8-C. The second component of negligence is breach of duty. Breach of duty may fall into one of three categories: malfeasance, misfeasance, or nonfeasance. Malfeasance is the performance of a wrongful or unlawful act. Misfeasance is the performance of a legal act in a way that is harmful. Nonfeasance is the failure to perform a required act.

9-A. To be found negligent, your action or inaction must be tied to injury or damages. Whether you acted (or failed to act) to willfully cause injury or harm is not at issue. Further, the patient does not have to prove monetary loss in order for you to be held accountable in a negligence case. To determine if your actions were appropriate, your performance would be measured against the "standard of care." Standard of care would compare your actions with the actions of a similarly trained EMT-Basic in a similar situation. Comparing your performance with the performance of a health care professional of higher training and certification (or licensure) would not be reasonable.

10-B. Implied consent is used when a patient needs emergency intervention but is unable to expressly consent to treatment due to mental, physical, or emotional complications. This patient is unconscious and in need of medical treatment. Implied consent is extended until the patient no longer needs emergency medical treatment or regains decision-making competence. The line between impairment and competence is wide and gray. When in doubt, err in favor of helping the patient and contact medical direction as soon as possible for advice.

11-C. Expressed consent is the form of consent every conscious, mentally competent adult must give before care or the continuation of care. Since this patient is now competent, expressed consent must be sought. Minors (nonemancipated persons younger than 18 years of age) may be treated without consent of the patient's guardian if the patient needs life-saving emergency care and the guardian is not available to give consent. Consent for mentally incompetent adults is handled in much the same way as consent for minors. An advance directive is a written document specifying the patient's health care wishes when the patient is no longer able to make decisions for him or herself. A "living will" is one type of advance directive.

12-B. Making physical contact with an individual without consent constitutes battery. Assault occurs when an individual is threatened with battery. Negligence is deviation from the standard of care that results in injury or damages. Abandonment is the inappropriate termination of care.

13-D. A mentally competent adult may refuse treatment at any time, despite prior consent. Be careful! Ensure that the patient refusing care is aware of all treatment or transportation options and is aware of the possible complications of refusing assistance. If you feel the patient does not fully understand his or her options, take the time to explain them. Give the patient the "worst-case scenario" of refusing treatment. For example, "Mr. _____, you are having chest pain that is consistent with a heart attack. We would like to treat you and transport you to an appropriate medical facility. Do you understand that by refusing our care, you may die from the heart attack we believe you are experiencing? What can we do to change your mind about refusing care?"

14-D. If the patient is competent to refuse care and you subsequently detain him, you have falsely imprisoned him. False imprisonment may also occur if you restrain a patient without proper cause or authority.

15-A. Abandonment is the termination of care without reasonable notice or turning the patient over to a less qualified health care professional. Although the patient is in the emergency department, you have abandoned the patient by turning him over to a person with less medical training (the unit clerk) than yourself. You must provide for the smooth transition of care to an equally or more qualified health care professional.

BIBLIOGRAPHY

Crosby LA, Lewallen DG (eds): *Emergency Care and Transportation of the Sick and Injured*, 6th ed. Rosemont, IL, American Academy of Orthopaedic Surgeons, 1995.

Grant HD, Murray RH Jr, Bergeron JD: *Emergency Care*, 7th ed. Englewood Cliffs, NJ, Prentice-Hall, 1995.

Hafen BQ, Karren KJ, Mistovich JJ: *Prehospital Emergency Care*, 5th ed. Upper Saddle River, NJ, Prentice-Hall, 1996.

McSwain NE, White RD, Paturas JL, et al (eds): *The Basic EMT: Comprehensive Prehospital Patient Care*. St. Louis, Mosby-Year Book, 1996.

Pozgar GD: *Legal Aspects of Health Care Administration*, 5th ed. Gaithersburg, Maryland, Aspen Publishers, 1993.

Stoy WA: *Mosby's EMT-Basic Textbook*. St. Louis, Mosby-Year Book, 1996.

United States Department of Transportation, National Highway Traffic Safety Administration. *Emergency Medical Technician: Basic. National Standard Curriculum*, 1994.

4 THE HUMAN BODY

OBJECTIVES

*4-1 Describe the anatomical position.

*4-2 List each body cavity and the primary structures contained within each cavity.

*4-3 Describe the body planes.

4-4 Define the following topographic terms:

a. Medial
b. Lateral
c. Proximal
d. Distal
e. Superior
f. Inferior
g. Cranial
h. Caudal
i. Anterior
j. Posterior
k. Right
l. Left
m. Bilateral
n. Midline
o. Midaxillary line
p. Midclavicular line

4-5 Describe the following body positions:

a. Supine
b. Prone
c. Fowler's position
d. Lateral recumbent
e. Shock position
f. Trendelenburg position

MOTIVATION FOR LEARNING

Patient assessment is an important skill the EMT-Basic must learn. An understanding of normal human anatomy and physiology is essential to understanding a patient's physical assessment findings. Knowledge of medical terminology is important in written and oral communication with other health care professionals.

4-6 Describe the anatomy and general functions of the following major body systems:

a. Skeletal
b. Muscular
c. Respiratory
d. Cardiac
e. Nervous
f. Integumentary
g. Endocrine
h. Digestive
i. Urinary
j. Reproductive

ANATOMICAL TERMS

ANATOMICAL POSITION

The **anatomical position** is standing erect, facing forward, with the arms at the sides and legs parallel; head, palms, and toes are facing forward.

BODY CAVITIES (FIGURE 4-1; TABLE 4-1)

1. **Definition.** A **body cavity** is a hollow space in the body that contains organs.
2. **Ventral (toward the front of the body) cavity**
   a. **Thoracic (chest) cavity**
      (1)   The **thoracic cavity** is located in the trunk between the **diaphragm** (the dome-shaped muscle used in breathing) and the neck.

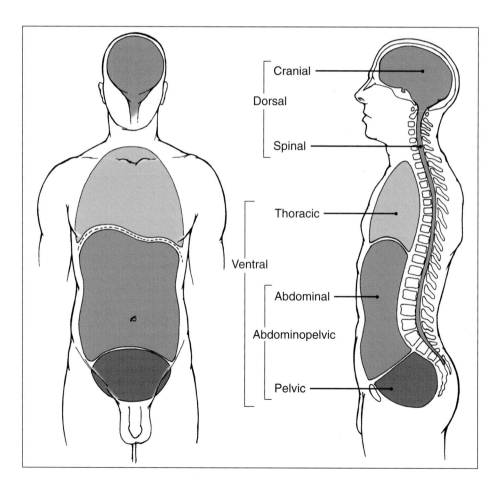

Fig. 4-1. Body cavities.

Table 4-1. Body Cavities and Their Contents

Cavity	Contents
Ventral (toward the front of the body)	
Thoracic	Mediastinum, pleural cavities
Abdominal	Stomach, large and small intestines, liver, gallbladder, pancreas, spleen
Pelvic	Urinary bladder, reproductive organs, rectum
Dorsal (toward the back of the body)	
Cranial	Brain
Spinal	Spinal cord

    (2) It contains the **mediastinum** and pleural cavities.
       (a) The mediastinum is the area between the lungs that extends from the sternum to the vertebral column.
       (b) The mediastinum includes all of the contents of the thoracic cavity (except the lungs), including the esophagus, trachea, heart, and large blood vessels.
       (c) The right lung is located in the right pleural cavity; the left lung is located in the left pleural cavity.
    (3) The thoracic cavity is protected by the rib cage and the upper portion of the spine.
  b. Abdominopelvic cavity
    (1) Abdominal cavity
       (a) The **abdomen** is the part of the body trunk below the ribs and above the pelvis.
       (b) The abdominal cavity contains the stomach, intestines, liver, gallbladder, pancreas, and spleen.
    (2) Pelvic cavity
       (a) The pelvis is the lowest part of the body trunk.
       (b) The pelvic cavity contains the urinary bladder, rectum, and reproductive organs.
3. Dorsal (toward the back of the body) cavity
  a. Cranial cavity
    (1) The cranial cavity is located in the head.
    (2) It contains the brain and is protected by the skull.
  b. Spinal cavity
    (1) The spinal cavity extends from the bottom of the skull to the lower back.
    (2) It contains the spinal cord and is protected by vertebrae.

BODY PLANES (SECTIONS) (FIGURE 4-2)

1. The **frontal plane** is the lengthwise field that passes through the body from side to side, dividing the body into anterior (ventral) and posterior (dorsal) parts.
2. The **sagittal plane** is the lengthwise field that passes through the body from front to back, dividing the body into right and left sections.
  a. In a sagittal cut, the right and left sides do not have to be equal.
  b. The midsagittal plane is the sagittal field that divides the body into two equal halves.
3. The **transverse (horizontal) plane** is the crosswise field that divides the body into superior (upper) and inferior (lower) sections.

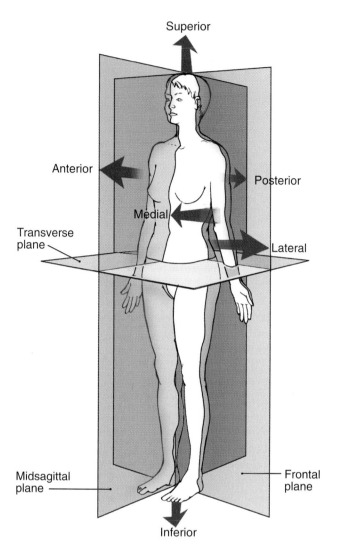

Fig. 4-2. Anatomical planes and directional terms.

DIRECTIONAL TERMS *(FIGURE 4-3)*

1. **Medial** is toward the midline or middle.
2. **Lateral** is away from the midline or middle; toward the side.
3. **Proximal** is nearest the point of reference; toward or nearest the trunk.
4. **Distal** is farthest from the point of reference; away from or farthest from the trunk.
5. **Superior** is above, upper, toward the head.
6. **Inferior** is below, lower, toward the feet.
7. **Cranial** (cephalic) is toward the head.
8. **Caudal** is toward the tail (lower end of the spine).
9. **Anterior** (ventral) is toward the front of the body.
10. **Posterior** (dorsal) is toward the back of the body.
11. **Right and left** always refers to the *patient's* right and left.
12. **Bilateral** means pertaining to both sides.
13. **Midline** refers to an imaginary line drawn vertically through the middle of the

body from the nose to the umbilicus (navel), which divides the body into right and left halves.

14. **Midaxillary line** refers to an imaginary line drawn vertically from the middle of the patient's armpits to the ankle, which divides the body into anterior and posterior sections.

15. **Midclavicular line** refers to an imaginary line drawn vertically in the middle of the clavicle, parallel to the midline.

BODY POSITIONS *(FIGURE 4-4)*

1. **Supine** is lying flat on the back; face up.
2. **Prone** is lying face down and flat.
3. **Fowler's position** is lying on the back with the upper body elevated at a 45° to 60° angle.
4. **Lateral recumbent** is lying in a horizontal position on either the right or left side.
5. **Recovery position** is lying on the left or right side. In prehospital care, the patient is usually placed on the left side so he or she is facing the EMT-Basic during transport.
6. **Shock position** is lying on the back with the feet elevated approximately 8–12 inches.
7. **Trendelenburg position** is lying on the back with the head of the bed lowered and the feet raised in a straight incline.

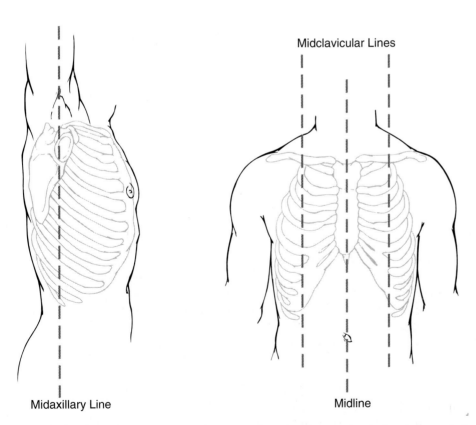

Fig. 4-3. Midline, midaxillary line, and midclavicular line. The midline is an imaginary line drawn vertically through the middle of the body from the nose to the umbilicus (navel). The midaxillary line is an imaginary line drawn vertically from the middle of the patient's armpits to the ankle. The midclavicular line is an imaginary line drawn vertically in the middle of the clavicle, parallel to the midline.

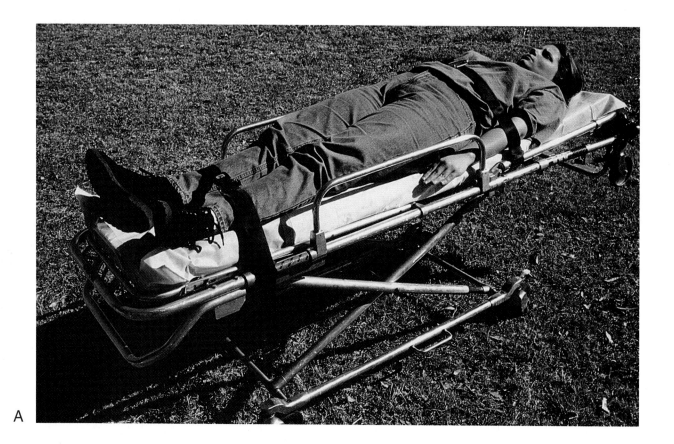

A

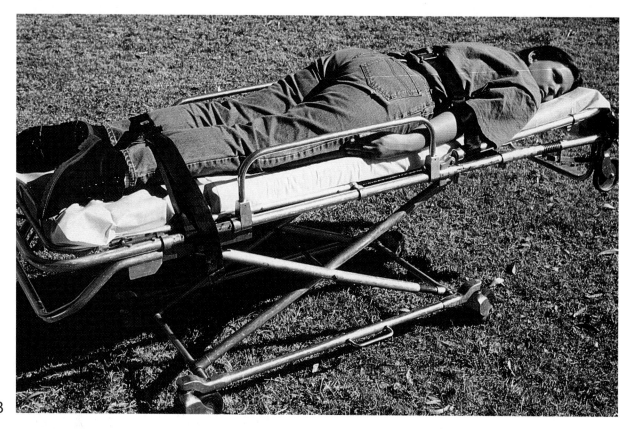

B

Fig. 4-4. Body positions. *(A)* Supine. *(B)* Prone. *(C)* Fowler's position. *(D)* Lateral recumbent. *(E)* Shock position. *(F)* Trendelenburg position.

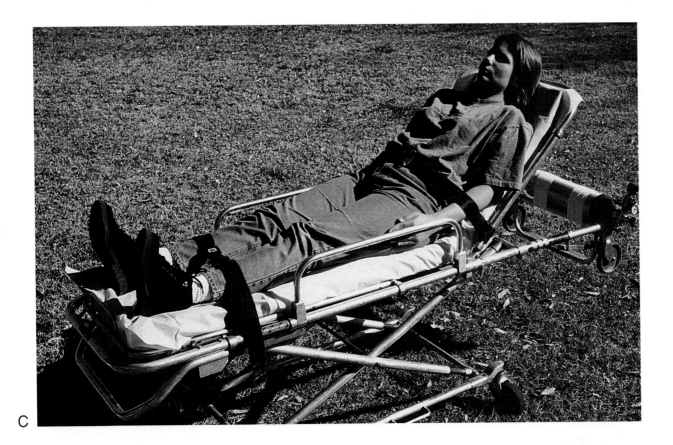

C

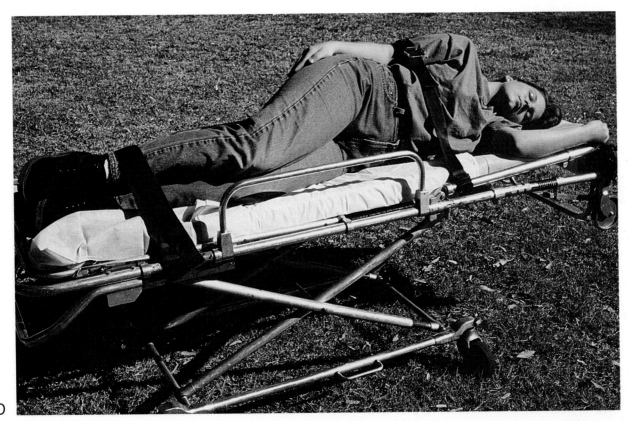

D

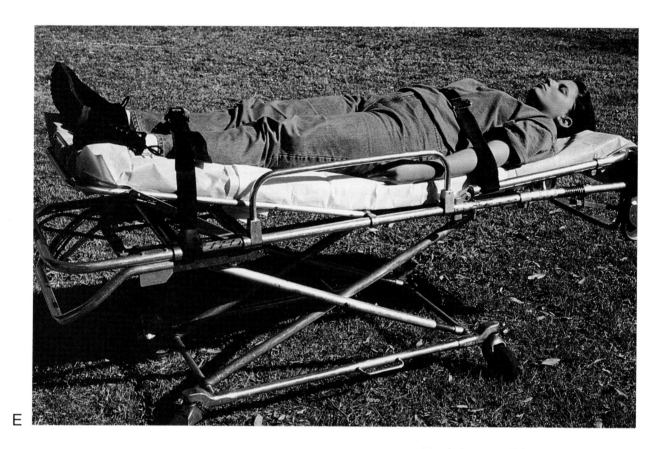

E

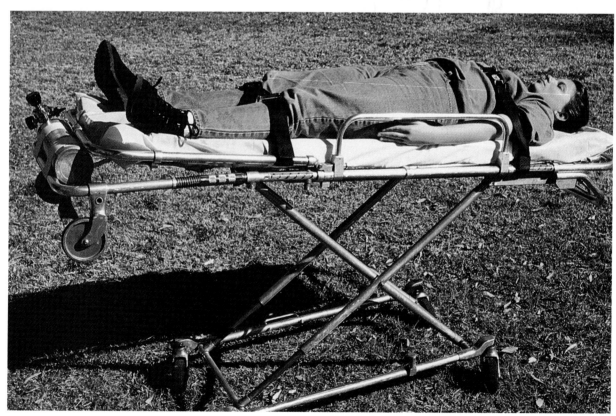

F

BODY STRUCTURE

The body is constructed of smaller units: cells, tissues, organs, and systems (*Figure 4-5*).

CELLS

1. Cells are the smallest living unit in the body.
2. They are the basic unit of all living tissue.

TISSUES

Tissues are collections of cells with similar features or functions.

ORGANS

1. An organ is a collection of different types of tissues.
2. "Vital organs" are those organs with functions that are essential to life (e.g., brain, heart, lungs).

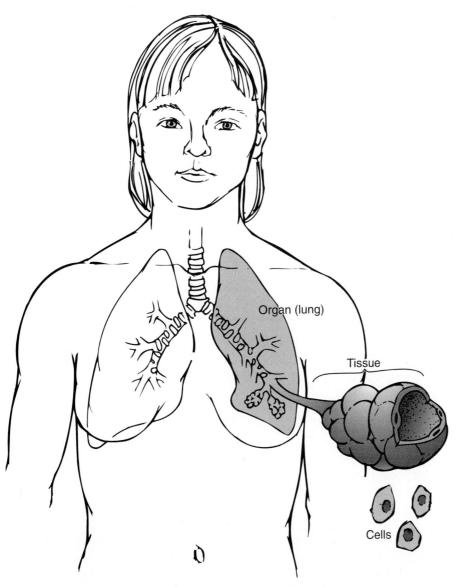

Fig. 4-5. Body cells form tissues. Tissues form organs, and organs make up body systems.

SYSTEMS

Systems are composed of many different types of organs that work together to carry out a complex function or functions.

SKELETAL SYSTEM (FIGURE 4-6)

FUNCTION

The **skeletal system** gives the body shape, support, and form; protects vital internal organs; works with muscles to provide for body movement; stores minerals (calcium, phosphorus); and produces red blood cells.

DIVISIONS OF THE SKELETON (TABLE 4-2)

1. The **axial skeleton** consists of the bones of the skull, spine, and chest and the hyoid bone.
2. The **appendicular skeleton** is composed of the bones of the upper extremities (shoulder girdles, arms, wrists, and hands) and lower extremities (pelvic girdles, legs, ankles, and feet).

SKULL

1. **Function.** The **skull** houses and protects the brain.
2. **Components**
   a. The **cranium** contains eight bones:

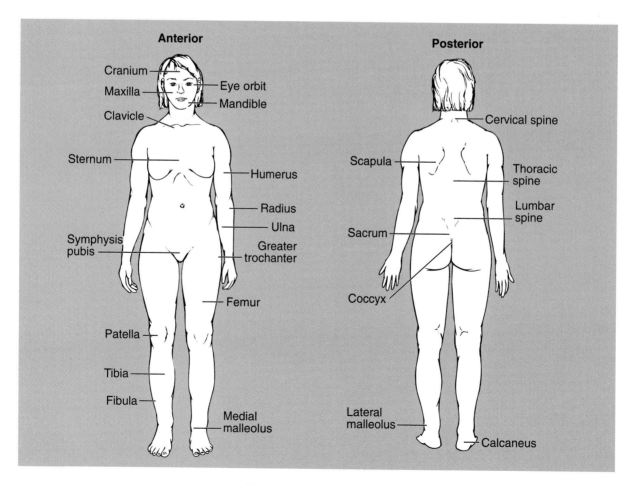

Fig. 4-6. Topographic anatomy.

Table 4.2 Divisions of the Skeleton

Components	Bones	Number of Bones
Axial skeleton		
Skull	Cranium	8
	Facial bones	4
	Ear bones	6
Thorax	Sternum	1
	Ribs	24
Spine	Vertebrae	26 (adult)
Hyoid bone	Hyoid bone	1
	Subtotal	80
Appendicular skeleton		
Upper extremities	Shoulder girdle	4
	Arms, wrists, hands	60
Lower extremities	Pelvic girdle	2
	Legs, ankles, feet	60
	Subtotal	126

(1)   Frontal (forehead) bone
(2)   Two parietal (top sides of cranium) bones
(3)   Two temporal (lower sides of cranium) bones
(4)   Occipital (back of skull) bone
(5)   Sphenoid (central part of floor of cranium) bone
(6)   Ethmoid (floor of cranium, nasal septum) bone
b. The face contains 14 bones:
   (1)   Orbits (eye sockets)
   (2)   Nasal bones (upper bridge of nose)
   (3)   Maxilla (upper jaw)
   (4)   Mandible (lower jaw)
      (a)   The mandible is the largest and strongest bone of the face.
      (b)   It is the only movable bone of the face.
   (5)   Zygomatic bones (cheek bones)
c. The ear contains six bones, which are located in the middle ear and are called the auditory ossicles.

HYOID BONE

1. The hyoid bone is the only bone in the body that does not connect to another bone.
2. The tongue is anchored to the hyoid bone.

SPINAL (VERTEBRAL) COLUMN

The **spinal column** consists of 33 separate but connected bones (vertebrae). These vertebrae are organized into the following regions:
1. Seven cervical (neck) vertebrae
   a. The first cervical vertebra supports the skull and is called the atlas.
   b. The second cervical vertebra is called the axis.
2. Twelve thoracic (upper back) vertebrae
3. Five lumbar (lower back) vertebrae
4. Five sacral (back wall of the pelvis) vertebrae (which fuse into one vertebra in adults)
5. Four coccyx (tailbone) vertebrae (which fuse into one vertebra in adults)

THORAX (CHEST)

The **thorax** contains the ribs and sternum.
1. Ribs
   a. There are 12 pairs of **ribs.**

  b. All of the ribs are attached posteriorly by ligaments to the thoracic vertebrae.

   (1) Pairs 1–10 are attached anteriorly to the sternum. Pairs 1–7 are attached anteriorly to the sternum by cartilage and are also called **true ribs.**

   (2) Pairs 8–10 are attached to the cartilage of the seventh ribs; these ribs are also called **false ribs.**

   (3) Pairs 11 and 12 are not attached to the sternum anteriorly; these ribs are called floating ribs.

 2. The **sternum (breastbone)** consists of three sections.

  a. The **manubrium** is the superior portion; it connects with the clavicle and first rib.

  b. The body is the middle portion.

  c. The **xiphoid process** is a piece of cartilage that makes up the inferior portion.

 3. The thorax contains the following major organs and blood vessels:

  a. Heart

  b. Lungs

  c. Diaphragm

  d. Aorta

  e. Superior and inferior vena cavae

PELVIS

The **pelvis** is a bony ring formed by three separate bones that fuse to become one in an adult.

 1. The **iliac crest** forms the wings of the pelvis.

 2. The **pubis** is the anterior portion of the pelvis. The two pubic bones join at the pubic symphysis.

 3. The **ischium** is the inferior portion of the pelvis and is the lower, posterior portion on which we sit.

UPPER EXTREMITIES

 1. Shoulder girdle

  a. The shoulder girdle connects the upper extremity to the torso.

  b. It is formed largely by the **clavicle** and **scapula.** The clavicle + scapula = shoulder girdle.

   (1) The clavicle is the collar bone.

   (2) The scapula is the shoulder blade.

    (a) The scapula anchors some muscles that move the upper arm.

    (b) Acromion process of scapula = tip of shoulder.

 2. Humerus (superior portion of arm)

  a. The **humerus** is the largest bone of the upper extremity.

  b. It is the second longest bone in the body.

 3. Radius

  a. In the anatomical position, the **radius** is the lateral bone of the forearm.

  b. It runs parallel to the ulna on the thumb side of the forearm.

 4. Ulna

  a. In the anatomical position, the **ulna** is the medial bone of the forearm.

  b. The ulna is the longer of the two bones of the forearm.

  c. The ulna runs parallel to the radius on the little finger side of the forearm.

 5. The **olecranon** is the elbow.

 6. Carpals

  a. The **carpals** are the wrist bones (carpus = wrist).

  b. Each hand contains eight carpal bones.

 7. Metacarpals

  a. The **metacarpals** form the support for the palm of the hand.

  b. Each hand contains five metacarpals.

8. **Phalanges**
   a. The **phalanges** are the finger bones.
   b. Each hand contains 14 phalanges.
      (1)   Each finger is made up of three phalanges.
      (2)   The thumb consists of two phalanges.

LOWER EXTREMITIES

1. **Hip joint**
   a. The lower extremity is attached to the pelvis at the hip joint.
   b. The hip joint is formed by the **acetabulum** (socket of the hip bone) and the head of the femur.
2. **Femur (thigh)**
   a. The **femur** is the longest, heaviest, and strongest bone of the body.
   b. The **greater trochanter** is the large, bony prominence on the lateral shaft of the femur to which the buttock muscles are attached.
   c. The head of the femur is the upper end of the bone and is shaped like a ball.
3. The **patella (kneecap)** is the largest joint in the body.
4. **Tibia (shinbone)**
   a. The **tibia** is the larger of the two bones of the lower leg.
   b. At its distal aspect, it forms the inner ankle prominence (medial malleolus).
5. **Fibula**
   a. The **fibula** runs parallel to the tibia along the lateral side of the lower leg.
   b. At its distal aspect, it forms the outer ankle prominence (lateral malleolus).
6. **Tarsals**
   a. The **tarsals** form the heel and back part of the foot.
   b. Each foot contains seven tarsals.
   c. The largest tarsal is the calcaneus.
7. **Metatarsals**
   a. The **metatarsals** form the part of the foot to which the toes attach.
   b. Each foot contains five metatarsals.
8. **Phalanges**
   a. The **phalanges** are the toe bones.
   b. Each foot contains 14 phalanges.
      (1)   Each big toe has two phalanges.
      (2)   Each of the remaining toes has three phalanges.

JOINTS

1. **Definition.** A joint is the place where two bones meet; also called an articulation.
2. **Types** (*Figure 4-7*)
   a. **Ball-and-socket joint**
      (1)   A ball-and-socket joint allows movement in all directions.
      (2)   Examples include the hip (pelvic bone and femur) and the shoulder (scapula and humerus).
   b. **Hinge joint**
      (1)   A hinge joint allows movement in only one plane.
      (2)   Examples include the elbow (humerus and ulna), knee (femur and tibia), and the joints between phalanges.

MUSCULAR SYSTEM

FUNCTION

1. The muscular system provides for movement.
   a. Muscle cells (fibers) shorten (contract) when stimulated by a nerve impulse.

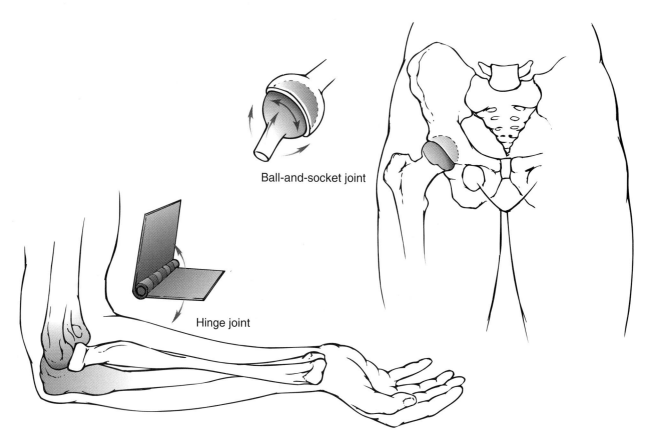

Ball-and-socket joint

Hinge joint

Fig. 4-7. Types of joints: Ball-and-socket and hinge.

      b. Muscle cells shorten by converting energy obtained from food (chemical energy) into movement (mechanical energy).

      c. Muscles produce motion of bones to which they are attached and produce movement within the body's internal organs.

  2. Other functions of muscles are to give the body shape, protection of internal organs, and heat production.

TYPES OF MUSCLE

Types of muscle include **skeletal (voluntary), smooth (involuntary),** and **cardiac** *(Figure 4-8; Table 4-3).*

  1. Skeletal muscle

    a. Description

      (1)   Skeletal muscle is also called striated or voluntary muscle.

        (a) Mature skeletal muscle cells possess crosswise stripes or striations.

        (b) Skeletal muscles form the major muscle mass of the body.

        (c) Their actions are under conscious control of the nervous system and brain, i.e., skeletal muscles can be contracted and relaxed at will.

        (d) They produce rapid, forceful contractions.

      (2)   **Parts of a skeletal muscle**

        (a) The origin is the stationary attachment of the muscle to a bone.

        (b) The insertion is the movable attachment to a bone.

        (c) The body is the main part of the muscle.

    b. Location. Muscles are attached to bones by tendons.

      (1)   **Tendons** are strong cords of fibrous connective tissue that stretch across joints.

      (2)   Tendons create a pull between bones when muscles contract.

    c. Function. Skeletal muscles move the skeleton, produce heat that helps maintain a constant body temperature, and maintain the posture.

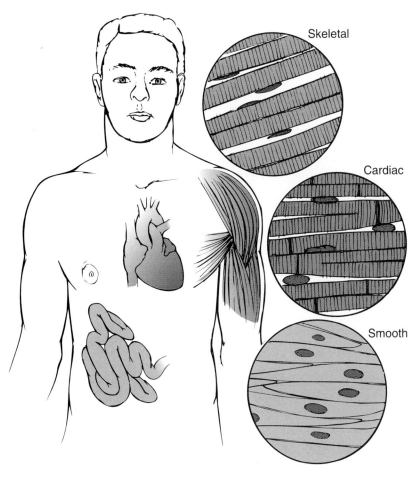

Fig. 4-8. Types of muscle. *(A)* Skeletal. *(B)* Smooth. *(C)* Cardiac.

2. **Smooth muscle**
   a. **Description.** Smooth muscle is also called visceral or involuntary muscle.
   (1)   Smooth muscle cells are smooth, tapered, and have no stripes (striations).
   (2)   Their contraction is not under voluntary control.
   (3)   Smooth muscles handle the work of all internal organs except the heart.
      (a)   The diaphragm can be voluntarily controlled, yet an individual cannot indefinitely hold his or her breath.
      (b)   The diaphragm is both a voluntary and involuntary muscle.
   (4)   Smooth muscle contractions are strong and slow.
   (5)   They respond to stimuli such as stretching, heat, and cold.

Table 4-3. Types of Muscle Tissue

Type	Appearance	Location	Function
Skeletal (voluntary)	Striated	Attached to bones	Moves skeleton Produces heat Maintains posture
Smooth (involuntary)	Smooth, tapered muscle fibers with no striations	Blood vessels Walls of hollow organs Walls of tubular structures	With contraction, reduces the length and circumference of hollow structures
Cardiac (involuntary)	Smooth with striations	Found only in the heart	Produces heartbeat Pumps blood

      b. Location
         (1)   Smooth muscle is found in blood vessels, the walls of hollow organs, and in the walls of tubular structures.
         (2)   Examples of structures that contain smooth muscle include:
            (a)   Iris of eye
            (b)   Walls of hollow organs of the gastrointestinal (GI) tract
            (c)   Ureters and urinary bladder
            (d)   Bronchi and bronchioles
            (e)   Uterus
   c. Function. Contraction of smooth muscle results in a reduction in the length and circumference of hollow structures.
         (1)   In blood vessels, smooth muscle helps maintains blood pressure.
         (2)   In the iris of the eye, smooth muscle regulates pupil size.
         (3)   In the stomach and intestines, smooth muscle is responsible for peristalsis, the waves of contraction that move food through the GI tract.
         (4)   In the ureters and urinary bladder, smooth muscle moves urine through the urinary tract.
         (5)   In the bronchi and bronchioles, constriction of smooth muscle may result in impaired breathing.

3. Cardiac muscle
   a. Description
         (1)   Cardiac muscle has its own supply of blood through the coronary artery system.
         (2)   It can tolerate interruption of blood supply for only very short periods.
         (3)   Cardiac muscle can contract on its own without stimulation from an outside source (such as a nerve). This property is called automaticity.
         (4)   Cardiac muscle contractions are strong and rhythmic.
   b. Location. Cardiac muscle is found only in the heart (forms the walls of the heart).
   c. Function. Cardiac muscle produces the heartbeat and pumps blood.

RESPIRATORY SYSTEM

FUNCTION

The **respiratory system** supplies oxygen from inhaled air to body cells and transports carbon dioxide produced by body cells for exhalation from the body.

DIVISIONS (FIGURE 4-9)

1. Upper respiratory tract
   a. The **upper respiratory tract** consists of parts outside the chest cavity, i.e., the nose, pharynx, and larynx.
   b. Function. The upper respiratory tract filters, warms, and humidifies the air, protecting the surfaces of the lower respiratory tract.

2. Lower respiratory tract
   a. The **lower respiratory tract** consists of parts found almost entirely within the chest cavity, i.e., the trachea and lungs (including the bronchial tree and alveoli).
   b. Function. The lower respiratory tract conducts air to the alveoli where gas exchange occurs.

STRUCTURES OF THE UPPER RESPIRATORY TRACT

1. Nose and nasal cavity
   a. Function. The **nose** and **nasal cavity** warms and moistens inhaled air, contains sense organs of smell, and aids in speech.

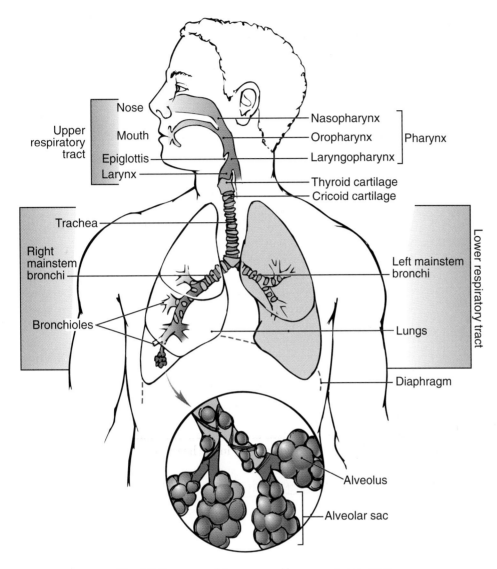

Fig. 4-9. Structures of the upper and lower respiratory tract.

b. Structure

    (1)   Air normally enters the respiratory system through the nostrils.

        (a)   The nostrils are also called the **external nares.**

        (b)   The nostrils open into the nasal cavity.

    (2)   Air is warmed, moistened, and filtered as it moves over the damp, sticky lining (**mucous membrane**) of the nose.

    (3)   The nasal **septum** [a wall (partition) that divides two cavities] divides the nasal cavity into right and left portions.

    (4)   The floor of the nasal cavity is bony and is called the **hard palate.**

    (5)   The **soft palate** is fleshy and extends behind the hard palate. It marks the boundary between the nasopharynx and the rest of the pharynx.

    (6)   Four **sinuses** (spaces or cavities inside some cranial bones) drain into the nose.

        (a)   Sinuses produce mucus and trap bacteria; they can become infected when bacteria become entrapped in the sinus tissues.

        (b)   Because they are filled with air, sinuses lighten the weight of the bones that make up the skull.

(c)   They provide additional surface area to nasal passages for warming and humidifying air.

(d)   They also serve as resonant chambers in speech production.

(7)   Each side of the nose has bones shaped like two inverted cones **(turbinates).**

    (a)   As air moves within the turbinates, it is warmed, humidified, and filtered.

    (b)   They protect structures of the lower airway from foreign body contamination.

2. **Pharynx**

  a. **Function.** The **pharynx** serves as a passageway for food, liquids, and air. It is common to both the respiratory and digestive tracts.

  b. **Structure.** The pharynx is a muscular tube, approximately 5 inches long, that starts at the internal nares and extends to the level of the cricoid cartilage.

    (1)   **Nasopharynx**

      (a)   The **nasopharynx** is located directly behind the nasal cavity.

      (b)   It serves as a passageway for air only.

      (c)   The tissues of the nasopharynx are extremely delicate and vascular. Improper or aggressive placement of tubes or airway adjuncts may result in significant bleeding.

    (2)   **Oropharynx**

      (a)   The **oropharynx** is the middle portion of the pharynx.

      (b)   It opens into the mouth and serves as a passageway for both food and air.

      (c)   It is separated from the nasopharynx by the soft palate.

      (d)   The **uvula** hangs down from the middle of the lower border of the soft palate.

    (3)   **Laryngopharynx**

      (a)   The **laryngopharynx** is the most inferior portion of the pharynx.

      (b)   It surrounds the openings of the esophagus and larynx.

      (c)   It opens anteriorly into the larynx and posteriorly into the esophagus.

      (d)   It serves as a passageway for both food and air.

3. **Larynx (voice box)**

  a. **Function**

    (1)   The **larynx** connects the pharynx with the trachea.

    (2)   It functions in voice production; the length and tension of the vocal cords determine voice pitch.

    (3)   It provides a passageway for air to and from the lungs.

  b. **Structure.** The larynx consists of nine cartilages connected to each other by muscles and ligaments.

    (1)   **Thyroid cartilage (Adam's apple)**

      (a)   The **thyroid cartilage** is the largest cartilage of the larynx and is shaped like a shield.

      (b)   It can be felt on the anterior surface of the neck.

      (c)   It is usually more prominent in males than females.

    (2)   **Epiglottis**

      (a)   The **epiglottis** is the uppermost cartilage and is shaped like a leaf.

      (b)   It is attached along the interior anterior border of the thyroid cartilage in a hinge-like fashion.

      (c)   It covers the opening to the larynx during swallowing, preventing food and liquids from entering the airway.

    (3)   **Cricoid cartilage**

      (a)   The **cricoid cartilage** is the most inferior of the cartilages of the larynx.

      (b)   It forms the base of the larynx on which the other cartilages rest.

(4)   **Vocal cords**

(a)   The **vocal cords** stretch across the interior of the larynx.

(b)   The space between the vocal cords is called the **glottis.**

STRUCTURES OF THE LOWER RESPIRATORY TRACT

1. **Trachea (windpipe)**
   a. **Function.** The **trachea** or **windpipe** serves as a passageway for air to and from the lungs.
   b. **Structure**
   (1)   The trachea is an elongated tube approximately 4–5 inches [10–12 centimeters (cm)] long.
   (2)   It is kept permanently open by C-shaped cartilaginous rings. The open part of each C-shaped cartilage faces the esophagus, allowing the esophagus to expand slightly into the trachea during swallowing.
   (3)   It extends from the larynx at approximately the sixth cervical vertebra to the fifth thoracic vertebra, where it divides into two primary bronchi.
2. **Bronchi and bronchioles**
   a. **Function.** The **bronchi** and **bronchioles** serve as passageways for air to and from the alveoli.
   b. **Structure**
   (1)   The trachea divides into two primary (mainstem) bronchi (right and left).
   (2)   The right primary bronchus is shorter, wider, and straighter than the left.
   (3)   The point at which the trachea divides into two primary bronchi forms an internal ridge called the **carina.** The mucous membrane of the carina is one of the most sensitive areas of the respiratory system and is associated with the cough reflex.
   (4)   Bronchi divide into smaller and smaller tubes, eventually leading to bronchioles. Cartilage is not present in the walls of the bronchioles.
   (5)   Bronchioles subdivide and end in microscopic tubes called **alveolar ducts.**
3. **Alveoli**
   a. **Function. Alveoli** are the sites where gases—oxygen and carbon dioxide—are exchanged between the air and blood. They are thus considered the functional units of the respiratory system.
   b. **Structure**
   (1)   Each alveolar duct ends in several alveolar sacs.
   (a)   Alveolar sacs are the air sacs of the lungs.
   (b)   Each sac resembles a cluster of grapes.
   (2)   The walls of the alveolar sacs are made up of alveoli.
   (3)   The structure of the alveoli is suited to gas exchange.
   (a)   Each alveolus is surrounded by a network of pulmonary capillaries.
   (b)   The wall of an alveolus consists of a single layer of cells.
   (c)   A thin film of **surfactant** coats each alveolus and prevents the alveoli from collapsing.
4. **Lungs**
   a. **Function. Lungs** bring air into contact with blood so oxygen and carbon dioxide can be exchanged in the alveoli.
   b. **Structure**
   (1)   Lungs are spongy, air-filled organs bound superiorly by the clavicles and inferiorly by the diaphragm.
   (2)   Primary bronchi and pulmonary blood vessels are bound by connective tissue and form the root of the lung. The root of the lung is the only real connection the lungs have with the body itself.
   (3)   The lungs are divided into lobes.
   (a)   The right lung has three lobes. The right lung is shorter than the left because the diaphragm is higher on the right to accommodate the liver that lies below it.

        (b) The left lung has two lobes. Because two-thirds of the heart lies to the left of the midline of the body, the left lung contains a notch to accommodate the position of the heart.

        (c) The lobes or lungs may be removed due to disease.

   (4) The **pleura** is the serous (oily) double-walled membrane that encloses each lung.

        (a) The **parietal pleura** is the outer lining and lines the wall of the thoracic cavity (rib cage, diaphragm, and mediastinum).

        (b) The **visceral pleura** is the inner layer and covers the surface of the lungs.

        (c) The **pleural space** is a space between the visceral and parietal pleura filled with a small amount of serous (oily) fluid that allows the lungs to glide easily against each other as the lungs fill and empty during breathing.

        (d) Inflammation of the pleura (**pleurisy**) results in painful breathing.

        (e) If either the parietal or visceral pleura is torn, the capability for normal expansion of the lungs is lost.

c. Terminology

   (1) The apex of the lung is the uppermost portion of the lung; reaches above the first rib.

   (2) The base of the lung is the portion of the lung resting on the diaphragm.

   (3) The mediastinum is part of the space in the middle of the chest, between the lungs.

        (a) The mediastinum extends from the sternum (breastbone) to the spine.

        (b) It contains all of the organs of the thorax except the lungs (heart, great vessels, esophagus, trachea, nerves).

MECHANICS OF BREATHING

1. Definitions

  a. Breathing (pulmonary ventilation) is the mechanical process of moving air into and out of the lungs.

  b. Inspiration (inhalation) is the process of breathing in and moving air into the lungs.

  c. Expiration (exhalation) is the process of breathing out and moving air out of the lungs.

  d. Respiration is the exchange of gases between a living organism and its environment.

2. Muscles of breathing

  a. Diaphragm

   (1) The diaphragm is the dome-shaped muscle below the lungs.

   (2) It is the primary muscle of respiration.

   (3) It separates the thoracic cavity from the abdominal cavity.

  b. The external **intercostal muscles** are located between the ribs.

  c. The internal intercostal muscles and abdominal muscles may be used during forceful expiration.

3. Breathing (*Figure 4-10*)

  a. When the diaphragm and external intercostal muscles contract, the chest cavity enlarges and fills with air.

   (1) This process is called inspiration.

   (2) Inspiration is an active process (requires muscle contraction).

  b. When the diaphragm and external intercostal muscles relax, the chest cavity becomes smaller, the lungs are compressed, and air is forced out.

   (1) This process is called expiration.

   (2) Expiration is normally a passive process.

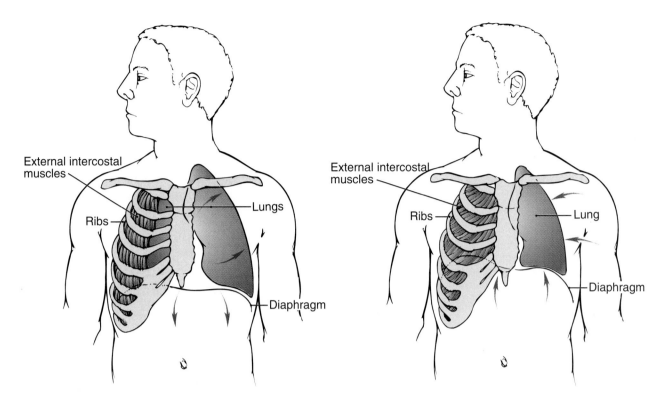

Fig. 4-10. Mechanism of breathing. (*A*) During inspiration, the diaphragm contracts and moves downward and the external intercostal muscles pull the ribs upward and outward. The pressure within the lungs falls below atmospheric pressure and air rushes into the lungs. (*B*) During expiration, the diaphragm and external intercostal muscles relax. The pressure within the lungs rises above atmospheric pressure and air rushes out of the lungs.

    c. The mechanics of breathing can be compared with a bellows: when it is open, air enters; as it closes, air is forced out.

RESPIRATORY PHYSIOLOGY

1. Alveolar/capillary exchange
    a. Oxygen-rich air enters the alveoli during each inspiration.
    b. Oxygen-poor blood in the capillaries passes into the alveoli.
    c. Oxygen enters the capillaries as carbon dioxide enters the alveoli.
2. Capillary/cellular exchange
    a. Cells give up carbon dioxide to the capillaries.
    b. Capillaries give up oxygen to the cells.

INFANT AND CHILD ANATOMY

1. Nose and mouth. In general, all structures are smaller and more easily obstructed than in adults.
2. Pharynx. The tongue takes up proportionally more space in the mouth than in an adult.
3. Trachea (windpipe)
    a. The trachea is softer and more flexible in infants and children.
    b. A narrower trachea is more easily obstructed by swelling.
3. Cricoid cartilage. Like other cartilage in the infant and child, the cricoid cartilage is less developed and less rigid.
4. Diaphragm
    a. The chest wall is softer.
    b. Infants and children depend more heavily on the diaphragm for breathing.

RESPIRATORY ASSESSMENT

1. **Adequate breathing**
   a. Normal rates are as follows:
      (1) Adults: 12–20 breaths/minute
      (2) Children: 15–30 breaths/minute
      (3) Infants: 25–50 breaths/minute
   b. **Regular rhythm**
   c. **Quality**
      (1) Breath sounds are present and equal bilaterally.
      (2) Chest expansion is adequate and equal with each breath.
      (3) No excess effort is required for breathing, i.e., no excessive use of accessory muscles during inspiration or expiration.
   d. **Adequate depth (tidal volume)**
      (1) **Tidal volume** is the amount of air inhaled and exhaled during normal breathing.
      (2) In the average adult, tidal volume is approximately 500 milliliters (mL).
         (a) Only about 350 mL of the tidal volume actually reaches the alveoli.
         (b) The other 150 mL remains in the air spaces of the nose, pharynx, larynx, trachea, bronchi, and bronchioles.
2. **Inadequate breathing**
   a. Respiratory rate is outside the normal range.
   b. Breathing pattern is irregular.
   c. Breath sounds are diminished or absent.
   d. Chest expansion is unequal or inadequate.
   e. Effort of breathing is increased.
      (1) Individual (usually infants and children) may use accessory muscles in breathing, as evidenced by retractions above the clavicles (between the ribs and below the rib cage). Retractions are usually seen in children.
      (2) Nasal flaring may be present, especially in children.
      (3) In infants, "seesaw" breathing, in which the chest and abdomen move in opposite directions, may be present.
   f. Depth (tidal volume) may be inadequate/shallow.
   g. Skin is pale, cyanotic (blue), cool, and clammy.
   h. Agonal respirations (occasional gasping breaths) may be seen just before death.
   i. An altered level of consciousness is an early sign of hypoxia.

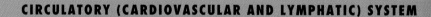

CIRCULATORY (CARDIOVASCULAR AND LYMPHATIC) SYSTEM

FUNCTION

1. **Transport**
   a. Blood carries oxygen, food, hormones, minerals, and other essential substances to all parts of the body.
   b. Blood carries carbon dioxide and other waste material from the body's cells to the lungs, kidneys, or skin for elimination.
2. **Maintenance of body temperature.** Blood vessels constrict and dilate as needed to retain or dissipate heat at the skin's surface.
3. **Protection.** The blood and lymphatic system protect the body against invasion by foreign microorganisms through the immune (defense) system (*Figure 4-11*).

COMPONENTS

1. The **cardiovascular system** consists of the heart, blood vessels, and blood.
2. The lymphatic system consists of lymph, lymph nodes, lymph vessels, tonsils, spleen, and thymus gland.

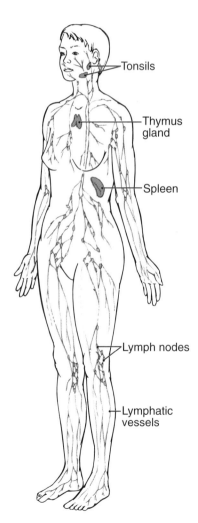

Tonsils

Thymus gland

Spleen

Lymph nodes

Lymphatic vessels

Fig. 4-11. The lymphatic system protects the body against invasion by foreign microorganisms through the immune (defense) system.

3. Organs that form and store blood are also associated with the circulatory system and include the spleen, liver, and bone marrow.

HEART

1. **Structure**
   a. The **heart** lies in the thoracic cavity (mediastinum) behind the sternum and between the lungs; approximately two-thirds of the heart's mass lies to the left of the body's midline.
   b. The heart is attached to the thorax through the great vessels (**pulmonary arteries** and veins, aorta, superior and inferior vena cavae).
2. **Heart layers**
   a. The pericardium is a double-walled membranous sac that encloses the heart.
   b. The myocardium (heart muscle) is the middle and thickest layer of the heart.
   c. The endocardium is the inner layer of the heart.
3. **Heart chambers** *(Figure 4-12)*
   a. The two upper chambers are the right and left atria.
      (1) **Atria** are thin-walled, low-pressure chambers that receive blood from the systemic circulation and lungs.
      (2) Atria are separated by a wall of myocardium called the **interatrial septum.**
      (3) The superior and inferior vena cavae deliver oxygen-poor blood from the body to the right atrium.
      (4) The right atrium pumps oxygen-poor blood through the tricuspid valve to the right ventricle.
      (5) The left atrium receives oxygen-rich blood from the pulmonary veins (lungs) and pumps the blood through the mitral (bicuspid) valve to the left ventricle.
   b. The two lower chambers are the right and left ventricles.
      (1) The ventricles pump blood to the lungs and systemic circulation (body).
         (a) The right ventricle pumps blood to the lungs.
         (b) The left ventricle pumps blood to the body.
      (2) The ventricles are larger and thicker walled than the atria.
         (a) The left ventricle is a high-pressure chamber.
         (b) It is approximately three times thicker than the right ventricle.
      (3) The right and left ventricles are separated by a wall of myocardium called the interventricular septum.
4. **Heart valves.** Heart valves prevent backflow of blood and keep blood moving in one direction *(see Figure 4-12)*.
   a. **Atrioventricular (AV) valves**
      (1) The tricuspid valve is located between the right atrium and right ventricle.
      (2) The mitral (**bicuspid**) valve is located between the left atrium and left ventricle.
   b. **Semilunar valves**
      (1) The pulmonic valve is located at the junction of the right ventricle and pulmonary artery.
      (2) The aortic valve is located at the junction of the left ventricle and aorta.
5. **Conduction system** *(Figure 4-13)*
   a. Specialized electrical (pacemaker) cells in the heart are arranged in a system of pathways called the conduction system.
   b. Normal pathway for electrical impulse: the impulse begins in the sinoatrial (SA) node → atrioventricular (AV) node (located between the atria and ventricles) → bundle of His → right and left bundle branches → Purkinje fibers.
   c. Electrical stimulation normally results in contraction of the heart's muscle fibers.
   d. Blood is then pumped to the lungs and through the aorta to the body.

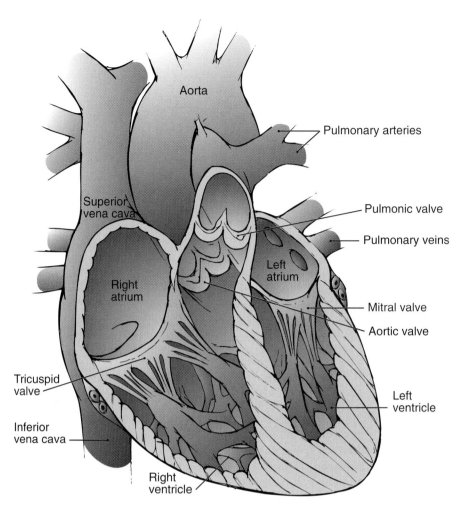

Fig. 4-12. Heart chambers, valves, and major vessels.

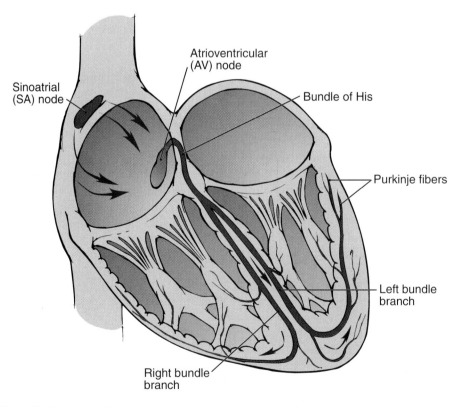

Fig. 4-13. Specialized cells in the heart are arranged in a system of pathways called the conduction system.

BLOOD VESSELS

1. Arteries
   a. Function. Arteries carry blood away from the heart and help maintain blood pressure.
   b. Arteries are high-pressure vessels.
   c. All arteries, except the pulmonary arteries, carry oxygen-rich blood.
   d. Major arteries
      (1) Aorta
         (a) The aorta is the major artery originating from the heart.
         (b) It lies in front of the spine in the thoracic and abdominal cavities.
         (c) It divides at the level of the navel into the iliac arteries.
      (2) Coronary arteries supply the heart with blood.
      (3) Carotid artery
         (a) The carotid artery is the major artery of the neck.
         (b) It supplies the head with blood.
         (c) Its pulsation can be palpated on either side of the neck.
         (d) The right and left carotid arteries should never be palpated at the same time because doing so can cause severe lowering of the heart rate.
      (4) Femoral artery
         (a) The femoral artery is the major artery of the thigh.
         (b) It supplies the lower extremity with blood.
         (c) Pulsation can be palpated in the groin area (the crease between the abdomen and thigh).
      (5) The pulsation of the **posterior tibial artery** can be palpated on the posterior surface of the medial malleolus.
      (6) Dorsalis pedis artery
         (a) The dorsalis pedis artery is the artery in the foot.
         (b) Pulsation can be palpated on the superior surface of the foot.
      (7) Brachial artery
         (a) The brachial artery is the artery of the upper arm.
         (b) Pulsation can be palpated on the inside of the arm between the elbow and shoulder.
         (c) This artery is used when determining a blood pressure (BP) using a blood pressure cuff and stethoscope.
      (8) Radial artery
         (a) The radial artery is the major artery of the lower arm.
         (b) Pulsation can be palpated at the wrist, thumb side.
      (9) Pulmonary arteries
         (a) Pulmonary arteries originate at the right ventricle of the heart.
         (b) They carry oxygen-poor blood from the right ventricle to the lungs.
2. Arterioles are the smallest branches of arteries leading to the capillaries.
3. Capillaries
   a. Capillaries are microscopic vessels that are one cell thick.
   b. They serve as vessels for exchange of wastes, fluids, and nutrients between the blood and tissues.
   c. They connect arterioles and venules.
   d. All tissues except cartilage, hair, nails, and the cornea of the eye contain capillaries.
4. Veins
   a. Veins collect blood for transport back to the heart.
   b. They are low-pressure vessels.
   c. They contain valves to prevent backflow of blood.
   d. All veins, except the pulmonary veins, carry deoxygenated (oxygen-poor) blood.
   e. Major veins
      (1) Pulmonary veins carry oxygen-rich blood from the lungs to the left atrium.

(2) Venae cavae return blood to the right atrium.
   (a) The superior vena cava carries blood from the head and upper extremities.
   (b) The inferior vena cava carries blood from the torso and lower extremities.
5. Venules are the smallest branches of veins leading to the capillaries.

COMPOSITION OF BLOOD

1. **Components**
   a. Formed elements are the cellular components of blood and include:
      (1) Red blood cells (erythrocytes)
      (2) White blood cells (leukocytes)
      (3) Platelets (thrombocytes)
   b. Plasma is the liquid component of blood.
2. **Red blood cells**
   a. Red blood cells transport oxygen to body cells.
      (1) Each red blood cell contains hemoglobin.
      (2) Hemoglobin is an iron-containing protein that chemically bonds with oxygen. Thus, hemoglobin is the part of the red blood cell that carries oxygen from the lungs to the tissues.
      (3) Hemoglobin is red and gives blood its red color.
   b. Red blood cells also transport carbon dioxide away from body cells.
3. White blood cells defend the body from microorganisms, such as bacteria and viruses, that have invaded the bloodstream or tissues of the body.
4. **Platelets**
   a. Platelets are essential for the formation of blood clots.
   b. They function to stop bleeding and repair ruptured blood vessels.
5. **Plasma**
   a. Plasma is the clear, straw-colored liquid component of blood (blood minus its formed elements).
   b. It carries nutrients to the cells and waste products from the cells.

PHYSIOLOGY OF CIRCULATION

1. **Pulse**
   a. When the left ventricle contracts, a wave of blood is sent through the arteries causing the arteries to expand and recoil.
   b. A **pulse** is the regular expansion and recoil of an artery caused by the movement of blood from the heart as it contracts.
   c. A pulse can be felt anywhere an artery simultaneously passes near the skin surface and over a bone.
   d. Central pulses are located close to the heart, e.g., **carotid** and **femoral pulses** (*Figure 4-14*).
   e. Peripheral pulses are located farther from the heart, e.g., **radial, brachial, posterior tibial,** and **dorsalis pedis pulses** (*see Figure 4-14*).
2. **Blood pressure**
   a. Blood pressure is the force exerted by the blood on the inner walls of the heart and blood vessels.
   b. **Systolic blood pressure** is the pressure exerted against the walls of the arteries when the left ventricle contracts.
   c. **Diastolic blood pressure** is the pressure exerted against the walls of the arteries when the left ventricle is at rest.
3. **Perfusion**
   a. **Definition. Perfusion** is the circulation of blood through an organ or a part of the body.
   b. **Hypoperfusion (shock)**

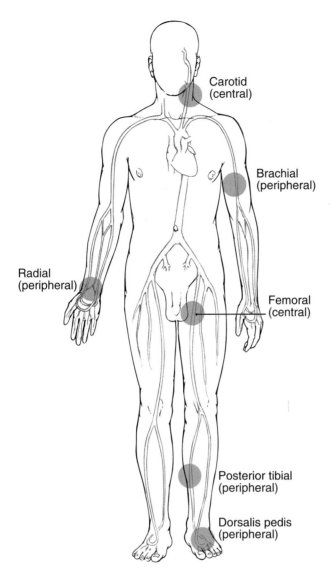

Fig. 4-14. Central and peripheral pulses.

(1) **Definition. Hypoperfusion** is the inadequate circulation of blood through an organ or a part of the body; a state of profound depression of the vital processes of the body.

(2) Hypoperfusion is characterized by the following signs and symptoms:

 (a) Pale, cyanotic, cool, clammy skin

 (b) Rapid, weak pulse

 (c) Rapid, shallow breathing

 (d) Restlessness, anxiety, or mental dullness

 (e) Nausea and vomiting

 (f) Reduction in total blood volume

 (g) Low or decreasing blood pressure

 (h) Subnormal temperature

NERVOUS SYSTEM

FUNCTION

The **nervous system** controls the voluntary and involuntary activities of the body.

DIVISIONS

The nervous system is divided into the **central nervous system** (CNS) and the **peripheral nervous system** (PNS).

CENTRAL NERVOUS SYSTEM

The CNS consists of the brain and spinal cord *(Figure 4-15)*.

1. **Brain**
    a. Protective coverings of the brain include:
    (1) The skull
    (2) **Meninges** (literally, membranes), which are three layers of connective tissue coverings that surround the brain and spinal cord.
    (a) The **pia mater** (literally, "gentle mother") forms the delicate inner layer that clings gently to the brain and spinal cord; it contains many blood vessels that supply the nervous tissue.
    (b) The **arachnoid** (literally, "resembling a spider's web") layer is the middle meningeal layer with delicate fibers resembling a spider's web; it contains few blood vessels.

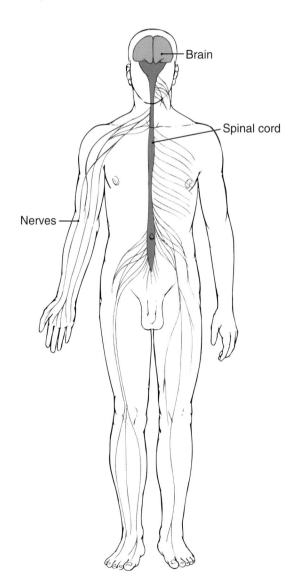

Fig. 4-15. The central nervous system (CNS) consists of the brain and spinal cord. The peripheral nervous system (PNS) consists of cranial and spinal nerves.

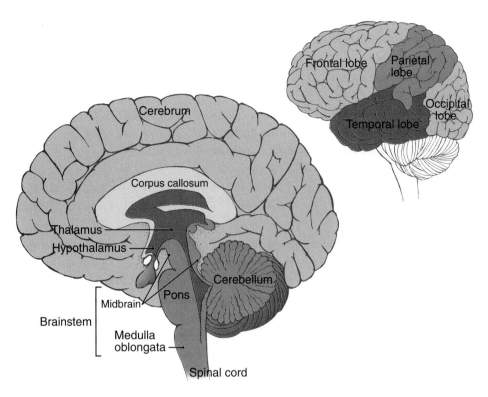

Fig. 4-16. Sagittal view of the brain.

    (c) The **dura mater** (literally, "hard" or "tough mother") is the tough, durable, outermost layer that adheres to the inner surface of the cranium.

b. Cerebrospinal fluid surrounds the brain and spinal cord

    (1) Cerebrospinal fluid acts as a shock-absorber for the central nervous system.

    (2) It provides a medium for exchange of nutrients and wastes among the blood, brain, and spinal cord.

c. Cerebrum *(Figure 4-16)*

    (1) The **cerebrum** is the largest part of the human brain.

    (2) It consists of two cerebral hemispheres; the **corpus callosum** joins the two hemispheres.

    (3) Each cerebral hemisphere has four lobes.

        (a) The frontal lobe controls motor function.

        (b) The parietal lobe receives and interprets nerve impulses from sensory receptors.

        (c) The occipital lobe controls eyesight.

        (d) The temporal lobe controls hearing and smell.

d. Cerebellum

    (1) The **cerebellum** is the second largest part of the human brain.

    (2) It is responsible for precise control of muscle movements, maintenance of posture, and maintaining equilibrium.

e. Brain stem

    (1) **Midbrain**

        (a) The midbrain connects the pons and cerebellum with the cerebrum.

        (b) It acts as a relay for auditory and visual impulses.

    (2) **Pons** (literally, "bridge")

        (a) The pons connects parts of the brain with one another by means of tracts.

        (b) It influences respiration.

      (3) Medulla oblongata
        (a) The medulla oblongata extends from the pons and is continuous with the upper portion of the spinal cord.
        (b) It is involved in the regulation of heart rate, blood vessel diameter, respiration, coughing, swallowing, and vomiting.
   2. Spinal cord
     a. The spinal cord is the center for many reflex activities of the body.
     b. It transmits impulses to and from the brain.
       (1) **Sensory nerves** transmit impulses to the brain.
       (2) **Motor nerves** transmit impulses from the brain.
     c. It extends from the medulla of the brain stem to the level of the upper border of the second lumbar vertebra in an adult.
       (1) The spinal cord is approximately 16–18 inches in length (adult).
       (2) It is approximately three-fourths of an inch in diameter in the midthorax (adult).

PERIPHERAL NERVOUS SYSTEM *(SEE FIGURE 4-15)*

  1. Components. The PNS consists of all nervous tissue found outside the brain and spinal cord.
    a. Cranial nerves
      (1) There are 12 pairs of **cranial nerves.**
      (2) They connect the brain with the neck and structures in the thorax and abdomen.
    b. Spinal nerves
      (1) There are 31 pairs of **spinal nerves.**
      (2) Sensory nerves transmit messages to the brain and spinal cord from the body.
      (3) Motor nerves transmit messages from the brain and spinal cord to the body.
  2. Divisions. The PNS has two divisions; both divisions contain sensory (afferent) and motor (efferent) nerves.
    a. Somatic (voluntary) division
      (1) The somatic division has receptors and nerves concerned with the external environment.
      (2) It influences the activity of the musculoskeletal system.
    b. Autonomic (involuntary) division
      (1) The autonomic division has receptors and nerves concerned with the internal environment.
      (2) It controls the involuntary system of glands and smooth muscle and functions to maintain a steady state in the body.
      (3) The autonomic division is further divided into the sympathetic division and parasympathetic division.
        (a) The sympathetic division mobilizes energy, particularly in stressful situations (i.e., the "fight-or-flight" response). Its effects are widespread throughout the body.
        (b) The parasympathetic division conserves and restores energy; its effects are localized in the body.

THE INTEGUMENTARY SYSTEM (SKIN)

FUNCTION

  1. The skin performs many protective functions; it is the first line of defense against bacteria and other organisms, ultraviolet rays from the sun, harmful chemicals, cuts, and tears.

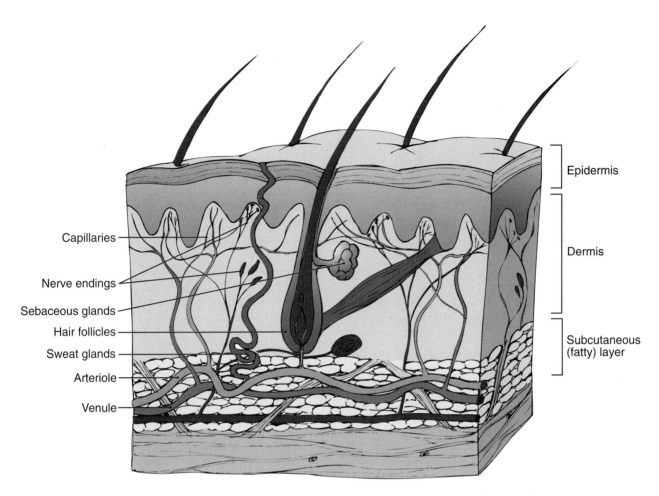

Fig. 4-17. Anatomy of the skin.

2. It helps regulate body temperature.
3. It senses heat, cold, touch, pressure and pain and transmits this information to the brain and spinal cord.
4. It is the site of vitamin D synthesis.
5. Sweat glands excrete excess water and some wastes (urea and uric acid).

LAYERS (FIGURE 4-17)

1. **Epidermis**
   a. The epidermis is the outermost skin layer.
   b. It consists of four or five layers.
   (1) New cells are continuously formed in the deeper layers of the epidermis.
   (2) Older cells are pushed upward and sloughed off.
   c. The epidermis contains keratin, a waterproofing protein.
2. The dermis is deeper and thicker layer of skin containing sweat and sebaceous glands, hair follicles, blood vessels, and nerve endings.
3. **Subcutaneous (fatty) layer**
   a. The subcutaneous layer helps conserve body heat.
   b. Fat can be used as an energy source when adequate food is not available.

ACCESSORY STRUCTURES

Accessory structures include hair, nails, sweat glands, and sebaceous (oil) glands.

ENDOCRINE SYSTEM

FUNCTION

The **endocrine system** is a system of ductless glands that secrete chemicals, such as **insulin** and **adrenalin,** that regulate and influence body activities and functions (*Figure 4-18*).

COMPONENTS

1. **Thyroid gland**
   a. The **thyroid gland** lies in the neck, just below the larynx.
   b. It regulates metabolic rate.
2. **Parathyroid glands**
   a. The **parathyroid glands** are located on the back of the thyroid gland.
   b. They control calcium and phosphorus metabolism and activate vitamin D.
3. **Adrenal glands**
   a. **Adrenal glands** are located on top of each kidney.
   b. They release epinephrine in response to stress.
4. **Pituitary gland**
   a. The **pituitary gland** is buried deep in the cranial cavity at the base of the brain.
   b. It is the "master gland" of the body.
   c. It regulates growth and controls other endocrine glands.
5. **Islets of Langerhans**
   a. The **islets of Langerhans** are located in the pancreas.

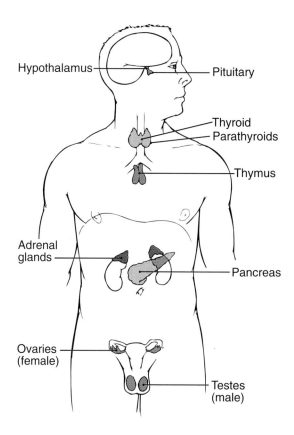

Fig. 4-18. The endocrine system.

    b. Alpha cells secrete **glucagon,** which increases blood glucose concentration.

    c. Beta cells secrete insulin, which decreases blood glucose concentration.

6. **Ovaries** secrete female sex hormones.
7. **Testes** secrete male sex hormones.
8. The hypothalamus produces hormones released by the pituitary.
    a. Antidiuretic hormone decreases the volume of urine.
    b. Oxytocin stimulates uterine contraction in pregnancy.
9. The thymus promotes development of immune system cells.

DIGESTIVE (GASTROINTESTINAL) SYSTEM

FUNCTION

The **digestive system** performs the following functions:
1. **Ingestion.** The digestive system brings nutrients, water, and electrolytes into the body.
2. **Digestion.** It chemically breaks down food into small parts so absorption can occur.
3. **Absorption.** It moves nutrients, water, and electrolytes into the circulatory system so they can be used by body cells.
4. **Defecation.** It eliminates undigested waste.

COMPONENTS (FIGURE 4-19)

1. The primary organs of the digestive system are the mouth, pharynx, esophagus, stomach, small intestine, large intestine, rectum, and anal canal.
2. The **accessory organs** are the teeth and tongue, salivary glands, liver, gallbladder, and pancreas.

PERISTALSIS

Peristalsis is the involuntary wavelike contraction of smooth muscle that moves material through the digestive tract.

MOUTH, TEETH, AND SALIVARY GLANDS

1. The mouth, teeth, and **salivary glands** begin the process of digestion.
2. The tongue manipulates food for chewing and swallowing.
3. The salivary glands dissolve food chemicals and moisten and lubricate food so it can be swallowed.
4. The teeth mince food into small pieces so it can be swallowed when mixed with saliva.

ESOPHAGUS

1. Swallowing moves food from the pharynx into the **esophagus.**
2. The esophagus transports food from the pharynx to the stomach by peristalsis.

STOMACH

1. The **stomach** stores food.
2. The stomach mixes food with gastric juices and breaks it down into chyme.
3. It moves food (chyme) into the small intestine.

SMALL INTESTINE

1. The small intestine is approximately 20 feet (7 meters) long.
2. It is smaller in diameter than the large intestine.

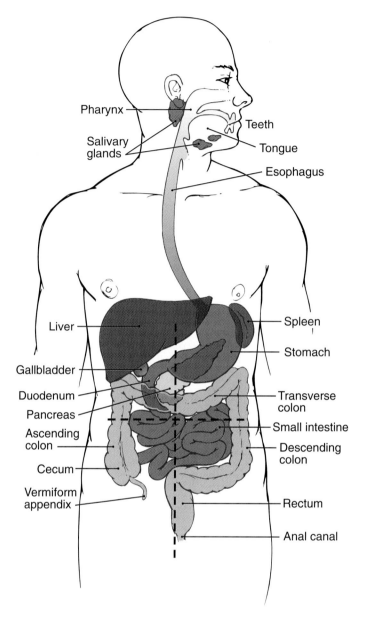

Fig. 4-19. The digestive system.

3. It receives food from the stomach and secretions from the pancreas and liver.
4. It completes the digestion of food that began in the mouth and stomach.
   a. Most digestion and absorption occurs here.
   b. It selectively absorbs nutrients that can be used by the body.
5. It is composed of three sections (listed in the order in which food passes through them):
   a. Duodenum
   b. Jejunum
   c. Ileum

LARGE INTESTINE (COLON)

1. The **large intestine** is approximately 5 feet (1.5 meters) in length.
2. It absorbs water and electrolytes from the remaining chyme and changes it from a fluid to a semisolid mass.

3. It excretes waste as feces.
4. The large intestine is subdivided into the following sections (listed in the order in which food passes through them): **cecum, ascending colon, transverse colon, descending colon, sigmoid colon, rectum,** and **anal canal.**

LIVER, GALLBLADDER, AND PANCREAS

1. **Liver**
   a. The **liver** produces bile, which breaks up (emulsifies) fats.
   b. It stimulates the gallbladder to secrete stored bile into the small intestine.
   c. It stores minerals and fat-soluble vitamins (A, D, E, and K).
   d. It stores blood (approximately 30% of cardiac output).
2. The **gallbladder** stores bile until it is needed by the small intestine.
3. The pancreas secretes juices that contain enzymes for protein, carbohydrate, and fat digestion into the small intestine.

URINARY SYSTEM

FUNCTION

The **urinary system** produces and excretes urine from the body.

COMPONENTS (FIGURE 4-20)

1. The **kidneys** produce urine, maintain water balance, aid in regulation of blood pressure, and regulate levels of many chemicals in the blood.

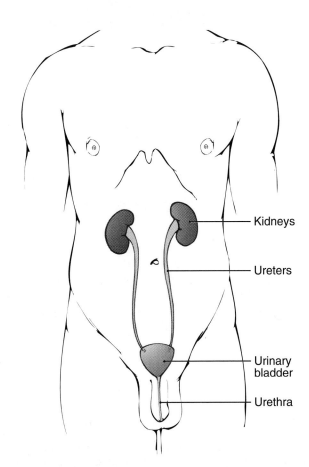

Kidneys

Ureters

Urinary bladder

Urethra

Fig. 4-20. The urinary system.

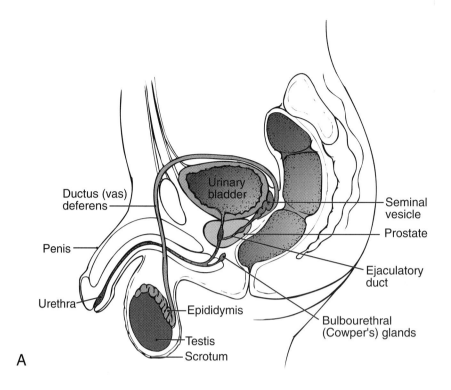

A

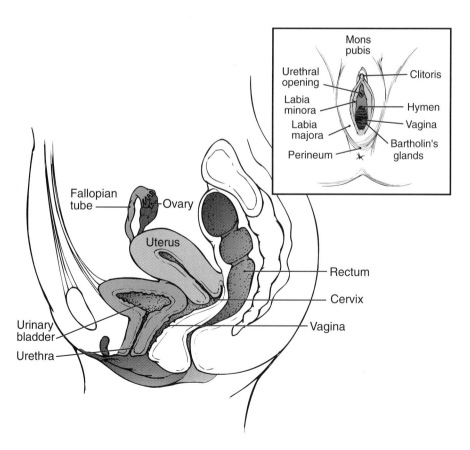

B

Fig. 4-21. *(A)* Male reproductive organs. *(B)* Female reproductive organs.

2. The **ureters** drain urine from the kidneys to the urinary bladder.
3. The **urinary bladder** serves as a temporary storage site for urine.
4. **Urethra**
   a. The **urethra** transports urine from the urinary bladder to the outside of the body.
   b. In males, the urethra transports semen from the body.
   c. The male urethra is longer than that of females.

REPRODUCTIVE SYSTEM

FUNCTION

The reproductive system functions in the perpetuation of the human species.

COMPONENTS

1. **Male** *(Figure 4-21A)*
   a. Gonads (testes) produce sperm and the hormone testosterone.
   b. Reproductive ducts allow passage of sperm. Ducts include:
      (1) Epididymis
      (2) Ductus (vas) deferens
      (3) Ejaculatory duct
      (4) Urethra
   c. **Accessory glands**
      (1) Seminal vesicles secrete fluid that nourishes and protects sperm.
      (2) The prostate gland secretes fluid that enhances sperm motility and neutralizes the acidity of the vagina during intercourse.
      (3) Bulbourethral (Cowper's) glands secrete mucuslike fluid.
   d. **External genitalia**
      (1) The penis serves as the outlet for sperm and urine.
      (2) The scrotum is the loose sac of skin that houses the testes.
2. **Female** *(Figure 4-21B)*
   a. Gonads (ovaries) produce the hormones estrogen and progesterone.
   b. Fallopian tubes (oviducts) receive and transport the ovum to the uterus after ovulation.
   c. The uterus is a hollow, muscular organ in which a fertilized ovum implants and receives nourishment until birth.
   d. The vagina (birth canal) receives the penis during intercourse and serves as a passageway for menstrual flow and delivery of an infant.
   e. Accessory organs include the mammary glands (breasts), which function in milk production after delivery of an infant.
   f. **External genitalia**
      (1) External genitalia include mons pubis, clitoris, urethral opening, Bartholin's gland, vagina, labia minora, labia majora, and hymen.
      (2) The perineum is the area between the vaginal opening and anus.

REVIEW QUESTIONS

Directions: Each of the numbered items or incomplete statements in this section is followed by answers or by completions of the statement. Select the ONE lettered answer or completion that is BEST in each case.

1. The xiphoid process is in what relationship to the body of the sternum?

   (A) Inferior
   (B) Superior
   (C) Posterior
   (D) Trendelenburg

2. The human body must produce an astounding 2.4 million new red blood cells per second to sustain normal body function. The system responsible for production of red blood cells is the

   (A) cardiovascular system
   (B) skeletal system
   (C) respiratory system
   (D) lymphatic system

3. Which of the body systems is responsible for providing movement, giving the body shape, protecting internal organs, and producing heat?

   (A) Skeletal
   (B) Muscular
   (C) Lymphatic
   (D) Integumentary

4. Your rescue crew is called to the local elementary school for a 10-year-old female patient who has fallen from the monkey bars. Your patient is in the nurse's office complaining of severe right wrist pain. During your physical exam, you gently palpate the affected limb. Which of the following correctly lists the order of the bones in the arm from proximal to distal?

   (A) Frontal, parietal, temporal, occipital, sphenoid
   (B) Phalanges, metacarpals, carpals, ulna and radius, humerus
   (C) Humerus, radius and ulna, carpals, metacarpals, phalanges
   (D) Femur, patella, tibia and fibula, tarsals, metatarsal, and phalanges

5. Blood pressure is maintained by the dilation and contraction of the vessels of the cardiovascular system. To lower blood pressure, these vessels dilate; to increase pressure, these vessels constrict. The walls of these vessels are composed of

   (A) tendons
   (B) ligaments
   (C) smooth muscle
   (D) striated muscle

6. The respiratory system is responsible for introducing atmospheric oxygen into the body and ridding the body of gaseous waste (mainly carbon dioxide). The exchange of oxygen and carbon dioxide occurs

   (A) in the alveoli
   (B) in the trachea
   (C) in the bronchioles
   (D) throughout the respiratory system

7. To prevent the aspiration of food or liquids, a flap of tissue closes over the trachea when swallowing. This tissue is called the

   (A) larynx
   (B) bronchi
   (C) epiglottis
   (D) pericardium

8. In the cardiovascular system, systemic circulation is responsible for delivering oxygenated blood to all body cells and picking up metabolic waste products. Which of the following are components of the systemic circulation?

    (A)   Right and left atria
    (B)   Right and left ventricles
    (C)   Left atrium and left ventricle
    (D)   Right atrium and right ventricle

9. In the cardiovascular system, pulmonary circulation is responsible for returning oxygen-poor blood to the respiratory tract for reoxygenation. Which of the following are components of the pulmonary circulation?

    (A)   Right and left atria
    (B)   Right and left ventricles
    (C)   Left atrium and left ventricle
    (D)   Right atrium and right ventricle

10. Preventing the backflow of blood is the responsibility of which of the following?

    (A)   Arteries and veins
    (B)   Septum
    (C)   Valves
    (D)   Pericardium

11. The _____ carry blood away from the heart. The _____ carry blood toward the heart.

    (A)   veins, arteries
    (B)   arteries, veins
    (C)   atria, ventricles
    (D)   capillaries, septum

12. Vision, speech, auditory skills, and cognitive movement are all controlled by the central nervous system. The area of the brain responsible for these skills is the

    (A)   cerebrum
    (B)   meninges
    (C)   brain stem
    (D)   cerebellum

13. During a perceived threat, the autonomic nervous system increases the body's energy level. This response is sometimes called the "fight-or-flight" response. The division of the autonomic nervous system responsible for this action is the

    (A)   medulla oblongata
    (B)   somatic nervous system
    (C)   sympathetic nervous system
    (D)   parasympathetic nervous system

14. The sweat glands, hair follicles, blood vessels, sebaceous glands, and nerve endings are located in which layer of the skin?

    (A)   Dermis
    (B)   Urethra
    (C)   Epidermis
    (D)   Subcutaneous fat

15. The endocrine system is a system of glands that secrete hormones to help regulate body function. Insulin, the hormone that regulates blood sugar levels, is one such hormone. Insulin is produced in the islets of Langerhans in which organ?

    (A) Colon
    (B) Spleen
    (C) Pancreas
    (D) Pituitary gland

16. The process of bringing nutrients, water, and electrolytes into the body is called

    (A) ingestion
    (B) defecation
    (C) absorption
    (D) digestion

17. Food is moved through the tubular passages of the gastrointestinal tract by

    (A) cilia
    (B) gravity
    (C) osmosis
    (D) peristalsis

18. The majority of digestion and absorption takes place in the

    (A) liver
    (B) stomach
    (C) small intestine
    (D) large intestine

19. The body system that regulates water, salt, and other chemicals is the

    (A) urinary system
    (B) digestive system
    (C) circulatory system
    (D) integumentary system

20. In the female reproductive system, the production of estrogen and progesterone takes place in the

    (A) uterus
    (B) ovaries
    (C) pituitary gland
    (D) mammary glands

21. Which of the following is common to both male and female anatomy?

    (A) The testes
    (B) The urethra
    (C) The scrotum
    (D) The perineum

22. The cerebrum is

    (A) the largest part of the human brain
    (B) responsible for maintenance of equilibrium
    (C) is located in the neck, just below the larynx
    (D) responsible for respiration, heart rate, and blood vessel diameter

23. Which of the following correctly lists the sections of the small intestine and the order in which food passes through them?

    (A)   Ilium, ischium, pubis
    (B)   Sigmoid, rectum, anus
    (C)   Duodenum, jejunum, ileum
    (D)   Ascending, transverse, descending colon

24. The axial skeleton consists of the

    (A)   shoulder, arm, and hand
    (B)   clavicle, skull, and fibula
    (C)   skull, vertebral column, and thorax
    (D)   scapula, vertebral column, and femur

> **Directions:** Each of the numbered items or incomplete statements in this section is negatively phrased, as indicated by a capitalized word such as NOT, LEAST, or EXCEPT. Select the ONE lettered answer or completion that is BEST in each case.

25. Which of the following is NOT a bone that forms the pelvis?

    (A)   Pubis
    (B)   Ischium
    (C)   Iliac crest
    (D)   Duodenum

26. Which of the following is NOT a component of blood?

    (A)   Platelets
    (B)   Pia mater
    (C)   Red blood cells
    (D)   White blood cells

27. Which of the following is NOT a component of the male reproductive system?

    (A)   Urethra
    (B)   Testes
    (C)   Oviducts
    (D)   Prostate gland

> **Directions:** Each of the numbered questions or incomplete statements in this section refers to a scenario that precedes them. The numbered questions or incomplete statements are followed by answers or by completions of the statement. Select the answer or completion of the statement that is BEST in each case.

Your rescue squad is called to the scene of a stabbing. Additional information at the time of dispatch reveals that law enforcement personnel have secured the scene and are on scene with a 14-year-old male patient.

Questions 28–31

28. As you approach the patient, you note he is lying face down in a parking lot. This body position is termed

    (A) supine
    (B) prone
    (C) Fowler's
    (D) lateral recumbent

29. The patient has a six-inch kitchen knife buried in his back, medial to his left scapula. In other words, the knife is between the

    (A) shoulder blade and the femur
    (B) shoulder blade and the spine
    (C) clavicle and the humerus
    (D) clavicle and the ischium

30. This knife wound is _____ to the patient's occipital region of the cranium.

    (A) caudal
    (B) anterior
    (C) posterior
    (D) proximal

31. Due to the estimated depth of the injury, the knife probably punctured the double-walled membrane that surrounds the lungs. This membrane is called the

    (A) pleura
    (B) meninges
    (C) diaphragm
    (D) pericardium

Your ambulance crew is dispatched to the scene of a motor vehicle collision for a 27-year-old female patient complaining of head and neck pain. After ensuring scene safety and taking appropriate body substance precautions, you begin assessing your patient. Conscious and alert, your patient is sitting in the driver's seat of a compact car.

Questions 32–35

32. While examining this patient, you palpate her vertebrae from the base of the skull to the buttocks. Which of the following is the order in which you will examine the vertebrae?

    (A) Thoracic, lumbar, maxilla, sternum, coccyx
    (B) Cervical, thoracic, lumbar, sacral, coccyx
    (C) Clavicle, thoracic, lumbar, occipital, coccyx
    (D) Coccyx, thoracic, lumbar, sacral, and cervical

33. The patient states she was not wearing her seat belt and struck her chest on the steering wheel. She is complaining of tenderness at the "breast bone." This bone is known to health care professionals as the

    (A) ulna
    (B) patella
    (C) clavicle
    (D) sternum

34. To assess this patient's distal sensory status, you would ask this patient about sensation

(A)   at the sight of the neck pain
(B)   in the hands and feet
(C)   at the cerebrum
(D)   at the sternum

35. While evaluating motor function, you ask the patient to form a fist with both hands and to push her feet against resistance. The ability to move the extremities on verbal command evaluates the coordinated effort between the nervous system and the

(A)   reflexes
(B)   cardiac muscle
(C)   striated muscles
(D)   smooth muscles

ANSWERS AND RATIONALES

1-A. The xiphoid process is the cartilaginous prominence inferior to (below) the body of the sternum. The manubrium is located superior to (above) the body of the sternum. The manubrium and body of the sternum are fused in an adult (the suture of the manubrium and body of the sternum is called the angle of Louis). In Trendelenburg position, the patient is lying on the back with the head lower than the feet.

2-B. Besides production of red blood cells, the skeletal system is responsible for giving the body shape, support, and form, protecting internal organs, providing support for the body, and storing minerals.

3-B. The muscular system is responsible for these functions. The lymphatic system is a series of vessels and nodes that act as the body's filter and drainage system. The integumentary system is the body's first line of defense against organism invasion. The components of the integumentary system include the hair, skin, and nails.

4-C. When examining from proximal to distal, one would start at a point closest to the body and move out a given extremity. The humerus is the bone of the upper arm. The radius and ulna compose the lower arm (forearm). The carpals and metacarpals make up the hand. The phalanges are the bones of the fingers (and toes).

5-C. Smooth (involuntary) muscles compose the walls of the vessels of the cardiovascular system. Tendons connect muscle to bone. Ligaments connect bones to bones and maintain the alignment of joints.

6-A. The exchange of gases does not occur until air reaches the alveoli, the terminal air sacs of the respiratory tree.

7-C. The epiglottis is the leaf-shaped structure that closes over the trachea to prevent aspiration of food or liquid. The larynx is the voice box. The bronchi are the large air passages that branch off the trachea. The point at which the trachea bifurcates into the right and left primary bronchi is called the carina. The pericardium is the tough, fibrous sac that surrounds the heart.

8-C. The left side of the heart (the left atrium and left ventricle) is responsible for systemic circulation. The systemic circulation delivers oxygen-rich blood to all cells of the body.

9-D. The right side of the heart (the right atrium and right ventricle) is responsible for pulmonary circulation. Pulmonary circulation is the delivery of deoxygenated blood to the alveolar-capillary membrane in the lung cavity. At the alveolar-capillary membrane, the blood is reoxygenated and returned to the left side of the heart for delivery to all cells of the body.

10-B. There are four valves in the heart: tricuspid, pulmonary, mitral (bicuspid), and aortic. These valves prevent blood from flowing backward during contraction (systole). The veins of the body also contain valves to prevent backflow of blood.

11-B. Arteries carry blood away from the heart. Veins carry blood toward the heart. In the systemic circulation, arteries carry oxygenated blood to the cells and veins carry oxygen-poor blood back to the heart. On the pulmonary side, arteries carry oxygen-poor blood to the lungs and veins carry oxygen-rich blood back to the heart.

12-A. The cerebrum is the largest division of the brain. It is responsible for the body's higher functions. The cerebellum, which is inferior to the cerebrum, is responsible for control of muscle movements, posture, and equilibrium. The brain stem is responsible for maintaining the body's several vital body functions such as heart rate, blood pressure, and respiratory rate. The meninges are the protective membranes of the brain and spinal cord.

13-C. The sympathetic and parasympathetic divisions of the autonomic nervous system work together to maintain the body's steady state. The sympathetic division mobilizes energy during stressful situations while the parasympathetic division conserves and restores energy. The somatic nervous system is also called the voluntary nervous system and is responsible for voluntary movement. The medulla oblongata is one of the three divisions of the brain stem (the other two are the midbrain and pons).

14-A. The dermis is the middle layer of the skin and contains the majority of the skin's organs such as the hair follicles, nerve endings, and blood vessels. The epidermis is the outermost layer of the skin. The subcutaneous fat layer is the deepest layer and varies in depth. The urethra is the passageway for urine to exit the body from the bladder.

15-C. The pancreas, located in the left upper quadrant of the abdomen posterior to the stomach, is responsible for producing insulin, glucagon, and pancreatic juices. The colon is another term for the large intestine. The spleen, also located in the left upper quadrant, is the primary organ of the lymphatic system. The pituitary, located at the base of the brain, is the master gland of the body. The pituitary gland regulates growth and controls the other glands of the endocrine system.

16-B. Absorption is the process of bringing nutrients, water, and electrolytes into the body. Digestion is the breakdown of food into parts that can be absorbed. Absorption is the movement of nutrients, water, and electrolytes so they can be used by the body cells. Defecation is the elimination of undigested waste.

17-D. Peristalsis is the wavelike contraction of the gastrointestinal tract. Smooth muscles that line the passages of the gastrointestinal tract contract and relax in a coordinated effort to move the contents through.

18-C. The small intestine, which measures approximately 20 feet long, receives chyme (partially digested food) from the stomach. The majority of digestion takes place in the small intestine. The liver produces bile to aid in the digestion of fats. Bile is stored in the gallbladder and transported to the small intestine via bile ducts. The large intestine absorbs the remaining water and electrolytes from the chyme after it leaves the small intestine.

19-A. Composed of two kidneys, two ureters, a urinary bladder, and a urethra, the urinary system produces urine, maintains water and chemical balance, and assists in regulating blood pressure.

20-B. The ovaries produce the hormones progesterone and estrogen. The uterus is the hollow, muscular organ in which the fertilized ovum implants and matures to birth. The pituitary gland is the master gland of the endocrine system. The mammary glands (breasts) are responsible for lactation after delivery of an infant.

21-B. The urethra is the passageway for urine out of the body from the bladder in both the male and female. In the male, the urethra is also used for the passage of sperm during ejaculation. The testes (gonads) and scrotum (sac that houses the testes) are specific to the male. The perineum is the area between the vagina and the anus.

22-A. The cerebrum is the largest part of the human brain. It consists of two cerebral hemispheres connected by a collection of fibers called the corpus callosum. The cerebrum is responsible for voluntary control of movements, consciousness, memory, and sensation.

23-C. The small intestine is made up of three sections. Food first passes through the duodenum, then the jejunum, and finally the ileum. The ilium, ischium, and pubis are bones of the pelvis. The ascending, transverse, and descending colon are portions of the large intestine as are the sigmoid colon, rectum, and anus.

24-C. The axial skeleton consists of the skull (cranial and facial bones), vertebral column, and thorax. The appendicular skeleton is made up of the bones of the upper and lower extremities. The upper extremity is composed of the scapula, clavicle, shoulder, arm, and hand. The lower extremity is composed of the hip, femur, tibia, fibula, and foot.

25-D. The duodenum is one of the three sections of the small intestine. The other two sections are the jejunum and ileum. The pubis, ischium, and iliac crest are bones of the pelvis.

26-B. The formed elements of the blood include red blood cells (erythrocytes), white blood cells (leukocytes), and platelets (thrombocytes). The pia mater is one of three meninges that protect the central nervous system (the brain and spinal cord). It is a thin membrane that adheres to the outer surface of the brain. The middle meningeal layer is the arachnoid membrane. The outermost membrane is the dura mater.

27-C. The oviducts (also known as the fallopian tubes) are part of the female reproductive system. The oviducts allow the passage of the produced ovum (egg) to the uterus for implantation if fertilized. The urethra is the passageway for sperm from the male body. The testes (gonads) produce sperm and the hormone testosterone. The prostate gland secretes prostate fluid that enhances sperm motility.

28-B. Lying flat, face down is the prone position. Supine would be lying flat face up. Fowler's position is lying on the back with the upper body elevated to a 45° to 60° angle. Lateral recumbent would be lying flat on one's side (right or left).

29-B. Another term for scapula is the "shoulder blade." Medial refers to a direction closer to midline. The femur is the thigh bone. The clavicle is the collar bone, which is on the anterior (front) aspect of the body. The ischium, with the pubis and iliac crest, form the pelvic girdle.

30-A. The occipital region is the posterior (back) aspect of the cranium (skull). Caudal is the direction toward the tail or lower end of the spine. Anterior refers to the front of the body. Posterior refers to the back of the body. Proximal refers to something that is closer to the given point of reference (e.g., the elbow is more proximal to the shoulder than is the hand).

31-A. The pleura is the double-walled membrane that surrounds the lungs. It allows the lungs to expand and contract within the chest cavity with minimal friction. The meninges are the membranes that protect the brain and spinal cord. There are three layers of meninges: the dura mater, the arachnoid layer, and the pia mater. The diaphragm is the flat muscle at the inferior (bottom) aspect of the lung cavity. When it contracts and pulls down, air is drawn into the lungs. The pericardium is the membrane that lines the abdominal cavity and helps keep the abdominal organs in their correct position.

32-B. The correct descending order of the vertebrae is cervical, thoracic, lumbar, sacral, and coccyx. The maxilla is the upper jaw bone. The sternum is the breast bone. The clavicle is the collar bone, and the occipital is the back region of the cranium.

33-D. The sternum is the medical name for the breast bone. The ulna is one of the bones that make up the forearm. The ulna is on the "pinkie" side of the arm while the radius is on the thumb side. The patella is the knee cap, and the clavicle is the collar bone.

34-B. Distal refers to a point farthest from the point of reference. If no point of reference is given, assume the point of reference is the trunk.

35-C. Striated muscles, also known as voluntary muscles, are responsible for deliberate movements. Smooth muscles, also known as involuntary muscles, handle the work of all internal organs, except the heart. Cardiac muscle performs the work of the heart and is different from other muscles in appearance and automaticity (the ability to generate its own electrical impulse independent of the nervous system).

BIBLIOGRAPHY

Anderson KN, Anderson LE, Glanze WD (eds): *Mosby's Medical, Nursing, & Allied Health Dictionary*, 4th ed. St. Louis, Mosby-Year Book, 1994.

Caroline NL: *Emergency Care in the Streets*, 4th ed. Boston, Little, Brown, 1991.

Crosby LA, Lewallen DG (eds): *Emergency Care and Transportation of the Sick and Injured*, 6th ed. Rosemont, IL, American Academy of Orthopaedic Surgeons, 1995.

Sloane E: *Anatomy and Physiology: An Easy Learner*. Boston, Jones and Bartlett, 1994.

Solomon EP and Phillips GA: *Understanding Human Anatomy and Physiology*. Philadelphia, WB Saunders, 1987.

Thibodeau GA, Patton KT: *The Human Body in Health and Disease*. St. Louis, Mosby-Year Book, 1992.

Tortora GJ, Grabowski SR: *Principles of Anatomy and Physiology*, seventh ed. New York, HarperCollins, 1993.

United States Department of Transportation, National Highway Traffic Safety Administration: *Emergency Medical Technician: Basic. National Standard Curriculum*, 1994.

Yvorra JG (ed): *Mosby's Emergency Dictionary Quick Reference for Emergency Responders*. St. Louis, Mosby-Year Book, 1989.

5 BASELINE VITAL SIGNS AND SAMPLE HISTORY

OBJECTIVES

5-1 Differentiate between a sign and a symptom.

*5-2 Define the terms "vital signs" and "baseline vital signs."

*5-3 Explain why vital signs are measured.

5-4 Identify the elements of vital signs.

5-5 Identify the attributes that should be evaluated when assessing breathing.

5-6 Describe how to assess a patient's breathing rate.

*5-7 Discuss factors that influence respiratory rate.

*5-8 Describe normal respiratory rates for an adult, child, and infant.

5-9 Differentiate between shallow, labored, and noisy breathing.

*5-10 Describe abnormal respiratory sounds, including snoring, wheezing, gurgling, and crowing.

*5-11 Differentiate between adequate and inadequate breathing.

*5-12 Discuss the locations of central and peripheral pulses.

*5-13 Discuss factors that influence the pulse rate.

5-14 Discuss how to assess a patient's pulse.

5-15 Identify the attributes that should be evaluated when assessing a patient's pulse.

*5-16 Describe average pulse rates for an adult, child, and infant.

5-17 Differentiate among an absent, weak, strong, and bounding pulse.

5-18 Differentiate between a regular and irregular pulse.

5-19 Identify the attributes that should be evaluated when assessing the skin.

5-20 Describe normal and abnormal findings when assessing skin color.

5-21 Describe normal and abnormal findings when assessing skin temperature.

5-22 Describe normal and abnormal findings when assessing skin condition.

5-23 Describe how capillary refill is assessed in infants and children.

MOTIVATION FOR LEARNING

An EMT-Basic must be able to accurately assess and record a patient's vital signs. Assessment and recording of vital signs are performed in order to recognize changes in the patient's condition. In addition to vital signs, the EMT-Basic should obtain a SAMPLE history in the event the patient loses consciousness.

5-24 Describe normal and abnormal findings when assessing skin capillary refill in the infant and child patient.

5-25 Describe the method used to assess the pupils.

5-26 Describe normal and abnormal pupil size.

5-27 Differentiate between dilated (big) and constricted (small) pupil size.

＊5-28 Define the term "reactivity" as it relates to assessment of the pupils.

5-29 Differentiate between reactive and nonreactive pupils and equal and unequal pupils.

5-30 Define the terms blood pressure, systolic pressure, diastolic pressure, and pulse pressure.

＊5-31 Describe factors that influence blood pressure.

＊5-32 Identify the four major parts of a stethoscope.

5-33 Describe the methods used to assess blood pressure.

5-34 Explain the difference(s) between auscultation and palpation for obtaining a blood pressure.

5-35 Identify normal blood pressure ranges for an adult, child, and infant.

5-36 Identify common errors in blood pressure measurement.

5-37 Discuss the frequency with which vital signs should be reassessed in the stable and unstable patient.

5-38 Identify the elements of the SAMPLE history.

5-39 Discuss the need to search for additional medical identification.

BASELINE VITAL SIGNS

TERMINOLOGY

1. A **sign** is any medical or trauma condition displayed by the patient and identifiable by the EMT-Basic. For example, the EMT-Basic can *see* bleeding and pale skin, *hear* noisy respirations, and *feel* cold skin.

2. A **symptom** is any condition described by the patient, e.g., shortness of breath, nausea, and dizziness.

3. **Vital signs** are assessments of breathing, pulse, skin, pupils, and blood pressure.
   a. Measurement of vital signs is an important part of every patient assessment.
   b. Vital signs are measured to detect changes in normal body function and determine a patient's response to interventions.
   c. When possible, two or more sets of vital signs should be taken. Two sets of vital signs allow the EMT-Basic to note changes in the patient's condition and response to treatment.

4. **Baseline vital signs** are an initial set of vital sign measurements against which succeeding measurements can be compared. They include:
   a. Respirations
   b. Pulse
   c. Skin
   d. Pupils
   e. Blood pressure

RESPIRATIONS

1. **Respiratory assessment.** Assessment of a patient's breathing includes:
   a. Respiratory rate
   b. Depth and equality of respiration
   c. Rhythm of respiration
   d. Alterations in respiration, including abnormal respiratory sounds

2. **Respiratory rate**
   a. **Procedure for assessment of respiratory rate**
      (1) Hold the patient's wrist as if you are assessing the radial pulse and observe the rise and fall of the chest.
          (a) Do not inform the patient you are counting his or her respiratory rate.
          (b) Patients subconsciously vary their respirations if they know they are being counted.
      (2) Begin counting when the chest rises.
          (a) Count each rise and fall of the chest as one respiration.
          (b) Observe if respirations are regular and if the chest rises equally.
      (3) Count respirations for 30 seconds and multiply the number by 2 to determine the rate for 1 minute. If the patient's respirations are irregular, count the rate for 1 full minute.
      (4) Observe the depth, rhythm, and effort of breathing.
      (5) Listen for any abnormal respiratory noises.
   b. **Factors that influence respiratory rate**
      (1) Exercise increases respiratory rate.
      (2) Stress/anxiety increases respiratory rate.
      (3) Increased altitude lowers oxygen concentration and increases respiratory rate.
      (4) **Medications**
          (a) Stimulants, such as cocaine, increase respiratory rate.
          (b) Narcotics and sedatives decrease respiratory rate.
      (5) Pain increases respiratory rate.
      (6) Injury to the brainstem decreases respiratory rate (and rhythm).
   c. **Special considerations in infants**
      (1) In infants, it is often easier to observe the rise and fall of the abdomen to determine respiratory rate.
      (2) Count an infant's respirations for 1 full minute.
   d. **Normal respiratory rates are as follows:**
      (1) Adult: 12–20 breaths/minute
      (2) Child: 15–30 breaths/minute
      (3) Infant: 25–50 breaths/minute
3. **Respiratory quality** can be evaluated while determining the respiratory rate.
   a. **Depth** and **equality** are assessed by observing the amount of movement of the chest wall.
      (1) In normal respirations, the average chest wall motion is observed and the chest expands symmetrically.
      (2) **Shallow respirations**
          (a) A small volume of air is exchanged.
          (b) Ventilatory movement is difficult to see; may involve only slight chest or abdominal wall motion.
      (3) **Deep respirations**
          (a) A large volume of air is exchanged.
          (b) Lungs fully expand.
   b. **Respiratory rhythm**
      (1) Normal respirations are evenly spaced.
      (2) Infants and young children tend to breathe less regularly than adults.
      (3) If an irregular (not constant) rhythm is observed in an adult, count the rate for 1 full minute (occasional sighing is normal).
      (4) Irregular breathing patterns may be associated with conditions such as a diabetic emergency or head injury, among other conditions.
   c. **Respiratory effort**
      (1) Normal breathing is relaxed and effortless.
      (2) **Labored breathing** is an increase in the effort of breathing.

(a) It may include grunting and stridor.

   (i) **Grunting** is the sound created when the patient forcefully exhales against a closed glottis; grunting traps air and keeps the alveoli open.

   (ii) **Stridor** is a harsh, high-pitched sound associated with severe upper airway obstruction; most often heard during inspiration.

(b) It is often characterized by the use of accessory muscles *(Figure 5-1)*.

(c) Nasal flaring, supraclavicular, and intercostal retractions may be present in infants and children.

   (i) **Nasal flaring** is excessive widening of the nostrils with respiration.

   (ii) **Retractions** are a visible "sinking in" of the soft tissues of the chest between and around the cartilage and ribs *(Figure 5-2)*.

(d) Gasping may be present.

d. Respiratory sounds

  (1) Normal breathing is quiet.

  (2) Abnormal respiratory sounds include:

    (a) **Snoring,** which results from partial obstruction of the upper airway by the tongue

    (b) **Wheezing,** which is a continuous, high-pitched musical sound heard on inspiration or expiration that suggests a narrowed or partially obstructed airway

    (c) **Gurgling,** which is the sound heard as air passes through moist secretions in the airway

    (d) **Crowing,** which is a long, high-pitched sound heard on inspiration

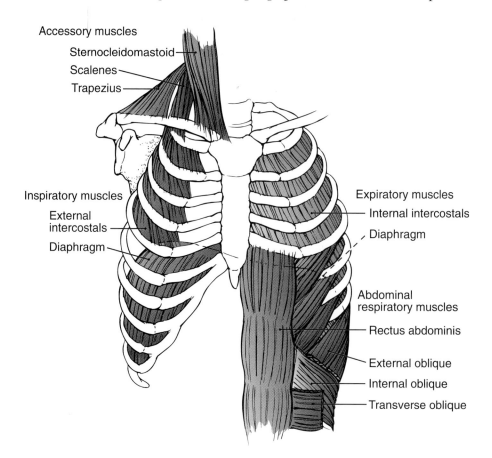

Fig. 5-1. Normal breathing uses specific muscle groups. The diaphragm and external intercostal muscles are used during inspiration. The internal intercostal and abdominal muscles may be used during expiration when movement of air out of the lungs is impeded, or during inspiration to draw more air into the lungs.

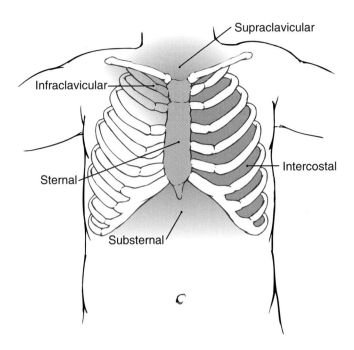

Fig. 5-2. Retractions usually begin in the intercostal spaces. Supraclavicular and infraclavicular retractions may be seen if more effort is needed to fill the lungs. Because of the pliability of an infant's chest, sternal retractions may be seen with only a slight increase in respiratory effort.

e. Signs of adequate breathing
  (1) Breathing is quiet and effortless breathing and does not involve the use of accessory muscles.
  (2) The respiratory rate is within normal limits for age.
  (3) The respiratory rhythm is regular with symmetrical chest expansion.
  (4) Respiratory depth is adequate.
f. Signs of inadequate breathing
  (1) The respiratory rate is outside normal ranges for age.
  (2) The breathing pattern is irregular.
  (3) Breath sounds are diminished or absent.
  (4) Chest expansion is unequal or inadequate.
  (5) Breathing effort is increased.
    (a) Inadequate breathing involves the use of accessory muscles, predominantly in infants and children. Retractions above the clavicles, between the ribs and below the rib cage, may be present, especially in children.
    (b) Nasal flaring may be present, especially in children.
    (c) In infants, **"seesaw" breathing** may be present (the chest and abdomen move in opposite directions).
  (6) Respiratory depth is inadequate (shallow respirations).
  (7) The skin is pale, cyanotic (blue), cool, and clammy.
  (8) Agonal respirations (occasional gasping breaths) may be seen just before death.

PULSE

1. Definition. The **pulse** is the expansion and contraction of an artery produced by pressure waves caused by the ejection of blood by the heart. The pulse can normally be felt anywhere an artery passes over a bone and lies near the skin.
2. Central pulse locations *(Figure 5-3)*
  a. The **carotid pulse** is located on either side of the neck.
    (1) Avoid excess pressure in the elderly patient.

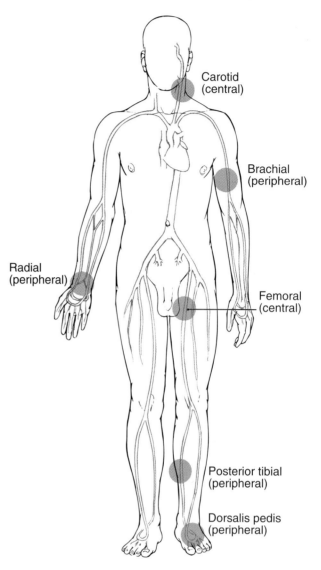

Fig. 5-3. Location of central pulses (carotid and femoral) and peripheral pulses (radial, brachial, posterior tibial, and dorsalis pedis).

     (2)   Never assess the carotid pulse on both sides at the same time.
   b. The **femoral pulse** is located in the fold between the thigh and pelvis.
     (1)   This pulse is infrequently used due to presence of clothing.
     (2)   It may require more pressure to adequately palpate than other sites.
3. **Peripheral pulse locations** *(see Figure 5-3)*
   a. The **radial pulse** is located proximal to the thumb on the wrist.
   b. The **brachial pulse** is located on the medial aspect of the upper arm, midway between the shoulder and elbow.
   c. The **posterior tibial pulse** is located posterior to the ankle bone.
   d. The **dorsalis pedis pulse** is located on the top surface of the foot.
4. **Initial pulse assessment**
   a. Initially, a radial pulse should be assessed in all patients 1 year of age or older.
   b. In patients younger than 1 year of age, a brachial pulse should be assessed.
   c. If a pulse is present, assessment should include the pulse rate and quality.
5. Factors that influence pulse rate include:
   a. Age
   b. Physical condition

    c. Presence of fever

    d. Medications

    e. Fear, stress, anger, pain

    f. Blood loss

    g. Position changes

6. Assessment of pulse rate

    a. The pulse rate is the number of heartbeats felt per minute.

    b. Procedure for assessment of pulse rate

      (1) Using the pads of the second and third fingers, apply moderate pressure to the artery.

        (a) The pads on the distal aspects of the finger are the most sensitive areas for detecting a pulse.

          (i) If excessive pressure is used, the pulse may be obliterated.

          (ii) If too little pressure is used, the pulse may not be detected.

        (b) The thumb should not be used to assess a pulse since it has a prominent pulse of its own and could be mistaken for the patient's pulse.

      (2) Count the number of beats for 30 seconds and multiply the number by 2 to determine the number of beats per minute.

        (a) If the pulse is irregular, it should be counted for 1 full minute.

        (b) In an adult, a rate of less than 60 beats per minute is called **bradycardia,** and a rate greater than 100 beats per minute is called **tachycardia.**

    c. Average pulse rates (in beats per minute)

      (1) Teenagers and adults (12 years of age and older): 60–100 (usually 60–80)

      (2) School-age children (6–12 years of age): 70–110

      (3) Toddlers and preschoolers (2–6 years of age): 80–120

      (4) Infants (4 weeks to 1 year of age): 80–130

      (5) Newborns (birth to 4 weeks of age): 70–170

7. Assessment of pulse quality

    a. Pulse strength refers to the force of the pressure wave as blood is pumped through the body.

      (1) Pulse may be absent (not discernible).

      (2) It may be difficult to feel.

        (a) This kind of pulse is called a "weak" or "feeble" pulse.

        (b) A weak, rapid pulse is called a "thready" pulse.

      (3) A normal pulse is readily detected, obliterated by strong pressure, and the pressure is equal for each beat. This kind of pulse is called a "strong" or "full" pulse.

      (4) An extremely strong pulse that is difficult to obliterate with pressure is called a "bounding" pulse.

    b. Pulse rhythm is the pattern of beats and the interval between the beats.

      (1) In a normal pulse, the time lapses between beats are equal (regular and constant).

      (2) In an irregular pulse, beats are skipped or are unevenly spaced.

        (a) An irregular pulse is not constant.

        (b) A pulse with an irregular rhythm is called a **dysrhythmia** or **arrhythmia.**

    c. Equality of pulses is determined by assessing and comparing pulses on both sides of the body.

      (1) Pulses are normally equal bilaterally.

      (2) Pulses may be unequal in strength due to extremity injury or clot formation, among other causes.

SKIN

1. Assessment of a patient's skin should include:

    a. Skin color

    b. Skin temperature

    c. Skin condition (moisture)

    d. Capillary refill in infants and young children

2. Color

    a. Normal skin color for a Caucasian is pink.

    b. Skin color can be assessed by examining specific sites.

        (1) Nail beds

            (a) Nail beds are an unreliable site to assess skin color.

            (b) They are easily affected by air temperature and many medical conditions.

        (2) Oral mucosa (mucous membranes of the mouth)

        (3) Conjunctiva (mucous membrane that lines the inner surface of the eyelid)

    c. In infants and children, assess the palms of the hands and soles of the feet.

    d. Abnormal skin color

        (1) Pale skin suggests poor perfusion (impaired blood flow) due to shock or fright, among other causes.

        (2) Cyanotic (blue-gray) skin suggests inadequate oxygenation or poor perfusion. Cyanosis often appears first in the fingertips or around the mouth (circumoral cyanosis).

        (3) Flushed (red) skin suggests exposure to heat or carbon monoxide poisoning or high blood pressure.

        (4) Jaundiced (yellow) skin suggests liver disease or hepatitis.

3. Skin temperature

    a. Procedure for assessment of skin temperature

        (1) Place the back of your hands or fingers against the patient's skin. The back surfaces of the hands and fingers are most sensitive to temperature.

        (2) This procedure provides a rough estimate of skin temperature.

    b. Normal skin temperature is warm [98.6° F (37.0° C) when measured orally].

    c. Abnormal skin temperatures

        (1) Hot skin temperature suggests fever or heat exposure.

        (2) Cool skin temperature suggests inadequate circulation or exposure to cold.

        (3) Cold skin temperature suggests extreme exposure to cold.

        (4) Clammy (cool and moist) skin suggests shock, among many other conditions.

4. Skin condition (moisture)

    a. Normal skin is dry.

    b. Wet or moist skin may indicate shock (hypoperfusion), a heat-related illness, or diabetic emergency.

    c. Excessively dry skin may indicate dehydration.

5. Capillary refill

    a. Capillary refill in infants and children is assessed by pressing on the patient's skin or nailbeds and determining the time for return to initial color.

        (1) Normal capillary refill in infants and children is less than 2 seconds.

        (2) Delayed (greater than 2 seconds) capillary refill suggests circulatory compromise.

    b. Capillary refill is most reliable as an indicator of circulatory function in infants and children younger than 6 years of age. In adults, other factors may affect capillary refill such as cold weather, medications, and smoking.

PUPILS

1. Pupils are assessed by briefly shining a light into the patient's eyes and assessing:

    a. Size

    b. Equality

    c. Reactivity

2. Normal findings are pupils that are normally equal in size, round, and equally reactive to light.

3. Abnormal findings

   a. Size

   (1) Dilated (very big) pupils can result from trauma, eye medications, neurologic disorders, or glaucoma.

   (2) Constricted (small) pupils may be caused by medications or inflammation of the iris.

   b. Equality

   (1) A small number of patients have pupils of unequal sizes, a condition called **anisocoria.**

   (2) In most patients, unequal pupils suggest a head injury, a stroke, or the possibility of an artificial eye.

   c. Reactivity

   (1) Reactivity refers to whether or not the pupils change in response to light.

   (2) Normally, a light shown into the pupil of one eye will cause pupil constriction of both eyes.

   (3) Nonreactive pupils do not change when exposed to light, which may occur because of medications, cardiac arrest, or central nervous system injury.

   (4) Unequally reactive pupils (one pupil reacts but the other does not) may occur because of a head injury or stroke.

BLOOD PRESSURE

1. Definitions

   a. Blood pressure is the force exerted by the blood against the wall of an artery as the ventricles of the heart contract and relax.

   b. Systolic blood pressure is the force exerted against the wall of an artery when the ventricles contract.

   c. Diastolic blood pressure is the force exerted against the wall of an artery when the heart is in the filling or relaxed state.

   d. Pulse pressure is the difference between the systolic and diastolic pressures.

2. Overview

   a. Blood pressure is measured in millimeters of mercury (mm Hg).

   b. The average blood pressure of a healthy adult at rest is 120/80 mm Hg.

   c. Blood pressure should be measured in all patients older than 3 years of age.

   d. In infants and young children, the general appearance and physical assessment findings are more valuable than vital sign numbers.

3. Factors that influence blood pressure

   a. Anxiety, fear, pain, and emotional stress increase blood pressure.

   b. Obesity increases blood pressure.

   c. Blood loss decreases blood pressure.

   d. Fever increases blood pressure.

   e. Some medications can directly or indirectly affect blood pressure.

   f. African-American males over 35 years of age have higher blood pressures than European-American males of the same age.

   g. Blood pressure is typically lowest in the early morning, gradually rises during the day, and peaks in the late afternoon or evening.

   h. Diseases affecting the viscosity (thickness) of the blood, arteries, or cardiac output affect blood pressure.

4. Equipment. Blood pressure measurement requires the use of a **sphygmomanometer** (blood pressure cuff) and, usually, a stethoscope.

   a. Measurement of the blood pressure by **auscultation** ("auscultation" refers to listening assessments) requires the use of a stethoscope.

   b. A stethoscope is not used if the blood pressure is measured by palpation.

   c. Electronic sphygmomanometers, which do not require the use of a stethoscope, are also available.

5. **Using a stethoscope**
   a. **Parts of a stethoscope**
      (1) **Earpieces**
          (a) Earpieces should fit snugly but comfortably in the ears.
          (b) For the best sound reception, the earpieces should follow the shape of the ear canal, i.e., the earpieces should normally point toward the face as the stethoscope is put on.
      (2) **Binaurals** (metal pieces of the stethoscope that connect the earpieces to the plastic or rubber tubing) should be angled so the earpieces remain in the ears without causing discomfort.
      (3) Plastic or rubber tubing should be flexible and approximately 12–18 inches in length (longer tubing decreases sound wave transmission).
      (4) **Chest piece**
          (a) The diaphragm is the circular, flat portion of the chest piece that has a thin plastic disk on the end.
              (i) It is used to detect high-pitched sounds such as breath sounds.
              (ii) The diaphragm should be firmly held against the patient's skin.
          (b) The bell has a deep, hollow, cuplike shape.
              (i) It is used to detect low-pitched sounds such as murmurs and in blood pressure measurement.
              (ii) The bell should be lightly held against the patient's skin, just enough to form a seal.
              (iii) Pressing harder causes the skin to act as a diaphragm, reducing sound amplification.
   b. When possible, the stethoscope should be placed directly on the patient's skin because clothing will obscure sounds.
6. **Parts of a sphygmomanometer**
   a. The sound dial's needle points to the calibrations.
   b. A rubber hand bulb with a pressure control (release) valve inflates and deflates the bladder.
   c. A cuff with an inflatable bladder is wrapped around the patient's arm extremity.
      (1) Cuffs come in a variety of sizes because the bladder must be the correct length and width for the patient's arm.
      (2) Correct cuff size ensures equal pressure will be exerted around the extremity, resulting in an accurate measurement.
      (3) The cuff width should not exceed two-thirds the length of the upper arm.
      (4) The cuff length should not completely wrap around or overlap the extremity but should ideally cover three-fourths of the circumference of the extremity.
7. **Procedure for assessing blood pressure**
   a. **By auscultation**
      (1) Expose the patient's upper arm.
      (2) Wrap the blood pressure cuff evenly around the patient's upper arm at least one inch above the elbow, placing the arrow on the cuff over the patient's brachial artery.
      (3) Locate the patient's radial artery.
      (4) Inflate the cuff until you can no longer feel the radial pulse.
      (5) Inflate the cuff 30 mmHg beyond the point at which you last felt the pulse.
      (6) Place the stethoscope over the brachial artery. If your stethoscope is so equipped, use the bell instead of the diaphragm (the bell is better suited for low-pitched sounds).
      (7) Deflate the cuff slowly and evenly at a rate of 2 to 3 mm Hg per second.
      (8) Note the point on the gauge where you hear the first sound. This point

marks the systolic pressure and should be near the point where the radial pulse disappeared.

   (9) Continue to deflate the cuff, noting the point where the sound disappears. This point marks the diastolic pressure.

   (10) Deflate the cuff completely.

   (11) Record the patient's blood pressure.

   (a) The blood pressure is recorded as the systolic pressure over the diastolic pressure.

   (b) The blood pressure is recorded as an even number since most gauges have a scale marked in increments of 2 mm Hg, e.g., 114/76.

   (c) Readings between the patient's arms may vary by as much as 10 mm Hg.

   (12) Wait 15–30 seconds before reinflating the cuff to allow blood trapped in the veins to dissipate.

b. By palpation

   (1) Expose the patient's upper arm.

   (2) Wrap the blood pressure cuff evenly around the patient's upper arm at least one inch above the elbow, placing the arrow on the cuff over the patient's brachial artery.

   (3) Locate the patient's radial artery.

   (4) Inflate the cuff until you can no longer feel the radial pulse.

   (5) Inflate the cuff 30 mm Hg beyond the point at which you last felt the pulse.

   (6) Deflate the cuff slowly and evenly at a rate of 2 to 3 mm Hg per second while continuing to palpate the radial artery.

   (7) Note the point on the gauge when you feel the return of the radial pulse.

   (a) This point is the systolic pressure and should be near the point where the radial pulse disappeared.

   (b) The diastolic pressure cannot be accurately measured by palpation.

   (8) Deflate the cuff completely.

   (9) Record the patient's blood pressure. When the blood pressure is obtained by palpation, the systolic pressure is recorded over a capital "P," e.g., 110/P.

8. Variations in blood pressure by age (in mm Hg):

   a. Adult: 120/80

   b. Age 14: 120/80

   c. Age 10: 102/62

   d. Age 6: 95/57

   e. Age 1: 90/55

   f. Newborn: 73/55

9. Common errors in blood pressure measurement

   a. Errors that produce a falsely low reading

   (1) The patient's arm is above level of heart.

   (2) The cuff is too wide.

   (3) The stethoscope tubing is too long.

   b. Errors that produce a falsely high reading

   (1) The cuff is deflated too slowly.

   (2) The patient's arm is unsupported.

   (3) The cuff is too narrow.

   (4) The cuff is wrapped too loosely or unevenly.

   c. Errors that produce either falsely high or low readings

   (1) Repeating blood pressure assessment too quickly may produce a falsely high systolic or low diastolic reading.

   (2) Deflating the cuff too quickly may produce a falsely low systolic and high diastolic reading.

VITAL SIGN REASSESSMENT

1. **Stable patient.** At a minimum, vital signs should be assessed and recorded every 15 minutes in a stable patient. Remember, a stable patient can become unstable very quickly—reassess frequently!
2. **Unstable patient.** Vital signs should be assessed and recorded every 5 minutes in the unstable patient.
3. **Interventions.** Vital signs should be assessed following every medical intervention.

SAMPLE HISTORY

OVERVIEW

1. The patient history is information gathered by the EMT-Basic concerning the patient's current medical problem (chief complaint) and previous medical history.
2. The SAMPLE acronym serves to remind the EMT-Basic of the information that should be gathered. SAMPLE stands for **s**igns and **s**ymptoms, **a**llergies, **m**edications, pertinent **p**ast medical history, **l**ast oral intake, and **e**vents leading to the injury or illness.

SIGNS AND SYMPTOMS

"Why did you call us today?" OPQRST is an acronym that may help identify the type and location of the patient's complaint.
1. **Onset:** "What were you doing when the problem started?"
2. **Provocation:** "What makes the problem better or worse?"
3. **Quality:** "What does the pain feel like (dull, sharp, pressure, tearing)?"
4. **Region/Radiation**
   a. "Where is the pain?"
   b. "Is the pain in one area or does it move?"
   c. "Is the pain located in any other area?"
5. **Severity:** "On a scale of 1 to 10, with 1 being the least and 10 being the worst, what number would you assign your pain or discomfort?"
6. **Time**
   a. "How long ago did the problem/discomfort begin?"
   b. "Have you ever had this pain before?"
      (1) "When?"
      (2) "How long did it last?"

ALLERGIES

1. "Do you have any allergies to medications?"
2. "Do you have any food allergies or allergies to pollen, dust, grass?"
3. Check for medical identification insignia.

MEDICATIONS

1. "Do you take any prescription or over-the-counter medications?"
2. "Do you take any illegal drugs?"
3. "Have you recently started taking any new medications?"
4. "Have you recently stopped taking any medications?"
5. "Are you taking birth control pills?" (If applicable.)
6. Check for medical identification insignia.

PERTINENT PAST MEDICAL HISTORY

1. "Are you seeing a physician for any medical problems?"
2. "Do you have a history of heart problems, respiratory problems, kidney problems, liver problems, hypertension, diabetes, or epilepsy?"

3. "Have you had any recent surgery?"
4. Check for medical identification insignia. The patient may be wearing a bracelet or necklace or carry a card that identifies a serious medical condition, such as allergies, or medications he or she is taking.

LAST ORAL INTAKE

1. "When was the last time you had anything to eat or drink?"
2. Determine what was ingested, how much was ingested, and when.

EVENTS LEADING TO THE INJURY OR ILLNESS

"What were you doing just before this happened?"

REVIEW QUESTIONS

Directions: Each of the numbered items or incomplete statements in this section is followed by answers or by completions of the statement. Select the ONE lettered answer or completion that is BEST in each case.

1. When assessing pulses, it is important to evaluate pulse strength, rhythm, and equality. Equality refers to

    (A) the presence of pulses on both sides of the body
    (B) the pattern of beats and the interval between the beats
    (C) how the patient's pulse compares to the rescuer's pulse
    (D) the force of the pressure wave as blood is pumped through the body

2. What is the most reliable indicator of circulatory function in infants and children less than 6 years of age?

    (A) Pulse rate
    (B) Capillary refill
    (C) Blood pressure
    (D) Respiratory rate

3. During an examination of the pupils, shining a light in one eye should cause

    (A) both eyes to dilate
    (B) both eyes to pulsate
    (C) both eyes to constrict
    (D) one eye to constrict and one eye to dilate

4. The average blood pressure of a healthy adult at rest is 120/80 mm Hg. The "top" number (120) refers to

    (A) the pulse rate during auscultation of the blood pressure
    (B) the difference between the systolic and diastolic pressures
    (C) the systolic pressure; the force exerted by the blood when the heart is contracting
    (D) the diastolic pressure; the force exerted by the blood between contractions of the heart

5. The SAMPLE acronym assists health care providers in evaluating

    (A)   the patient's vital signs
    (B)   the condition of a newborn
    (C)   the patient's signs and symptoms
    (D)   the patient's medical history and chief complaint

6. When treating an unstable patient, vital signs should be assessed and recorded

    (A)   every 5 minutes
    (B)   every 15 minutes
    (C)   every 30 minutes
    (D)   only during the initial assessment and upon transfer of care

---

Directions: Each of the numbered questions or incomplete statements in this section refers to a scenario that precedes them. The numbered questions or incomplete statements are followed by answers or by completions of the statement. Select the answer or completion of the statement that is BEST in each case.

You are dispatched to the home of a 78-year-old man. You find the patient sitting upright on the edge of a chair complaining of severe difficulty breathing. His skin is cool, pale, and clammy and he is speaking in short sentences.

Questions 7–11

7. Which of the following is a "sign" of this patient's distress?

    (A)   The patient's skin is cool, pale, and clammy
    (B)   The patient states he was vomiting all night
    (C)   The patient has a history of difficulty breathing
    (D)   The patient complains he has been short of breath for 2 hours

8. Which of the following is a "symptom" of this patient's distress?

    (A)   The patient's nail beds are blue (cyanotic)
    (B)   The patient's feet are swollen (pedal edema)
    (C)   The patient is coughing up pink, frothy sputum
    (D)   The patient states his difficulty breathing becomes worse when he lies supine (on his back)

9. What equipment would you need to auscultate this patient's lung sounds?

    (A)   Stethoscope
    (B)   Oxygen regulator
    (C)   Sphygmomanometer
    (D)   Pulse oximetry device

10. When assessing the quality of respirations, it is important to note the depth, rhythm, sounds, effort, and rate of breathing. A normal respiratory rate for this patient, based on his age, is

    (A)   6–10 breaths/minute
    (B)   12–20 breaths/minute
    (C)   15–30 breaths/minute
    (D)   25–50 breaths/minute

11. While assessing this patient, you note he is becoming increasingly cyanotic (blue). His cyanosis is most likely a result of

    (A) high blood pressure
    (B) inadequate oxygenation
    (C) liver disease or hepatitis
    (D) carbon monoxide poisoning

You respond to a local elementary school for a 10-year-old female patient with a history of asthma. The school nurse informs you the patient was playing during recess when she experienced a sudden onset of difficulty breathing. The patient has used her asthma medication inhaler twice without relief.

Questions 12–15

12. Upon auscultation of lung sounds, you note the patient has a continuous, high-pitched musical sound on expiration. This sound is consistent with

    (A) snoring
    (B) crowing
    (C) gurgling
    (D) wheezing

13. While assessing pulses, your partner notes the patient does not have a palpable radial pulse; however, a strong brachial pulse is present. Brachial pulses are felt by palpating

    (A) on either side of the throat
    (B) proximal to the thumb on the wrist
    (C) in the crease between the pelvis and thigh
    (D) on the medial aspect of the upper arm, midway between the shoulder and elbow

14. During inhalation, you note the skin between the patient's ribs appears to "sink in." This sign is called

    (A) grunting
    (B) gastric distention
    (C) intercostal retractions
    (D) subcutaneous emphysema

15. Upon further examination of this patient, you note she is using her abdominal muscles to assist with exhalation and the shoulder and neck muscles to assist with inhalation. This finding is called

    (A) a pneumothorax
    (B) gastric distention
    (C) accessory muscle usage
    (D) paradoxical chest wall movement

ANSWERS AND RATIONALES

1-A. Equality of pulses refers to comparing the pulses on both sides of the patient's body. An example would be to compare radial pulses (at the wrist) or posterior tibial pulses (at the ankle). It would NOT be correct to compare the patient's left radial pulse with his or her right posterior tibial pulse. The pattern of beats and the interval between the beats refer to the pulse *rhythm*. Comparing the patient's pulse to the rescuer's pulse is of no value. The force of the pressure wave as blood is pumped through the body refers to the pulse *strength*.

2-B. Capillary refill is the most reliable indicator of circulatory function in infants and children. To assess capillary refill, blanch (press) the nail bed and determine the amount of time required for return of initial color. A capillary refill time of more than 2 seconds suggests inadequate perfusion.

3-C. Both eyes should constrict (become smaller) when a light is shown into one eye. The term given this finding is PERL (pupils equal and reactive to light).

4-C. Blood pressure readings record the pressure in the artery during contraction of the heart (systole) over the pressure in the artery during relaxation (diastole).

5-D. SAMPLE is a tool to remind health care providers of the pertinent questions to ask patients. SAMPLE stands for **s**igns and symptoms, **a**llergies, **m**edications, pertinent **p**ast medical history, **l**ast oral intake, and **e**vents leading up to the injury or illness. The OPQRST acronym may be used to evaluate a patient's symptoms (**o**nset of illness/injury, **p**rovoking factors, **q**uality/description of the illness or injury, **r**egion/radiation of the injury or illness, **s**everity of the discomfort, and **t**ime of discomfort).

6-A. The vital signs (pulse, blood pressure, skin condition, respiratory rate) of an unstable patient should be assessed and recorded every 5 minutes. Stable patients should be reevaluated every 15 minutes.

7-A. A "sign" is a condition displayed by the patient that the health care provider observes by methods such as seeing, hearing, or feeling. Responses B, C, and D refer to conditions that are described by the patient. These responses are called "symptoms."

8-D. A "symptom" is something the patient describes to the health care provider. Responses A, B, and C are conditions displayed by the patient. These responses are called "signs."

9-A. Auscultate refers to listening assessments. A stethoscope is a listening device. An oxygen (pressure) regulator is a device used to control the pressure in an oxygen cylinder. A sphygmomanometer is a blood pressure cuff. A pulse oximeter is a device used to assess the amount of gases (such as oxygen) carried by red blood cells.

10-B. The "normal" range of respirations for an adult at rest is 12–20 breaths per minute. Children have an average respiratory rate of 15 to 30 breaths per minute. Infants have an average rate of 25 to 50 breaths per minute.

11-B. Cyanosis, a blue-gray appearance of the skin, is generally attributed to inadequate oxygenation or poor perfusion. Flushed (red) skin may occur as a result of exposure to heat or carbon monoxide or high blood pressure.

12-D. Wheezing is the sound created by air whistling through narrowed bronchioles. Snoring occurs when the upper airway is partially obstructed by the tongue. Crowing is a long, high-pitched sound heard on inspiration. Gurgling is a sound created by air as it moves through moist respiratory secretions. (Caution: The absence of wheezing in a previously distressed, wheezing patient is not necessarily a good sign. Wheezing may subside if the narrowing of the airway is reversed *or* if the patient is no longer moving enough air in and out of the lungs to make the narrowed airway whistle. The absence of wheezing can, in the latter example, be an ominous sign.)

13-D. The brachial pulse is located on the medial aspect of the mid-upper arm. It can generally be found by palpating the "groove" between the biceps muscle and the humerus bone. The carotid pulse is found in the neck on either side of the throat. The radial pulse is located on the thumb-side of the wrist. The femoral pulse is located in the crease between the pelvis and the thigh.

14-C. Intercostal ("inter" = between; "costal" = pertaining to the ribs) retractions is the term given to this finding. Grunting is the sound created by air forced against a closed glottis in an attempt to keep the alveoli expanded. Gastric distention occurs when air enters the stomach. Gastric distention is a concern when ventilating a patient and is the reason why ventilations should be delivered slowly (over 1.5 to 2 seconds) in apneic patients. Subcutaneous emphysema is the presence of air in the subcutaneous tissue.

15-C. Accessory muscle usage occurs when the primary muscles of respiration, the diaphragm and intercostals, do not provide sufficient mechanical support to meet the body's oxygen demand. Additional muscles throughout the abdomen, shoulders, neck, face, and back may assist the ventilatory effort. A pneumothorax is the presence of air in the pleural space (the space created by the double-walled sac that surrounds the lungs). Gastric distention is the presence of air in the stomach. Paradoxical chest wall movement occurs when a "floating" section of broken ribs moves in a direction opposite the rest of the chest wall during breathing.

BIBLIOGRAPHY

Butman AM, Martin SW, Vomacka RW, et al (eds): *Comprehensive Guide to Pre-Hospital Skills: A Skills Manual for EMT-Basic, EMT-Intermediate, EMT-Paramedic.* Akron, Ohio, Emergency Training, 1995.

Crosby LA, Lewallen DG (eds): *Emergency Care and Transportation of the Sick and Injured*, 6th ed. Rosemont, IL, American Academy of Orthopaedic Surgeons, 1995.

Grant HD, Murray RH Jr, Bergeron JD: *Emergency Care*, 7th ed. Englewood Cliffs, NJ, Prentice-Hall, 1995.

Hafen BQ, Karren KJ, Mistovich JJ: *Prehospital Emergency Care*, 5th ed. Upper Saddle River, NJ, Prentice-Hall, 1996.

Jarvis C: *Pocket Companion for Physical Examination and Health Assessment*, 2nd ed. Philadelphia, WB Saunders Company, 1996.

Kozier B, Erb G, Blais K, et al: *Fundamentals of Nursing: Concepts, Process, and Practice*, 5th ed. Redwood City, CA, Addison-Wesley, 1995.

McSwain NE, White RD, Paturas JL, et al (eds): *The Basic EMT: Comprehensive Prehospital Patient Care*. St. Louis, Mosby-Year Book, 1996.

McSwain NE, Paturas JL, Wertz EM (eds): *EMT and Paramedic Quick Reference*. Westport, Connecticut, Concepts in Emergency Care, 1994.

Potter PA, Perry AG: *Fundamentals of Nursing: Concepts, Process, and Practice*, 3rd ed. St. Louis, Mosby-Year Book, 1993.

Seidel HM, Ball JW, Davis JE, et al: *Mosby's Guide to Physical Examination*, 3rd ed. St. Louis, Mosby-Year Book, 1996.

Stoy WA: *Mosby's EMT-Basic Textbook*. St. Louis, Mosby-Year Book, 1996.

United States Department of Transportation, National Highway Traffic Safety Administration: *Emergency Medical Technician: Basic. National Standard Curriculum*, 1994.

6 LIFTING AND MOVING PATIENTS

OBJECTIVES

6-1 Define body mechanics.

*6-2 Describe the three basic elements of body mechanics.

*6-3 Define the terms body alignment, body balance, center of gravity, base of support, and friction.

6-4 Discuss the guidelines and safety precautions that need to be followed when lifting a patient.

6-5 Describe the procedure for safe lifting of cots and stretchers.

*6-6 Describe the power (squat) lift.

*6-7 Describe the power grip.

6-8 Describe the guidelines and safety precautions for carrying patients and/or equipment.

6-9 Discuss one-handed carrying techniques.

6-10 Describe correct and safe carrying procedures on stairs.

6-11 State the guidelines for safe reaching and their application.

6-12 Describe correct reaching for log rolls.

6-13 State the guidelines for safe pushing and pulling.

6-14 Discuss the general considerations for moving patients.

*6-15 Discuss the differences among an emergency move, an urgent move, and a non-urgent move.

6-16 State three situations that may require the use of an emergency move.

*6-17 Describe three types of emergency moves.

*6-18 State three situations that may require the use of an urgent move.

*6-19 Describe the procedure for rapid extrication.

*6-20 Describe four types of non-urgent moves.

6-21 Identify the following patient equipment:
  a. Wheeled stretcher

MOTIVATION FOR LEARNING

Many EMT-Basics are injured each year due to improper lifting and bending techniques. Understanding proper body mechanics is essential to injury prevention.

  b. Portable stretcher

  c. Stair chair

  d. Long backboard

  e. Short backboard

  f. Scoop (orthopedic) stretcher

  g. Flexible stretcher

  h. Basket stretcher

*6-22 Discuss proper patient positioning for the following situations:

  a. Unresponsive patient

  b. Patient complaining of chest pain, nausea, or difficulty breathing

  c. Patient with suspected spine injury

  d. Patient with signs and symptoms of shock

  e. Pregnant patient with hypotension

  f. Infants and children

  g. Elderly

BODY MECHANICS

DEFINITION

1. **Body mechanics** is the field of physiology that studies muscular actions and the function of muscles in maintaining the posture of the body.
2. This term is also used to describe the coordinated effort of the musculoskeletal and nervous systems to maintain proper balance, posture and body alignment during lifting, bending, moving, and other activities of daily living.

BASIC ELEMENTS OF BODY MECHANICS

Basic elements of body mechanics are **body alignment** (posture), balance (stability), and **coordinated body movement.**

1. **Body alignment (posture)**
   a. Body alignment refers to the positioning of the body's parts in relation to one another while in a standing, sitting, or lying position.
   b. Proper body alignment is synonymous with good posture.
      (1) It reduces strain on the structures of the musculoskeletal system.
      (2) It contributes to balance.
      (3) It maintains adequate muscle tone.
   c. **Terminology**
      (1) **Center of gravity** is the point at which the mass of an object is centered.
      (2) The **line of gravity** is an imaginary vertical line drawn through an object's center of gravity.
      (3) The **base of support** is the foundation on which an object rests.
   d. Body balance is achieved when the line of gravity passes through the body's center of gravity and the center of gravity is balanced over a wide, stable base of support (*Figure 6-1*). Proper body alignment is essential to body balance.
   e. Body balance can be enhanced by:
      (1) Broadening the base of support (e.g., separating the feet to a comfortable distance)
      (2) Lowering the center of gravity in order to bring it closer to the base of support (e.g., bending the knees and flexing the hips to achieve a squatting position)

2. **Coordinated body movement**
   a. **Friction** is a force that resists the motion of two objects in contact.
   b. Friction must be overcome when moving a patient.

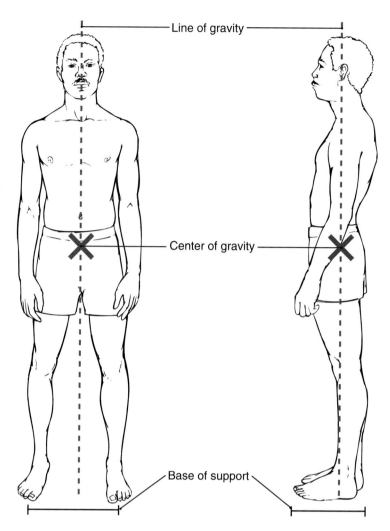

Fig. 6-1. Body balance is achieved when the line of gravity passes through the body's center of gravity and the center of gravity is balanced over a wide, stable base of support.

> **(1)** Use of a draw sheet reduces friction because the patient is more easily moved across a bed's surface.
>
> **(2)** Before moving a patient, place his or her arms across the chest to decrease surface area and reduce friction.

LIFTING TECHNIQUES

1. General guidelines for safe lifting

  a. Before lifting:

    (1) Consider the weight of the patient

    (2) Request additional help if necessary

    (3) Know your physical ability and limitations

  b. Position the feet approximately a shoulder's width apart, one foot slightly in front of the other.

    (1) Placing the feet slightly apart broadens the base of support and helps maintain body balance, reducing the risk of injury.

    (2) Place your feet in the direction in which the movement will occur. This foot placement:

      (a) Prevents twisting of the spine

      (b) Promotes effective use of major muscle groups

    (3) Wear proper footwear to protect your feet and maintain a firm footing.

   c. Stand as close as possible to the object to be moved. Standing close to the object:
      (1) Moves your center of gravity closer to the object
      (2) Helps maintain balance and reduces muscle strain
   d. Lower your center of gravity to the object to be lifted. Lowering your center of gravity:
      (1) Increases body balance
      (2) Enables muscle groups to work together effectively
   e. Before moving an object, contract (tense) your gluteal, abdominal, leg, and arm muscles while keeping your shoulders aligned over the spine and pelvis. Contracting these muscles:
      (1) Reduces the amount of energy required to move the object
      (2) Lessens the likelihood of muscle strain and injury
   f. When working with objects below your center of gravity, bend at your knees and hips, keeping the back straight. Use the muscles of your buttocks and legs, rather than the muscles of your back, to lift.
   g. Communicate clearly and frequently with your partner (and patient).

2. Guidelines for safe lifting of cots and stretchers
   a. Know or find out the weight to be lifted.
      (1) Consider the weight of the patient and the weight of the equipment being used.
      (2) Know or find out the weight limitations of the equipment being used.
      (3) Know what to do with patients who exceed the weight limitations of the equipment.
   b. Make sure that enough help is available.
      (1) Use at least two people to lift.
      (2) If possible, always use an even number of people to lift to maintain balance.
   c. When possible, use a stair chair instead of a stretcher, if medically appropriate.
   d. Plan how you will move the patient and where you will move him or her. Make sure the area is free of obstructions.
   e. Communicate clearly and frequently with your partner (and patient) throughout the lift.

3. Power (squat) lift
   a. The **power lift** is the recommended technique for lifting.
   b. It is useful for persons with weak knees or thighs.
   c. Power lift technique
      (1) Stand with your feet a comfortable distance apart.
      (2) Bend your knees to bring your center of gravity closer to the object to be lifted.
      (3) Tense your abdominal muscles to lock your back in a slight inward curve.
      (4) Keep your back as straight as possible, avoid bending at the waist, and keep your head facing forward.
      (5) Straddle the object.
      (6) Keep your feet flat with your weight evenly distributed to the balls of your feet or just behind them.
      (7) Use the **power grip** to get maximum force from your hands.
         (a) The power grip is used to get maximum force from your hands and should always be used in lifting.
         (b) Place hands at least 10 inches apart.
         (c) The palms should face up and palm and fingers should be in complete contact with the stretcher, with all fingers bent at the same angles.
      (8) Return to a standing position by locking your back in and raising your upper body before your hips.
      (9) Reverse these steps when lowering the stretcher or other object.

CARRYING PATIENTS AND EQUIPMENT

1. **Guidelines for safe carrying**
   a. Whenever possible, transport patients on devices that can be rolled.
   b. Know or find out the weight to be lifted.
   c. Know your physical abilities and limitations and that of your crew.
   d. Work in a coordinated manner and communicate frequently with your partner and the patient.
   e. Keep the weight as close to the body as possible.
   f. Keep your back in a locked-in position and avoid twisting.
   g. Flex at the hips, not at the waist, and bend at the knees.
   h. Do not hyperextend the back (do not lean back from the waist).
   i. Whenever possible, partners should be of similar height and strength.
   j. When carrying a stretcher or backboard with only two crew members, face each other from either the sides or ends of the stretcher.
2. **One-handed carrying technique**
   a. Pick up and carry with the back in a locked-in position.
   b. Avoid leaning to either side to compensate for the imbalance.
3. **Carrying procedure on stairs**
   a. When possible, use a stair chair instead of a stretcher.
   b. Make sure that the stairway is free of obstructions.
   c. Have another rescuer act as a guide or "spotter," especially if going down the stairs.
   d. Ensure that the patient is secured to the stair chair before lifting.
   e. Carry patients head first up the stairs and feet first down the stairs.
   f. Keep your back in a locked-in position.
   g. Flex at the hips, not at the waist, and bend at the knees.
   h. Keep the weight and your arms as close to your body as possible.

REACHING

1. **Guidelines for safe reaching**
   a. Keep your back in a locked-in position.
   b. When reaching overhead, avoid stretching or leaning back from the waist (hyperextending).
   c. Avoid twisting while reaching.
   d. Avoid reaching more than 15 to 20 inches in front of your body.
   e. Avoid situations where prolonged (more than a minute) strenuous effort is needed to avoid injury.
2. **Correct reaching for log rolls**
   a. Keep your back straight while leaning over the patient.
   b. Lean from the hips.
   c. Use your shoulder muscles to help with the roll.

GUIDELINES FOR PUSHING AND PULLING

1. Push, rather than pull, whenever possible.
   a. When pushing an object, broaden your base of support by moving your front foot forward.
   b. When pulling an object, broaden your base of support by moving your rear leg back (if you are facing the object) or moving the front foot forward (if you are facing away from the object).
2. Keep your back in a locked-in position.
3. Keep the line of pull through the center of the body by bending your knees.
4. Keep the weight close to your body.
5. Push from the area between the waist and shoulder.
6. If the weight is below waist level, use a kneeling position.
7. If possible, avoid pushing or pulling from an overhead position.
8. Keep your elbows bent with your arms close to your sides.

PRINCIPLES OF MOVING PATIENTS

EMERGENCY MOVES

1. **Indications.** In general, a patient should be moved **immediately** only where there is an immediate danger to the patient if he or she is not moved, such as in the following situations.
   a. Fire or danger of fire
   b. Danger of, or exposure to, explosives or other hazardous materials
   c. Inability to protect the patient from other hazards at the scene
   d. Inability to gain access to other patients who need life-saving care
   e. Inability to provide life-saving care due to location or position
   f. Any other situation that has the potential for causing injury, such as rapidly rising water or a structure in danger of collapse
2. **General guidelines**
   a. The greatest danger in moving a patient quickly is the possibility of aggravating a spine injury.
   b. Every effort should be made to pull the patient in the direction of the long axis of the body to provide as much protection to the spine as possible.
   c. Removing a patient from a vehicle quickly may aggravate an existing spinal injury. If possible, apply an interim immobilization during extrication.
3. **Types of emergency moves**
   a. In a **clothing drag,** the rescuer pulls on the patient's clothing in the neck and shoulder area.
   b. In a **blanket drag,** the rescuer places the patient on a blanket and drags the blanket.
   c. In a **bent-arm drag,** the rescuer puts his or her hands under the patient's armpits (from the back), grasps the patient's forearms, and drags the patient.

URGENT MOVES (RAPID EXTRICATION)

1. **Indications.** A patient should be moved **quickly** (urgent move) when there is an immediate threat to life, such as in the following situations.
   a. Altered mental status
   b. Inadequate breathing
   c. Shock (hypoperfusion)
2. **General guidelines**
   a. Rapid extrication must be accomplished quickly, without compromise or injury to the spine.
   b. One EMT-Basic positions himself or herself behind the patient. This EMT-Basic then places his or her hands on either side of the patient's head, bringing the cervical spine into a neutral in-line position and providing manual immobilization. At the same time, the EMT-Basic begins evaluation of the patient's airway.
   c. A rapid initial assessment is performed and a cervical immobilization device is applied by a second EMT-Basic.
   d. A third EMT-Basic simultaneously places a long backboard near the door and then moves to the passenger seat.
   e. The second EMT-Basic supports the patient's chest and back as the third EMT-Basic frees the patient's legs from the pedals and floor panels.
   f. At the direction of the first or second EMT-Basic, the patient is rotated in several short, coordinated moves until the patient's back is in the open doorway and his or her feet are on the passenger seat.
   g. Because the first EMT-Basic cannot usually support the patient's head any longer, another available EMT-Basic or emergency worker supports the patient's head as the first EMT-Basic gets out of the vehicle and takes support of the head outside the vehicle.

h. The end of the long backboard is placed on the seat next to the patient's but-tocks. Assistants support the other end of the board as the first EMT-Basic and the second EMT-Basic lower the patient onto it.

i. The second and third EMT-Basics slide the patient into proper position on the board in short, coordinated moves.

NON-URGENT MOVES

1. **Indications.** If no threat to life exists, the patient should be moved when ready for transportation (non-urgent move).
2. **Types of non-urgent moves**
   a. Direct ground lift (no suspected spine injury)
   (1) Two or three rescuers line up on one side of the patient.
   (2) Each rescuer kneels on one knee (preferably the same knee for all res-cuers).
   (3) The patient's arms are placed on his or her chest, if possible.
   (4) The rescuer at the head places one arm under the patient's neck and shoulder and cradles the patient's head.
   (5) The rescuer's other arm is placed under the patient's lower back.
   (6) The second rescuer places one arm under the patient's knees and one arm above the buttocks.
   (7) If a third rescuer is available, he or she places both arms under the waist. The other two rescuers then slide their arms either up to the mid-back or down to the buttocks as appropriate.
   (8) On a signal from the first rescuer, the rescuers lift the patient to their knees and roll the patient in toward their chests.
   (9) On a signal from the first rescuer, the rescuers stand and move the patient to the stretcher.
   (10) To lower the patient, the steps are reversed.

   b. Extremity lift (no suspected spine or extremity injury)
   (1) The first rescuer kneels at the patient's head. A second rescuer kneels at the patient's side by the knees.
   (2) The first rescuer places one hand under each of the patient's shoulders while the second rescuer grasps the patient's wrists.
   (3) The first rescuer slips his or her hands under the patient's arms and grasps the patient's wrists.
   (4) The second rescuer slips his or her hands under the patient's knees.
   (5) Both rescuers move up to a crouching position.
   (6) On a signal from the first rescuer, both rescuers stand simultaneously and move with the patient to a stretcher.

   c. Transfer of a supine patient to a bed or stretcher: direct carry (no sus-pected spine injury)
   (1) Position the stretcher at a right angle (perpendicular) to the bed with the head end of the stretcher at the foot of the bed.
   (2) Prepare the stretcher by unbuckling the straps and removing other items and lowering the closest railing.
   (3) Both rescuers stand between the bed and stretcher, facing the patient.
   (4) The rescuer at the head slides one arm under the patient's neck and shoulders, cupping the far shoulder with his or her hand and cradling the patient's head.
   (5) The second rescuer slides one hand under the patient's hip and lifts slightly.
   (6) The rescuer at the head slides his or her other arm under the patient's back.
   (7) The second rescuer places his or her arms underneath the patient's hips and calves.
   (8) Both rescuers slide the patient to edge of bed.

(9) The patient is lifted and curled toward the rescuers' chests.

(10) Both rescuers rotate and place the patient gently onto the stretcher.

d. Transfer of a supine patient to a bed or stretcher: draw sheet method

(1) Loosen the bottom sheet or draw sheet on the patient's bed.

(2) Position the stretcher so that it is parallel to and touching the bed.

(3) Prepare the stretcher by adjusting height, lowering rails, and unbuckling straps.

(4) Reach across the stretcher and grasp the sheet firmly at the patient's head, chest, hips, and knees.

(5) Slide the patient gently onto the stretcher.

EQUIPMENT

WHEELED STRETCHER

1. Overview

a. The wheeled stretcher is the most commonly used device by rescuer personnel.

b. Whenever possible, move patients by rolling them on a wheeled stretcher.

2. Types

a. The **two-person stretcher** (lift-in stretcher) requires two rescuers on each side when loading and unloading from the ambulance.

b. One-person stretcher (roll-in stretcher)

(1) The **one-person stretcher** has special loading wheels at the head, allowing it to be rolled in and out of the ambulance by one person.

(2) Despite its name, many agencies recommend using two rescuers when loading and unloading this stretcher from the ambulance.

c. Features

(1) Most wheeled stretchers are designed to accommodate weights of up to 400 pounds.

(2) Most wheeled stretchers can be adjusted to different heights to ease patient transfers.

(3) The head of the stretcher can be adjusted to several different angles.

(4) Wheeled stretchers have handles used for lifting and rolling.

(5) Some stretchers are equipped to hold additional items such as oxygen devices and intravenous lines.

(6) Side bars and straps should be used to secure the patient.

d. Guidelines for safe moving

(1) Never leave the patient unattended.

(2) The wheeled stretcher should only be used on smooth terrain.

(3) The stretcher should be pulled from the foot end while a second rescuer pushes and guides the head end.

(4) In narrow spaces, it is possible for two rescuers to carry the stretcher.

(a) This procedure requires more strength.

(b) The stretcher may become easily unbalanced.

(c) Rescuers should face each other from opposite ends of the stretcher.

(5) Four rescuers should be used to move a wheeled stretcher over rough terrain.

(a) Use of four rescuers provides more stability and requires less strength.

(b) One rescuer should be positioned at each corner.

e. Loading the ambulance

(1) Use sufficient lifting power.

(2) Load hanging and portable stretchers before a wheeled stretcher.

(3) Follow the manufacturer's directions.

(4) Ensure all patients and stretchers are secured before moving the ambulance.

PORTABLE STRETCHER

1. The **portable stretcher** is used as a secondary stretcher.
2. It is generally available in three styles:
   a. Basic model
   b. Basic model with folding wheels and posts
   c. Breakaway
3. The portable stretcher can be:
   a. Suspended from the ceiling of the ambulance by special brackets
   b. Secured to the squad bench
   c. Placed on the ambulance floor next to the main stretcher
4. It is usually folded in half for storage.
5. It may be used for carrying patients down stairs, downhill, or over rough terrain; removing patients from spaces too confined or narrow for a wheeled stretcher; or in multiple casualty incidents.
6. The portable stretcher is carried end to end.

STAIR CHAIR

1. The **stair chair** is designed for patients who can assume a sitting position while being carried to the ambulance.
2. The stair chair is useful for moving patients:
   a. Up or down stairs
   b. Through narrow corridors and doorways
   c. Into small elevators
   d. In narrow aisles in aircraft or buses
3. Do not use if:
   a. Neck or spinal injury is suspected
   b. The patient is unconscious or has an altered level of consciousness
   c. Lower extremity injury is suspected
4. Before moving a patient in a stair chair:
   a. Secure all belts and straps
   b. Instruct the patient to cross his or her arms over the chest to prevent injury
5. Upon arrival at the ambulance, transfer the patient to the main stretcher before transporting.

BACKBOARDS

1. **Long backboard**
   a. **Features**
      (1) The **long backboard** is available in a variety of styles. They are commonly made of wood, metal, or plastic.
      (2) Long backboards usually have holes spaced along the head and foot ends and sides of the board for handholds and insertion of straps.
      (3) They are 6–7 feet long.
   b. **Uses.** The long backboard is used for:
      (1) Patients found standing or lying down who require immobilization
      (2) Lifting and moving patients
      (3) To provide secondary support when a short backboard or orthopedic stretcher is used
      (4) As a firm surface on which to perform cardiopulmonary resuscitation (CPR)
2. **Short backboard**
   a. **Features**
      (1) The **short backboard** is also called a "half-backboard."
      (2) It is 3–4 feet long.

(3) It may be made of wood, aluminum, or plastic.

(4) The vest-type short backboard is wrapped around the patient; straps are sewn into the device.

b. Uses

(1) The short backboard serves as an intermediate device for immobilizing noncritical patients found in a sitting position.

(2) It must be used in conjunction with a long backboard for full spinal immobilization.

SCOOP (ORTHOPEDIC) STRETCHER

1. Features

a. The **scoop stretcher** is also called a split litter.

b. It is made of metal.

c. Currently available devices consist of four sections.

(1) Two sections support the upper body.

(2) Two sections support the lower body.

d. This stretcher is designed to be separated in the center of the head and foot ends into two long halves.

(1) Use of this stretcher requires that all sides of the patient be accessible.

(2) Each half is inserted under the patient from each side.

(3) The halves are then reconnected to form the completed "scoop."

2. Uses

a. In the absence of spinal injury, the scoop stretcher may be used to carry a supine patient up or down stairs or in other confined spaces.

b. If spinal injury is suspected, the patient and scoop stretcher should be secured to a long backboard for immobilization. Check local protocols regarding the use of this device.

FLEXIBLE STRETCHER

1. Features

a. The **flexible stretcher** is also called a Reeves stretcher.

b. It is made of canvas or synthetic flexible material with carrying handles.

c. Some flexible stretchers have wooden slats sewn into pockets.

2. Uses

a. The flexible stretcher is particularly useful when space is limited to access the patient, such as in:

(1) Narrow hallways

(2) Stairs

(3) Cramped corners

b. It should not be used for patients with suspected spinal injury.

BASKET STRETCHER

1. Features

a. The **basket stretcher** is also called the Stokes basket.

b. It is shaped like a long basket and can accommodate a scoop stretcher or a long backboard.

c. It is usually made of plastic.

2. Uses

a. The basket stretcher is used for moving patients over rough terrain.

b. It is often used in water rescues or high-angle rescues.

EQUIPMENT MAINTENANCE

Follow the manufacturer's directions for inspection, cleaning, repair, and maintenance.

PATIENT POSITIONING

UNRESPONSIVE PATIENT

An unresponsive patient **without** suspected head, neck, or spinal injury should be placed in the recovery position during transport *(Figure 6-2)*.
1. In the recovery position, the patient is placed on his or her left side to face the EMT-Basic.
2. The recovery position aids drainage of secretions from the patient's mouth and reduces the risk of aspiration in case of vomiting.

CHEST PAIN, DIFFICULTY BREATHING, OR NAUSEA/VOMITING

1. If hypotension (low blood pressure) is not present, a patient complaining of chest pain, discomfort, nausea, or difficulty breathing should be allowed to assume a position of comfort.
2. Do not permit a patient complaining of chest pain or difficulty breathing to walk to the ambulance.

SUSPECTED SPINE INJURY

1. Any patient with a suspected spine injury should be fully immobilized on a long backboard.
2. Ensure that suction is readily available should vomiting occur.

SHOCK

1. A patient with signs and symptoms of shock (hypoperfusion) should be placed in a supine position with his or her feet elevated 8–12 inches *(Figure 6-3)*.
2. This position should not be used if:
   a. The patient has sustained injuries to the head or neck, chest, abdomen, pelvis, spine, or lower extremities.
   b. The patient is exhibiting signs or symptoms of respiratory distress.

PREGNANCY

1. The pregnant patient with hypotension should be positioned on her left side.
2. This position moves the weight of the baby off the large blood vessels in the abdomen, increasing blood return to the heart.

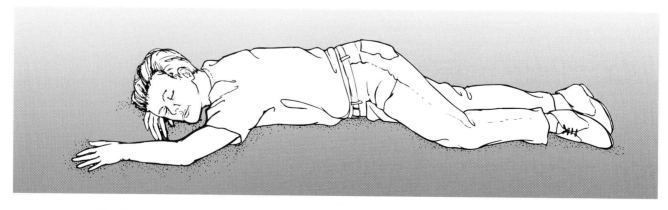

Fig. 6-2. An unresponsive patient without suspected head, neck, or spinal injury should be placed in the recovery position.

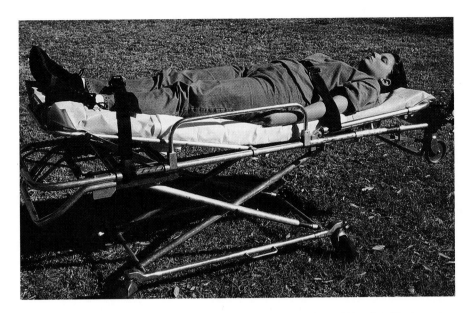

Fig. 6-3. A patient with signs and symptoms of shock (hypoperfusion) should be placed in the supine position with the feet elevated 8–12 inches.

INFANTS AND CHILDREN

1. When possible, consider immobilizing an infant or child in his or her own safety seat.
2. If the infant or child was not already in a safety seat and requires immobilization, immobilize on a backboard.

ELDERLY

1. Body functions slow and become less efficient.
2. Physical changes associated with aging, illness, and disease make some tasks difficult or impossible.
   a. Bones may become brittle and break easily.
   b. Joints become stiff and painful.
3. Patience, tolerance, and kindness are essential when working with the elderly.
4. Unless dictated otherwise by the patient's condition, allow the patient to assume a position of comfort.
5. Additional padding may be needed to maintain proper body alignment.

REVIEW QUESTIONS

Directions: Each of the numbered items or incomplete statements in this section is followed by answers or by completions of the statement. Select the ONE lettered answer or completion that is BEST in each case.

1. When lifting and moving patients, proper body alignment is imperative. Proper alignment

   (A) is more important when lifting conscious patients
   (B) ensures that the rescuer will be able to lift the patient
   (C) reduces the strain on the rescuer's musculoskeletal system
   (D) is achieved by moving the rescuer's center of gravity higher

2. A rescuer's balance may be enhanced by

    (A) bringing the feet close together
    (B) bending at the knees and hips to a squatting position
    (C) assuming a heel–toe stance with the right foot forward
    (D) bending at the lower back and lifting with the arms extended

3. Friction occurs when two objects rub together. When moving patients, rescuers should attempt to reduce friction. Which of the following would reduce the friction involved when moving a bedridden patient onto a stretcher?

    (A) Vest-type short backboard
    (B) Draw sheet
    (C) Traction splint
    (D) Short wooden backboard

4. In which of the following scenarios would you need to move a patient immediately?

    (A) A patient in severe shock
    (B) A patient threatened by a fire
    (C) A patient with an altered mental status
    (D) A patient with inadequate ventilations

5. Which of the following is considered an emergency move?

    (A) The foot drag
    (B) The head drag
    (C) The hand drag
    (D) The clothing drag

6. The first step in extricating a patient from a vehicle is

    (A) applying a cervical collar
    (B) positioning a backboard at the patient's side
    (C) having the patient release his or her seat belt
    (D) manual immobilization of the cervical spine in a neutral position

7. When moving a patient with suspected spinal compromise, the rescuer at the _____ is responsible for coordinating all movement.

    (A) feet
    (B) head
    (C) chest
    (D) pelvis

8. When moving a stretcher over rough terrain

    (A) use two rescuers to carry the stretcher
    (B) use four rescuers positioned at the four corners of the stretcher
    (C) having a conscious patient walk over rough terrain is better than carrying the patient
    (D) position one rescuer at the head, one rescuer at the foot, and one rescuer at the patient's side

9. As a rule of thumb, most wheeled stretchers are rated to carry

    (A) a patient of any size
    (B) up to 300 pounds
    (C) up to 400 pounds
    (D) up to 500 pounds

10. Patients in shock without suspected spinal compromise should be carried

    (A) in a prone position
    (B) fully immobilized to a long backboard
    (C) supine with the feet elevated 8–12 inches
    (D) with the head elevated at a 45° angle

11. The preferred position for transporting a pregnant patient is

    (A) in a prone position
    (B) in a supine position
    (C) with the patient positioned on her left side
    (D) in the Trendelenburg position

12. Your rescue crew responds to the scene of a motor vehicle accident. You are assigned responsibility for immobilizing an eighteen-month-old female patient. You should first consider immobilizing the patient with

    (A) a long backboard
    (B) a scoop stretcher
    (C) a short backboard
    (D) a child restraint seat

Directions: Each of the numbered questions or incomplete statements in this section refers to a scenario that precedes them. The numbered questions or incomplete statements are followed by answers or by completions of the statement. Select the answer or completion of the statement that is BEST in each case.

Your ambulance crew is dispatched to an adult care center for an 87-year-old male patient requesting transport to his weekly dialysis appointment. Your patient is in no apparent distress. He lives on the second floor, and the care center has no elevator.

Questions 13–15

13. The best device to move this patient down the stairs is

    (A) a short backboard
    (B) a long backboard
    (C) a draw sheet
    (D) a stair chair

14. When carrying the patient down the stairs, your crew should carry the patient

    (A) in a prone position
    (B) feet first
    (C) head first
    (D) in the anatomical position

15. After dialysis, your crew returns this patient to his room at the care center. When carrying the patient upstairs, your crew should carry the patient

    (A) in a supine position
    (B) feet first
    (C) head first
    (D) in the anatomical position

ANSWERS AND RATIONALES

1-C. Proper body alignment will reduce the strain on the rescuer's body, thus decreasing the chance of injury. Lowering the rescuer's center of gravity enhances body alignment. Proper alignment is imperative regardless of patient's level of consciousness. Proper alignment does not, however, guarantee that the rescuer will be able to lift the patient.

2-B. Bending at the knees and hips reduces the stress on the lower back and allows the major muscle groups to help in lifting. Bringing the feet closer together narrows the rescuer's balance and increases the strain on the body. The feet should be positioned apart at a comfortable distance, approximately shoulder's width. The lower back should be kept as straight as possible.

3-B. A draw sheet is ideal for reducing friction when helping patients on and off beds or stretchers. The sheet is placed under the patient, and the patient is simply pulled across. A vest-type short backboard helps with maintaining spinal immobilization on patients before application of a long backboard. A traction splint is used to stabilize long bone fractures, and a short wooden backboard is used to secure a patient's upper body while preparing for full spinal immobilization.

4-B. Patients should be immediately moved when their physical position places them in danger of further harm (e.g., fire, explosion, structural collapse, and rising floodwater). Patients in severe shock, with an altered mental status, or with inadequate ventilatory status should be moved urgently to ensure expedient treatment.

5-D. The clothing drag, blanket drag, and bent-arm drag are examples of emergency moves. When moving a patient in an emergency situation, every effort should be made to pull the patient in the long axis of the body to minimize spinal manipulation. Dragging by a hand or foot would twist the spine, and dragging by the head can cause damage to the spine or airway compromise.

6-D. The first step in dealing with a patient with suspected spinal compromise is to immobilize the cervical spine to prevent further injury. Immobilization is accomplished in conjunction with establishing and maintaining a patent airway. Application of a cervical collar should be done only after a visual and tactile examination of the entire neck. Having the patient release his or her seat belt is not advisable because it may require the patient to move the head and neck. Positioning the backboard should be done only after the patient has been manually immobilized.

7-B. Since the rescuer at the head is responsible for maintaining cervical spine alignment and airway patency, this rescuer is responsible for coordinating all movement of the patient. Movement between rescuers should be coordinated to ensure smooth movement of the patient.

8-B. Positioning a rescuer at each corner of the stretcher maximizes stability (more rescuers can be used if necessary and available). Having a patient walk over rough terrain is not appropriate.

9-C. While 400 pounds is a good rule of thumb, rescuers should know the specific limitations of all their equipment.

10-C. Placing the patient supine with the feet elevated helps blood to return from the lower extremities to the body's core. The increased blood returning to the core helps slow the progression of shock. Placing a patient in a prone position makes monitoring of the patient's airway more difficult. Patients without suspected spinal compromise need not be fully immobilized. Elevating the head and upper body has the reverse effect of raising the legs: it allows more blood to drain into the legs and requires more work by the heart.

11-C. Positioning pregnant patients on their left side moves the weight of the fetus off the mother's inferior vena cava. If the inferior vena cava is compressed, the return of blood to the heart is decreased, thus decreasing the amount of blood the heart can pump.

12-D. Frequently, a child restraint seat is the most appropriate device to use when transporting a young patient. In some circumstances, however, the restraint seat should not be used as an immobilization device (e.g., if CPR were required). A long backboard or short backboard can be used in these situations. Small children may slide around excessively in a scoop stretcher.

13-D. A stair chair is ideal for moving a patient without spinal injury down a flight of stairs. The long and short backboard would be used if spinal compromise were suspected. A draw sheet is appropriate for sliding a patient from one horizontal surface to another.

14-B. Carrying patients down stairs feet first greatly decreases patient anxiety. All other positions increase patient apprehension and should be avoided.

15-C. Moving the patient up the stairs in a head-first position decreases patient anxiety by allowing the patient to assume a more natural position. Whenever possible, patient comfort should be considered when moving patients.

BIBLIOGRAPHY

Anderson KN, Anderson LE, Glanze WD (eds): *Mosby's Medical, Nursing, & Allied Health Dictionary*, 4th ed. St. Louis, Mosby-Year Book, 1994.

Butman AM, Martin SW, Vomacka RW, et al (eds): *Comprehensive Guide to Pre-Hospital Skills: A Skills Manual for EMT-Basic, EMT-Intermediate, EMT-Paramedic*. Akron, Ohio, Emergency Training, 1995.

Crosby LA, Lewallen DG (eds): *Emergency Care and Transportation of the Sick and Injured*, 6th ed. Rosemont, IL, American Academy of Orthopaedic Surgeons, 1995.

Grant HD, Murray RH Jr, Bergeron JD: *Emergency Care*, 7th ed. Englewood Cliffs, NJ, Prentice-Hall, 1995.

Hafen BQ, Karren KJ, Mistovich JJ: *Prehospital Emergency Care*, 5th ed. Upper Saddle River, NJ, Prentice-Hall, 1996.

Kozier B, Erb G, Blais K, et al: *Fundamentals of Nursing: Concepts, Process, and Practice*, 5th ed. Redwood City, CA, Addison-Wesley, 1995.

McSwain NE, White RD, Paturas JL, et al (eds): *The Basic EMT: Comprehensive Prehospital Patient Care*. St. Louis, Mosby-Year Book, 1996.

O'Toole M (ed): *Miller-Keane Encyclopedia and Dictionary of Medicine, Nursing, and Allied Health*. Philadelphia, WB Saunders, 1992.

Potter PA, Perry AG: *Fundamentals of Nursing: Concepts, Process, and Practice*, 3rd ed. St. Louis, Mosby-Year Book, 1993.

Stoy WA: *Mosby's EMT-Basic Textbook*. St. Louis, Mosby-Year Book, 1996.

United States Department of Transportation, National Highway Traffic Safety Administration: *Emergency Medical Technician: Basic. National Standard Curriculum*, 1994.

TWO

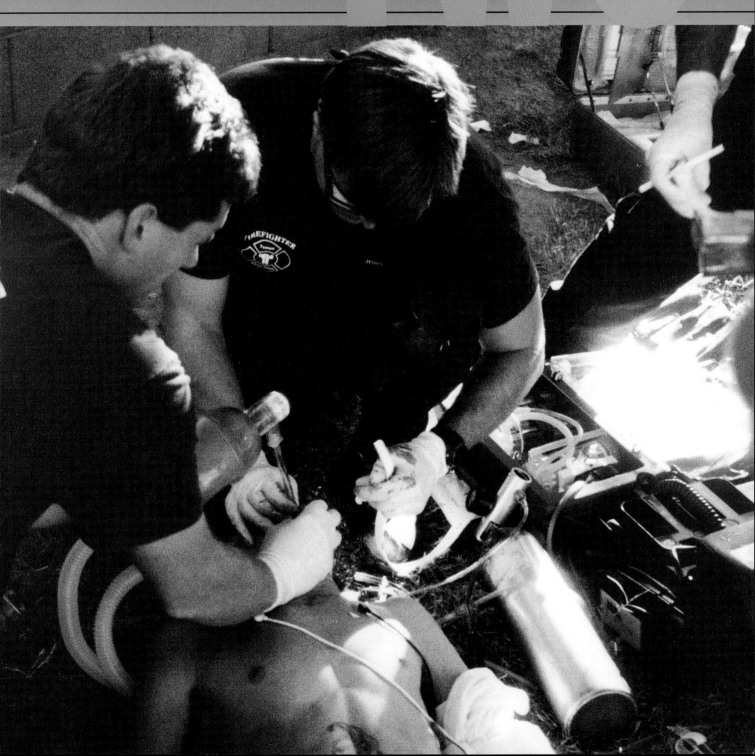

7 AIRWAY

OBJECTIVES

7-1 Name and label the following structures of the respiratory system: nose, mouth, nasopharynx, oropharynx, laryngopharynx, epiglottis, trachea, thyroid cartilage, cricoid cartilage, larynx, right and left mainstem bronchi, lungs, alveoli, diaphragm.

7-2 List the signs of adequate breathing.

*7-3 List factors that result in an increased respiratory rate.

*7-4 List factors that result in a decreased respiratory rate.

7-5 List the signs of inadequate breathing.

*7-6 List the signs and symptoms of partial or complete obstruction caused by a foreign body.

7-7 Describe the steps in performing the following manual airway maneuvers:
   a. Opening the mouth
   b. Head-tilt, chin-lift maneuver
   c. Jaw-thrust maneuver

7-8 Relate the mechanism of injury to opening the airway.

7-9 State the importance of having a suction unit ready for immediate use when providing emergency care.

*7-10 Describe types of suction equipment including:
   a. Mounted suction devices
   b. Battery-powered portable suction devices
   c. Hand-powered portable suction devices

MOTIVATION FOR LEARNING

All living cells of the body require oxygen and produce carbon dioxide. Oxygen is particularly important to cells of the nervous system because without it, brain cells begin to die within 4 to 6 minutes. A nonbreathing patient or a patient with difficulty breathing is a true emergency. To prevent death, the EMT-Basic must learn to detect early signs of respiratory difficulty and how to intervene. Proper performance of airway management skills may mean the difference between the patient's life and death.

*7-11 Describe the following types of suction devices:
    a. Rigid suction catheter
    b. Soft (flexible) suction catheter
    c. Bulb syringe

7-12 Describe the technique of suctioning.

*7-13 Describe the indications for insertion of an oropharyngeal airway.

7-14 Describe how to measure and insert an oropharyngeal airway.

*7-15 Describe the indications for insertion of a nasopharyngeal airway.

7-16 Describe how to measure and insert a nasopharyngeal airway.

*7-17 List, in order of preference, the methods for ventilating a patient by the EMT-Basic.

7-18 Describe how to artificially ventilate a patient with a pocket mask.

7-19 List the parts of a bag-valve-mask system.

7-20 Describe the steps in performing the skill of artificially ventilating a patient with a bag-valve mask for one and two rescuers.

7-21 Describe the steps in performing the skill of artificially ventilating a patient with a bag-valve mask while using the jaw thrust.

7-22 Describe the signs of adequate artificial ventilation using the bag-valve mask.

7-23 Describe the signs of inadequate artificial ventilation using the bag-valve mask.

7-24 Describe the steps in artificially ventilating a patient with a flow-restricted, oxygen-powered ventilation device.

*7-25 Describe the purpose of applying cricoid pressure (Sellick maneuver).

*7-26 Describe the technique of applying cricoid pressure.

*7-27 Describe the steps in providing bag-valve-device-to-tracheostomy-tube ventilation.

7-28 Describe the steps in providing bag-valve mask-to-stoma ventilation.

7-29 Define the components of an oxygen delivery system.

7-30 Identify a nonrebreather face mask and state the oxygen flow requirements for its use.

7-31 Describe the indications for using a nasal cannula versus a nonrebreather face mask.

7-32 Identify a nasal cannula and state the flow requirements for its use.

REVIEW OF THE RESPIRATORY SYSTEM

FUNCTION OF THE RESPIRATORY SYSTEM

1. The respiratory system supplies oxygen from the atmosphere to body cells.
2. It transports carbon dioxide produced by body cells to the atmosphere.

ANATOMY REVIEW (FIGURE 7-1)

1. Nose and mouth
    a. Air normally enters the body through the nostrils. The air is warmed, moistened, and filtered as it flows over the mucous membrane lining of the nose.
    b. Air entering the mouth is not filtered or warmed as efficiently as air entering the nostrils.
2. **Pharynx**
    a. Air entering the nose or mouth or food entering the mouth is moved to the pharynx (throat).

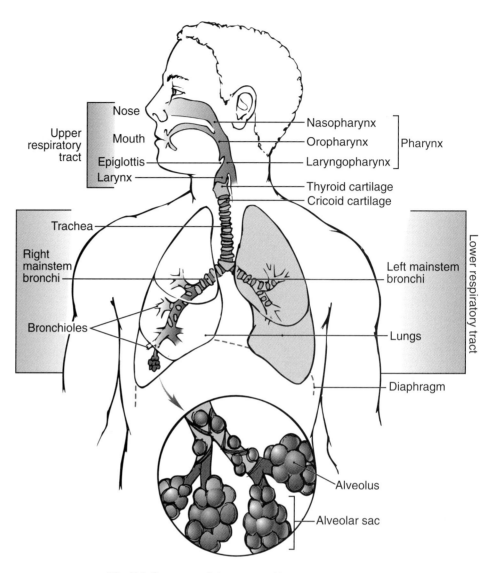

Fig. 7-1. Structures of the upper and lower respiratory tract.

   b. At the base of the pharynx are two passageways.
      (1)   Air is moved to the trachea (windpipe) which conducts air to the lungs.
      (2)   Food is moved to the esophagus and then to the stomach.
   c. The epiglottis is a leaf-shaped flap of elastic cartilage that is attached on one end to the anterior portion of the thyroid cartilage.
      (1)   During swallowing, the epiglottis covers the opening of the larynx and prevents food or liquids from entering it.
      (2)   Choking may result if the epiglottis fails to close, allowing food or liquids to enter the airway.
      (3)   Infection of the epiglottis (epiglottitis) may result in swelling. Swelling may close the glottis, resulting in suffocation.
3. Larynx and trachea
   a. The larynx contains the vocal cords.
      (1)   The space between the vocal cords is called the glottis.
      (2)   The largest cartilage of the larynx is thyroid cartilage.
         (a)   The thyroid cartilage is also called the Adam's apple.
         (b)   The narrowest diameter of the adult airway is at the vocal cords.
      (3)   The cricoid cartilage is the most inferior of the cartilages of the larynx.

The narrowest diameter of the airway in infants and children older than 10 years of age is at the cricoid cartilage.

b. The trachea is the passageway for air to and from the lungs.

   (1) The trachea is held open by C-shaped rings of cartilage.

   (2) Obstruction of the trachea will cause death if not corrected within minutes.

4. Lungs and bronchi

  a. The trachea branches into two smaller tubes, called the right and left mainstem (primary) bronchi.

    (1) The right mainstem bronchus enters the right lung, and the left mainstem bronchus enters the left lung.

    (2) The right mainstem bronchus is shorter, wider, and straighter than the left.

      (a) An endotracheal tube that is inserted too far is more likely to enter the right mainstem bronchus.

      (b) Foreign material that is aspirated is more likely to enter the right mainstem bronchus than the left.

  b. Each bronchus branches into smaller and smaller tubes eventually leading to bronchioles (Figure 7-2).

    (1) The bronchi of the lungs can be compared to a tree.

    (2) The bronchioles leading to the alveoli are the branches of the tree.

  c. Bronchioles end in millions of tiny air sacs called alveoli.

    (1) The alveoli are the leaves of the tree.

    (2) Oxygen passes through the thin walls of the alveoli to capillaries.

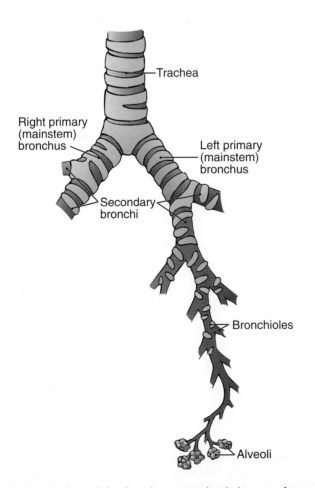

Fig. 7-2. The bronchi, bronchioles, and alveoli can be compared with the parts of a tree. The bronchi are the tree, the bronchioles are the branches, and the alveoli are the leaves.

(3) Carbon dioxide passes from the capillaries to the alveoli and is breathed out into the atmosphere.

MECHANICS OF BREATHING

1. **Definitions**
   a. **Breathing (pulmonary ventilation)** is the mechanical process of moving air into and out of the lungs.
   b. **Inspiration** (inhalation) is the process of breathing in and moving air into the lungs.
   c. **Expiration** (exhalation) is the process of breathing out and moving air out of the lungs.
   d. **Respiration** is the exchange of gases between a living organism and its environment.
2. **Muscles of breathing**
   a. **Diaphragm**
      (1) The diaphragm is a dome-shaped muscle located below the lungs.
      (2) It is the primary muscle of respiration.
      (3) It separates the chest cavity from the abdominal cavity.
   b. External **intercostal muscles** are located between the ribs.
   c. Internal intercostal muscles and abdominal muscles may be used during forceful expiration.
3. **Inspiration** (Figure 7-3)
   a. Inspiration is an active process (requires muscle contraction).
   b. Motor impulses are received from the medulla in the brain stem.
      (1) Impulses travel along phrenic and intercostal nerves.

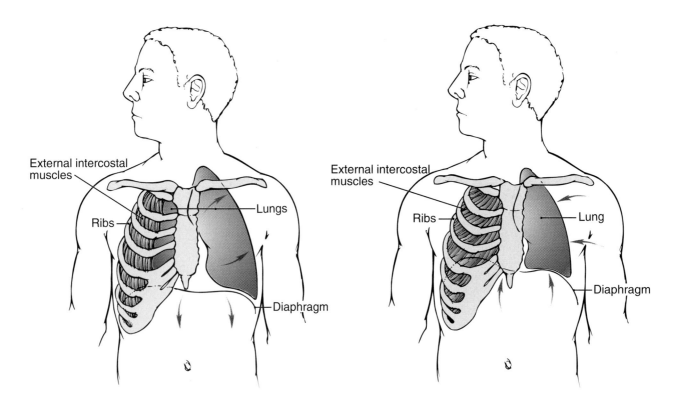

Fig. 7-3. Mechanism of breathing. *(A)* During inspiration, the diaphragm contracts and moves downward, and the external intercostal muscles pull the ribs upward and outward. The pressure within the lungs falls below atmospheric pressure, and air rushes into the lungs. *(B)* During expiration, the diaphragm and external intercostal muscles relax. The pressure within the lungs rises above atmospheric pressure, and air rushes out of the lungs.

    (2) Phrenic nerves stimulate the diaphragm.

    (3) Intercostal nerves stimulate external intercostal muscles.

  c. The diaphragm contracts (flattens out) and moves downward; this movement increases the diameter of the chest from top to bottom.

  d. The external intercostal muscles increase the size of the chest cavity by pulling ribs upward and outward; this movement increases the diameter of the chest from side to side and front to back.

  e. As the size of the chest cavity increases, the pressure within the lungs falls below the atmospheric pressure and air rushes into the lungs.

  f. Air continues to enter the lungs until the pressure within the lungs is equal to atmospheric pressure.

4. Expiration (see Figure 7-3)

  a. Expiration is normally a passive process.

  b. Motor impulses from the medulla decrease, resulting in relaxation of the inspiratory muscles (diaphragm and external intercostals).

  c. Lungs are compressed as the respiratory muscles relax; elastic lung tissue recoils and compresses the alveoli.

  d. As the size of the chest cavity decreases, the pressure within the lungs rises above atmospheric pressure and air rushes out of the lungs.

  e. Air continues to leave the lungs until the pressure within the lungs is equal to atmospheric pressure.

RESPIRATORY PHYSIOLOGY

1. Alveolar/capillary exchange (exchange of gases in the lungs)

  a. Blood pumped from the right ventricle of the heart enters the pulmonary artery and eventually enters the lungs.

  b. The blood then flows through the lung capillaries that are close to the alveoli.

    (1) The blood from the right heart is low in oxygen (oxygen-poor) and high in carbon dioxide.

      (a) Oxygen is continuously used by the cells of the body.

      (b) Carbon dioxide is a waste product of cellular work.

    (2) Air entering the alveoli from the atmosphere during inspiration is rich in oxygen (oxygen-rich) and contains little carbon dioxide.

  c. Oxygen-rich air enters the alveoli and passes through the capillary walls into the bloodstream.

  d. Carbon dioxide passes from the blood through the capillary walls into the alveoli and leaves the body in exhaled air.

2. Capillary/cellular exchange (exchange of gases in tissues)

  a. Oxygen-rich blood moves out of the tissue capillaries and into the tissue cells.

    (1) Tissue cells use oxygen.

    (2) Carbon dioxide, a waste product, is produced.

  b. Carbon dioxide moves from the tissue cells into the tissue capillaries and is transported to the lungs for removal from the body.

INFANT AND CHILD ANATOMY

1. Nose and mouth

  a. In general, all structures of the nose and mouth are smaller and more easily obstructed than in adults.

  b. The teeth are either absent or very delicate.

2. Pharynx

  a. The tongue takes up proportionally more space in the mouth than in an adult. The large tongue and shorter distance between the tongue and hard palate increase the risk of upper airway obstruction.

  b. The epiglottis is large and floppy.

3. Trachea

    a. The trachea is softer and more flexible in infants and children.

    b. The trachea is funnel-shaped due to narrow, undeveloped cricoid cartilage; the cricoid cartilage is the narrowest portion of the airway in children younger than 10 years of age.

    c. A small change in airway size results in a significant increase in airway resistance.

4. Chest wall

    a. Ribs and cartilage are softer.

        (1) The chest wall of the infant and young child is flexible because it is composed of more cartilage than bone.

        (2) Because of the flexibility of the ribs, children are more resistant to rib fractures than adults.

            (a) The force of the injury, however, is readily transmitted to the lungs.

            (b) Chest injury may result in bruising of the lungs (pulmonary contusion) or more significant injury.

    b. Infants and children depend more heavily on the diaphragm for breathing. Effective respiration may be compromised when movement of the diaphragm is limited because the chest wall cannot compensate.

RESPIRATORY ASSESSMENT

SIGNS OF ADEQUATE BREATHING

1. The respiratory rate is normal.

    a. Normal resting respiratory rates are:

        (1) Adults: 12–20 breaths/minute

        (2) Children: 15–30 breaths/minute

        (3) Infants: 25–50 breaths/minute

    b. Factors that may result in an increased respiratory rate include fever, pain, anxiety, and insufficient oxygen.

    c. Factors that may result in a decreased respiratory rate include sleep and depressant drugs.

2. The rhythm is regular.

3. The quality is normal.

    a. Breath sounds are present and equal bilaterally.

    b. Chest expansion is adequate and equal with each breath.

    c. Breathing at rest is effortless; patient does not excessively use accessory muscles during inspiration or expiration.

4. Depth (tidal volume) is adequate.

    a. Tidal volume is the amount of air inhaled and exhaled during normal breathing.

    b. In the average adult, tidal volume is approximately 500 milliliters (mL).

5. The skin is pink (in Caucasians), warm, and dry.

SIGNS OF INADEQUATE BREATHING

1. The respiratory rate is the outside normal range for age.

    a. Tachypnea is an excessively rapid rate of breathing.

    b. Bradypnea is an excessively slow rate of breathing.

    c. Agonal respirations (occasional gasping breaths) may be seen just before death.

2. Rhythm is irregular.

    a. The patient has an irregular breathing pattern.

    b. An irregular breathing pattern is significant until proven otherwise.

3. Quality is abnormal.

    a. Breath sounds are diminished or absent.

    b. Chest expansion is unequal or inadequate.

    c. Breathing effort is increased.
        (1) Patient may be restless or anxious.
        (2) Patient may use accessory muscles.
            (a) The diaphragm and neck muscles may be used in inhalation.
            (b) The abdominal muscles may be used in exhalation.
            (c) Retractions may be seen above the clavicles, between the ribs and below the rib cage, especially in children.
        (3) Nasal flaring may be present, especially in children.
        (4) Infants may have **"seesaw" breathing,** in which the chest and abdomen move in opposite directions.
    d. Patients often compensate by changing position.
        (1) Patients frequently avoid supine position.
        (2) They usually prefer to sit up.
4. Depth (tidal volume) is inadequate or shallow.
5. Skin is pale or cyanotic (grayish-blue) and feels cool and/or clammy.

BASIC LIFE SUPPORT

AIRWAY OBSTRUCTION

1. Obstruction by the tongue
    a. In an unconscious patient, the jaw relaxes and the tongue can fall back and obstruct the airway.
    b. The tongue is the most common cause of upper airway obstruction in unconscious patients.
    c. Partial airway obstruction is associated with snoring respirations.
    d. Airway obstruction caused by the tongue is corrected with proper airway positioning.
2. Obstruction by a foreign body
    a. A foreign body may cause partial or complete obstruction.
    b. Signs and symptoms may include:
        (1) Choking
        (2) Gagging
        (3) Stridor
        (4) Dyspnea
        (5) Inability to speak
    c. In cases of complete obstruction, management depends on:
        (1) Age of victim
        (2) If victim is conscious or unconscious

OPENING THE MOUTH

The **crossed-finger technique** may be used to open the mouth of an **unconscious** patient (Figure 7-4).
1. Kneel above and behind the patient.
2. Cross the thumb and forefinger of one hand.
3. Place the thumb on the patient's lower incisors and your forefinger on the upper incisors.
4. Use a scissors motion or finger-snapping motion to open the mouth.

OPENING THE AIRWAY

1. Head-tilt, chin-lift maneuver
    a. The **head-tilt, chin-lift maneuver** should be used to open the airway when:
        (1) The patient is unresponsive
        (2) The patient is unable to protect his or her own airway

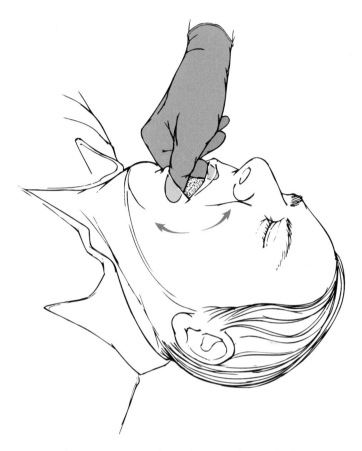

Fig. 7-4. The crossed-finger technique may be used to open the mouth of an unconscious patient.

(3) Cervical spine injury is **not** suspected
  b. **Technique**
    (1) Place the patient in a supine position.
    (2) Tilt the patient's head back by placing one hand on the forehead, gently extending the patient's neck.
    (3) Place the fingers of the other hand under the patient's chin and pull gently upward. Do not compress the soft tissues under the chin; compression of these structures may result in airway obstruction.
  c. An advantage of this maneuver is that it does not require special equipment.
  d. **Disadvantages**
    (1) The head-tilt, chin-lift maneuver does not protect the airway from aspiration.
    (2) An additional rescuer is needed to perform bag-valve-mask ventilation.
    (3) It is difficult to maintain for a prolonged period.
2. **Jaw-thrust maneuver**
  a. The **jaw-thrust maneuver** should be used to open the airway when:
    (1) The patient is unresponsive
    (2) The patient is unable to protect his or her own airway
    (3) Cervical spine injury is suspected
  b. **Technique**
    (1) While maintaining cervical spine immobilization, grasp the angles of the patient's lower jaw with both hands, one on each side.
    (2) Using upward pressure, thrust the patient's lower jaw forward, lifting the tongue out of the pharynx.
  c. **Advantages**
    (1) The jaw-thrust maneuver does not require special equipment.

(2)   It may be used in cases of suspected cervical spine injury.

d. Disadvantages

(1)   It does not protect the airway from aspiration.

(2)   An additional rescuer is needed to perform bag-valve-mask ventilation.

(3)   The jaw thrust cannot be maintained if the patient becomes responsive or combative.

(4)   It is difficult to maintain for a prolonged period.

(5)   It is difficult to maintain with bag-valve-mask ventilation.

SUCTIONING

1. The purpose of suctioning is to remove oral secretions, blood, other liquids, or food particles from the airway.

a. Suction immediately if a gurgling sound is heard with artificial ventilation.

b. Body substance isolation (BSI) precautions are essential when suctioning; use a high-efficiency particulate air (HEPA) respirator if tuberculosis is suspected.

2. Suction devices

a. Mounted suction devices

(1)   **Mounted suction devices** are also called fixed suction units.

(2)   These devices are mounted (built-in) in ambulances and are usually powered by the vehicle's battery.

(3)   **Advantages**

(a)   The vacuum is strong and adjustable.

(b)   The components of the device that come in contact with body fluids are disposable.

(4)   **Disadvantages**

(a)   The mounted device is not portable.

(b)   It cannot be used with an alternative power source.

b. Portable suction devices

(1)   **Battery-operated devices**

(a)   **Advantages**

(i)   Battery-operated devices are lightweight and portable.

(ii)   They have good suction power.

(b)   **Disadvantages**

(i)   These devices have more complicated mechanics than hand-powered devices.

(ii)   The battery may lose integrity over time.

(iii)   Batteries must be kept charged and checked daily.

(iv)   Some of the components that come in contact with body fluids are not disposable.

(2)   **Hand-powered devices**

(a)   **Advantages**

(i)   Hand-powered devices are lightweight, portable, and reliable.

(ii)   They are mechanically simple.

(iii)   They are inexpensive.

(b)   **Disadvantages**

(i)   The devices are manually powered.

(ii)   They have limited volume.

(iii)   The components that come in contact with body fluids are not disposable.

3. Suction catheters

a. Rigid catheters (Yankauer; tonsil-tip)

(1)   These catheters are used to clear the mouth and oropharynx of an unresponsive patient.

(a)   Their use in conscious or semiconscious patients may cause vomiting.

(b)   These catheters are able to rapidly suction large amounts of fluid.

(2) Technique
- **(a)** Take BSI precautions.
- **(b)** Preoxygenate the patient if possible.
- **(c)** Turn on the suction unit. If the unit is equipped with a pressure gauge, be sure it can generate a vacuum of 300 millimeters of mercury (mm Hg).
- **(d)** Attach the catheter to the suction unit.
- **(e)** Insert the suction device into the mouth WITHOUT applying suction.
  - **(i)** It should be inserted only as far as you can see.
  - **(ii)** Do not insert past the base of the tongue.
- **(f)** Once the suction tip is in contact with secretions, apply suction for no more than 5 seconds in infants and children and 15 seconds in adults.
  - **(i)** In infants and children, avoid touching the back of the throat.
  - **(ii)** Stimulation of the back of the throat may result in slowing of the heart rate.
- **(g)** Periodically rinse the catheter and tubing with water to ensure patency.
- **(h)** Administer oxygen after suctioning.

b. Flexible plastic catheter (soft; whistle-tip; French)
- **(1)** These catheters are used to clear the oropharynx and nasopharynx and to remove secretions from an endotracheal tube in intubated patients.
  - **(a)** They are available in many sizes.
  - **(b)** The inside diameter of flexible catheters is smaller than that of rigid catheters.
- **(2) Technique**
  - **(a)** Take BSI precautions.
  - **(b)** Preoxygenate the patient if possible. If suctioning an intubated patient, preoxygenation is essential.
  - **(c)** Measure the catheter from the tip of the nose to the tip of the ear and do not insert past the base of the tongue (in patients without an endotracheal tube in place).
  - **(d)** Turn on the suction unit. If the unit is equipped with a pressure gauge, be sure it can generate a 300-mm Hg vacuum.
  - **(e)** Attach the catheter to the suction unit.
  - **(f)** Insert the catheter WITHOUT applying suction.
  - **(g)** Apply intermittent suction by closing the side opening while withdrawing the catheter in a side-to-side motion.
  - **(h)** Apply suction for no more than 5 seconds in infants and children and 15 seconds in adults.
  - **(i)** Periodically rinse the catheter and tubing with water to ensure patency.
  - **(j)** Administer oxygen after suctioning.

c. Bulb syringe
- **(1)** The bulb syringe is used to clear secretions from the mouth and/or nose of infants.
- **(2) Technique**
  - **(a)** Take BSI precautions.
  - **(b)** Preoxygenate if possible.
  - **(c)** Depress the bulb syringe before inserting to remove air in the syringe.
  - **(d)** With the syringe depressed, insert into the nose or mouth and release.
  - **(e)** Allow syringe to fill.

(**f**) Remove syringe and expel contents.

(**g**) Apply suction for no more than 5 seconds.

(**h**) Administer oxygen after suctioning.

4. Complications of suctioning include:

a. Hypoxia

b. Trauma to the oropharynx or nasopharynx

c. Stimulation of the gag reflex resulting in bradycardia

5. **Special considerations**

a. If emesis or secretions cannot be removed quickly and easily by suctioning, the patient should be logrolled and the oropharynx should be cleared manually.

b. If the patient produces large amounts of frothy secretions, suction for 15 seconds, provide artificial ventilation for 2 minutes, suction for 15 seconds.

(**1**) Continue this sequence until the airway is cleared of secretions.

(**2**) Consult medical direction in this situation.

AIRWAY ADJUNCTS

OROPHARYNGEAL AIRWAY (ORAL AIRWAY, OPA)

1. **Description and indications**

a. An oropharyngeal airway is a semicircular device made of hard plastic designed to hold the tongue away from the back of the throat.

b. It is used to maintain an open airway in unresponsive patients without a gag reflex. Use in responsive or semiresponsive patients may stimulate the gag reflex when the back of the tongue or throat is touched, resulting in vomiting.

2. **Sizing**

a. Place the airway on the side of the patient's face.

b. Select an airway that extends from the corner of the mouth to the bottom of the earlobe or angle of the jaw.

3. **Insertion—Adults** (Figure 7-5)

a. Take BSI precautions.

b. Select airway and determine proper size.

c. Open the patient's mouth.

d. Remove visible obstructions.

e. Insert the airway with the distal tip facing upward (pointing toward the roof of the patient's mouth).

f. Gently advance the airway until the distal tip reaches the soft palate.

g. Rotate the airway 180° and advance it until the flange rests on the patient's lips or teeth.

4. **Insertion—Infants and children** (and alternate method for adults) [Figure 7-6]

a. Take BSI precautions.

b. Select airway and determine proper size.

c. Open the patient's mouth.

d. Use a tongue depressor to push the tongue down and out of the way.

e. Insert the airway with the distal tip pointing downward (toward the patient's feet).

f. Gently advance the airway until the flange rests comfortably on the patient's lips or teeth.

5. **Special considerations**

a. Use of an oropharyngeal airway does not eliminate the need for maintaining proper head position.

b. An airway of the wrong length or an airway that is improperly inserted may push the tongue back into the pharynx, resulting in airway obstruction.

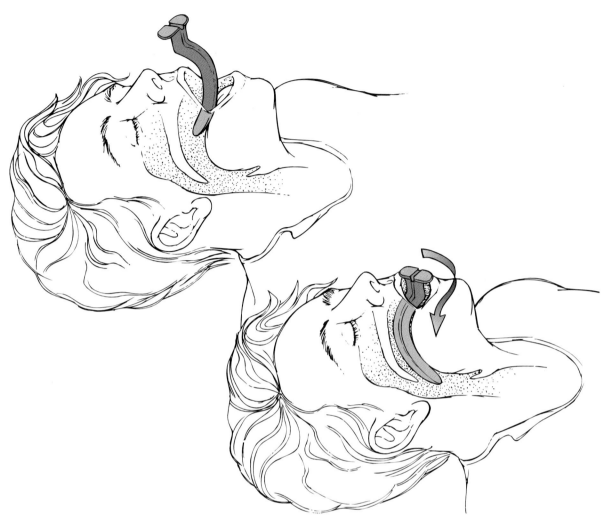

Fig. 7-5. Insertion of the oropharyngeal airway in an adult. *(A)* Insert the airway with the distal tip pointing toward the roof of the patient's mouth. (B) Rotate the airway 180° until the flange rests on the patient's lips or teeth.

NASOPHARYNGEAL AIRWAY (NASAL AIRWAY, NPA, NASAL TRUMPET)

1. **Description and indications**
   a. A nasopharyngeal airway is a curved, hollow tube approximately 6 inches long made of soft rubber or plastic with a flange at the top end and a bevel tip at the distal end.
   b. It is used in the following situations:
      (1) Unresponsive patient
      (2) Responsive patient who is not alert enough to maintain his or her own airway adequately
2. **Sizing.** Measure from the tip of the patient's nose to the tip of the patient's ear.
3. **Insertion**
   a. Take BSI precautions.
   b. Select airway and determine proper size.
   c. Lubricate the airway with a water-soluble lubricant.
   d. Hold the airway so that its curvature follows that of the floor of the nasal cavity.
   e. Insert the airway with the bevel toward the nasal septum.
   f. Gently advance the airway along the floor of the nasal cavity parallel to the mouth until the flange is flush against the opening of the nostril (Figure 7-7).
      (1) Do not direct the airway upward.

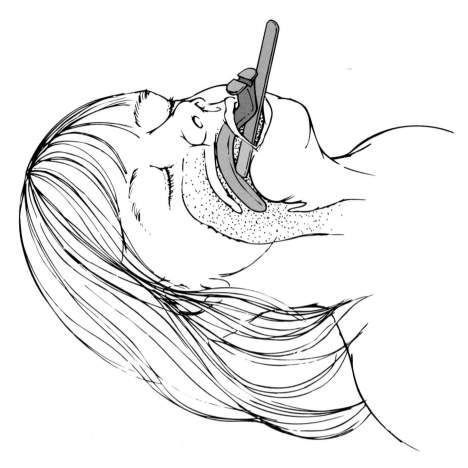

Fig. 7-6. Oropharyngeal airway insertion in infants and children. Use a tongue depressor to push the tongue down and out of the way. Insert the airway with the distal tip pointing downward (toward the patient's feet). Gently advance the airway until the flange rests comfortably on the patient's lips or teeth.

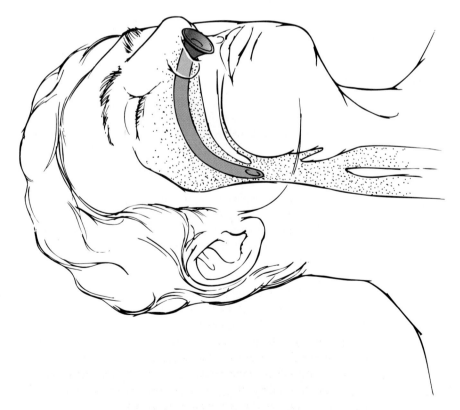

Fig. 7-7. The nasopharyngeal airway in proper position.

(2) Do not force.

g. Assess placement by feeling for air coming from the device.

4. **Special considerations**

a. If the nasopharyngeal airway cannot be inserted into one nostril, try the other nostril.

b. Forceful insertion may cause abrasions or lacerations of the nasal mucosa and result in significant bleeding.

c. If the tube is too long, it may enter the esophagus, causing gastric distention and inadequate ventilation.

d. It should not be used in situations involving trauma to the nose or suspected basilar skull fracture (blood or clear fluid coming from the nose). Check local protocol in these situations.

e. Use of the nasopharyngeal airway does not eliminate the need for maintaining proper head position.

f. Use of the nasopharyngeal airway does not prevent aspiration.

ARTIFICIAL VENTILATION TECHNIQUES

ORDER OF PREFERENCE FOR VENTILATING A PATIENT

1. Mouth-to-mask ventilation
2. Two-person, bag-valve-mask ventilation
3. Flow-restricted, oxygen-powered ventilation device
4. One-person, bag-valve-mask ventilation

MOUTH-TO-MASK VENTILATION (POCKET MASK)

1. The pocket mask allows the delivery of oxygen to a nonbreathing patient.

2. **Inspired oxygen concentration**

a. Exhaled air (mouth to mask) = 16%–17%

b. 10 liters (L) per minute = 50%

c. 15 L per minute = 80%

3. **Desirable mask features**

a. The mask should be made of transparent material to allow detection of vomitus or other secretions.

b. It should fit tightly on the patient's face.

c. It should be equipped with an oxygen inlet to allow for high-concentration oxygen delivery [15 liters per minute (LPM)]

d. It is available in one average size for adults, with additional sizes for infants and children.

e. It should be equipped with a one-way valve at the ventilation port.

4. **Advantages.** Mouth-to-mask ventilation is the preferred method of ventilation in the prehospital setting because:

a. The pocket mask provides a physical barrier between the rescuer and the patient's nose, mouth, and secretions.

(1) It reduces the risk of infectious disease exposure.

(2) Use of a one-way valve at the ventilation port eliminates exposure to patient's exhaled air.

b. If the patient resumes spontaneous breathing, the mask can be used as a simple face mask to deliver 40%–60% oxygen by administering supplemental oxygen through the oxygen inlet on the mask.

c. A greater tidal volume can be delivered with a pocket mask than with a bag-valve-mask device.

(1) Both of the rescuer's hands can be used to hold the mask in place while simultaneously maintaining proper head position.

      (2) Proper head positioning results in greater lung ventilation and less gastric distention.

   d. With mouth-to-mask ventilation, the rescuer can feel the resistance of the patient's lungs.

4. Technique

   a. Take BSI precautions.

   b. Connect a one-way valve to ventilation port on the mask.

   c. Connect oxygen tubing to the oxygen inlet on the mask.

   d. Set oxygen flow rate for 15 LPM.

   e. Open the airway with a head-tilt, chin-lift maneuver, or if trauma is suspected, perform the jaw-thrust maneuver.

   f. Insert an oropharyngeal or nasopharyngeal airway if needed to maintain an open airway.

   g. Position yourself at the top of the supine patient's head.

   h. Place the mask on the patient's face.

      (1) Apply the apex (narrow portion) of the mask over the bridge of the patient's nose and hold it in place with your thumbs.

      (2) Lower the mask over the patient's face and mouth.

      (3) Use the remaining fingers of both hands to maintain proper head position and stabilize the broad portion of the mask in place over the cleft of the chin (indentation beneath the lower lip).

   i. Place your mouth around the one-way valve and deliver slow, steady breaths.

      (1) Each breath should be delivered over 1.5 to 2 seconds for an adult.

      (2) Each breath should be delivered over 1 to 1.5 seconds for an infant or child.

   j. If an assistant is available, cricoid pressure should be applied.

      (1) Cricoid pressure helps prevent inflation of the stomach during ventilation.

      (2) It reduces the possibility of vomiting and aspiration.

   k. Observe the rise and fall of the patient's chest with each ventilation.

   l. Stop ventilation when adequate chest rise is observed and allow the patient to exhale between breaths.

   m. Ventilate the patient at an age-appropriate rate:

      (1) Once every 3 seconds for an infant or child

      (2) Once every 5 seconds for an adult

BAG-VALVE-MASK VENTILATION

1. Desirable bag-valve-mask features

   a. The bag should be self-refilling and either disposable or easily cleaned and sterilized.

   b. It should have a nonjam valve system that allows a minimum oxygen inlet flow of 15 LPM.

   c. It should not have a pop-off (pressure-release) valve or, if a pop-off valve is present, it should be one that can be manually disabled. Failure to disable a pop-off valve may result in inadequate artificial ventilation.

   d. It should have standard 15-mm/22-mm fittings.

   e. It should have an oxygen inlet and reservoir for delivering high concentrations of oxygen.

   f. It should have a true nonrebreathing valve.

   g. It should perform satisfactorily under all common environmental conditions and temperature extremes.

   h. It should be available in adult, child, and infant sizes.

2. Oxygen delivery

   a. The volume of most commercially available adult bag-valve-mask devices is 1600 mL.

   b. Ideally, bag-valve-mask ventilation is a two-rescuer operation.

    c. Tidal volume delivered should be 10–15 mL per kilogram of body weight (mL/kg).

    d. Inspired oxygen concentration

        (1) Bag-valve mask without supplemental oxygen = 21% oxygen (room air)

        (2) Bag-valve mask with supplemental oxygen at 12 LPM = 40%–60% oxygen

        (3) Bag-valve mask with supplemental oxygen at 12 LPM and a reservoir = 90% oxygen

3. Technique—unresponsive patient, no trauma suspected (Figure 7-8)

    a. Take BSI precautions.

    b. Open the airway using a head-tilt, chin-lift maneuver.

    c. Size and insert an oropharyngeal or nasopharyngeal airway.

    d. Select correct mask size (adult, infant, or child).

    e. Create a face-to-mask seal.

        (1) Position thumbs over top half of mask, index and middle fingers over bottom half.

        (2) Place apex of mask over bridge of nose, then lower mask over mouth and upper chin.

        (3) If mask has a large, round cuff surrounding a ventilation port, center port over mouth.

        (4) Use ring and little fingers to bring jaw up to mask.

        (5) If alone, form a "C" around the ventilation port with thumb and index finger; use middle, ring, and little fingers under jaw to maintain chin lift and complete the seal.

    e. Connect bag to mask if not already done.

    f. Have assistant squeeze bag with two hands until chest rises.

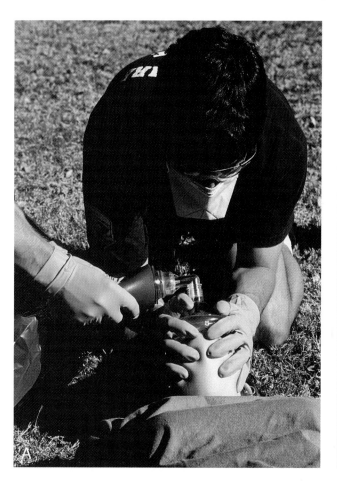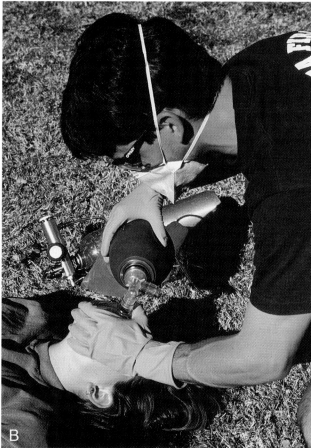

Fig. 7-8. Bag-valve-mask ventilation. *(A)* Two-rescuer technique. *(B)* Single-rescuer technique.

g. Connect bag to oxygen at 15 LPM and attach reservoir.

h. Observe rise and fall of the patient's chest with each ventilation.
   (1) Stop ventilation when adequate chest rise is observed.
   (2) Allow the patient to exhale between breaths.

i. Ventilate the patient:
   (1) Once every 3 seconds for an infant or child
   (2) Once every 5 seconds for an adult

4. **Technique—unresponsive patient with suspected trauma**

   a. Take BSI precautions.

   b. Immobilize the patient's head and neck. Have an assistant hold head manually or use your knees to prevent movement.

   c. Open the airway using the jaw-thrust maneuver.

   d. Select correct mask size (adult, infant, or child).

   e. Create a face-to-mask seal.
   (1) Position thumbs over top half of mask, index and middle fingers over bottom half.
   (2) Place apex of mask over bridge of nose, then lower mask over mouth and upper chin.
   (3) If mask has a large, round cuff surrounding a ventilation port, center port over mouth.
   (4) Use ring and little fingers to bring jaw up to mask without tilting the head or neck.

   f. Connect bag to mask if not already done.

   g. Have assistant squeeze bag with two hands until chest rises.

   h. Connect bag to oxygen at 15 LPM and attach reservoir.

   i. Observe rise and fall of the patient's chest with each ventilation.
   (1) Stop ventilation when adequate chest rise is observed.
   (2) Allow the patient to exhale between breaths.

   j. Ventilate the patient:
   (1) Once every 3 seconds for an infant or child
   (2) Once every 5 seconds for an adult

   k. Maintain manual in-line stabilization until the patient is completely immobilized to a backboard.

ADEQUATE AND INADEQUATE ARTIFICIAL VENTILATION

1. Artificial ventilation is adequate when:
   a. The chest rises and falls with each artificial ventilation
   b. The rate is sufficient. Sufficient rates are:
      (1) Approximately 12 times per minute for adults (once every 5 seconds)
      (2) Approximately 20 times per minute for infants and children (once every 3 seconds)
   c. The heart rate returns to normal

2. Artificial ventilation is inadequate when:
   a. The chest does not rise and fall with artificial ventilation
   b. The rate is too slow or too fast
   c. The heart rate does not return to normal with artificial ventilation

3. **Problems with bag-valve-mask ventilation**
   a. If chest does not rise and fall, reevaluate the patient.
      (1) Reassess head position; reposition the airway and reattempt to ventilate.
      (2) Inadequate tidal volume may be the result of an improper mask seal or incomplete bag compression.
         (a) If air is escaping from under the mask, reposition fingers and mask.
         (b) Reevaluate effectiveness of bag compression.
      (3) Check for obstruction.
   b. If the chest still does not rise, select an alternative method of artificial ventilation, e.g., pocket mask or flow-restricted, oxygen-powered ventilation device.

FLOW RESTRICTED OXYGEN-POWERED VENTILATION DEVICE
(DEMAND-VALVE DEVICE)

1. **Desirable features of the flow-restricted, oxygen-powered ventilation device**
   a. The device should provide a constant flow rate of 100% oxygen at less than 40 LPM.
   b. It should have an inspiratory pressure relief valve that opens at pressure of 50 to 60 centimeters of water (cm H_2O) and vents any remaining oxygen to the atmosphere or ceases gas flow.
   c. An audible alarm should sound when the relief valve pressure is exceeded to alert the rescuer that the patient requires high inflation pressures and may not be receiving adequate ventilatory volumes.
   d. It should perform satisfactorily under common environmental conditions and temperature extremes.
   e. It should have a trigger positioned so that both hands of the rescuer remain on the mask to hold it in position.
2. **Technique (NOTE: This device should only be used in adults.)**
   a. Take BSI precautions.
   b. Open the airway.
      (1) If no trauma is suspected, use a head-tilt, chin-lift maneuver.
      (2) If trauma is suspected:
         (a) Immobilize head and neck
         (b) Have an assistant hold head manually or use your knees to prevent movement
         (c) Maintain manual in-line stabilization until the patient is completely immobilized to a backboard
         (d) Open the airway using a jaw-thrust maneuver
   c. Size and insert an oropharyngeal or nasopharyngeal airway.
   d. Attach the adult mask.
   e. Create face-to-mask seal.
      (1) Position thumbs over top half of mask, index and middle fingers over bottom half.
      (2) Place apex of mask over bridge of nose, then lower mask over mouth and upper chin.
      (3) Use ring and little fingers to bring jaw up to mask. In cases of suspected trauma, do not tilt the head or neck.
   f. Connect device to mask if not already done.
   g. Trigger device until chest rises.
   h. Ventilate the patient once every 5 seconds.
3. Complications include:
   a. Gastric distention in patients who are not intubated
   b. Barotrauma to the lungs, including pneumothorax and subcutaneous emphysema
4. **Contraindications.** This device should not be used for pediatric patients.

CRICOID PRESSURE (SELLICK MANEUVER)

1. **Purpose**
   a. The Sellick maneuver minimizes gastric distention and aspiration.
   b. It aids placement of an endotracheal tube into the tracheal opening.
2. **Technique**
   a. Locate the cricoid cartilage.
   b. Apply firm pressure on the cricoid cartilage with the thumb and index or middle finger, just lateral to the midline.

   c. Maintain pressure until:
       (1) The patient begins breathing spontaneously,
       (2) The patient is intubated, or
       (3) The patient becomes responsive by moving, coughing, or gagging

SPECIAL ARTIFICIAL VENTILATION SITUATIONS

DEFINITIONS

1. A **stoma** is an artificial opening.
2. A **tracheal stoma** is an opening in the neck that opens the trachea to the atmosphere.
3. A **laryngectomy** is the surgical removal of the larynx.
4. A **tracheostomy** is the surgical formation of an opening into the trachea.

BAG-VALVE-DEVICE-TO-TRACHEOSTOMY-TUBE VENTILATION

1. **Technique**
   a. Take BSI precautions.
   b. If present, remove any garment (scarf, necktie) covering the tracheostomy tube.
   c. Connect the bag-valve device to the tracheostomy tube.
   d. Squeeze the bag over 2 seconds until the chest rises.
   e. Allow the patient to exhale passively .
2. **Problem solving.** If you are unable to ventilate through the tracheostomy tube:
   a. Suction the tracheostomy tube with a flexible suction catheter and reattempt ventilation
   b. Seal the patient's nose and mouth and reattempt ventilation; release the seal to permit exhalation

BAG-VALVE-MASK-TO-STOMA VENTILATION

1. **Technique** (Figure 7-9)
   a. Take BSI precautions.
   b. If present, remove any garment (scarf, necktie) covering the stoma.
   c. Connect a child or infant mask to the bag-valve device.
   d. Center the mask over the stoma.
   e. Make an airtight seal with the mask against the neck.
   f. Squeeze the bag over 2 seconds until the chest rises.
   g. Allow the patient to exhale passively.
2. **Problem solving.** If the chest does not rise and fall:
   a. Seal the patient's mouth and nose and reattempt ventilation; release the seal to permit exhalation
   b. Suction the stoma with a flexible suction catheter if foreign matter is present and reattempt ventilation

INFANTS AND CHILDREN

1. Place head in neutral position for an infant and slightly extended position for a child. Hyperextension of the head may result in airway obstruction.
2. Avoid excessive bag pressure.
   a. Use only enough pressure to make chest rise.
   b. Gastric distention is common when ventilating infants and children.
3. Ventilate with bag-valve mask until the chest rises adequately.

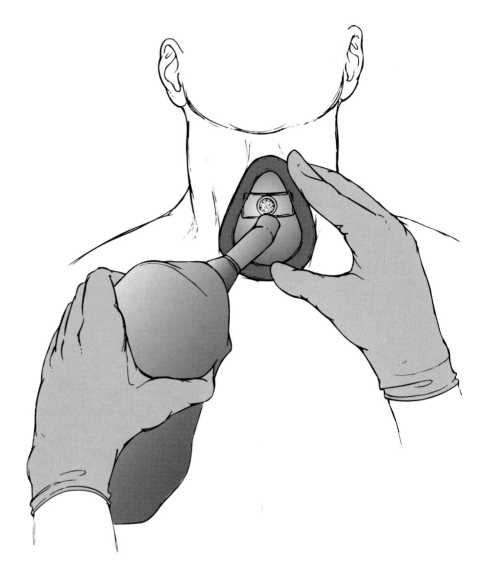

Fig. 7-9. Bag-valve-mask-to-stoma ventilation.

    a. Do not use a pop-off valve.
    b. If a pop-off valve is present, it must be disabled (placed in closed position) for adequate ventilation.
4. An oropharyngeal or nasopharyngeal airway may be considered when other procedures fail to provide a clear airway.

SUPPLEMENTAL OXYGEN—OXYGEN CYLINDERS

DESCRIPTION

1. Oxygen is stored in steel or aluminum cylinders.
2. Oxygen cylinders may be green in color or silver or chrome with green around the valve stem.
3. The tank pressure of a fully pressurized cylinder is approximately 2000 pounds per square inch (psi), but tank pressure varies with the ambient temperature.
    a. Tank pressure increases with increased temperature.
    b. Tank pressure decreases with decreased temperature.

CYLINDER SIZES

1. D cylinder contains 350 L.
2. E cylinder contains 625 L.
3. M cylinder contains 3000 L.
4. G cylinder contains 5300 L.
5. H cylinder contains 6900 L.

SAFETY CONSIDERATIONS

1. Handle cylinders carefully because their contents are under pressure.
2. Tanks should be positioned to prevent falling and blows to the valve-gauge assembly.
3. Tanks should be secured during transport.
4. Keep combustible materials away from oxygen equipment.
5. Never position any part of your body over the cylinder.

PRESSURE REGULATORS

1. A pressure regulator reduces pressure in the oxygen cylinder to a safe range.
2. The attached flowmeter controls liters delivered per minute.
3. An oxygen humidifier (container of sterile water) can be attached to regulator.
   a. An oxygen humidifier is needed only for a patient on oxygen for a long time.
   b. Dry oxygen is not harmful in short term.
   c. It is generally not needed for prehospital care.

OPERATING PROCEDURES

1. Place the cylinder in an upright position and position yourself to the side of the cylinder.
2. Remove protective seal.
3. Quickly open, then shut, the valve to remove dust and debris.
4. Attach the regulator-flowmeter to tank
5. Attach the oxygen device to the flowmeter.
6. Open flowmeter to desired setting
7. Apply the oxygen device to the patient.
8. When complete, remove the device from the patient, turn off the valve, and remove all pressure from the regulator.

EQUIPMENT FOR OXYGEN DELIVERY

NONREBREATHER MASK

1. **Description and function**
   a. The nonrebreather mask is the preferred method of oxygen delivery in the prehospital setting.
      (1) It permits delivery of high-concentration oxygen to a spontaneously breathing patient.
      (2) At 15 LPM, the oxygen concentration delivered is approximately 90%.
   b. A one-way valve allows exhaled air to escape but prevents room air from being inspired.
2. **Special considerations**
   a. Fill the reservoir bag with oxygen before placing the mask on the patient.
   b. After placing the mask on the patient, adjust the flow rate so the bag does not completely deflate when the patient inhales (usually 15 LPM). Sufficient supplemental oxygen must be available for each breath.

   c. Patients who are cyanotic with cool and clammy skin or who are short of breath need oxygen.

     (1) Concerns about the dangers of giving too much oxygen to patients with history of chronic obstructive pulmonary disease and infants and children have not been shown to be valid in the prehospital setting.

     (2) Patients with chronic obstructive pulmonary disease and infants and children who require oxygen should receive high-concentration oxygen.

   d. Nonrebreather masks are available in adult, child, and infant sizes.

     (1) Select the correct size mask.

     (2) Ensure that the mask fits snugly.

NASAL CANNULA

1. Description and function

   a. A nasal cannula is rarely the best method of delivering adequate oxygen in the prehospital environment.

   b. It should be used only when patients will not tolerate a nonrebreather mask despite coaching.

   c. It can deliver an oxygen concentration of 24% to 44% at 1 to 6 LPM.

2. Special considerations

   a. Flow rates of more than 6 LPM are irritating to the nasal mucosa.

   b. Use of a nasal cannula is contraindicated in patients who are:

     (1) Apneic

     (2) Severely hypoxic

     (3) Breathing primarily through the mouth

     (4) Exhibiting poor respiratory effort

REVIEW QUESTIONS

Directions: Each of the numbered items or incomplete statements in this section is followed by answers or by completions of the statement. Select the ONE lettered answer or completion that is BEST in each case.

1. The exchange of gases in the respiratory system occurs at the alveolar–capillary membrane. The primary gases exchanged during normal respiration are

   (A) oxygen and plasma
   (B) oxygen and hemoglobin
   (C) oxygen and carbon dioxide
   (D) oxygen and carbon monoxide

2. Which of the following correctly identifies a difference between the airway of an adult and the airway of a child or infant?

   (A) The infant's trachea is more rigid
   (B) The adult's tongue is proportionally larger
   (C) The infant's chest wall is more unyielding to pressure
   (D) The narrowest portion of the infant's airway is the cricoid cartilage

3. To size an oropharyngeal airway correctly, you would measure from the

   (A) center of the patient's mouth to the suprasternal notch
   (B) corner of the patient's mouth to the bottom of the earlobe

(C)   patient's nasal septum to the Adam's apple (thyroid cartilage)
(D)   center of the patient's mouth to the Adam's apple (thyroid cartilage)

4. When delivering artificial ventilations by bag-valve mask, adequate ventilations are achieved when

   (A)   the oxygen reservoir collapses
   (B)   the patient slowly becomes more cyanotic
   (C)   the patient's chest wall rises and falls with each ventilation
   (D)   the bag-valve mask becomes progressively more difficult to compress with each ventilation

5. An advantage of the nasopharyngeal airway (NPA) over the oropharyngeal airway (OPA) is that the NPA

   (A)   does not cause trauma during insertion
   (B)   is better tolerated by semiresponsive patients
   (C)   allows for delivery of greater oxygen concentrations
   (D)   does not require sizing because one size fits all patients

6. Which of the following is a disadvantage to opening the airway with the modified jaw thrust?

   (A)   Decreases oxygen delivery to the alveoli
   (B)   Cannot be maintained during suctioning
   (C)   Compromises the integrity of the cervical spine
   (D)   An additional rescuer is needed to perform bag-valve-mask ventilations

7. When delivering artificial ventilations by means of a pocket mask, rescuers can successfully deliver approximately _____ oxygen **without** the use of supplemental oxygen.

   (A)   16%
   (B)   21%
   (C)   50%
   (D)   80%

8. When delivering artificial ventilations by means of a bag-valve mask, rescuers can successfully deliver approximately _____ oxygen **without** the use of supplemental oxygen.

   (A)   16%
   (B)   21%
   (C)   50%
   (D)   80%

9. Cricoid pressure (Sellick maneuver)

   (A)   minimizes gastric distention and aspiration
   (B)   should not be used in unconscious patients
   (C)   may be used instead of the modified jaw thrust
   (D)   will hamper attempts at endotracheal intubation

10. Which of the following statements regarding oxygen-powered ventilation devices is FALSE?

   (A)   The device can deliver up to 100% oxygen
   (B)   The device should only be used in children or infants
   (C)   The device may cause barotrauma (trauma to the lungs)
   (D)   The device may increase gastric distention in nonintubated patients

11. The airways of infants and children differ from the airways of adults. To properly open the airway of an infant you must

    (A)   tilt the head to one side
    (B)   place the head in a neutral position
    (C)   hyperextend the head and neck more than that of an adult
    (D)   place the infant's chin on his or her chest and open the mouth as wide as possible

12. Improper sizing and insertion of an oropharyngeal airway may cause

    (A)   barotrauma
    (B)   cardiac tamponade
    (C)   complete airway obstruction
    (D)   delivery of a higher concentration of oxygen than desired

13. Oxygen regulators are designed to

    (A)   prevent explosion or fire
    (B)   humidify the oxygen for greater patient comfort
    (C)   sound an alarm when oxygen levels drop below 2000 psi
    (D)   reduce the oxygen pressure to a therapeutic pressure and flow

14. The flow-restricted, oxygen-powered ventilation device may also be called a

    (A)   nasal cannula
    (B)   bag-valve mask
    (C)   tracheostomy
    (D)   demand valve

15. The reservoir of a nonrebreather mask should be filled with oxygen before the mask is placed on the patient.

    (A)   True
    (B)   False

Directions: Each of the numbered questions or incomplete statements in this section refers to a scenario that precedes them. The numbered questions or incomplete statements are followed by answers or by completions of the statement. Select the answer or completion of the statement that is BEST in each case.

Your rescue crew is called to the scene of an 87-year-old man in severe respiratory distress. The patient has a past medical history of emphysema and is a two-pack a day cigarette smoker. Due to his distress and fatigue, he has a very difficult time speaking with you.

Questions 16–20

16. You determine this patient is breathing at a rate of 30 times per minute. The term used to describe this respiratory rate is

    (A)   bradypnea
    (B)   tachypnea
    (C)   tachycardia
    (D)   hypertension

17. The patient's skin is cool, clammy, and cyanotic. Cyanotic skin is _____ in appearance.

(A) red
(B) pale
(C) blue
(D) yellow

18. The patient's mouth is full of frothy sputum. A guideline to follow for suctioning this patient is

(A) suction for no more than 30 seconds
(B) suction up to, but not including, the bronchi
(C) suction on insertion and removal of the suction catheter
(D) preoxygenate the patient before suctioning, if possible

19. After suctioning the airway, you insert a nasopharyngeal airway and administer supplemental oxygen by means of a nonrebreather mask. Which of the following statements correctly reflects the proper oxygen liter flow and oxygen percentage delivered by this device?

(A) 2 liters per minute (LPM) delivers approximately 24% oxygen
(B) 6 LPM delivers approximately 44% oxygen
(C) 10 LPM delivers approximately 65% oxygen
(D) 15 LPM delivers approximately 90% oxygen

20. While en route to the hospital, the patient's respiratory rate increases to 40 breaths per minute with very low tidal volume. His mental status is diminishing. You decide to assist his respiratory effort with supplemental oxygen by bag-valve mask. You should deliver slow ventilations (approximately two seconds per ventilation) at a rate of

(A) one ventilation every 3 seconds
(B) one ventilation every 5 seconds
(C) one ventilation every 10 seconds
(D) one ventilation every 12 seconds

Your ambulance crew is called to the scene of a local restaurant for a 43-year-old man possibly choking. Upon arrival, you find your patient collapsed in his booth seat. He is unconscious, cyanotic, and apneic. Your crew moves the patient to the floor to begin assessment and treatment.

Questions 21–24

21. To open this patient's airway, you should perform the

(A) head-tilt, chin-lift maneuver
(B) head-tilt, neck-lift maneuver
(C) head-tilt, jaw-thrust maneuver
(D) head-tilt, tongue-lift maneuver

22. If you found this patient unconscious on the ground (rather than seated), you would suspect cervical spine damage from a fall. To open a patient's airway with spinal precautions involves which technique?

(A) Jaw-thrust maneuver
(B) Neck-thrust maneuver
(C) Head-tilt, chin-lift maneuver
(D) Head-tilt, neck-thrust maneuver

23. After evaluating the airway and attempting ventilations, you conclude that the patient's airway is obstructed. Your partner straddles the patient's lower body and delivers subdiaphragmatic abdominal thrusts. A large piece of steak pops out, and the patient begins vomiting. What type of suction device are you mostly likely to use while in the restaurant?

(A) Bulb syringe
(B) Mounted device
(C) Hand-powered device
(D) Two-stroke, gas-powered device

24. After reassessing this patient, you find that he is breathing at a rate of 24 breaths per minute with a good, deep, tidal volume and regular rhythm. His skin is slightly pale. He can answer some questions but appears sleepy. Further treatment for this patient during transport should include

(A) insert a nasopharyngeal airway (NPA) and deliver oxygen via pocket mask
(B) insert an oropharyngeal airway (OPA) and deliver oxygen via nasal cannula
(C) insert an NPA and deliver oxygen via nonrebreather mask
(D) insert an OPA and have the patient breathe into a paper bag

Your rescue crew is called to the local high school for a 15-year-old girl complaining of difficulty breathing. Upon arrival in the nurse's office, you find your patient in moderate to severe distress, crying and complaining of chest pain and difficulty breathing. Her lung sounds are clear, and her respiratory rate is 30 breaths per minute. The nurse informs you the patient "got in an argument with her boyfriend and is probably hyperventilating."

Questions 25–28

25. Immediate treatment for this patient should include

(A) oxygen therapy
(B) having the patient breathe into a paper bag
(C) no treatment until the patient's guardian can be contacted
(D) having the nurse monitor the patient and call you again if the situation worsens

26. While continuing your assessment of this patient, you ask your partner to put the patient on supplemental oxygen by nasal cannula. An appropriate flow range that should be used with this device is

(A) 1–6 liters per minute (LPM)
(B) 5–10 LPM
(C) 6–12 LPM
(D) 15–20 LPM

27. As you are assessing this patient, her level of distress increases. She has no past medical history. The patient takes oral contraceptives and is a pack-a-day smoker. She is becoming increasingly cyanotic with a respiratory rate of 30 breaths per minute, good tidal volume, and clear lung sounds. Based on your patient's condition, which of the following should be used to increase the concentration of oxygen delivered to this patient?

(A) Pocket mask
(B) Bag-valve mask
(C) Nonrebreather mask
(D) Oxygen-powered ventilation device

28. While en route to the hospital, the patient goes into cardiopulmonary arrest. During cardiopulmonary resuscitation, you should deliver ventilations with the bag-valve mask

(A)   as fast as possible
(B)   over 3 to 5 seconds
(C)   over 1.5 to 2 seconds
(D)   between each chest compression

ANSWERS AND RATIONALES

1-C.   Oxygen and carbon dioxide are the two primary gases exchanged in the alveoli. Hemoglobin aids the transport of oxygen on the red blood cell. Carbon monoxide is an odorless, colorless, tasteless, poisonous gas that binds to hemoglobin more readily than oxygen. Plasma is the fluid in which red blood cells are suspended as they flow throughout the body.

2-D.   Although the narrowest portion of the adult airway is at the level of the vocal cords, the narrowest part of the young child and infant's airway is at the level of the cricoid cartilage. The infant and child's trachea and chest wall are more pliable than that of an adult. The tongue is larger in proportion to the airway in the infant and child than in the adult.

3-B.   The correct technique for measuring the oropharyngeal airway is from the corner of the mouth to the bottom of the earlobe. The oropharyngeal airway is positioned in an adult's mouth by inserting it upside down, then rotating it right-side up as the tip of the device follows the hard palette (roof of the mouth). Improper sizing can lead to disastrous complications. An oversized airway may push the epiglottis over the trachea and occlude the airway. An undersized airway may terminate prematurely to ensure a patent airway.

4-C.   The most reliable indicator of ventilation adequacy is the rise and fall of the chest wall. Remember, gas exchange does not take place until fresh air reaches the alveolar-capillary membrane. If the bag-valve-mask oxygen reservoir collapses with each ventilation, it may indicate that the oxygen flow is too low or the ventilation rate is too rapid. If the bag-valve mask becomes progressively more difficult to squeeze when ventilating a patient, assess the need to suction, ensure that proper airway opening procedures are in use, suspect that there may be excessive air in the stomach (anticipate vomiting), and suspect a possible collapsed lung (pneumothorax).

5-B.   The oropharyngeal airway should only be used in patients without a gag reflex; however, the nasopharyngeal airway may be tolerated in semiresponsive patients. Both devices may cause minor trauma on insertion and, if properly sized, will allow for equal oxygen concentrations to be delivered. Both devices must be sized according to the patient. The nasopharyngeal airway is sized by measuring from the tip of the nose to the bottom of the earlobe. Improper sizing may lead to stimulation of the gag reflex.

6-D.   The modified jaw thrust is the technique to use for patients with possible spinal compromise. In the apneic (nonbreathing) patient, the modified jaw thrust requires two rescuers to manage the airway. One rescuer opens the airway using both hands to displace jaw anteriorly without manipulating the spine. The other rescuer applies the bag-valve mask to the face and delivers ventilations. The jaw thrust can and should be maintained during suctioning to ensure that the spine is not manipulated.

7-A. The atmospheric air we breathe contains approximately 21% oxygen. We exhale 16%–17% oxygen. When using a pocket mask without supplemental oxygen, rescuers deliver the percent of oxygen in their expired air. With 15 liters per minute of supplemental oxygen attached to the oxygen inlet on the pocket mask, the device can deliver up to 80% oxygen.

8-B. Unlike the pocket mask, the bag-valve mask delivers atmospheric air (not expired air). Since atmospheric air contains 21% oxygen, a bag-valve mask without supplemental oxygen will deliver 21% oxygen. With 12 to 15 liters per minute supplemental oxygen, the bag-valve mask can deliver approximately 90% oxygen.

9-A. Cricoid pressure decreases the chance of vomiting since the esophagus is closed, decreases the amount of gastric distention associated with assisted ventilation, and aids endotracheal intubation (intubation is to be performed only by those trained and authorized to perform this procedure). Cricoid pressure should be maintained until the patient regains spontaneous respirations, intubation is accomplished, or the patient becomes responsive.

10-B. Oxygen-powered ventilation devices are contraindicated in children or infants. These devices can deliver up to 100% oxygen. Complications associated with the use of oxygen-powered ventilation devices include barotrauma and increased gastric distention in nonintubated patients.

11-B. The airway of a child is more pliable than the airway of an adult. To open the airway of an infant or child, place the patient in a supine position with the head in a neutral (looking straight forward) position. Hyperextending the neck may cause the trachea to kink (much like a drinking straw bent too far). Placing the chin on the chest and opening the mouth as wide as possible are not acceptable techniques.

12-C. Improper sizing and insertion of the oropharyngeal airway may cause airway obstruction. Barotrauma would not result since barotrauma occurs in the lower airway. Cardiac tamponade occurs when blood leaks into the sac surrounding the heart and is not associated with oropharyngeal airway use. Oxygen concentrations would, since the airway is obstructed, drop if the oropharyngeal airway were inserted incorrectly.

13-D. Oxygen is compressed to approximately 2000 psi. A regulator is necessary to reduce this pressure to a therapeutic range. Regulators do not prevent oxygen's interaction with fire or combustibles. Finally, a separate water-filled chamber must be added to provide humidified oxygen. Humidified oxygen is generally not necessary for prehospital care.

14-D. The flow-restricted, oxygen-powered ventilation device (demand valve) consists of a high-pressure tubing connecting the oxygen supply and a valve activated by a lever or push button. When the valve is open, oxygen flows into the patient and permits positive-pressure ventilation with 100% oxygen. The device can be attached to a face mask, endotracheal tube, esophageal airway, or tracheostomy tube and may be used in an apneic or spontaneously breathing adult patient.

15-A. The reservoir bag of a nonrebreather mask must be filled with oxygen before placing the mask on the patient. After placing the mask on the patient, adjust the flow rate so the bag does not completely deflate when the patient inhales. An oxygen flow rate of 15 liters per minute is usually needed to ensure proper inflation of the reservoir bag.

16-B. "Tachy" refers to a faster than normal pace, and "pnea" refers to breathing; therefore, tachypnea is fast breathing. A normal respiratory rate for an adult at rest is 12–20 respirations per minute. Bradypnea refers to a slow respiratory rate ("brady" = slow). Tachycardia refers to a faster than normal heart rate ("cardio" = heart). Finally, hypertension refers to high blood pressure ("hyper" = above/excess; "tension" refers to pressure).

17-C. Cyanosis is the bluish appearance generally associated with poor oxygenation or perfusion. A red appearance may be referred to as flushed, and a yellowish appearance may be referred to as jaundiced. A flushed appearance may be associated with hypertension, high ambient temperature, use of certain drugs, or carbon monoxide poisoning (a late sign). A jaundiced appearance is often associated with liver dysfunction.

18-D. If the patient's airway is patent (open) and a need for suction has been identified, attempt to provide high-flow oxygen before suctioning. Preoxygenating the patient is important because oxygen levels will drop during suctioning. The maximum length of time allowed for suctioning an adult is 15 seconds and 5 seconds in children and infants. The suction catheter should be inserted before applying suction. Suction should be applied only as the catheter is removed. This technique decreases the length of time of oxygen deprivation associated with suctioning.

19-D. A nonrebreather mask is a "high-concentration" oxygen delivery device. With the oxygen flow regulator set at 15 liters per minute, an oxygen concentration of approximately 90% can be delivered. A nasal cannula is a "low-concentration" oxygen delivery device. At 6 liters per minute, a nasal cannula can deliver an oxygen concentration of approximately 44%. Oxygen is stored as a compressed gas, and oxygen cylinders are pressurized to approximately 2000 psi.

20-B. The normal respiratory rate for an adult is 12 respirations per minute (once every 5 seconds). Therefore, when assisting ventilations, rescuers should attempt to match this rate. For children and infants, the normal respiratory rate is 20 respirations per minute (once every 3 seconds) or more. Newborns may require ventilation rates as fast as 40 to 60 times per minute.

21-A. When there is no indication of spinal compromise, the head-tilt, chin-lift maneuver is the preferred method of opening the airway. Since this patient was found still in his seat, it can be assumed that the patient's spine has not been compromised.

22-A. In this situation, you must assume that the spine may be compromised. In cases of possible spinal compromise, the jaw-thrust maneuver is recommended. The jaw thrust allows the rescuer to displace the tongue from the airway without manipulating the spine.

23-C. A hand-powered device is a good, portable option for suctioning. Bulb syringes are generally only used in infants. A mounted device may deliver more power and options than the hand-powered device, but mounted devices are not portable.

24-C. Because this patient's level of consciousness has not fully returned, a nasopharyngeal airway may be tolerated. An oropharyngeal airway would cause a semiconscious patient to cough and gag. Since the patient is hypoxic and unconscious, you should attempt to deliver as much oxygen as possible. Since the patient has a "good" tidal volume, a nonrebreather mask is a better option than a pocket mask.

25-A. Attributing this patient's discomfort to her emotional status would be easy; however, this assumption is improper. Any patient complaining of chest pain should be given a therapeutic level of supplemental oxygen. Even if this patient is experiencing discomfort due to emotional stress, your compassion and treatment may ease her anxious state and reduce her symptoms. Asking a patient to breathe into a paper bag is not an acceptable practice. If you suspect your patient is hyperventilating, remove all negative stimuli (in this case, the boyfriend) and calmly attempt to coach your patient in controlling her respiratory rate. Although you must temper your treatment for minors to suit the desires of their guardian, do not withhold reasonable or life-saving treatment in the absence of the guardian's expressed consent. As for leaving the patient with the school nurse, the following guideline applies: if you are unable to relieve a patient's medical complaint, contact medical direction before terminating your encounter with the patient.

26-A. At 1 to 6 liters per minute, a nasal cannula delivers an oxygen concentration of approximately 24% to 44%. At flow rates higher than 6 liters per minute, the oxygen concentration does not improve and the patient's discomfort increases.

27-C. A nonrebreather mask is ideal for delivering high-flow oxygen to patients with an acceptable tidal volume. Tidal volume is the amount of air that the patient can inhale and exhale. If the patient's tidal volume were to decrease, you might consider using a bag-valve mask or pocket mask with supplemental oxygen. An oxygen-powered ventilation device may be considered in an adult patient with low or absent tidal volume.

28-C. Aren't you glad you decided to treat and transport this patient rather than assuming her presentation was based on an emotional state? When ventilating a patient, ventilations should be slow and full, approximately 1.5 to 2 seconds per ventilation. Delivering ventilations too rapidly may cause air to enter the stomach and frequently leads to aspiration of stomach contents. Because the proper two-rescuer compression-to-ventilation ratio is 5:1, delivering a ventilation between each compression would be improper.

BIBLIOGRAPHY

Aehlert BJ: *ACLS Quick Review Study Guide*. St. Louis, Mosby-Year Book, 1994.

Butman AM, Martin SW, Vomacka RW, et al (eds): *Comprehensive Guide to Pre-Hospital Skills: A Skills Manual for EMT-Basic, EMT-Intermediate, EMT-Paramedic*. Akron, Ohio, Emergency Training, 1995.

Caroline NL: *Emergency Care in the Streets*, 4th ed. Boston, Little, Brown, 1991.

Chameides L, Hazinski MF (eds): *Textbook of Pediatric Advanced Life Support*. Dallas, American Heart Association, 1994.

Crosby LA, Lewallen DG (eds): *Emergency Care and Transportation of the Sick and Injured*, 6th ed. Rosemont, IL, American Academy of Orthopaedic Surgeons, 1995.

Cummins RO (ed): *Textbook of Advanced Cardiac Life Support*. Dallas, American Heart Association, 1994.

Cummins RO, Graves J: *ACLS Scenarios: Core Concepts for Case-Based Learning*. St. Louis, Mosby-Year Book, 1996.

Grant HD, Murray RH Jr, Bergeron JD: *Emergency Care*, 7th ed. Englewood Cliffs, NJ, Prentice-Hall, 1995.

Hafen BQ, Karren KJ, Mistovich JJ: *Prehospital Emergency Care*, 5th ed. Upper Saddle River, NJ, Prentice-Hall, 1996.

Martini FH: *Fundamentals of Anatomy and Physiology*, 3rd ed. Englewood Cliffs, NJ, Prentice-Hall, 1995.

McSwain NE, White RD, Paturas JL, et al (eds): *The Basic EMT: Comprehensive Prehospital Patient Care*. St. Louis, Mosby-Year Book, 1996.

Seeley RR, Stephens TD, Tate P: *Anatomy and Physiology*, 3rd ed. St. Louis, Mosby-Year Book, 1996.

Stoy WA: *Mosby's EMT-Basic Textbook*. St. Louis, Mosby Year Book, 1996.

United States Department of Transportation, National Highway Traffic Safety Administration: *Emergency Medical Technician: Basic. National Standard Curriculum*, 1994.

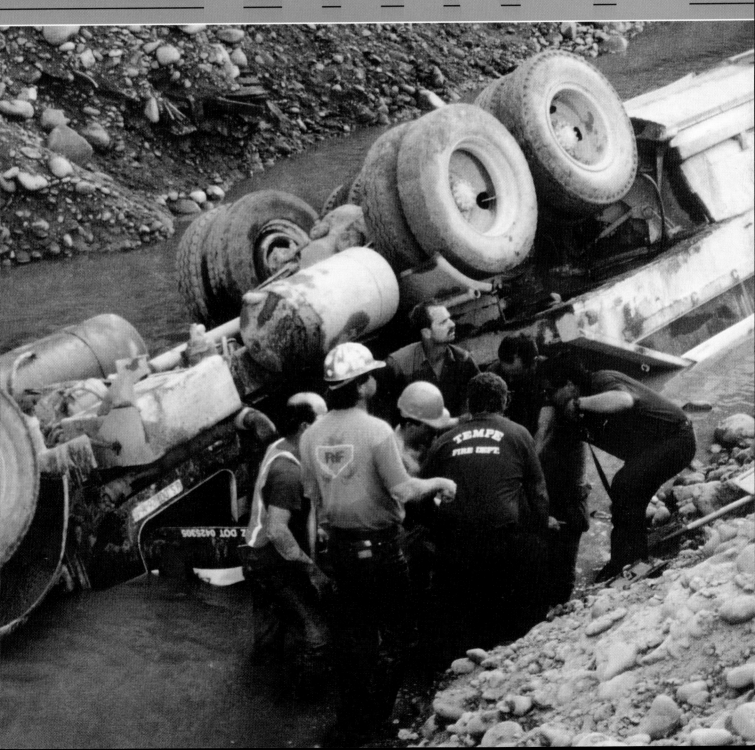

8 SCENE SIZE-UP

OBJECTIVES

8-1 Recognize hazards and potential hazards.

8-2 Describe common hazards found at the scene of a trauma and a medical patient.

8-3 Differentiate a safe from an unsafe scene.

8-4 Discuss common mechanisms of injury/nature of illness.

8-5 Discuss the reason for identifying the total number of patients at the scene.

8-6 Explain the reason for identifying the need for additional help or assistance.

COMPONENTS OF SCENE SIZE-UP

Scene size-up includes body substance isolation (BSI) precautions, evaluation of scene safety, determining the mechanism of injury or nature of the patient's illness, determining the total number of patients, and determining the need for additional resources.

BODY SUBSTANCE ISOLATION (BSI)—REVIEW

WHEN TO CONSIDER BSI PRECAUTIONS

Before beginning the scene size-up, consider the need for BSI precautions.

ELEMENTS OF BSI PRECAUTIONS

BSI precautions include using eye protection, gloves, gown, and mask necessary for a particular scene.

MOTIVATION FOR LEARNING

Scene size-up is the first and most important aspect of patient assessment. Scene size-up begins as the EMT-Basic approaches the scene. During this phase, the EMT-Basic surveys the scene to determine if any threats may cause injury to the EMT-Basic. This evaluation also allows the EMT-Basic to determine the nature of the call and obtain additional resources as necessary.

Scene Size-Up

Take body substance isolation precautions
Determine scene safety
Determine mechanism of injury/nature of illness
Determine number of patients
Request additional help if necessary

Initial Assessment

Form general impression of patient
Determine chief complaint/apparent life threats
Assess mental status (AVPU)
Assess airway
Assess breathing
Assess circulation
–Pulse
–Major bleeding
–Skin color, temperature, condition
Identify priority patients
Make transport decision

Focused History and Physical Examination

Perform focused physical examination or, if indicated, complete rapid assessment
(DCAP-BTLS)
Obtain baseline vital signs
Obtain SAMPLE history
Reevaluate transport decision

Detailed Physical Examination

DCAP-BTLS
Reassess vital signs

Ongoing Assessment

Repeat initial assessment
Reassess vital signs
Repeat focused assessment regarding patient complaint or injuries
Reevaluate interventions

EVALUATION OF SCENE SAFETY

DEFINITION

Evaulation of **scene safety** involves an assessment of the scene to ensure the well-being of the EMT-Basic, the crew, the patient(s), and bystanders (Figure 8-1).

GENERAL GUIDELINES

1. Do not enter unsafe scenes.
2. Scenes may be dangerous even if they seem safe.
3. If the scene is unsafe, make it safe. Otherwise, do not enter.

PERSONAL (AND CREW) SAFETY

Study the scene and determine if it is safe to approach the patient.

1. **Crash/rescue scenes**
   a. Look to see if the area is marked by flares or safety lights.

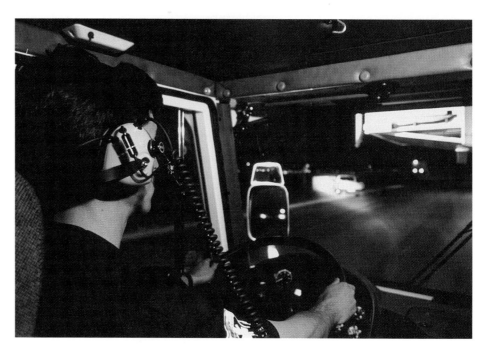

Fig. 8-1. Study the scene and determine if it is safe to approach the patient.

    b. Observe traffic flow.

    c. Observe the stability of the vehicle(s), aircraft, or machinery.

    d. Look for downed power lines.

    e. Look for flammable liquids.

    f. Look for fires or potential fire hazards.

    g. Look for entrapped victims.

2. **Toxic substances and low-oxygen areas**

    a. Obvious hazards will be present at some scenes; at others, the hazards may not be as obvious.

    b. Look for clues that suggest the presence of hazardous materials, such as:

        (1) Signs (placards) on railroad cars, storage facilities, or vehicles

        (2) Vapor clouds or heavy smoke

        (3) Unusual odors

        (4) Spilled solids or liquids

        (5) Leaking containers, bottles, or gas cylinders

        (6) Chemical transport tanks or containers

    c. Low-oxygen areas may include:

        (1) Mines

        (2) Wells

        (3) Unreinforced trenches

    d. Call for specially trained personnel as needed.

3. **Crime scenes/hostile situations**

    a. Assess the potential for violence. Clues incude:

        (1) Knowledge of prior violence at a particular location

        (2) Evidence of alcohol or other substance use

        (3) Weapons visible or in use

        (4) Loud voices, fighting, or potential for fighting

    b. Assess the crowd and look for hostile bystanders.

    c. Do not enter a known crime scene or potentially violent scene until it has been secured by law enforcement personnel.

4. **Unstable surfaces and slopes.** Call for specially trained personnel as needed.

5. **Water and ice**

(a) Call for specially trained personnel as needed.

(b) Do not enter a body of water unless you have been trained in water rescue.

(c) Do not enter fast-moving water or venture out on ice unless you have been trained in this type of rescue.

PATIENT SAFETY

1. Protect the patient from curious onlookers.
2. Assess for traffic and other hazards.
3. Protect the patient from glass and other debris during extrication procedures.
4. Protect the patient from environmental temperature extremes.

BYSTANDER SAFETY

1. Look for bystanders who may be in danger.
    a. Help bystanders avoid becoming patients by preventing them from getting too close to the scene.
    b. Bystanders may become so engrossed in the situation that they fail to watch out for themselves.
2. Look for bystanders who may endanger your safety or that of the patient.

MECHANISM OF INJURY/NATURE OF ILLNESS

MECHANISM OF INJURY

In trauma situations, look for the **mechanism of injury** and determine the number of patients.

1. **Definition.** Mechanism of injury refers to the manner in which an injury occurs and the forces involved in producing the injury.
2. Determine from the patient, family or bystanders, and inspection of the scene what is the mechanism of injury.
3. Significant mechanisms of injury include:
    a. Ejection from a vehicle
    b. Dead occupant in the same passenger compartment
    c. Falls over 20 feet (or three times body height)
    d. Rollover of vehicle
    e. High-speed vehicle collision
    f. Vehicle–pedestrian collision
    g. Motorcycle crash
    h. Unresponsive or altered mental status
    i. Penetrations of the head, chest, or abdomen
    j. Hidden injuries from seat belts or air bags
4. Significant mechanisms of injury for infants and children include (Figure 8-2):
    a. Falls over 10 feet in infants and children (or three times body height)
    b. Bicycle collision
    c. Vehicle collision at a medium speed
    d. Any vehicle collision in which the infant or child was unrestrained
5. Determine the total number of patients.
    a. If there are more patients than you or your crew can effectively handle, call for additional resources.
        (1) Be alert for patients in addition to the first patient you observe at the scene.
        (2) Look for clues that other patients may be present (e.g., toys, diapers, bottles, school books, purse, child safety seat).
    b. Obtain additional help BEFORE contact with patients (the EMT-Basic is less

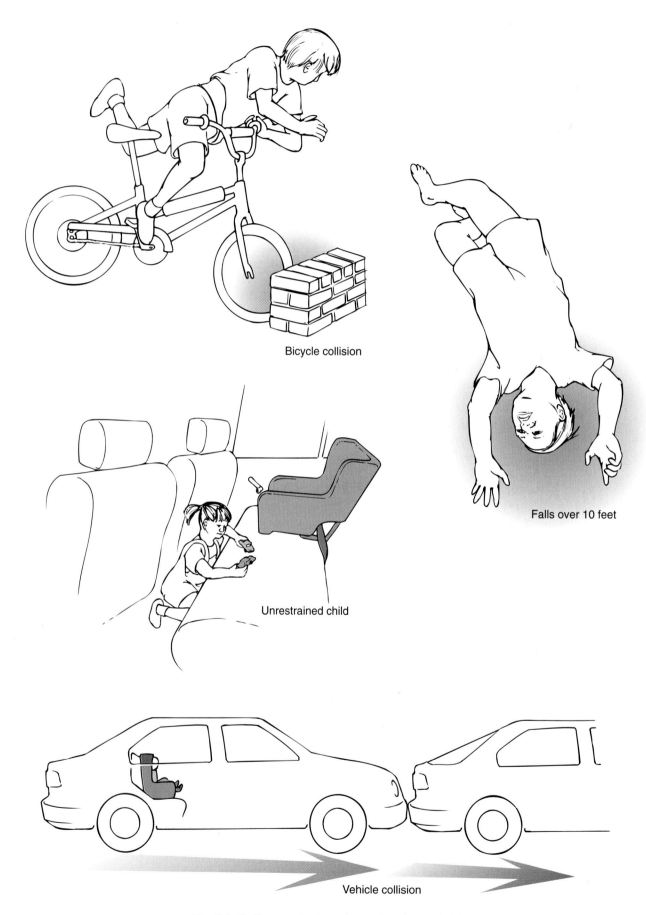

Bicycle collision

Falls over 10 feet

Unrestrained child

Vehicle collision

Fig. 8-2. Significant mechanisms of injury for infants and children.

likely to call for help when involved in patient care). Help includes law enforcement; fire, rescue, and advanced-life-support personnel; and utility company.
  c. Begin triage.
  d. If you and your crew can manage the situation, consider spinal precautions and continue care.

NATURE OF ILLNESS

In medical situations, look for the **nature of the illness** and determine the number of patients.
  1. **Definition.** Nature of the illness includes the cause, or signs and symptoms, of the patient's problem.
  2. Determine the nature of the illness from the patient, family, or bystanders.
  3. Determine the total number of patients.
     a. If there are more patients than you and your crew can effectively handle, call for additional resources.
     b. Obtain additional help BEFORE contact with patients (the EMT-Basic is less likely to call for help if involved in patient care). Help includes law enforcement; fire, rescue, and advanced-life-support personnel; and utility company.
     c. Begin triage.

REVIEW QUESTIONS

Directions: Each of the numbered items or incomplete statements in this section is followed by answers or by completions of the statement. Select the ONE lettered answer or completion that is BEST in each case.

1. Which of the following is a component of scene size-up and assessment?

   (A) Body substance isolation precautions
   (B) Containing hazardous chemical leaks
   (C) Assessing baseline vital signs on all patients
   (D) Opening the airway of all unconscious patients

2. Your crew is dispatched to the scene of a drive-by shooting. Additional information at the time of dispatch says there are multiple gunshot victims in front of the local movie theater. The suspects are believed to still be in the area. One of your patients has been reportedly shot in the chest and is not breathing. Your immediate action should be to

   (A) drive into the scene and quickly remove all patients
   (B) drive into the scene and remove only those patients that are in critical condition
   (C) park a safe distance from the scene and wait for law enforcement personnel to tell you that the scene is safe
   (D) drive to the scene but not get out of your vehicle until law enforcement personnel tell you the scene is safe

3. Your ambulance crew is called to the local flood control for a child trapped on an island of debris. Your patient was rafting down the wash when he became stuck on an accumulation of tree branches. He does not appear to be in distress. Your immediate action should be to

   (A) go upstream and float down to the child
   (B) wade out in the water and bring the child to shore
   (C) throw the child a rescue ring and pull him back to the shore with a rope
   (D) wait until specially trained personnel arrive on the scene to rescue the child

4. Mechanism of injury refers to

   (A) the patient's past medical history
   (B) the forces involved with traumatic injury
   (C) the signs and symptoms of the patient's problem
   (D) the sorting of patients based on severity of injury

5. Your rescue crew is dispatched to the scene of a car versus train collision. En route you are given information that a passenger van has collided with a freight train carrying unknown chemicals. Which of the following should be included in your scene size-up?

   (A) Stabilizing all derailed train cars
   (B) Triaging seriously injured patients
   (C) Initiating cardiopulmonry resuscitation on all cardiac arrest victims
   (D) Calling for a hazardous materials response team

6. Which of the following is a hazard you may encounter at the scene of a motor vehicle collision?

   (A) Traffic hazards
   (B) Downed power lines
   (C) Hazardous materials
   (D) All of the above may be encountered

7. Which of the following best indicates that hazardous materials may be involved at the scene of a motor vehicle accident?

   (A) The time of day
   (B) The location of the accident
   (C) The color of the involved vehicles
   (D) The presence of chemical placards on involved vehicles

8. On multiple patient incidents, after completing the scene size-up, the first responding EMT-Basics should

   (A) triage all patients
   (B) begin treating the most seriously injured patient
   (C) "scoop and run" to the hospital with the most seriously injured patient
   (D) stage away from the scene until additional rescuers arrive to assist with treatment

9. Rescuers should call for additional resources needed at the scene

   (A) only as the need arises
   (B) during the scene size-up
   (C) after crews at the scene request a break
   (D) when existing resources become overwhelmed

10. Wearing the appropriate level of contamination protection (gloves, mask, goggles, etc.) is called _____ and must be addressed during scene size-up so there is no unnecessary delay in patient treatment and transport.

(A) triage
(B) mechanism of injury
(C) body substance isolation
(D) hazardous material containment

ANSWERS AND RATIONALES

1-A. Proper personal protective measures [body substance isolation (BSI)] must be addressed in the scene size-up. Furthermore, your level of protection must be in response to each individual scenario. Err in favor of overprotecting yourself. Containing hazardous chemical leaks is not a size-up task and is not generally the responsibility of the first responders. However, calling for the resources necessary to deal with a hazardous leak would be appropriate during your scene size-up. Assessment of vital signs should take place after the size-up and after triage. Opening the airway of all unconscious patients may be a task performed during triage (or according to your local protocol).

2-C. Rescue personnel should not enter a potentially violent scene until law enforcement personnel ensure that the scene is safe. Parking a safe distance away allows you to be out of harm's way. Additionally, rescuers should park far enough away that they are not motioned into an unsecured scene by bystanders.

3-D. You need to be a part of the solution, not a part of the problem. There are many hazards associated with water rescues, hence the development of specially trained swift-water rescue teams. A rescue ring or other flotation device would place the patient back in the running water and may rapidly worsen the situation. Because the patient in this scenario is in no apparent distress, your efforts should be limited to calling for the additional resources needed for rescue, establishing an area in which evaluate and treat the patient after the rescue is performed, and reassuring the patient that the appropriate help is on the way.

4-B. Mechanism of injury, identifying the manner in which an injury occurs and the forces involved in the injury, is an important part of scene size-up. By evaluating the mechanism of injury, rescuers can get an idea of the resources necessary on the scene and anticipate the types of injuries they may encounter.

5-D. Calling any additional resources necessary to secure the hazard and treat and transport the injured is a critical component of the scene size-up. The other tasks listed are performed by appropriate personnel after the scene size-up.

6-D. The hazards that may be encountered at vehicle collision scenes are too numerous to list. Remember, safety precautions come before treatment procedures. If rescuers are not safe, they run the risk of compounding the problem by becoming injured themselves. Stop, look around, and think during the initial size-up and throughout the incident.

7-D. This question illustrates that hazardous materials can complicate a scene regardless of time of day, day of week, location, or information given by dispatchers. Some areas (e.g., heavy industrial complexes) may be more prone to hazardous materials incidents (also known as "HazMat" incidents). However, rescuers are generally more alert for the presence of hazardous materials in an industrial setting. At incidents in rural areas, on side roads, or in residential areas, rescuers may fail to recognize the presence of hazardous materials until it is too late.

8-A. Triage, sorting the patients according to injury, should follow size-up in multiple patient incidents. Triage allows the initial crew to prioritize treatment and make meaningful, organized assignments to the additional responding units. Treating the most seriously injured patient first may end up costing the lives of several less seriously injured patients. Follow your local triage protocols. Scooping up the most seriously injured patient for rapid transport not only leaves the other patients without treatment, but also neglects the needed scene structure and direction for additional responding units.

9-B. Call for additional resources EARLY. Waiting until on-scene resources are overwhelmed or tired is poor scene management and may jeopardize patient care. Do not wait until you have specific tasks outlined for each additional unit before you call for help. Remember that it takes time to get additional resources to the scene. If you end up not needing the extra help, you can always release the extra units/crews.

10-C. Body substance isolation (BSI) refers to measures taken to protect oneself from contamination due to patient interaction. BSI precautions may include using supplemental equipment such as medical gloves, mask and goggles (for face and eye protection), and gowns (for extremity and trunk protection). Triage is the method by which patients are categorized according to injury. Mechanism of injury refers to the manner in which patients are injured.

BIBLIOGRAPHY

Butman AM, Martin SW, Vomacka RW, et al (eds): *Comprehensive Guide to Pre-Hospital Skills: A Skills Manual for EMT-Basic, EMT-Intermediate, EMT-Paramedic.* Akron, Ohio, Emergency Training, 1995.

Caroline NL: *Emergency Care in the Streets*, 4th ed. Boston, Little, Brown, 1991.

Crosby LA, Lewallen DG (eds): *Emergency Care and Transportation of the Sick and Injured*, 6th ed. Rosemont, IL, American Academy of Orthopaedic Surgeons, 1995.

Grant HD, Murray RH Jr, Bergeron JD: *Emergency Care*, 7th ed. Englewood Cliffs, NJ, Prentice-Hall, 1995.

Hafen BQ, Karren KJ, Mistovich JJ: *Prehospital Emergency Care*, 5th ed. Upper Saddle River, NJ, Prentice-Hall, 1996.

McSwain NE, White RD, Paturas JL, et al (eds): *The Basic EMT: Comprehensive Prehospital Patient Care*. St. Louis, Mosby-Year Book, 1996.

Stoy WA: *Mosby's EMT-Basic Textbook*. St. Louis, Mosby-Year Book, 1996.

United States Department of Transportation, National Highway Traffic Safety Administration: *Emergency Medical Technician: Basic. National Standard Curriculum*, 1994.

9 INITIAL ASSESSMENT

OBJECTIVES

*9-1 List the components of an initial assessment.

*9-2 State the purpose of an initial assessment.

9-3 Explain the purpose of forming a general impression of a patient.

*9-4 Define the term "chief complaint."

9-5 Discuss methods of assessing altered mental status.

9-6 Describe the differences among the assessments of altered mental status in the adult, child, and infant.

*9-7 Describe how to document a patient's mental status.

9-8 Discuss methods of assessing the airway in the adult, child, and infant.

*9-9 State signs and symptoms associated with complete or partial airway obstruction.

9-10 State the reasons for management of the cervical spine once the patient has been determined to be a trauma patient.

9-11 Compare the methods of providing airway care to the adult, child, and infant.

9-12 Distinguish among methods of assessing breathing in the adult, child, and infant.

*9-13 State the normal respiratory rates for an adult, child, and infant.

9-14 Differentiate between adequate and inadequate breathing.

9-15 State what care should be provided to the adult, child, and infant with adequate breathing.

9-16 State what care should be provided to the adult, child, and infant with inadequate breathing.

9-17 Differentiate between obtaining a pulse in an adult, child, and infant.

*9-18 Discuss the need for assessing the patient for external bleeding.

*9-19 Define perfusion.

9-20 Describe normal and abnormal findings when assessing skin color.

MOTIVATION FOR LEARNING

The EMT-Basic will encounter patients who require emergency medical care. It is important for the EMT-Basic to identify those patients who require rapid assessment, critical interventions, and immediate transport and those who require on-scene stabilization.

9-21 Describe normal and abnormal findings when assessing skin temperature.

9-22 Describe normal and abnormal findings when assessing skin condition.

9-23 Describe normal and abnormal findings when assessing skin capillary refill in the infant and child.

9-24 Explain the reason for prioritizing a patient for care and transport.

9-25 List nine examples of priority patients.

INITIAL ASSESSMENT

COMPONENTS

Components of the initial assessment include forming a general impression; assessing mental status, airway, breathing, and circulation; and determining patient priorities.

PURPOSE

The purpose of the initial assessment is to:
1. Identify life-threatening problems
2. Begin interventions
3. Identify priority patients
4. Determine whether immediate transport is necessary

GENERAL GUIDELINES FOR GATHERING INFORMATION DURING THE INITIAL ASSESSMENT

The initial assessment involves gathering information using most of the senses.
1. Seeing (inspection) = Look
2. Hearing (auscultation) = Listen
3. Touch (palpation) = Feel
4. Smell

FORMING A GENERAL IMPRESSION

PURPOSE

The purpose of forming a general impression is to determine priority of care. The general impression is based on the EMT-Basic's immediate assessment of the environment and the patient's chief complaint.

CHIEF COMPLAINT AND NATURE OF THE ILLNESS/MECHANISM OF INJURY

1. Determine the patient's **chief complaint.**
   a. The chief complaint is the reason EMS was called, usually in the patient's own words. The EMT-Basic may ask, "Why did you call 9-1-1 today?"
   b. If the patient is unable to answer, the family or bystanders may be able to provide information. The EMT-Basic may ask, "Can you tell me what happened?"
2. Determine if the patient is ill (medical) or injured (trauma).
   a. If the patient is ill, identify the nature of the illness.
   b. If the patient is injured, identify the mechanism of injury. If the mechanism of injury suggests spinal injury, maintain in-line stabilization of the cervical spine.
3. Determine the patient's age, gender, and race.

Scene Size-Up

Take body substance isolation precautions
Determine scene safety
Determine mechanism of injury/nature of illness
Determine number of patients
Request additional help if necessary

Initial Assessment

Form general impression of patient
Determine chief complaint/apparent life threats
Assess mental status (AVPU)
Assess airway
Assess breathing
Assess circulation
–Pulse
–Major bleeding
–Skin color, temperature, condition
Identify priority patients
Make transport decision

Focused History and Physical Examination

Perform focused physical examination or, if indicated, complete rapid assessment
(DCAP-BTLS)
Obtain baseline vital signs
Obtain SAMPLE history
Reevaluate transport decision

Detailed Physical Examination

DCAP-BTLS
Reassess vital signs

Ongoing Assessment

Repeat initial assessment
Reassess vital signs
Repeat focused assessment regarding patient complaint or injuries
Reevaluate interventions

4. Assess the patient and determine if the patient has a life-threatening condition.
   a. If a life-threatening condition is found, treat immediately.
   b. Examples of life-threatening situations include:
       (1) Airway obstruction
       (2) Respiratory arrest
       (3) Cardiac arrest
       (4) Major bleeding

ASSESSING MENTAL STATUS

SPINAL IMMOBILIZATION DURING ASSESSMENT OF MENTAL STATUS

It is important to maintain spinal immobilization during assessment of mental status, if needed.

HOW TO BEGIN MENTAL STATUS ASSESSMENT

Begin the assessment of mental status by speaking to the patient.
1. State your name.
2. Tell the patient you are an emergency medical technician.
3. Explain that you are there to help.

LEVELS OF MENTAL STATUS

Four different levels of mental status can be differentiated by using the mnemonic **AVPU.**
1. **A = alert**
    a. Patient is awake and responds appropriately to questions.
    b. An awake patient may be disoriented.
    c. Evaluate the awake patient's orientation to:
        (1) Person (the patient can tell you his name)
        (2) Place (the patient can tell you where he is)
        (3) Time (the patient can tell you day, date, or time)
        (4) Event (the patient can tell you what happened)
    d. A patient who is oriented to person, place, time, and event is said to be "alert and oriented × ('times') 4" or "A and O × 4."
2. **V = responds to verbal stimuli**
    a. The patient is not awake but responds appropriately when spoken to.
    b. For example, the patient will respond correctly to a request such as "squeeze my fingers."
3. **P = responds to painful stimuli.** The patient responds only to a painful stimulus, such as a pinch.
4. **U = unresponsive**
    a. The patient does not respond, even to a painful stimulus.
    b. The patient has no gag or cough reflex.

INFANTS AND CHILDREN

1. An alert infant or young child (younger than 3 years of age):
    a. Smiles
    b. Orients to sound
    c. Follows objects with his or her eyes
    d. Interacts
2. As the infant or young child's mental status decreases, the following changes may be observed (in order of decreasing status):
    a. The child may cry but can be comforted
    b. The child may exhibit inappropriate, persistent crying
    c. The child may become irritable, agitated, and restless
    d. The child may have no response (unconscious)
3. Assessment of mental status for a child older than 3 years of age is the same as that for an adult.

CHANGES IN MENTAL STATUS

1. During the initial assessment, note the patient's mental status.
2. As the assessment continues, it is important to note any changes in the patient's mental status.
    a. Communicate any changes in mental status to medical personnel at the receiving facility.
    b. Document any changes in mental status in the prehospital care report.
3. Document the patient's response to a specific stimulus.
    a. "The patient opened her eyes on command."
    b. "The patient moaned in response to a pinch on the wrist."

   c. "The patient knows his name but does not know the date, where he is, or what happened."

4. Avoid terms such as "obtunded," "lethargic," or "semiresponsive"; these terms are subject to interpretation and their meaning varies from one individual to another.

ASSESSING THE PATIENT'S AIRWAY STATUS

RESPONSIVE PATIENT

Is the patient alert and talking clearly or crying without difficulty?

1. If yes, assess the adequacy of breathing.

2. If no, further evaluation of the airway is essential.

   a. Assess for complete or partial airway obstruction.

   b. Signs and symptoms of complete or partial airway obstruction are:

      (1) Inability to speak, cry, cough, or make any other sound

      (2) Cyanosis

      (3) Restlessness, anxiety

      (4) Difficult or labored breathing

      (5) Decreased or no air movement

      (6) Hoarseness

      (7) Noisy breathing: **crowing, snoring, gurgling, wheezing**

UNRESPONSIVE PATIENT

Is the airway open and clear?

1. Inspect for actual or potential obstruction, such as:

   a. A foreign body

   b. Blood

   c. Vomitus

   d. Teeth

   e. Tongue

2. The airway may be opened and maintained using any (or all) of the following techniques.

   a. Manual airway maneuvers

      (1) For medical patients, perform the head-tilt, chin-lift maneuver.

      (2) For trauma patients or those with an unknown nature of illness, the cervical spine should be stabilized and the jaw-thrust maneuver performed.

      (3) Do not hyperextend the neck when opening the airway of an infant or child.

   b. Suctioning

   c. Airway adjuncts

      (1) Nasopharyngeal airway

      (2) Oropharyngeal airway

   d. Obstructed airway maneuvers

      (1) Abdominal thrusts (Heimlich maneuver) for children and adults

      (2) Chest thrusts and back blows for infants

ASSESSING THE PATIENT'S BREATHING

LOOK, LISTEN, AND FEEL

Breathing is assessed by looking, listening, and feeling for air movement.

1. Look for:

   a. Rise and fall of the chest

      (1) Note the respiratory rate.

      (2)   Note the depth and equality of breathing.
      (3)   Note the rhythm of respirations.
   b. Signs of increased work of breathing (respiratory effort)
   c. Signs of chest trauma
   d. Patient's position
2. Listen for air movement and note if respirations are absent, quiet, or noisy.
3. Feel for:
   a. Air movement against your hand or cheek
   b. Depth and equality of breathing

NORMAL RESPIRATORY RATES

1. Adult: 12–20 breaths/minute.
2. Child: 15–30 breaths/minute.
3. Infant: 25–50 breaths/minute.

SIGNS OF ADEQUATE BREATHING

1. Breathing is quiet and effortless with no use of accessory muscles.
2. The respiratory rate is within the normal limit for age.
3. The rhythm is regular with symmetrical chest expansion.
4. The respiratory depth is adequate.

MANAGEMENT—ADEQUATE BREATHING

1. If breathing is adequate and the patient is responsive, oxygen may be indicated.
2. If the patient is unresponsive and the breathing is adequate, open and maintain the airway and provide high-concentration oxygen at 15 liters per minute (LPM) by nonrebreather mask.

SIGNS OF INADEQUATE BREATHING

1. The respiratory rate is outside normal range for age.
2. The breathing pattern is irregular.
3. Breath sounds are diminished or absent.
4. Chest expansion is unequal or inadequate.
5. Effort of breathing is increased.
   a. Patient may use accessory muscles, especially infants and children. Retractions above the clavicles, between the ribs and below the rib cage, may be present, especially in children.
   b. Nasal flaring may be present, especially in children.
   c. In infants, "seesaw" breathing may be present (the chest and abdomen move in opposite directions).
6. Depth is inadequate (shallow respirations).
7. Skin is pale, cyanotic (blue), cool, and clammy.
8. Agonal respirations (occasional gasping breaths) may be seen just before death.

MANAGEMENT—INADEQUATE BREATHING

1. All responsive patients breathing more than 24 breaths per minute or less than 8 breaths per minute should receive high-flow oxygen at 15 LPM by nonrebreather mask
2. If the patient is not breathing, or is unresponsive and breathing is inadequate:
   a. Open and maintain the airway by using:
      (1)   Head-tilt, chin-lift maneuver (no trauma suspected)
      (2)   Jaw-thrust maneuver (trauma suspected)
      (3)   Nasopharyngeal airway
      (4)   Oropharyngeal airway
   b. Assist the patient's breathing with a ventilatory adjunct such as:

      (1) Pocket mask
      (2) Bag-valve mask
      (3) Flow-restricted, oxygen-powered ventilation device
    c. In all cases, oxygen should be used.
3. Infants and children
    a. The priorities for assessing breathing and providing necessary treatment for infants and children are the same as for adults.
    b. The normal respiratory rates for infants and children are faster than for adults. In infants, observing the rise and fall of the abdomen to determine respiratory rate is often easier.

ASSESSING THE PATIENT'S CIRCULATION

PULSE

1. In adults and children older than 1 year of age, circulation is assessed by feeling for a radial pulse. In infants, palpate a brachial pulse.
2. If no radial pulse is felt, palpate the carotid pulse.
3. In adults, the presence of a pulse at specific sites may be used to estimate the patient's systolic blood pressure.
    a. Palpable carotid pulse: systolic blood pressure 60 millimeters of mercury (mm Hg)
    b. Palpable femoral pulse: systolic blood pressure 70 mm Hg
    c. Palpable radial pulse: systolic blood pressure 80 mm Hg
4. If pulseless, begin cardiopulmonary resuscitation (CPR).
    a. For a medical patient older than 8 years old, start CPR and apply automated external defibrillator (AED).
    b. For a medical patient younger than 8 years old, start CPR.
    c. For a trauma patient, start CPR.

BLEEDING

1. Look from head to toes for signs of significant external bleeding.
2. Control major bleeding by:
    a. Applying direct pressure
    b. Applying a pressure bandage
    c. Elevation
    d. Applying pressure to pressure points
    e. Applying a tourniquet (may be needed in rare situations)

PERFUSION

1. Overview
    a. Definition. Perfusion is the flow of blood through tissues.
    b. Perfusion requires:
      (1) A functioning pump (the heart)
      (2) Adequate blood volume (fluid)
      (3) Intact vascular system (container)
    c. Perfusion is assessed by evaluating the patient's:
      (1) Skin color
      (2) Skin temperature
      (3) Skin condition (moisture)
      (4) Capillary refill (in infants and children younger than 6 years of age)
2. Skin color
    a. Assessment
      (1) In Caucasians, normal skin color is pink.

    (2) Assess the patient's skin color in the nail beds, oral mucosa, and conjunctivae (the skin inside the eyelids).

    (3) In infants and children, assess the palms of the hands and soles of the feet.

  b. Abnormal skin color

    (1) Pale skin suggests poor perfusion (impaired blood flow) due to shock, fright, or other causes.

    (2) Cyanotic (blue-gray) skin suggests inadequate oxygenation or poor perfusion. It often appears first in the fingertips or around the mouth (circumoral cyanosis).

    (3) Flushed (red) skin suggests exposure to heat, carbon monoxide poisoning, or high blood pressure.

    (4) Jaundiced (yellow) skin suggests liver disease or hepatitis.

3. Skin temperature

  a. Normal skin temperature is warm.

  b. Assess skin temperature by placing the back of your hand against the patient's face, neck, or abdomen (Figure 9-1).

  c. Abnormal skin temperature

    (1) Hot skin suggests fever or heat exposure.

    (2) Cool skin suggests inadequate circulation or exposure to cold.

    (3) Cold skin suggests extreme exposure to cold.

    (4) Clammy (cool and moist) skin suggests shock, among many other conditions.

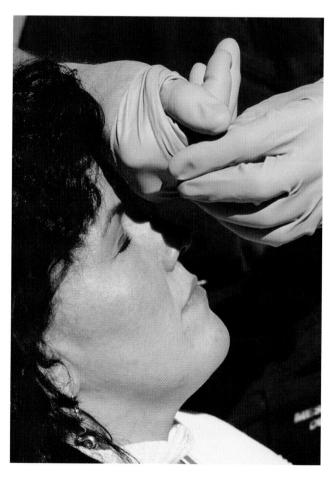

Fig. 9-1. Assess skin temperature by placing the back of your hand against the patient's face, neck, or abdomen.

4. **Skin condition (moisture)**
   a. Normal skin is dry.
   b. Wet or moist skin may indicate shock (hypoperfusion), a heat-related illness, or diabetic emergency.
   c. Excessively dry skin may indicate dehydration.
5. **Capillary refill**
   a. Normal capillary refill in infants and children is less than 2 seconds.
   b. Delayed (greater than 2 seconds) capillary refill suggests circulatory compromise.
   c. Capillary refill in adults is an unreliable indicator of perfusion because it is easily affected by medications, chronic medical conditions, cold weather, and smoking.

IDENTIFYING PRIORITY PATIENTS

AFTER COMPLETING THE INITIAL ASSESSMENT, DETERMINE IF THE PATIENT REQUIRES:

1. On-scene stabilization
2. Immediate transport with stabilization en route to a receiving facility

PATIENTS WHO REQUIRE IMMEDIATE TRANSPORT

Patients who require immediate transport include:
1. Poor general impression
2. Unresponsive patients (no gag or cough reflex)
3. Responsive patient who cannot follow commands
4. Difficulty breathing
5. Shock (hypoperfusion)
6. Complicated childbirth
7. Chest pain with systolic blood pressure less than 100 mm Hg
8. Uncontrolled bleeding
9. Severe pain anywhere

REVIEW QUESTIONS

Directions: Each of the numbered items or incomplete statements in this section is followed by answers or by completions of the statement. Select the ONE lettered answer or completion that is BEST in each case.

1. Forming a general impression is a critical component of the initial assessment. The general impression helps to determine the priority of care and is based on an assessment of

   (A) a predetermined set of guidelines
   (B) the information given at the time of dispatch
   (C) the environment and the patient's chief complaint
   (D) the information gathered during the detailed physical examination

2. While forming the general impression, which of the following injuries would be considered a life-threatening condition?

   (A) Major bleeding
   (B) Severe back pain
   (C) A fractured humerus
   (D) Shortness of breath/difficulty breathing

3. After the general impression is formed, rescuers should turn their attention to assessing the patient's mental status. The mnemonic for evaluating level of consciousness is

   (A) AVPU
   (B) APGAR
   (C) OPQRST
   (D) SAMPLE

4. An unresponsive patient is one who

   (A) does not respond to a painful stimulus
   (B) refuses to talk to you
   (C) is slow to answer questions
   (D) does not recognize others or interact appropriately

5. To evaluate the level of mental status of patients younger than 3 years of age, rescuers should assess the patient's

   (A) speech
   (B) vital signs
   (C) coordination
   (D) interaction with parent

6. Which of the following would cause you the most alarm when assessing a young child?

   (A) A child who cries persistently
   (B) A child who does not react to his or her surroundings
   (C) An irritable, agitated, restless child
   (D) A child who cries, but can be comforted

7. After forming a general impression of the patient and evaluating mental status, you should turn your attention to

   (A) splinting and bandaging
   (B) evaluating airway status
   (C) evaluating breathing status
   (D) evaluating circulation and perfusion

8. The proper technique to open the airway of an unconscious patient involved in a motor vehicle collision is the

   (A) head-tilt, chin-lift maneuver
   (B) head-lift, neck-thrust maneuver
   (C) jaw-thrust maneuver
   (D) neck-thrust maneuver

9. At what age is it considered appropriate to apply the automated external defibrillator to a pulseless patient?

   (A) All ages

(B) One year of age and older
(C) Eight years of age and older
(D) Eighteen years of age and older

10. After completing the initial assessment, you should

   (A) evaluate the patient's airway status
   (B) begin cardiopulmonary resuscitation
   (C) identify the patient's chief complaint
   (D) decide whether to begin on-scene stabilization or transport immediately

Directions: Each of the numbered items or incomplete statements in this section is negatively phrased, as indicated by a capitalized word such as NOT, LEAST, or EXCEPT. Select the ONE lettered answer or completion that is BEST in each case.

11. Perfusion is the flow of blood to the tissues of the body. Which of the following is a reliable indicator of perfusion in children and infants but NOT adults?

   (A) Skin color
   (B) Skin temperature
   (C) Skin condition (moisture)
   (D) Capillary refill

Directions: Each of the numbered questions or incomplete statements in this section refers to a scenario that precedes them. The numbered questions or incomplete statements are followed by answers or by completions of the statement. Select the answer or completion of the statement that is BEST in each case.

Your rescue crew responds to the home of a 65-year-old male patient. Dispatch information states that the patient was found unconscious by a family member and that he has a history of hypertension (high blood pressure). You arrive to find your patient unconscious and unresponsive in bed.

Questions 12–16

12. The proper method of opening this patient's airway is

   (A) head-tilt, chin-lift maneuver
   (B) head-lift, neck-thrust maneuver
   (C) jaw-thrust maneuver
   (D) neck-thrust maneuver

13. To maintain a patent airway in this patient, it would be appropriate to

   (A) insert a nasopharyngeal airway
   (B) begin oxygen therapy with a nasal cannula
   (C) begin oxygen therapy with a nonrebreather mask
   (D) begin ventilating with a bag-valve mask

14. Your general impression is that this patient is potentially in a critical condition and will require prompt stabilization and rapid transport. While assessing the patient's mental status, you observe that the patient is not alert, will not respond to verbal commands, and opens his eyes when a painful stimulus is applied. Which of the following would be the most appropriate way of recording this finding?

    (A) The patient is not alert
    (B) The patient is unresponsive
    (C) The patient responds to painful stimuli
    (D) The patient responds to painful stimuli by opening his eyes

15. After assessing that this patient's airway is patent and inserting a nasopharyngeal airway, you assess his respiratory status. The patient is breathing 16 times per minute with an adequate tidal volume. You should provide this patient supplemental oxygen by means of a

    (A) nasal cannula at 6 liters per minute (LPM)
    (B) nonrebreather mask at 15 LPM
    (C) bag-valve mask at 15 LPM
    (D) bag-valve mask at 6 LPM

16. After assessing breathing, you evaluate this patient's circulatory status. The patient has a weak carotid pulse of 120 beats per minute, and no radial pulse is palpable. Which of the following would be a correct assumption based on these findings?

    (A) The patient's systolic blood pressure is 0 millimeters of mercury (mm Hg)
    (B) You should begin cardiopulmonary resuscitation
    (C) The patient's systolic blood pressure is about 120 mm Hg
    (D) The patient's systolic blood pressure is between 60 and 80 mm Hg

ANSWERS AND RATIONALES

1-C. The general impression is formed by evaluating the patient's chief complaint and physical environment. The components of the general impression are the chief complaint, the nature of the illness (medical complaints), the mechanism of injury (traumatic complaints), and the presence of life-threatening injury or illness. A predetermined set of guidelines should not dictate your care priorities, because each scenario is different. While the information given at time of dispatch is helpful, this information must be confirmed at the scene with the patient. Your physical impression may be much different from the "phone" impression the dispatcher may have formed. Information gathered during the detailed physical examination may greatly influence your care priorities; however, the general impression is formed during the initial assessment that precedes the detailed physical exam.

2-A. Major bleeding is considered a life-threatening condition that can readily be recognized during the general impression phase. The other complaints will be evaluated in more detail during subsequent evaluations.

3-A. AVPU is used to evaluate the patient's level of consciousness. AVPU stands for **A**lert, **V**erbal, **P**ainful, and **U**nresponsive. Patients who are not fully alert should be categorized according to their response to a stimulus. For example, a patient who responds to a painful stimulus by moaning and pushing the stimulus away should be described as such. Simply saying that the patient responds to painful stimuli is not enough; the response must also be documented (in this case moaning and purposeful movement). APGAR is a scale used to evaluate the status of newborns. OPQRST is used for evaluating a patient's complaint of pain, and SAMPLE is a method of gathering information about the patient's chief complaint and past medical history.

4-A. An unresponsive patient does not respond to a painful stimulus and has no gag or cough reflex. The other options indicate the patient responds to the surroundings; however, the response may be inappropriate.

5-D. Perhaps the best indicator of a young child's mental status is the interaction (or lack of) between the child and a familiar face, especially the parent. It is important to document and treat accordingly when a parent tells you, "He is just not acting right." Because children go through such drastic developmental changes during their early years, assessing a child based solely on age is difficult for rescuers.

6-B. The usual progression in deteriorating mental status for a child is: the child cries but can be comforted; the child cries despite attempts to be comforted; the child becomes irritable, agitated, and restless; and finally the child does not react at all to his or her surroundings. Often, rescuers confuse a child with an altered mental status with a child who is simply "being good." It is not normal for a 2-year-old child to allow a stranger (the rescuer) to take him or her away from mom or dad. If the rescuer can take the child, ask the parent if the child normally allows strangers to hold him or her.

7-B. The next step in the initial assessment is determining airway status. Assessing the status of breathing and circulation follow. Splinting and bandaging interventions should be incorporated into the detailed physical examination that follows the initial assessment, unless control of life-threatening hemorrhage is necessary.

8-C. Maintaining spinal immobilization is critical for trauma patients with suspected spinal compromise. Suspect spinal compromise in patients complaining of traumatic head or neck pain, patients with head or neck trauma, unconscious patients of unknown etiology (cause), or in patients whose mechanism of injury suggests that spinal compromise may be present. The jaw-thrust maneuver allows the airway to be opened without manipulating the spine. It is accomplished by lifting the patient's jaw anteriorly while maintaining the head in a neutral position.

9-C. The automated external defibrillator may be used in pulseless patients 8 years of age and older.

10-D. After completing the initial assessment, you should have sufficient information to decide whether to stabilize your patient on-scene or begin immediate transport and stabilize en route to the receiving facility. Evaluating the patient's airway, beginning cardiopulmonary resuscitation (if necessary), and identifying the patient's chief complaint should be done during the initial assessment.

11-D. Capillary refill evaluates the time required for the return of a normal, pink appearance in the capillary beds after blanching (pinching). Normal refill time is less than 2 seconds. In adults, this technique is not completely reliable as capillary refill is easily affected by medications, chronic medical conditions, cold weather, and smoking.

12-A. Since this patient is found in bed and there are no signs of recent trauma, it is safe to assume that the head-tilt, chin-lift technique would be appropriate. In this case, the head-tilt, chin-lift maneuver is preferred since maintaining it is easier than the jaw thrust, and there is no sign that manipulating the cervical spine would be hazardous to this patient.

13-A. A nasopharyngeal airway helps in maintaining a patent (open) airway by creating a passageway from the tip of the nose to the base of the tongue. Oxygen therapy with a nasal cannula or nonrebreather mask does not assist in maintaining an open airway. Also, ventilatory support with a bag-valve mask does not ensure that the airway will stay open.

14-C. When documenting or communicating the patient's mental status, you should be as descriptive as necessary to convey the patient's actual presentation. The other responses, while not completely false, do not paint as accurate a picture.

15-B. Since this patient has an altered mental status with adequate respirations, high-flow oxygen via nonrebreather mask is most appropriate. A nasal cannula does not deliver high-concentration oxygen and a bag-valve mask is not necessary because the patient is breathing well on his own.

16-D. If the patient has a radial pulse, you may temporarily assume that his systolic blood pressure is 80 millimeters of mercury (mm Hg). Since no radial pulse is present, you should assume that the pressure is below 80 mm Hg. The presence of a carotid pulse suggests that the patient's systolic blood pressure is at least 60 mm Hg. Therefore, this patient's pressure can temporarily be assumed to be between 60 and 80 mm Hg. Additionally, if this patient has a femoral pulse, you can assume that his blood pressure is at least 70 mm Hg.

BIBLIOGRAPHY

Butman AM, Martin SW, Vomacka RW, et al (eds): *Comprehensive Guide to Pre-Hospital Skills: A Skills Manual for EMT-Basic, EMT-Intermediate, EMT-Paramedic.* Akron, Ohio, Emergency Training, 1995.

Caroline NL: *Emergency Care in the Streets*, 4th ed. Boston, Little, Brown, 1991.

Crosby LA, Lewallen DG (eds): *Emergency Care and Transportation of the Sick and Injured*, 6th ed. Rosemont, IL, American Academy of Orthopaedic Surgeons, 1995.

Cummins RO (ed): *Textbook of Advanced Cardiac Life Support.* Dallas, American Heart Association, 1994.

Grant HD, Murray RH Jr, Bergeron JD: *Emergency Care*, 7th ed. Englewood Cliffs, NJ, Prentice-Hall, 1995.

Hafen BQ, Karren KJ, Mistovich JJ: *Prehospital Emergency Care*, 5th ed. Upper Saddle River, NJ, Prentice-Hall, 1996.

Kidd PS, Stuart P (eds): *Mosby's Emergency Nursing Reference.* St. Louis, Mosby-Yearbook, 1996.

McSwain NE, White RD, Paturas JL, et al (eds): *The Basic EMT: Comprehensive Prehospital Patient Care.* St. Louis, Mosby-Yearbook, 1996.

Miller RH, Wilson JK: *Manual of Prehospital Emergency Medicine.* St. Louis, Mosby-Yearbook, 1992.

Stoy WA: *Mosby's EMT-Basic Textbook.* St. Louis, Mosby-Year Book, 1996.

United States Department of Transportation, National Highway Traffic Safety Administration: *Emergency Medical Technician: Basic. National Standard Curriculum*, 1994.

FOCUSED HISTORY AND PHYSICAL EXAMINATION: TRAUMA

OBJECTIVES

10-1   Discuss the reasons for reevaluating the mechanism of injury.

10-2   State the reasons for performing a rapid trauma assessment.

10-3   Recite examples and explain why patients should receive a rapid trauma assessment.

10-4   Describe the areas included in the rapid trauma assessment and discuss what should be evaluated.

10-5   Describe situations in which the rapid assessment may be altered to provide patient care.

10-6   Discuss the reason for performing a focused history and physical examination.

FOCUSED HISTORY AND PHYSICAL EXAMINATION: TRAUMA

COMPONENTS OF THE FOCUSED HISTORY AND PHYSICAL EXAMINATION

Components include physical examination, baseline vital signs, and SAMPLE history.

WHEN TO PERFORM THE FOCUSED HISTORY AND PHYSICAL EXAMINATION

The focused history and physical examination follow the initial assessment. After completion of the initial assessment, reevaluate the mechanism of injury.

1. Reevaluate the mechanism of injury to determine:
    a. Potential for life-threatening injuries
    b. Need for advanced-life-support (ALS) personnel
    c. Need for immediate transport

● MOTIVATION FOR LEARNING ●

The EMT-Basic will encounter seriously injured trauma patients who require a rapid (head-to-toes) trauma assessment and critical interventions. The EMT-Basic may also encounter less seriously injured trauma patients who can be managed using the focused physical examination. Using the mechanism of injury, chief complaint, and initial assessment findings, the EMT-Basic must be able to distinguish between these two types of trauma patients.

Scene Size-Up

Take body substance isolation precautions
Determine scene safety
Determine mechanism of injury/nature of illness
Determine number of patients
Request additional help if necessary

Initial Assessment

Form general impression of patient
Determine chief complaint/apparent life threats
Assess mental status (AVPU)
Assess airway
Assess breathing
Assess circulation
–Pulse
–Major bleeding
–Skin color, temperature, condition
Identify priority patients
Make transport decision

Focused History and Physical Examination

Perform focused physical examination or, if indicated, complete rapid assessment (DCAP-BTLS)
Obtain baseline vital signs
Obtain SAMPLE history
Reevaluate transport decision

Detailed Physical Examination

DCAP-BTLS
Reassess vital signs

Ongoing Assessment

Repeat initial assessment
Reassess vital signs
Repeat focused assessment regarding patient complaint or injuries
Reevaluate interventions

2. If there is no significant mechanism of injury (e.g., cut finger), proceed with a focused physical examination.
   a. Perform the focused physical examination based on:
      (1) The patient's chief complaint
      (2) The mechanism of injury
      (3) Initial assessment findings
   b. Assess baseline vital signs.
   c. Obtain SAMPLE history.
3. If there is a significant mechanism of injury, proceed with a **rapid trauma assessment** and perform critical interventions.
   a. Continue in-line spinal stabilization.
   b. Consider requesting ALS personnel.
   c. Reconsider transport decision.
   d. Reassess mental status.
   e. Perform rapid trauma assessment to determine life-threatening injuries. If the patient is responsive, ask about symptoms before and during the trauma assessment.
   f. Assess baseline vital signs.
   g. Obtain SAMPLE history.

TRAUMA PATIENT WITH SIGNIFICANT MECHANISM OF INJURY

SIGNIFICANT MECHANISMS OF INJURY

1. Significant mechanisms of injury include:
   a. Ejection from a vehicle
   b. Dead occupant in the same passenger compartment
   c. Falls from more than 20 feet (or three times body height)
   d. Rollover of a vehicle
   e. High-speed vehicle collision
   f. Vehicle–pedestrian collision
   g. Motorcycle crash
   h. Unresponsive or altered mental status
   i. Penetrations of the head, chest, or abdomen
   j. Hidden injuries from seat belts or air bags
      (1) **Seat belts**
          (a) If buckled, seat belts may have produced injuries.
          (b) A buckled seat belt does not mean that the patient does not have injuries.
      (2) **Air bags**
          (a) Air bags may not be effective without a seat belt.
          (b) The patient can hit wheel after deflation.
              (i) Lift the deployed air bag and look at the steering wheel for deformation.
              (ii) "Lift and look" under the bag after the patient has been removed.
          (c) Any visible deformity of the steering wheel should be regarded as an indicator of potentially serious internal injury.
2. Significant mechanisms of injury in infants and children include:
   a. Falls from more than 10 feet (or three times body height)
   b. Bicycle collision
   c. Vehicle collision at a medium speed
   d. Any vehicle collision in which the infant or child was unrestrained

IN-LINE SPINAL STABILIZATION

In-line spinal stabilization should be maintained until the patient is completely immobilized to a long backboard.

CONSIDERATION OF REQUEST FOR ALS PERSONNEL

Consider request for ALS personnel.
1. Consider requesting ALS personnel, air transport, or specialized resources.
2. Request help as soon as possible.

RECONSIDERATION OF TRANSPORT DECISION

Reconsider transport decision.
1. If a decision to transport immediately was not made at the end of the initial assessment, transport will occur after completion of the rapid or focused trauma assessment, baseline vital signs assessment, and gathering of the SAMPLE history.
2. If the patient appeared stable at the end of the initial assessment, but he or she becomes unstable during the focused examination, expedite patient transport to the closest appropriate medical facility.

REASSESSMENT OF MENTAL STATUS

1. An alert patient can direct the physical examination with his or her complaints and response.

   2. A patient who is not awake may still react during the physical examination.
   a. Patients may respond to voices.
   b. They may withdraw from pain.
      (1) Purposeful movement is displayed when the patient attempts to remove the stimulus.
      (2) Nonpurposeful movement is displayed when the patient does not attempt to remove the stimulus.
   c. Note any changes in the patient's mental status.
      (1) Communicate any changes in mental status to medical personnel at the receiving facility.
      (2) Document any changes in mental status in the prehospital care report.
      (3) It is important to document the patient's response to a specific stimulus.
         (a) "The patient responded to a painful stimulus by arching his back and pulling both arms toward his chest."
         (b) "The patient gagged when oropharyngeal airway insertion was attempted."

RAPID TRAUMA ASSESSMENT

Perform a rapid trauma assessment.
   1. The rapid trauma assessment is a head-to-toes physical examination performed to detect the presence of life-threatening injuries.
   2. A rapid trauma assessment (a head-to-toes examination) should be performed when:
   a. A significant mechanism of injury exists
   b. The EMT-Basic suspects additional injuries
   c. A critical injury is found during the focused physical examination
   d. A previously stable patient with no significant mechanism of injury becomes unstable during the focused physical examination
   3. Inspect (look), auscultate (listen), and palpate (feel) body areas to identify potential injuries.
   4. Use your sense of smell to identify unusual odors, such as alcohol on the patient's breath, body, or clothing, or the smell of gasoline at the scene.
   5. Identify obvious areas of injury using the mnemonic **DCAP-BTLS:**
   a. Deformities
   b. Contusions (bruises)
   c. Abrasions (scrapes)
   d. Punctures or **p**enetrating wounds
   e. Burns
   f. Tenderness to palpation
   g. Lacerations (cuts)
   h. Swelling
   6. Performing a rapid trauma assessment
   a. Head. Assess DCAP-BTLS plus the following:
      (1) Scalp and skull
         (a) Note any depressions, protrusions, or discoloration.
         (b) Periodically examine your gloves for the presence of blood.
         (c) Intervention. Dress open wounds.
      (2) Ears
         (a) Look for blood or clear fluid in the ears.
         (b) Look for bluish discoloration **(ecchymosis)** over the mastoid process (behind the ear) **[Battle's sign].** This sign suggests possible skull fracture.
         (c) Intervention. If fluid is observed in the ears, do not attempt to stop the flow; cover the ear with a loose sterile dressing.
      (3) Face. Assess DCAP-BTLS plus the following:
         (a) Look for singed facial hair.

      (b) Gently palpate the facial bones—orbits, nasal bones, cheek bones, maxilla (upper jaw bone), mandible (lower jaw bone)—for instability or tenderness.

      (c) Assess for **crepitation** (the grating sound heard or sensation felt when broken bone ends rub together).

      (d) Intervention

         (i) If the patient is unresponsive, insert an oropharyngeal airway to maintain an open airway.

         (ii) Suction as necessary.

         (iii) Do not insert a nasopharyngeal airway if the patient has known or suspected trauma to the mid-face; check local protocol.

  (4) Eyes. Assess DCAP-BTLS plus the following:

      (a) Look for bilateral bluish discoloration (ecchymosis) around the eyes **(raccoon eyes).** This sign suggest possible skull fracture.

      (b) Look for the presence of blood in the anterior chamber of the eye (hyphema).

      (c) Look for the presence of a foreign body.

      (d) Check pupil size, equality, and reaction to light. Unequal pupils in the presence of head trauma suggest cerebral swelling (edema).

  (5) Nose. Assess DCAP-BTLS plus the following:

      (a) Look for blood or fluid from the nose and singed nasal hairs.

      (b) Feel for stability of nasal bones.

  (6) Mouth. Assess DCAP-BTLS plus the following:

      (a) Look for foreign body, blood, vomitus, absent or broken teeth, and injured or swollen tongue.

      (b) Look at the color of the mucous membranes of the mouth.

      (c) Intervention

         (i) Suction as necessary.

         (ii) Administer high-flow oxygen.

b. Neck. Assess DCAP-BTLS plus the following:

  (1) Look for jugular venous distention (JVD).

      (a) The neck veins are normally slightly distended when a patient is supine.

      (b) Flat neck veins in a supine patient suggest decreased blood volume.

      (c) Distention of the neck veins when the patient is placed in a sitting position at a 45° angle suggests injury to the chest, lungs, or heart.

  (2) Check for the presence of a stoma (surgical opening in the neck).

  (3) Check for use of accessory muscles in the neck during breathing.

  (4) Look for open wounds.

  (5) Check for presence of medical identification device.

  (6) Note position of the trachea. Shifting of the trachea (deviation) from a midline position suggests a pneumothorax.

  (7) Check for air trapped beneath the skin **(subcutaneous emphysema).**

  (8) Assess tenderness of the cervical spine.

  (9) Assess for crepitation.

  (10) Intervention

      (a) If present, cover an open wound of the neck with an occlusive dressing.

      (b) Apply a cervical immobilization device.

      (c) Control significant bleeding if present.

c. Chest

  (1) Expose the chest.

  (2) Palpate the sternum, each rib, and both clavicles.

  (3) Assess DCAP-BTLS plus the following:

      (a) Check for **paradoxical motion** of a segment of the chest wall (part of the chest moves in an opposite direction during respiration).

(b) Evaluate ease of respiratory effort; check use of accessory muscles during breathing.

(c) Check for tenderness, instability, and crepitation.

(d) Check for the presence of subcutaneous emphysema.

(e) Check for the presence of a flail segment.

(f) Auscultate breath sounds. Listen to the chest in six places (Figure 10-1):

    (i) At the apices, midclavicular line bilaterally

    (ii) At the bases bilaterally

    (iii) In the midaxillary line bilaterally

    (iv) Compare from side to side

(g) Determine if breath sounds are:

    (i) Present, diminished, absent

    (ii) Equal or unequal

    (iii) Clear or noisy

(h) Intervention

    (i) Administer high-flow oxygen.

    (ii) If present, seal open chest wounds with an occlusive dressing.

    (iii) Stabilize a flail segment if present.

    (iv) Control significant bleeding if present.

d. Abdomen

(1) Assess the abdomen with the patient in a supine position.

(2) Assess DCAP-BTLS plus the following:

(a) Note **evisceration** (organs protruding through an open abdominal wound).

(b) Note the presence of abdominal distention (abdomen appears larger than normal). Distention is difficult to assess in obese patients.

(c) Assess firmness/hardness.

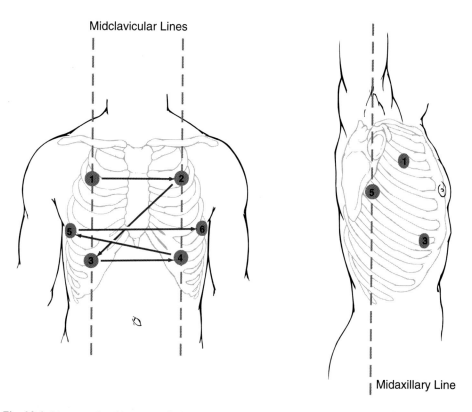

Fig. 10-1. Listen to the chest in six places: at the apices in the mid-clavicular line bilaterally, at the bases bilaterally, and in the midaxillary line bilaterally. Compare from side to side.

        (i) Feel all four quadrants for tenderness.

        (ii) Use the pads of your fingers to palpate the abdomen.

    (d) Check for the presence of any masses or pulsations.

    (e) **Intervention**

        (i) If present, cover exposed abdominal organs with a moist, sterile dressing.

        (ii) Control significant bleeding if present.

e. Pelvis. Assess DCAP-BTLS plus the following:

  (1) Gently compress over the symphysis pubis and push in laterally over the iliac crests.

    (a) Feel for tenderness, instability, and crepitation.

    (b) Do NOT rock the pelvis.

    (c) If the patient complains of pain in the pelvic region, or obvious deformity is present, do NOT palpate the pelvis.

    (d) Severe blood loss may occur from a break in the continuity of the pelvis.

  (2) **Intervention**

    (a) If tenderness, instability, or crepitation of the pelvis is present:

        (i) Administer high-flow oxygen

        (ii) Immobilize the patient with the pneumatic antishock garment (PASG) check local protocol].

        (iii) Secure the patient to a long backboard.

        (iv) Transport to the closest appropriate medical facility.

    (b) Control significant bleeding if present.

f. Extremities. Assess DCAP-BTLS plus the following:

  (1) Check for abnormal extremity position.

  (2) Check for presence of medical identification device.

  (3) Assess for tenderness, instability, and crepitation.

  (4) Assess distal **p**ulses, **m**otor function, and **s**ensation (PMS).

    (a) **Distal pulses**

        (i) Assess the dorsalis pedis or posterior tibial pulses in the lower extremity.

        (ii) Assess the radial pulse in the upper extremity.

        (iii) Compare injured extremity to uninjured extremity.

    (b) **Motor function.** If the patient is awake, ask if he or she can wiggle toes and squeeze your fingers.

    (c) **Sensation**

        (i) If the patient is awake, ask if he or she can feel you touch fingers and toes.

        (ii) If the patient is unconscious, note if he or she responds when you pinch fingers and toes.

  (5) Check for presence of femur injury.

    (a) A closed break of the femur may result in a loss of 1 liter of blood.

    (b) Injury to both femurs may cause life-threatening hemorrhage.

  (6) **Intervention**

    (a) **Bilateral femur injury**

        (i) Administer high-flow oxygen.

        (ii) Immobilize the patient on a long backboard.

        (iii) Transport to the closest appropriate medical facility.

    (b) **Other extremity injuries**

        (i) In the noncritical patient, immobilize the injured body part with an appropriate splint before transport.

        (ii) In the critical patient, splints should be applied during transport as time permits.

    (c) Control significant bleeding if present.

g. Posterior body

  (1) While maintaining in-line spinal stabilization, logroll the patient and assess the posterior body.

    (2) Assess DCAP-BTLS plus tenderness, instability, crepitation.
    (3) Intervention
        (a) Cover open wounds of the posterior chest with an occlusive dressing.
        (b) Control significant bleeding if present.
        (c) Immobilize the patient to a long backboard.

ASSESSMENT OF BASELINE VITAL SIGNS

Assess baseline vital signs; reassess and record vital signs at least every 5 minutes in the unstable trauma patient.

1. Assess respirations by evaluating:
   a. Rate
   b. Depth/equality
   c. Rhythm
   d. Alterations in respiration, including abnormal respiratory sounds
2. Assess pulse.
   a. Initially, a radial pulse should be assessed in all patients 1 year of age or older.
   b. In patients younger than 1 year of age, a brachial pulse should be assessed.
   c. If a pulse is present, assess:
      (1) Rate
      (2) Quality, including:
         (a) Strength [absent, weak, strong/full (normal), or bounding]
         (b) Rhythm
         (c) Equality
   d. Assess skin for:
      (1) Color
      (2) Temperature
      (3) Condition (moisture)
      (4) Capillary refill in infants and children younger than 6 years of age
   e. Assess pupils for size, equality, and reactivity.
   f. Assess blood pressure.
      (1) Blood pressure should be assessed in any patient older than 3 years of age.
      (2) Whenever possible, blood pressure should be assessed by auscultation.

SAMPLE HISTORY

Obtain a **SAMPLE** history.

1. **Signs and symptoms**
   a. Ask, "Why did you call us today?"
   b. The OPQRST acronym may help identify the type and location of the patient's complaint.
2. **Allergies**
   a. "Do you have any allergies to medications?"
   b. "Do you have any food allergies or allergies to pollen, dust, grass?"
3. **Medications**
   a. "Do you take any prescription or over-the-counter medications?"
   b. "Do you take any illegal drugs?"
   c. "Have you recently started taking any new medications?"
   d. "Have you recently stopped taking any medications?"
   e. "Are you taking birth control pills?" (If applicable)
4. **Pertinent past medical history**
   a. "Are you seeing a physician for any medical problems?"
   b. "Do you have a history of heart problems, respiratory problems, kidney problems, liver problems, hypertension, diabetes, or epilepsy?"
   c. "Have you had any recent surgery?"
5. **Last oral intake**
   a. "When was the last time you had anything to eat or drink?"
   b. Determine what was ingested, how much was ingested, and when.
6. **Events leading to the injury.** "What were you doing just before this happened?"

TRAUMA PATIENT WITH NO SIGNIFICANT MECHANISM OF INJURY

FOCUSED PHYSICAL EXAMINATION

Perform a focused physical examination.

1. The focused physical examination concentrates on the specific injury site based on what the patient states is wrong and the EMT-Basic's suspicions based on the mechanism of injury and initial assessment findings.
2. The focused physical examination is based on:
   a. Patient's chief complaint
   b. Mechanism of injury (e.g., cut finger, swollen ankle)
   c. Initial assessment findings

ASSESSMENT OF BASELINE VITAL SIGNS AND SAMPLE HISTORY

After completion of the focused physical examination:

1. Assess baseline vital signs
2. Obtain a SAMPLE history

REVIEW QUESTIONS

Directions: Each of the numbered items or incomplete statements in this section is followed by answers or by completions of the statement. Select the ONE lettered answer or completion that is BEST in each case.

1. The rapid trauma assessment

   (A) is valuable in adult patients only
   (B) is performed immediately following scene size-up
   (C) involves assessing the body to identify potential injuries
   (D) is only performed if life-threatening injuries are reported

2. The "P" in the SAMPLE acronym stands for

   (A) Pain
   (B) Perfusion
   (C) Patient's name, gender, and age
   (D) Pertinent past medical history

3. When evaluating the mechanism of injury, rescuers must recognize that certain circumstances pose a severe threat of significant bodily harm. For an adult patient, falls from greater than _____ are considered significant.

   (A) 6 feet or equal to the patient's height
   (B) 12 feet or equal to twice the patient's height
   (C) 20 feet or three times the patient's height
   (D) 50 feet or 10 times the patient's height

4. Your ambulance crew is treating a 45-year-old woman who fell while skating. Initially, your patient is in mild distress complaining of left hip pain and a slight headache. During your focused trauma assessment, the patient complains of "light-headedness and weakness." You should

(A) assure the patient that nothing is wrong
(B) reconsider your decision to delay transportation
(C) put smelling salts (ammonia capsules) under the patient's nose
(D) instruct the patient to put her head between her knees and breathe deeply

Directions: Each of the numbered items or incomplete statements in this section is negatively phrased, as indicated by a capitalized word such as NOT, LEAST, or EXCEPT. Select the ONE lettered answer or completion that is BEST in each case.

5. Which of the following is NOT a component of the focused history and physical examination for trauma patients?

(A) SAMPLE history
(B) Baseline vital signs
(C) Physical examination
(D) Identification of life-threatening injuries

Directions: Each of the numbered questions or incomplete statements in this section refers to a scenario that precedes them. The numbered questions or incomplete statements are followed by answers or by completions of the statement. Select the answer or completion of the statement that is BEST in each case.

Your rescue crew is dispatched to the scene of a motor vehicle collision. You find a 34-year-old man supine on the pavement. Bystanders state he was struck by a vehicle that has fled the scene. During your initial assessment, you identify that the patient is in moderate distress, complaining of right leg pain. His airway, breathing, and circulatory status seem within acceptable range. He is alert and answers questions appropriately.

Questions 6–11

6. For treatment purposes, reevaluating the mechanism of injury may indicate

(A) the need for advanced-life-support personnel
(B) that you should take down the names of all witnesses on the scene
(C) that you should concern yourself with getting a vehicle description from the bystanders
(D) that you should allow law enforcement personnel to speak with the patient before transporting him to the appropriate receiving facility

7. While stabilizing this patient, your crew takes measures to immobilize this patient's spine. Your partner begins manual in-line immobilization of the patient's head and neck. When may your partner release manual immobilization?

(A) After application of the cervical collar
(B) Upon arrival at the appropriate receiving facility
(C) After the patient is completely immobilized on a long backboard
(D) After you determine that the patient does not have head or neck pain

8. In this situation, the focused physical examination should address

(A) the patient's entire body
(B) only the patient's right leg
(C) only the lower half of the body
(D) only those areas where the patient complains of pain

9. Which of the following mnemonics would assist you in performing the rapid trauma assessment on this patient?

    (A)   ABC
    (B)   ALS
    (C)   DOT
    (D)   DCAP-BTLS

10. During your rapid assessment of this patient, you note that he has a one-inch laceration to the chin. An appropriate intervention for this finding would be to

    (A)   apply a first aid cream
    (B)   dress the wound with dry, sterile gauze
    (C)   attempt to close the wound with a "butterfly" bandage
    (D)   leave the wound alone so it can be properly evaluated in the emergency department

11. While assessing the patient's right leg, you find the thigh is angulated, suggesting a probable femur injury. This finding

    (A)   is common and not overly alarming
    (B)   does not necessitate any intervention
    (C)   is frequently associated with significant blood loss
    (D)   can be corrected in the field without the need for hospital intervention

Your rescue crew is called to the scene of an assault. Your patient is a 24-year-old man. Bystanders state that the patient was jumped by three men armed with bats and chains.

Questions 12–15

12. During the rapid trauma assessment, fluid is observed flowing from the patient's ears. Appropriate treatment should include

    (A)   cover the ears with an occlusive dressing
    (B)   pack the ears with dry, sterile gauze and change when soaked
    (C)   pack the ears with dry, sterile gauze and do not change when soaked
    (D)   cover the ears with dry, sterile gauze but do not attempt to stop the flow of fluid

13. While examining pupil response, you observe that the right pupil is dilated and does not react. The left pupil constricts when exposed to light. This sign may be indicative of

    (A)   shock
    (B)   massive blood loss
    (C)   severe hypothermia
    (D)   cerebral swelling (edema)

14. Which of the following findings may be indicative of a skull fracture in this patient?

    (A)   A chipped tooth
    (B)   Bruising behind the ears
    (C)   A large laceration over the mandible
    (D)   A low blood pressure that continues to fall

15. During your physical examination, you observe that the patient has a deep laceration over the anterior neck. Appropriate management of this injury should include

    (A)   covering the wound with an occlusive dressing
    (B)   covering the wound with a dry, sterile dressing
    (C)   wrapping the neck with a gauze roll to control bleeding
    (D)   immediately assisting ventilations with a bag-valve mask

ANSWERS AND RATIONALES

1-C. A rapid trauma assessment should be conducted on all patients who have a significant mechanism of injury, regardless of whether the injuries appear initially to be life threatening. The assessment should be performed on children and infants as well as adults. It is performed after the initial assessment (not immediately following the scene size-up).

2-D. SAMPLE is an acronym used for history gathering. The "P" stands for pertinent past medical history. Information may be obtained from the patient, family or friends, medical records found on the patient or at the facility, medical identification bracelet, or by obtaining a list of medications the patient takes (e.g., insulin would indicate a patient with a diabetic history).

3-C. Three times the body height for adults and children is the general rule of thumb. For children the height of significance is 10 feet; however, falls from a lesser height can also be significant. Many factors must be evaluated: the surface the patient landed on, the body position upon impact, the patient's presentation during the initial assessment and physical examination, and the patient's past medical history.

4-B. If your patient becomes unstable during assessment, you should immediately reconsider your transportation priority. Do not falsely assure a patient that nothing is wrong. Putting smelling salts under the nose of an injured patient is inappropriate. Having the patient put her head between her knees does not address the problem and complicates the situation since you cannot provide spinal immobilization with the patient in this position.

5-D. Life-threatening injuries should be identified during the initial assessment. The focused history and physical examination for trauma patients includes the physical examination, assessment of baseline vital signs, and the SAMPLE history.

6-A. A vehicle-pedestrian collision is a significant mechanism of injury. While legal ramifications certainly surround this collision, your attention should be on providing the appropriate level of stabilization for this patient. Given the mechanism of injury, advanced-life-support personnel should be called to the scene.

7-C. Not until the patient is completely immobilized can you release manual immobilization regardless of the patient's denial of head or neck pain. The mechanism of injury suggests that this patient may have spinal compromise, regardless of current physical status. The cervical collar by itself does not provide sufficient support to maintain spinal alignment.

8-A. Although the patient's complaint was initially limited to the right leg, the mechanism of injury (vehicle striking a pedestrian) suggests that other injuries may be present. Therefore, the entire body should be rapidly inspected (looked at), auscultated (listened to), and palpated (felt).

9-D. DCAP-BTLS is a mnemonic designed to assist rescuers in remembering what signs to look for on a trauma patient. It stands for **d**eformities, **c**ontusions (bruises), **a**brasions (scrapes), **p**unctures or **p**enetrating wounds, **b**urns, **t**enderness to palpation, **l**acerations (cuts), and **s**welling. ABC is a mnemonic for initial assessment: **a**irway, **b**reathing, and **c**irculation. ALS refers to Advanced Life Support (e.g, EMT-Intermediates and EMT-Paramedics). DOT stands for the Department of Transportation.

10-B. Dressing the wound is the appropriate action. Use a dry, sterile dressing when available. Creams should be avoided as the patient may have an adverse reaction to such products. Do not attempt to close open wounds unless it is necessary to control bleeding. Closing the wound before it is disinfected may increase the risk of infection.

11-C. Up to 1 liter of blood can be lost due to a femur fracture (roughly 20% of this patient's total blood volume). Intervention should include a full assessment of the extremity and application of the appropriate splint. This condition may be aided by on-scene stabilization; however, it is crucial that this patient be transported to an appropriate medical facility.

12-D. Fluid, either blood or clear fluid, leaking from the ears may be indicative of a skull fracture. Attempting to stop the flow may lead to an increase in intracranial pressure.

13-D. Unequal pupils in the presence of a head injury can be assumed to indicate swelling of the brain (cerebral edema). In this case, the right pupil does not respond because the cerebral edema is compressing the nerve that controls pupil response (to the right eye). If the swelling progresses, both eyes may exhibit dilated, nonreactive pupils.

14-B. Bruising behind the ears, called Battle's sign, is generally indicative of a skull fracture. A chipped tooth or laceration may be found on a patient with a skull fracture, but they are not suggestive of one. Contrary to a falling blood pressure, the blood pressure of a patient with a head injury will often be high.

15-A. Because the laceration may be deep enough to cut the trachea, an occlusive dressing should be used to form an air-tight seal. If air is drawn into the surrounding tissues of the neck, a condition known as subcutaneous emphysema may result. This condition is detected by pushing on the tissues and noting a crackling sensation (like "bubble packs" under the skin). Wrapping the neck with gauze may have the effect of a tourniquet on the head and should be avoided. If the patient is breathing well on his own, there is no need to assist ventilations with the bag-valve mask.

BIBLIOGRAPHY

Bledsoe BE, Porter RS, Shade BR: *Paramedic Emergency Care,* 3rd ed. Englewood Cliffs, NJ, Prentice-Hall, 1997.

Butman AM, Martin SW, Vomacka RW, et al (eds): *Comprehensive Guide to Pre-Hospital Skills: A Skills Manual for EMT-Basic, EMT-Intermediate, EMT-Paramedic.* Akron, Ohio, Emergency Training, 1995.

Campbell JE (ed): *Basic Trauma Life Support for Paramedics and Advanced EMS Providers,* 3rd ed. Englewood Cliffs, NJ, Prentice-Hall, 1995.

Caroline NL: *Emergency Care in the Streets,* 4th ed. Boston, Little, Brown, 1991.

Crosby LA, Lewallen DG (eds): *Emergency Care and Transportation of the Sick and Injured,* 6th ed. Rosemont, IL, American Academy of Orthopaedic Surgeons, 1995.

Grant HD, Murray RH Jr, Bergeron JD: *Emergency Care,* 7th ed. Englewood Cliffs, NJ, Prentice-Hall, 1995.

Hafen BQ, Karren KJ, Mistovich JJ: *Prehospital Emergency Care,* 5th ed. Upper Saddle River, NJ, Prentice-Hall, 1996.

McSwain NE, White RD, Paturas JL, et al (eds): *The Basic EMT: Comprehensive Prehospital Patient Care.* St. Louis, Mosby-Year Book, 1996.

Stoy WA: *Mosby's EMT-Basic Textbook.* St. Louis, Mosby-Year Book, 1996.

United States Department of Transportation, National Highway Traffic Safety Administration: *Emergency Medical Technician: Basic. National Standard Curriculum,* 1994.

11-1   Describe the unique needs for assessing an individual with a specific chief complaint with no known prior history.

11-2   Differentiate between the history and physical examination that are performed for a responsive patient with no known prior history and a responsive patient with a known prior history.

11-3   Describe the unique needs for assessing an individual who is unresponsive or has an altered mental status.

11-4   Differentiate between the assessment that is performed for a patient who is unresponsive or has an altered mental status and other medical patients requiring assessment.

FOCUSED HISTORY AND PHYSICAL EXAMINATION: MEDICAL—COMPONENTS

The focused history and physical examination of a medical patient are guided by the patient's chief complaint and presenting signs and symptoms.

RESPONSIVE MEDICAL PATIENT

1. Determine the history of the present illness.
    a. The chief complaint is determined during the initial assessment.
    b. The chief complaint is the reason EMS was called, usually in the patient's own words.
2. Gather a SAMPLE history.
3. Perform a focused physical examination based on the patient's chief complaint. Assess the following body areas, if necessary:

• MOTIVATION FOR LEARNING •

The emergency medical care for the patient by the EMT-Basic is based upon assessment findings. In the focused history and physical exam of a medical patient, the EMT-Basic concentrates on the patient's complaint and history, allowing for rapid emergency medical care.

Scene Size-Up

Take body substance isolation precautions
Determine scene safety
Determine mechanism of injury/nature of illness
Determine number of patients
Request additional help if necessary

Initial Assessment

Form general impression of patient
Determine chief complaint/apparent life threats
Assess mental status (AVPU)
Assess airway
Assess breathing
Assess circulation
–Pulse
–Major bleeding
–Skin color, temperature, condition
Identify priority patients
Make transport decision

Focused History and Physical Examination

Perform focused physical examination or, if indicated, complete rapid assessment (DCAP-BTLS)
Obtain baseline vital signs
Obtain SAMPLE history
Reevaluate transport decision

Detailed Physical Examination

DCAP-BTLS
Reassess vital signs

Ongoing Assessment

Repeat initial assessment
Reassess vital signs
Repeat focused assessment regarding patient complaint or injuries
Reevaluate interventions

---

    a. Head
    b. Neck
    c. Chest
    d. Abdomen
    e. Pelvis
    f. Extremities
    g. Posterior body
4. Obtain baseline vital signs.

UNRESPONSIVE MEDICAL PATIENT

1. Conduct a rapid, head-to-toes physical examination by assessing the following body areas:
    a. Head
    b. Neck
    c. Chest
    d. Abdomen

   e. Pelvis
   f. Extremities
   g. Posterior body
2. Obtain baseline vital signs.
3. Obtain the history of the present illness (OPQRST) from family members or bystanders.
4. Obtain a SAMPLE history from family members or bystanders.

RESPONSIVE MEDICAL PATIENT

HISTORY OF PRESENT ILLNESS

Obtain **history of the present illness** (OPQRST).
1. The history of the present illness (OPQRST) provides a complete description of the patient's current complaint. This is the "S" component of the SAMPLE history.
2. When possible, ask open-ended questions.
   a. Open-ended questions do not require a "yes" or "no" answer.
   b. Open-ended questions often begin with "what," "how," or "when."
3. **OPQRST**
   a. **Onset:** "What were you doing when the problem started?"
   b. **Provocation:** "What makes the problem better or worse?"
   c. **Quality:** "What does the pain feel like (dull, sharp, pressure, tearing)?"
   d. **Region/Radiation**
      (1) "Where is the pain?"
      (2) "Is the pain in one area or does it move?"
      (3) "Is the pain located in any other area?"
   e. **Severity:** "On a scale of 1 to 10, with 1 being the least and 10 being the worst, what number would you assign your pain or discomfort?"
   f. **Time**
      (1) "How long ago did the problem/discomfort begin?"
      (2) "Have you ever had this pain before?" If the answer is yes:
         (a) "When?"
         (b) "How long did it last?"

SAMPLE HISTORY

Obtain SAMPLE history.
1. **Sign and symptoms** (OPQRST)
2. **Allergies**
   a. "Do you have any allergies to medications?"
   b. "Do you have any food allergies or allergies to pollen, dust, or grass?"
3. **Medications**
   a. "Do you take any prescription or over-the-counter medications?"
   b. "Do you use illegal drugs?"
   c. "Have you recently started taking any new medications?"
   d. "Have you recently stopped taking any medications?"
   e. Are you taking birth control pills? (If applicable.)
4. **Pertinent past medical history**
   a. "Are you seeing a physician for any medical problems?"
   b. "Do you have a history of heart problems, respiratory problems, kidney problems, liver problems, hypertension, diabetes, or epilepsy?"
   c. "Have you had any recent surgery?"
5. **Last oral intake**
   a. "When was the last time you had anything to eat or drink?"
   b. Determine what was ingested, how much was ingested, and when.
6. **Events leading to the illness:** "What were you doing just before this happened?"

CHIEF COMPLAINT AND PRIOR HISTORY

1. **Patient with a specific chief complaint and no known prior history**
   a. After obtaining the patient's history, the EMT-Basic may learn that the patient's chief complaint is new; the patient has had no previous episodes of the present problem.
   b. In these situations, the patient is usually transported to a medical facility for evaluation.
2. **Patient with a specific chief complaint and a known prior history**
   a. After obtaining the patient's history, the EMT-Basic may learn that the patient's chief complaint is a recurring event.
      (1) The patient may be seeing a physician regularly for treatment.
      (2) The patient may be taking prescribed medications for his or her complaint.
         (a) In specific situations, the EMT-Basic may assist the patient in taking his or her own prescribed medications, such as:
            (i) Epinephrine autoinjector for severe allergic reaction
            (ii) Nitroglycerin for chest pain of cardiac origin
            (iii) Inhaler for difficulty breathing
         (b) Check local protocol.
   b. In these situations, the patient is usually transported to a medical facility for evaluation.

FOCUSED PHYSICAL EXAMINATION

Perform a focused physical examination.
1. The focused physical examination is guided by the patient's chief complaint and presenting signs and symptoms.
2. Assess the following body areas, if necessary:
   a. Head
   b. Neck
   c. Chest
   d. Abdomen
   e. Pelvis
   f. Extremities
   g. Posterior body

ASSESSMENT OF BASELINE VITAL SIGNS

Obtain baseline vital signs; reassess and record vital signs at least every 15 minutes in the stable patient.
1. Assess respirations by evaluating:
   a. Rate
   b. Depth/equality
   c. Rhythm
   d. Alterations in respiration, including abnormal respiratory sounds
2. Assess pulse.
   a. Initially, a radial pulse should be assessed in all patients 1 year of age or older.
   b. In patients younger than 1 year of age, a brachial pulse should be assessed.
   c. If a pulse is present, assess:
      (1) Rate
      (2) Quality, including:
         (a) Strength [volume, which can be described as absent, weak, strong/full (normal), or bounding]
         (b) Rhythm
         (c) Equality
   d. Assess skin for:
      (1) Color

      (2)   Temperature

      (3)   Condition (moisture)

      (4)   Capillary refill in infants and children younger than 6 years of age

  e. Assess pupils for size, equality, and reactivity.

  f. Assess blood pressure.

      (1)   Blood pressure should be assessed in any patient older than 3 years of age.

      (2)   Whenever possible, blood pressure should be assessed by auscultation.

UNRESPONSIVE MEDICAL PATIENT

RAPID MEDICAL ASSESSMENT

Perform a rapid medical assessment.

  1. Position the patient to protect the airway.

  2. Assess the head.

    a. Look and feel for signs of trauma from an earlier injury.

    b. Inspect the:

      (1)   Face for symmetry (does one side of the face appear to droop?)

      (2)   Color of the sclerae (whites of the eyes); yellow discoloration (jaundice) suggests liver disease

      (3)   Ears and nose for leakage of blood or fluid

      (4)   Pupils for size, reactivity, and equality

      (5)   Mouth for blood, vomitus, foreign body, or secretions

    c. Note the presence of any unusual odors on the patient's breath, body, or clothing.

  3. Assess the neck and look for:

    a. **Jugular venous distention** (JVD) [distention of the neck veins when the patient is placed in a sitting position at a 45° angle] suggests injury to the chest, lungs, or heart.

    b. Presence of a **stoma** (surgical opening in the neck).

    c. Use of accessory muscles in the neck during breathing.

    d. Presence of a medical identification device.

  4. Assess the chest.

    a. Look for:

      (1)   Ease of respiratory effort (use of accessory muscles during breathing)

      (2)   Symmetrical rise and fall

      (3)   Shape of the chest; a barrel-shaped chest suggests chronic lung disease

    b. Listen for breath sounds.

      (1)   Listen to the chest in six places (Figure 11-1):

         (a) At the apices, midclavicular line bilaterally

         (b) At the bases bilaterally

         (c) In the midaxillary line bilaterally

      (2)   Compare from side to side.

      (3)   Determine if breath sounds are:

         (a) Present, diminished, or absent

         (b) Equal or unequal

         (c) Clear or noisy

  5. Assess the abdomen.

    a. The abdomen is assessed with the patient in a supine position.

    b. Look for:

      (1)   Evidence of obvious pregnancy

      (2)   Presence of abdominal **distention** (abdomen appears larger than normal). This sign is difficult to assess in obese patients.

    c. Feel all four quadrants for tenderness.

      (1)   Use the pads of your fingers to palpate the abdomen.

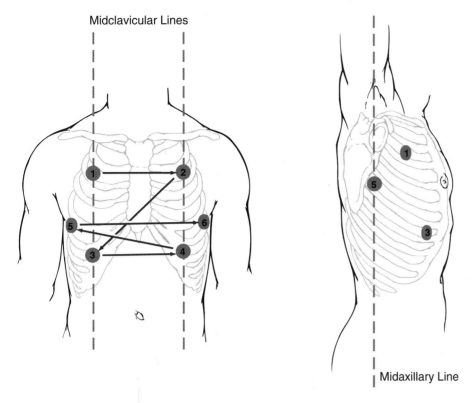

Midclavicular Lines

Midaxillary Line

Fig. 11-1. Listen to the chest in six places: at the apices in the midclavicular line bilaterally, at the bases bilaterally, and in the midaxillary line bilaterally. Compare from side to side.

        (2)   Begin palpating from the quadrant furthest away from the point of tenderness.

        (3)   Determine if the abdomen is soft or hard (rigid).

        (4)   Note the presence of any masses or pulsations.

        (5)   Observe the patient's face while palpating the abdomen; a grimace may indicate tenderness over a particular abdominal region.

6. Assess the pelvis. In the pregnant patient, observe the perineum for signs of imminent delivery.

7. Assess the extremities.

    a. Look for a medical identification device.

    b. Assess pulses, motor function, and sensation in each extremity.

    c. Look for swelling (edema) of the hands, feet, and ankles.

8. Assess the posterior body. Look for swelling in the sacral region; in patients confined to bed, fluid collects in the sacral region.

ASSESSMENT OF BASELINE VITAL SIGNS

Obtain baseline vital signs; reassess and record vital signs at least every 5 minutes in the unresponsive medical patient.

1. Assess respirations by evaluating:

    a. Rate

    b. Depth/equality

    c. Rhythm

    d. Alterations in respiration, including abnormal respiratory sounds

2. Assess pulse.

    a. Initially, a radial pulse should be assessed in all patients 1 year of age or older.

    b. In patients younger than 1 year of age, a brachial pulse should be assessed.

    c. If a pulse is present, assess:

      (1)   Rate
      (2)   Quality
3. Assess skin by evaluating:
   a. Color
   b. Temperature
   c. Condition (moisture)
   d. Capillary refill in infants and children less than 6 years of age
4. Assess pupil size, equality, and reactivity.
5. Assess blood pressure.
   a. Blood pressure should be assessed in any patient older than 3 years of age.
   b. Whenever possible, blood pressure should be assessed by auscultation.

PATIENT HISTORY

Obtain patient history.
1. Obtain the history of the present illness (OPQRST) from family members or bystanders.
2. Obtain a SAMPLE history from family members or bystanders.

REVIEW QUESTIONS

Directions: Each of the numbered items or incomplete statements in this section is followed by answers or by completions of the statement. Select the ONE lettered answer or completion that is BEST in each case.

1. The first step of the focused history and physical examination for an unresponsive patient is to

   (A)   obtain a baseline set of vital signs
   (B)   conduct a rapid physical examination
   (C)   obtain a SAMPLE history from family members or bystanders
   (D)   obtain a history of present illness from family members or bystanders

2. When treating a responsive patient with a medical complaint, the focused physical examination should be

   (A)   the same as for an unresponsive patient
   (B)   the same as for a traumatically injured patient
   (C)   conducted before obtaining a history of the present illness
   (D)   based on the patient's complaint and presenting signs and symptoms

3. One component of the SAMPLE history deals with the patient's medications ("M" for medications). Which of the following best describes the information you need to elicit about the patient's medications?

   (A)   Medications the patient is allergic to
   (B)   Medications related to the current complaint
   (C)   Prescription medications the patient is currently taking
   (D)   Prescription and over-the-counter medications the patient is currently taking or recently stopped taking

4. For an unresponsive patient, vital signs should be assessed at least every

   (A)   2 minutes
   (B)   5 minutes

    (C)   10 minutes

    (D)   20 minutes

5. Which of the following attributes should be evaluated during the respiratory assessment?

    (A)   Respiratory rate and lung sounds

    (D)   Respiratory rate, depth, rhythm, and lung sounds

    (C)   Respiratory rate, capillary refill, and lung sounds

    (D)   Respiratory rate, pulse rate, capillary refill, and lung sounds

6. While assessing pupil response in an unresponsive patient, particular attention should be paid to

    (A)   pupil size, equality, and reactivity

    (B)   iris color, size, equality, and reactivity

    (C)   pupil reactivity, equality, and tracking

    (D)   pupil size, equality, and response to pain

7. During assessment of baseline vital signs, pulses should be assessed. In patients younger than 1 year of age, where should pulses be assessed initially?

    (A)   Radial artery

    (B)   Carotid artery

    (C)   Femoral artery

    (D)   Brachial artery

8. Your ambulance crew responds to the home of a 65-year-old man complaining of severe shortness of breath. Upon arrival, you find the patient supine on the ground. He is conscious and in severe respiratory distress, speaking in one- to two-word sentences. During your focused history and physical examination, you note that this patient has a "barrel chest." This finding may indicate a past medical history of

    (A)   diabetes

    (B)   gallstones

    (C)   chronic lung disease

    (D)   cerebrovascular accident (CVA)

Directions: Each of the numbered questions or incomplete statements in this section refers to a scenario that precedes them. The numbered questions or incomplete statements are followed by answers or by completions of the statement. Select the answer or completion of the statement that is BEST in each case.

Your ambulance crew has been called to a restaurant for a 54-year-old female patient complaining of chest pain. On arrival, you note that the patient is awake, responsive, and speaking in full sentences without obvious difficulty.

Questions 9–13

9. The first step in this patient's focused history and physical examination should be to

    (A)   obtain a history of present illness

    (B)   conduct a rapid trauma assessment

    (C)   lay the patient supine on the ground

    (D)   open the patient's airway with a modified jaw thrust

10. Which of the following questions should you use when asking a patient about his or her discomfort?

(A) "Are you having chest pain?"
(B) "Have you had pain like this before?"
(C) "Are you having difficulty breathing?"
(D) "Would you describe how you are feeling?"

11. Which of the following acronyms would assist you in questioning the patient about the history of this present illness?

(A) NREMT
(B) OPQRST
(C) SAMPLE
(D) DCAP-BTLS

12. Which of the following acronyms would assist you in gathering information about the patient's past medical history?

(A) NREMT
(B) OPQRST
(C) SAMPLE
(D) DCAP-BTLS

13. When asked to describe her chest pain, the patient states, "I was sitting here having dinner when I all of a sudden got this chest pain. It's been going on for about the past 20 minutes. It feels very sharp on my left side and hurts more when I take a deep breath. It makes my shoulder ache, too." To complete your history of present illness questioning using the OPQRST acronym, what would be an appropriate question to ask this patient?

(A) "What medications are you allergic to?"
(B) "What medications are you currently taking?"
(C) "When is the last time you were seen by a physician?"
(D) "On a scale of 1 to 10 with 10 being the worst pain you have felt, how would you rate this pain?"

Your ambulance crew is called by concerned neighbors to check the welfare of a 64-year-old woman who has not been seen for several days. Upon arrival, you find the patient moaning unintelligibly in her bed. A shoe box full of medication bottles is on her nightstand. She does not respond to your or your crew. The scene is safe. The initial assessment reveals that the patient has a clear airway, is breathing adequately, has a weak radial pulse, and responds to painful stimuli by moaning more loudly.

Questions 14–17

14. Your next step should be to

(A) begin a rapid medical assessment
(B) attempt to contact the patient's next of kin
(C) examine and record the medications in the shoe box
(D) attempt to obtain information from the concerned neighbors about the patient's past medical history

15. While examining this patient, you attempt to check the symmetry of her face. Facial symmetry refers to

(A) the condition of the fontanelles
(B) the condition of the mucous membranes
(C) the presence of drainage from the nose or mouth
(D) comparing the muscle tone of one side of the face to the other

16. While assessing this patient's neck, you check for jugular venous distention (JVD). JVD is assessed by looking for distention of the neck veins with the patient in _____ position.

(A) prone
(B) supine
(C) Trendelenburg (head lower than the feet)
(D) semi-Fowler's (sitting up at a 45° angle)

17. Which of the following regarding evaluation of this patient's abdomen is correct?

(A) Evaluation of the abdomen is unnecessary because the patient is unresponsive
(B) Evaluation of the abdomen is useful since this patient may react if palpation of the abdomen elicits pain
(C) Evaluation of the abdomen is useful only if the patient has a past medical history of abdominal or pelvic problems
(D) Evaluation of the abdomen does not reveal anything about the medical patient and is only valuable in the trauma patient

Your crew is called to the home of a 2-year-old male patient "not acting normal" according to the child's mother. The mother states the child has had a runny nose for 2 weeks and for the last 2 nights he has been up all night coughing and wheezing. When questioned about his condition, the child states, "Gotta runny nose." He is currently taking children's Tylenol® and a children's strength decongestant.

Questions 18–20

18. A focused physical examination

(A) should not be performed as it would be a waste of time
(B) should be performed mainly to look for signs of child abuse
(C) should be limited to the nose and chest
(D) should include evaluation of the face, neck, chest, back, and abdomen

19. When obtaining baseline vital signs on this patient, a blood pressure

(A) should be palpated
(B) should be auscultated
(C) should be taken on the leg
(D) is not absolutely necessary

20. When assessing this patient's anterior (chest) breath sounds, you should listen with a stethoscope

(A) in two places
(B) in three places
(C) in five places
(D) in six places

ANSWERS AND RATIONALES

1-B. If a patient is unresponsive, it is impossible to obtain a history of present illness from the patient. Therefore, to gain a better understanding of the factors involved with the patient's condition, a rapid medical assessment must be performed. However, you may be able to obtain information about the patient's history of present illness from family members or bystanders. You may question family members and bystanders while conducting the rapid medical assessment as long as you are able to process both sets of information simultaneously.

2-D. Your physical examination should be guided by the patient's complaint and presenting signs and symptoms. However, this does NOT mean that you would only evaluate the area of pain. For example, a patient with chest pain may have significant physical findings in areas other than the chest (e.g., pedal edema, jugular venous distention). By identifying the chief complaint before the physical examination, a more meaningful and detailed exam can be performed.

3-D. You should attempt to obtain as complete a picture as possible. A complete picture of the patient's medications includes both prescription and over-the-counter medications that the patient is currently taking or has recently stopped taking. The medications that the patient is allergic to are addressed in SAMPLE ("A" for allergies). Because drugs may interact in many ways, it is important to list all of the patient's medications, not just those you suspect are related to the patient's current complaint.

4-B. Vital signs should be assessed at least every 5 minutes in unresponsive patients. If the patient's condition changes, vital signs should be reassessed, regardless of the time of the last vital signs. For example, if a patient who was moaning loudly suddenly stops moaning, you should immediately reassess the patient's airway, breathing, circulation, and mental status and then obtain a set of vital signs.

5-B. When evaluating respiratory status for baseline vital signs, it is important to note the rate of respirations, the depth (amount of air moved or tidal volume), the rhythm of respirations, and lung sounds. Capillary refill is assessed during assessment of skin condition. Pulse rate is also addressed during in vital signs but not as a component of the patient's respiratory status. An abnormal finding in one area may influence the response in another.

6-A. Proper pupil assessment should include the pupil size, equality, and reactivity. Some health care professionals refer to the pupil as the "window to the brain." The nerve that controls pupil response comes directly from the brain; therefore, changes in the condition of the central nervous system may be observed by abnormal pupil response (e.g., unequal or nonreactive pupils).

7-D. Brachial pulses should be initially assessed in patients under 1 year of age. Infants have necks that are short and stubby, making palpation of a carotid pulse difficult. Brachial pulses are initially more accessible than femoral pulses, and radial pulses may be difficult to locate.

8-C. A barrel chest is common in patients with a past medical history of chronic lung disease such as emphysema and bronchitis. Due to the chronic (long-term) nature of these diseases and the increased effort involved with breathing, it is not uncommon for the chest wall of these patients to change dimensions over time. A patient with a past medical history of diabetes may appear very thin and may be a partial amputee due to the destructive effect diabetes can have on the peripheral vasculature. A patient with a history of gallstones may present with a surgical scar over the right upper quadrant of the abdomen. Finally, a patient with a past medical history of a cerebrovascular accident (CVA) may present with neuromuscular deficits (e.g., partial paralysis, impaired speech, personality changes, and facial droop).

9-A. The first step in a focused history and physical evaluation for a responsive patient is to obtain a history of the present illness and the patient's chief complaint. The information gathered during the history taking will help guide and prioritize the actions that follow. A rapid trauma assessment would not be appropriate unless this patient's complaint stemmed from a traumatic event (i.e., vehicle collision). Putting the patient in a supine position may be appropriate in some cases; however, it is not a priority unless the patient shows signs that she may pass out and fall to the ground. Finally, the modified jaw thrust is used to open the airway of a potentially spinal-compromised patient. This patient is neither spinally compromised nor in need of assistance keeping her airway open.

10-D. While questioning the patient about her pain and breathing status is appropriate, it is best to use open-ended questions. Open-ended questions are those that cannot be answered with a "yes" or "no." By using open ended questions, you are assured that you will not be putting words or thoughts in the patient's mouth. You may still direct the patient's responses (many times patients will wander from pertinent information), but it is best to do so by allowing the patient to tell you her "story" about what is happening.

11-B. OPQRST is the correct response. Each letter of the OPQRST acronym represents a line of questioning about a different facet of this complaint. NREMT stands for National Registry of Emergency Medical Technicians, the agency that provides national EMT certification. SAMPLE is an acronym used to obtain information about the patient's past medical history (as opposed to the current complaint). DCAP-BTLS is the acronym used to recall the injuries to look for during a physical assessment of a trauma patient.

12-C. The SAMPLE acronym assists in obtaining information about the patient's past medical history. SAMPLE stands for **s**igns and **s**ymptoms, **a**llergies, **m**edications, pertinent **p**ast medical history, **l**ast oral intake, and **e**vents leading up to this illness.

13-D. In response to an initial open-ended question, this patient gave all the OPQRST information with the exception of "S," severity. The questions listed in "A" through "C" are all appropriate questions to ask. However, organizing the questions so that you deal with the current complaint followed by the patient's history is much less confusing to the patient. It is helpful to have one person asking questions of the patient, rather than having the patient answer questions from everyone on the scene. This allows a logical progression of questioning and also allows the patient to develop a rapport with the rescuer asking the questions.

14-A. Since this patient is unresponsive, you should IMMEDIATELY attempt to identify the factors influencing her condition through a rapid medical assessment. If you have sufficient personnel, you may want to send a crew member to find a neighbor knowledgeable about the patient's present illness and past medical history. If the information is readily available, notifying relatives (next of kin) may also assist in gaining insight into the patient's presentation. The types of medications in the shoe box may also assist you in gathering more information about the patient. Many receiving facilities prefer that these medications be brought with the patient.

15-D. Evaluating facial symmetry refers to checking for a difference in muscle tone on one side of the face compared to the other. A lack of symmetry is often referred to as "facial droop" and may be indicative of a cerebrovascular accident (CVA; stroke; "brain attack"). Checking for symmetry in a completely unresponsive patient may be impossible; however, since this patient is moaning, you may note a lack of symmetry about the mouth. Fontanels are "soft spots" in an infant's skull and are not present in adults (the bones fuse together at about 18 months of age). The condition of the mucous membranes of the mouth and eyes, whether moist or dry, may give you a good indication about how long the patient has been ill.

16-D. Jugular venous distention (JVD) is clinically evaluated with the body at a 45° angle. When the patient is prone, supine, or in a Trendelenburg position, JVD may be present merely due to gravity's effect on blood flow.

17-B. Since this patient is unresponsive, a rapid physical examination should be performed that includes an evaluation of all body regions and systems. When palpating the abdomen of a patient with an altered mental status, you should note the position the patient is in (fetal position may indicate abdominal pain). Visualize the abdomen for color, scars (indicating past abdominal surgery), or other abnormalities. Finally, palpate the abdomen while paying close attention to any response the patient may exhibit (tightening of the muscles, grimacing, increased moaning).

18-D. Resist the temptation to only evaluate the region of the medical complaint! While this patient's complaint centers on the respiratory system, many signs of respiratory compromise may be found throughout the body. It is necessary to evaluate this patient's chest, back, and abdomen for signs of accessory muscle use. Lung sounds may be auscultated at the chest and the back. With children, it is sometimes easier to evaluate lung sounds on the back because a parent can hold the patient to his or her chest during the examination.

19-D. In children younger than 3 years of age, blood pressure assessment is not absolutely necessary in the prehospital setting. These patients don't typically lend themselves to having their blood pressure taken. In a child, a falling blood pressure is an ominously late sign of compromise. By the time a child's blood pressure begins to drop, the child should have other physical signs (such as poor capillary refill, altered level of consciousness, persistent tachycardia) that indicate extreme illness. Check your local protocols about assessment of blood pressure in children under 3 years of age.

20-D. To adequately evaluate lung sounds, it is necessary to auscultate six regions of the chest: both apices at the midclavicular line, both bases, and both midaxillary lines. Compare the sounds from one side to the other, rather than top to bottom on the same side. For example, compare the sounds heard at the left lung base to the sounds heard at the right lung base.

BIBLIOGRAPHY

Bledsoe B: *Paramedic Emergency Care*, 3rd ed. Englewood Cliffs, NJ, Prentice-Hall, 1997.

Campbell J (ed): *Basic Trauma Life Support for Paramedics and Advanced EMS Providers*, 3rd ed. Englewood Cliffs, NJ, Prentice-Hall, 1995.

Caroline NL: *Emergency Care in the Streets*, 4th ed. Boston, Little, Brown, 1991.

Crosby LA, Lewallen DG (eds): *Emergency Care and Transportation of the Sick and Injured*, 6th ed. Rosemont, IL, American Academy of Orthopaedic Surgeons, 1995.

Grant HD, Murray RH Jr, Bergeron JD: *Emergency Care*, 7th ed. Englewood Cliffs, NJ, Prentice-Hall, 1995.

Hafen BQ, Karren KJ, Mistovich JJ: *Prehospital Emergency Care*, 5th ed. Upper Saddle River, NJ, Prentice-Hall, 1996.

McSwain NE, White RD, Paturas JL, et al (eds): *The Basic EMT: Comprehensive Prehospital Patient Care*. St. Louis, Mosby-Year Book, 1996.

Stoy, WA: *Mosby's EMT-Basic Textbook*. St. Louis, Mosby-Year Book, 1996.

United States Department of Transportation, National Highway Traffic Safety Administration: *Emergency Medical Technician: Basic. National Standard Curriculum*, 1994.

12-1   Discuss the components of the detailed physical examination.

12-2   State the areas of the body evaluated during the detailed physical examination.

12-3   Explain what additional care should be provided while performing the detailed physical examination.

12-4   Distinguish between the detailed physical examination performed on a trauma patient and that performed on a medical patient.

DETAILED PHYSICAL EXAMINATION—OVERVIEW

DEFINITION

1. The detailed examination is a head-to-toes examination.
   a. It repeats many steps performed in the rapid trauma or medical assessment in more depth.
   b. It may identify additional injuries or other information that will help determine the patient's illness or injury.
2. The **detailed physical examination** is patient and injury specific.
3. It is guided by the acronym **DCAP-BTLS.**
4. A patient with an isolated injury, such as a painful ankle, would not require a detailed physical examination.

MOTIVATION FOR LEARNING

The EMT-Basic makes decisions about the emergency medical care to be delivered based on his or her findings during assessment of the patient. The detailed physical examination is performed after the focused history and physical examination and after all critical interventions have been completed. Depending upon the severity of the patient's injury or illness, this assessment may not be completed. The detailed physical examination may identify additional injuries or other information that will help determine the patient's illness or injury.

Scene Size-Up

Take body substance isolation precautions
Determine scene safety
Determine mechanism of injury/nature of illness
Determine number of patients
Request additional help if necessary

Initial Assessment

Form general impression of patient
Determine chief complaint/apparent life threats
Assess mental status (AVPU)
Assess airway
Assess breathing
Assess circulation
–Pulse
–Major bleeding
–Skin color, temperature, condition
Identify priority patients
Make transport decision

Focused History and Physical Examination

Perform focused physical examination or, if indicated, complete rapid assessment (DCAP-BTLS)
Obtain baseline vital signs
Obtain SAMPLE history
Reevaluate transport decision

Detailed Physical Examination
DCAP-BTLS
Reassess vital signs

Ongoing Assessment

Repeat initial assessment
Reassess vital signs
Repeat focused assessment regarding patient complaint or injuries
Reevaluate interventions

PATIENTS WHO SHOULD RECEIVE A DETAILED PHYSICAL EXAMINATION

A detailed physical examination should be performed for:
1. Trauma patients with a significant mechanism of injury
2. Trauma patients with an unknown or unclear mechanism of injury
3. Unconscious patients or a patient with an altered mental status

WHEN TO PERFORM A DETAILED PHYSICAL EXAMINATION

The detailed physical examination is performed only after all critical interventions have been performed.
1. Depending on the severity of the patient's injury or illness, the detailed physical examination may not be completed.
2. Treatment of life-threatening conditions takes precedence over performance of the examination.

DETAILED PHYSICAL EXAMINATION—PROCEDURE

HEAD

1. **Scalp and skull.** Assess DCAP-BTLS plus crepitation, depressions, protrusions, and discoloration.
2. **Ears**
   a. Look for blood or clear fluid in the ears.
   b. Look for **Battle's sign.**
3. **Face.** Assess DCAP-BTLS plus singed facial hair, symmetry, instability, tenderness, and crepitation.
4. **Eyes**
   a. Assess DCAP-BTLS plus discoloration, presence of a foreign body, and blood in the anterior chamber of the eye (hyphema).
   b. Assess the pupils for size, equality, and reactivity to light.
5. **Nose.** Assess DCAP-BTLS plus blood or fluid from the nose, singed nasal hairs, and stability of nasal bones.
6. **Mouth**
   a. Assess DCAP-BTLS plus presence of a foreign body, blood, vomitus, unusual breath odor, absent or broken teeth, and injured or swollen tongue.
   b. Look at the color of the mucous membranes of the mouth.

NECK

Assess DCAP-BTLS plus:
1. Crepitation
2. Position of the trachea
   a. The trachea should be in a midline position.
   b. Note any deviation from this position.
3. Jugular venous distention (JVD)
4. Subcutaneous emphysema
5. Presence of a medical identification device
6. Presence of a stoma (surgical opening in the neck)
7. Use of accessory muscles in the neck during breathing

CHEST

Assess DCAP-BTLS plus:
1. Breath sounds
2. Shape of the chest
3. Symmetrical rise and fall
4. Ease of respiratory effort (use of accessory muscles during breathing)

ABDOMEN

Assess DCAP-BTLS plus:
1. Evidence of obvious pregnancy
2. Presence of abdominal distention, masses, pulsations, or evisceration
3. Firmness/hardness

PELVIS

Assess DCAP-BTLS plus (Figure 12-1):
1. Pain, motion, crepitation
2. In the pregnant patient, observe the perineum for signs of imminent delivery
3. Look for signs of bowel or bladder incontinence

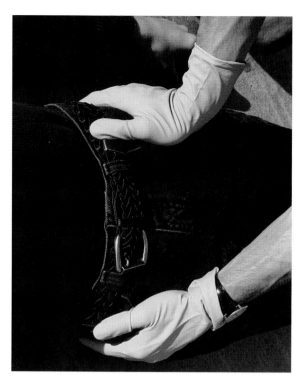

Fig. 12-1. Assess the stability of the pelvis noting the presence of tenderness, instability, and/or crepitation. If the patient complains of pain in the pelvic region, or obvious deformity is present, do NOT palpate the pelvis.

EXTREMITIES

Assess DCAP-BTLS plus:
1. Abnormal extremity position
2. Tenderness, instability, and crepitation
3. Presence of a medical identification device
4. Assess distal pulses, motor function, and sensation

POSTERIOR BODY

Assess DCAP-BTLS plus:
1. In bedridden patients, look for swelling in the sacral region
2. Tenderness, instability, and crepitation

REASSESSMENT OF VITAL SIGNS

Reassess vital signs.

ELEMENTS

Vital signs include:
1. Respirations
2. Pulse
3. Blood pressure
4. Pupils
5. Skin color, temperature, condition (moisture)
6. Capillary refill in infants and children younger than 6 years of age

STABLE PATIENT

In a stable patient, reassess and record vital signs at least every 15 minutes.

UNSTABLE PATIENT

In the unstable patient, reassess and record vital signs at least every 5 minutes.

COMPARISON OF VITAL SIGNS

Compare baseline vital signs with repeat measurements, noting any changes or trends.

CONTINUATION OF EMERGENCY CARE

LIFE-THREATENING CONDITIONS

Life-threatening conditions must be managed as soon as they are found.

LESS CRITICAL CONDITIONS

Less critical conditions can be managed as they are found during the detailed physical examination. Examples include:
1. Abrasions and lacerations: provide wound care
2. Swollen, discolored, deformed extremity: provide immobilization
3. Minor bleeding: control bleeding and provide wound care

TRAUMA PATIENT VERSUS MEDICAL PATIENT EXAMINATION

The detailed physical examination is patient and injury specific.

TRAUMA PATIENT

1. A patient with an isolated injury, such as a painful ankle or a cut finger, would not generally require a detailed physical examination.
2. A patient who has sustained trauma to more than one area of the body requires a detailed (head-to-toes) physical examination.

MEDICAL PATIENT

1. A responsive medical patient should receive a detailed physical examination based on the patient's history and focused physical examination findings.
2. For example, a patient with chest pain and difficulty breathing should receive a detailed (head-to-toes) physical examination.

UNRESPONSIVE PATIENTS

All unresponsive patients should receive a detailed physical examination.

REVIEW QUESTIONS

Directions: Each of the numbered items or incomplete statements in this section is followed by answers or by completions of the statement. Select the ONE lettered answer or completion that is BEST in each case.

1. Which of the following describes the detailed physical examination?

   (A)   A rapid assessment for life-threatening conditions
   (B)   An assessment of the patient's airway, breathing, circulatory status

    (C)   A head-to-toes examination to identify additional injuries or other information

    (D)   A quick assessment of the scene, safety concerns, and resource requirements

2. At what point is the detailed physical examination performed?

    (A)   Immediately with unconscious patients
    (B)   Before the focused history and physical examination
    (C)   Following the focused history and physical examination
    (D)   Before stabilization of life-threatening injuries or illnesses

3. Your ambulance crew is dispatched to the scene of a high-speed motor vehicle collision. You are assigned responsibility for a patient who was ejected from one of the vehicles. He has massive head and chest trauma. He is not breathing and does not have a pulse. The detailed physical examination

    (A)   should be performed before starting cardiopulmonary resuscitation (CPR)
    (B)   should be performed quickly while stopping CPR
    (C)   should be performed before leaving the scene of the collision
    (D)   may not be performed due to the extent of this patient's injuries

4. Your rescue crew is called to a local park for a 34-year-old male patient complaining of ankle pain. Upon arrival, you find your patient sitting on a bench seat with a shoe off and ice on his foot. He states he was playing tennis with his wife when he twisted his ankle. He did not fall to the ground. He denies any other complaint. The detailed physical examination

    (A)   should be performed immediately
    (B)   should be performed after scene size-up
    (C)   may be omitted due to the extent of this patient's injury
    (D)   should be performed in conjunction with the initial assessment

5. Which of the following correctly identifies when a detailed physical examination should be performed?

    (A)   Trauma patient with an unknown or unclear mechanism of injury
    (B)   Trauma patient with a significant mechanism of injury
    (C)   Unconscious patients or patients with an altered mental status
    (D)   All of the above

Directions: Each of the numbered questions or incomplete statements in this section refers to a scenario that precedes them. The numbered questions or incomplete statements are followed by answers or by completions of the statement. Select the answer or completion of the statement that is BEST in each case.

Your rescue crew is called for a 27-year-old male patient who is threatening suicide. You stage a safe distance from the scene until the local law enforcement agency informs you that the scene is safe. You arrive at the scene to find the patient covered with blood. He tells you he was in a fight last night and now he wants to die. He smells of alcohol, and an empty bottle of whiskey is on the nightstand. The following questions refer to the detailed physical examination.

Questions 6–10

6. While examining the patient's head, you look behind the patient's ears for bruising. If present, this finding is called

    (A)   Meningitis
    (B)   Battle's sign
    (C)   Hemothorax
    (D)   Raccoon's eyes

7. While examining the patient's neck, you should check for

    (A)   pupil response
    (B)   distal sensation
    (C)   jugular venous distention (JVD)
    (D)   the color of the mucous membranes

8. During your examination of the patient's chest, you note crepitus and pain on palpation of the lower left chest wall. Crepitus is the sound or sensation of

    (A)   air leaking into the pleura
    (B)   bone ends grinding together
    (C)   blood leaking into the pericardium
    (D)   blood leaking into the subdural space

9. After removing this patient's shirt to perform your examination, you note a loop of bowel protruding from an abdominal laceration. This finding is called

    (A)   an evisceration
    (B)   a placenta previa
    (C)   a uterine inversion
    (D)   an abdominal aortic aneurysm

10. When questioned about alcohol ingestion, the patient denies having had any alcoholic beverages in the last 24 hours. He smells of alcohol and is acting intoxicated. Which of the following would be a safe assumption?

    (A)   The patient is lying to avoid being arrested
    (B)   The patient is drunk and cannot remember the drinking incident
    (C)   The patient is severely intoxicated and may die as a result of alcohol poisoning
    (D)   Some other condition may be present that warrants more attention during the detailed physical examination

ANSWERS AND RATIONALES

1-C. The detailed physical examination is conducted to provide additional information about the patient's chief complaint. The additional information may be the presence of additional injuries or other signs related to the injury or illness. A rapid assessment for life-threatening injuries is part of the initial assessment, as is assessment of airway, breathing, and circulation. The quick assessment of the scene, safety factors, and resource requirements is part of scene size-up.

2-C. The detailed physical examination is performed after the focused history and physical examination. Stabilization of unconscious patients or potentially life-threatening conditions take precedence over the detailed physical examination. The focused history and physical examination also take precedence over the detailed physical examination.

3-D. The detailed physical examination is performed only after all critical interventions have been performed. Do not delay life-saving interventions such as cardiopulmonary resuscitation (CPR) or rapid transportation to perform a detailed physical examination.

4-C. Since this patient has an isolated, minor injury without complications, a detailed physical examination is not necessary. If the patient suffered a fall or appeared to have other injuries, a detailed examination would be performed after the focused history and physical examination.

5-D. While previous questions have stressed that a detailed physical examination is not always completed, this question illustrates the usefulness of the detailed physical examination to help "complete the picture." If the mechanism of injury is vague or suggests something more than what the patient is telling you, conduct a detailed physical examination. Also, if the patient is not able to express his or her complaint, conduct a detailed physical examination.

6-B. Battle's sign is the presence of bruising behind the ear at the mastoid process. This finding is suggestive of a basilar skull fracture. Meningitis is an inflammation of the meninges, the protective coverings of the central nervous system. Hemothorax is the presence of blood in the pleural space that surrounds the lungs. Raccoon's eyes is the presence of bilateral black eyes and can suggest the presence of a basilar skull fracture.

7-C. Jugular venous distention (JVD) is assessed at the neck with the patient sitting at a 45° angle. Pupil response refers to the reactivity of the eyes to light. Distal sensation assesses the presence of sensation in the extremities. The color of the mucous membranes may be assessed by examining the oropharynx.

8-B. Crepitus is the grinding sensation or sound created when bone ends rub together. Crepitus at the chest wall would suggest fractured ribs and possibly damage to the underlying organs. In this case, with crepitus to the lower left chest wall, you should be particularly concerned about the integrity of the lungs, heart, and spleen. Air leaking into the pleura is a pneumothorax. A pneumothorax may accompany this patient's injury. Blood leaking into the pericardium is called a pericardial tamponade. It, too, may accompany this patient's injury. Blood leaking into the subdural space is called a subdural hematoma. Based on the patient's altered mental status, a head injury must also be suspected.

9-A. Exposed abdominal contents is called an abdominal evisceration. If found, the abdominal organs should be kept clean, moist, and warm. Returning the organs to the abdominal cavity is the responsibility of a physician. Placenta previa and uterine inversion are complications of pregnancy. An abdominal aortic aneurysm is created by a weak spot in the aorta (major artery) as it passes through the abdomen. An abdominal aortic aneurysm can be life threatening.

10-D. This patient may be lying to you or may be too intoxicated to recognize the truth. You must investigate further to rule out any other problems. This patient may have diabetes and could be experiencing a diabetic emergency. In a diabetic emergency, the patient may have an altered mental status and may smell of alcohol. Beware of assumptions!

BIBLIOGRAPHY

Crosby LA, Lewallen DG (eds): *Emergency Care and Transportation of the Sick and Injured*, 6th ed. Rosemont, IL, American Academy of Orthopaedic Surgeons, 1995.

Grant HD, Murray RH Jr, Bergeron JD: *Emergency Care*, 7th ed. Englewood Cliffs, NJ, Prentice-Hall, 1995.

Hafen BQ, Karren KJ, Mistovich JJ: *Prehospital Emergency Care*, 5th ed. Upper Saddle River, NJ, Prentice-Hall, 1996.

McSwain NE, White RD, Paturas JL, et al (eds): *The Basic EMT: Comprehensive Prehospital Patient Care*. St. Louis, Mosby-Year Book, 1996.

Stoy, WA: *Mosby's EMT-Basic Textbook*. St. Louis: Mosby-Year Book, 1996.

United States Department of Transportation, National Highway Traffic Safety Administration: *Emergency Medical Technician: Basic. National Standard Curriculum*, 1994.

13

13-1   Discuss the reasons for repeating the initial assessment as part of the ongoing assessment.
13-2   Describe the components of the ongoing assessment.
13-3   Describe how to look for trends in assessment findings.

ONGOING ASSESSMENT

OVERVIEW

1. The **ongoing assessment** should be performed on EVERY patient.
2. It should be performed after completion of critical interventions.
3. It is performed after the detailed physical examination, if one is performed (in some situations, the patient's condition may prevent performance of the detailed physical examination).
4. It is often performed en route to the receiving facility; if transport is delayed, the ongoing assessment should be performed on the scene.

PURPOSE

1. The ongoing assessment allows the EMT-Basic to reevaluate the patient's condition.
2. It allows assessment of the effectiveness of emergency care interventions provided.
3. It can identify any missed injuries or conditions.
4. It allows the EMT-Basic to observe subtle changes or trends in the patient's condition.
5. It allows the EMT-Basic to alter emergency care interventions as needed.

● MOTIVATION FOR LEARNING ●

To assure appropriate care, the EMT-Basic must frequently reevaluate the patient. These reevaluations are called ongoing assessments. The length of time spent with the patient or the condition of the patient will assist in establishing how often the ongoing assessments will be conducted. It is important to accurately document all findings and interventions as well as the time at which this care is provided.

Scene Size-Up

Take body substance isolation precautions
Determine scene safety
Determine mechanism of injury/nature of illness
Determine number of patients
Request additional help if necessary

Initial Assessment

Form general impression of patient
Determine chief complaint/apparent life threats
Assess mental status (AVPU)
Assess airway
Assess breathing
Assess circulation
–Pulse
–Major bleeding
–Skin color, temperature, condition
Identify priority patients
Make transport decision

Focused History and Physical Examination

Perform focused physical examination or, if indicated, complete rapid assessment (DCAP-BTLS)
Obtain baseline vital signs
Obtain SAMPLE history
Reevaluate transport decision

Detailed Physical Examination
DCAP-BTLS
Reassess vital signs

Ongoing Assessment

Repeat initial assessment
Reassess vital signs
Repeat focused assessment regarding patient complaint or injuries
Reevaluate interventions

COMPONENTS OF THE ONGOING ASSESSMENT

1. Repeat the initial assessment in order to identify and treat life-threatening injuries.
2. Reassess and document vital signs and note changes or trends in the patient's condition.
3. Repeat the focused assessment.
4. Reevaluate emergency care interventions.

REPEATING THE INITIAL ASSESSMENT

REASSESSMENT OF MENTAL STATUS

Reassess mental status.
1. Note any changes in the patient's mental status.
2. For patients with an altered mental status, document the patient's response to a specific stimulus.

    a. Communicate any changes in mental status to medical personnel at the receiving facility.

    b. Document any changes in mental status in the prehospital care report (PCR).

REASSESSMENT OF THE PATIENT'S AIRWAY

Reassess the patient's airway.

  1. If the patient is able to talk clearly and without difficulty, assume his or her airway is open.

  2. If the patient is unresponsive, inspect the mouth for actual or potential obstruction (e.g., foreign body, blood, vomitus, teeth, tongue).

  3. Document and communicate any changes or trends to the staff at the receiving facility.

REASSESSMENT OF BREATHING

Reassess breathing.

  1. Reassess breathing rate and quality by noting:

    a. Rise and fall of the chest

    b. Respiratory rate

    c. Depth/equality of breathing

    d. Rhythm of respirations

    e. Signs of increased work of breathing (respiratory effort)

    f. Signs of chest trauma

    g. If respirations are absent, quiet, or noisy

  2. Provide appropriate treatment as necessary (e.g., administer oxygen, suction).

  3. Document and communicate any changes or trends to the staff at the receiving facility.

REASSESSMENT OF CIRCULATION

Reassess circulation.

  1. Reassess pulse rate and quality.

    a. In adults and children older than 1 year of age, feel for a radial pulse.

    b. In infants, palpate a brachial pulse.

    c. If pulseless, begin cardiopulmonary resuscitation (CPR).

  2. Reassess bleeding and control bleeding if present.

  3. Reassess perfusion status.

    a. Look for changes in skin color.

    b. Feel for changes in skin temperature and condition (moisture).

    c. Reassess capillary refill in infants and children younger than 6 years of age.

  4. Document and communicate any changes or trends to the staff at the receiving facility.

TRANSPORT DECISION

Reestablish patient's priority for transport.

  1. If the ongoing assessment is performed en route to the hospital and the patient's condition worsens, consider transport with lights and siren.

  2. If the ongoing assessment is performed on the scene, reconsider the transport decision based on assessment findings.

REASSESSMENT OF VITAL SIGNS

ELEMENTS

Vital signs include:

  1. Respiratory rate and quality

2. Pulse rate and quality
3. Blood pressure
4. Pupils
5. Perfusion status
    a. Skin color, temperature, and condition (moisture)
    b. Capillary refill in infants and children younger than 6 years of age

STABLE PATIENT

In a stable patient, the ongoing assessment should be repeated and the findings documented every 15 minutes.

UNSTABLE PATIENT

In an unstable patient, the ongoing assessment should be repeated and documented every 5 minutes.

TRENDS

Note any changes or trends and adjust emergency care interventions as necessary.

REPEATING THE FOCUSED ASSESSMENT

Repeat the focused assessment of the patient's specific complaint or injury. If the patient develops a new complaint or if there is a previously identified symptom change, perform a focused assessment on the area of complaint.

REEVALUATING EMERGENCY CARE INTERVENTIONS

AIRWAY AND BREATHING

Ensure adequacy of oxygen delivery or artificial ventilation.
1. Ensure the patient's airway is open.
2. If an oropharyngeal or nasopharyngeal airway has been inserted, ensure the adjunct is properly positioned.
3. If the patient is being ventilated with a bag-valve device:
    a. Ensure the device is connected to oxygen at 15 liters per minute (LPM).
    b. If a reservoir bag is used, ensure the reservoir is inflated.
    c. Reassess effectiveness of ventilation.
        (1) Ensure adequate rise and fall of the chest.
        (2) Ensure adequate face-to-mask seal.
        (3) Evaluate lung compliance (resistance to ventilation); increasing resistance suggests airway obstruction.
4. If oxygen is being delivered by nonrebreather mask:
    a. Ensure the mask is connected to oxygen at 15 LPM.
    b. Ensure the reservoir bag is not pinched off and remains inflated.
    c. Ensure the inhalation valve is not obstructed.
5. If oxygen is being delivered by nasal cannula:
    a. Ensure the oxygen flow rate is set at no more than 6 LPM.
    b. Ensure the prongs are properly placed in the patient's nose.
6. Ensure open chest wounds have been properly sealed with an occlusive dressing.
7. Ensure suction is readily available.

CIRCULATION

1. Ensure bleeding is controlled.
2. If CPR is performed, ensure pulses are produced with chest compressions.

3. Other interventions
   a. Ensure the trauma patient's cervical spine is adequately immobilized.
   b. Ensure injured extremities are effectively immobilized.
   c. Ensure the patient is adequately secured to a long backboard.
   d. Ensure open wounds are properly dressed and bandaged.

REVIEW QUESTIONS

Directions: Each of the numbered items or incomplete statements in this section is followed by answers or by completions of the statement. Select the ONE lettered answer or completion that is BEST in each case.

1. Which of the following best describes the type of patient who requires an ongoing assessment?

   (A)   A medically ill patient
   (B)   A traumatically injured patient
   (C)   A patient in cardiopulmonary arrest
   (D)   All patients should receive ongoing assessments

2. The ongoing physical exam should be performed

   (A)   only during transport
   (B)   immediately after the initial assessment
   (C)   only if you think the patient's condition has changed
   (D)   after the detailed physical exam and pertinent interventions

3. The purpose of the ongoing assessment is

   (A)   to initially assess the patient's chief complaint
   (B)   to provide proof that your initial actions were correct
   (C)   to initially identify and treat life-threatening conditions
   (D)   to reevaluate the patient's condition and ensure effective interventions are being performed

4. Your ambulance crew is transporting a 76-year-old male with an altered mental status. He has a history of previous cerebrovascular accidents (strokes) and hypertension. Initially this patient was slow to respond and could not speak. Reassessment of his mental status

   (A)   would be of no benefit in charting this patient's condition
   (B)   should focus on any changes from the initial presentation
   (C)   should not be performed since it has already been noted that the patient has an altered mental status
   (D)   should not be performed in the field; reassessment of mental status is the responsibility of the receiving facility physician

5. Your rescue crew is called to the scene of a motor vehicle collision. Your patient is a 27-year-old woman complaining of neck and lower back pain. As part of the ongoing assessment of this patient, you reassess the patient's airway. She is alert and speaking clearly. You should

   (A)   assume that the airway is patent (open)
   (B)   immediately being suctioning the airway

    (C)   open the airway with a jaw thrust

    (D)   open the airway with the head-tilt, chin-lift technique

6. When reassessing circulation for conscious patients older than 1 year of age, rescuers should check the rate and quality of the pulse at which location?

    (A)   Radial artery

    (B)   Brachial artery

    (C)   Femoral artery

    (D)   Posterior tibial artery

7. Capillary refill is an excellent tool for evaluating perfusion status. This statement applies to

    (A)   all patients

    (B)   patients younger than 6 years of age

    (C)   patients older than 6 years of age

    (D)   patients older than 1 year of age

8. Your ambulance crew is transporting a 57-year-old male patient complaining of severe chest pain. The initial assessment and focused history and physical examination have been performed. The patient is given oxygen at 15 liters per minute via nonrebreather mask. During your ongoing assessment in the back of the ambulance, you note the patient has a marked increase in level of distress. You should consider

    (A)   inserting an oropharyngeal airway

    (B)   having the patient breathe into a paper bag

    (C)   transporting the patient with lights and siren

    (D)   changing the patient's oxygen delivery device to a nasal cannula

9. Your rescue crew is called to the scene of a 14-year-old male patient complaining of wrist pain. The patient states his hand was slammed in a sliding door. Distal sensation, movement, and circulation are intact. For this stable patient, the ongoing assessment should be repeated and the findings documented every

    (A)   2 minutes

    (B)   5 minutes

    (C)   10 minutes

    (D)   15 minutes

10. You are dispatched to the scene of a major motor vehicle collision. Your rescue crew is assigned to treat and transport a 34-year-old male patient in cardiac arrest. The ongoing assessment of this patient

    (A)   would not be necessary

    (B)   may include checking for pulses during chest compressions

    (C)   may include ensuring the patient is kept cold to slow his metabolism

    (D)   may include ensuring that his nasal cannula flows at 6 liters per minute or less

11. Any changes in patient presentation observed during the ongoing assessment should be

    (A)   documented

    (B)   relayed immediately to medical direction

    (C)   cause for immediate transport with lights and siren

    (D)   documented and communicated to the receiving facility

Directions: Each of the numbered items or incomplete statements in this section is negatively phrased, as indicated by a capitalized word such as NOT, LEAST, or EXCEPT. Select the ONE lettered answer or completion that is BEST in each case.

12. Which of the following is NOT a component of the ongoing assessment?

   (A)   Reassess vital signs
   (B)   Repeat initial assessment
   (C)   Repeat contact with medical direction
   (D)   Reevaluate emergency care interventions

Directions: Each of the numbered questions or incomplete statements in this section refers to a scenario that precedes them. The numbered questions or incomplete statements are followed by answers or by completions of the statement. Select the answer or completion of the statement that is BEST in each case.

Your ambulance is dispatched to a long-term care facility for a 66-year-old female patient in severe respiratory distress. The patient is cool and pale with a respiratory rate of 28 breaths per minute. She speaks in short, choppy sentences and is coughing up white, foamy sputum.

Questions 13–15

13. For this patient, the ongoing assessment should be repeated and the findings documented every

   (A)   2 minutes
   (B)   5 minutes
   (C)   10 minutes
   (D)   15 minutes

14. This patient is given oxygen by nonrebreather mask at 15 liters per minute. While reevaluating your emergency care interventions for this patient, you should

   (A)   ensure the mask's reservoir is inflated
   (B)   ensure an oropharyngeal airway is in place
   (C)   ensure suction is turned on and left in the patient's mouth
   (D)   ensure the mask's reservoir deflates completely with each inspiration

15. This patient's mental status decreases until she is completely unresponsive. A carotid pulse is present at a rate of 120 beats per minute. Respirations are shallow at 30 respirations per minute. When reassessing the patient's airway, you should consider

   (A)   changing the patient's airway delivery device to a nasal cannula
   (B)   discontinuing the use of the nonrebreather mask for better lung sound auscultation
   (C)   inserting an oropharyngeal airway and assisting ventilations with a bag-valve mask
   (D)   not changing any of your emergency care interventions until a physician can evaluate the patient

ANSWERS AND RATIONALES

1-D. In any patient, a change in signs and symptoms or status may occur. Therefore, all patients should be continuously assessed until transfer of care is accomplished at the receiving facility. Stable patients may become unstable. Unstable patients may require further emergency care interventions. Closely monitoring patients allows the rescuer the opportunity to observe and document any trends in patient response. This information is valuable to both prehospital and hospital care providers.

2-D. The ongoing assessment should follow all initial assessments, examinations, and treatments. If transport is delayed, use that extra time to reevaluate the patient's status. Do not wait to perform an ongoing assessment until you suspect the patient's status has changed. If you are waiting for the obvious signs of change rather than evaluating for the presence of subtle changes, your emergency care interventions will be delayed. Subtle changes to watch for include any changes in mental status, vital signs, and level of distress.

3-D. The ongoing assessment provides an opportunity to evaluate the effectiveness of your efforts and chart trends in the patient's presentation and status. The ongoing assessment, by definition, is not an initial assessment; rather it retraces the steps of your initial assessment and intervention to gauge the patient's response. Based on the ongoing assessment, you may need to conduct a more detailed examination or change treatment and transport procedures (especially if the patient's condition is deteriorating). If you approach the ongoing assessment from the standpoint that you are attempting to prove that you were "right the first time," then your ongoing assessments will be prejudiced toward a fixed outcome. This approach is incorrect, as patient condition generally changes over time.

4-B. As stated before, all patients should receive ongoing assessments. Although this patient has an altered mental status, you should constantly reassess for any changes in the patient's condition. Ideally, you should be able to provide the receiving facility with a report (written and verbal) that addresses the patient's progress while under your care.

5-A. Since the patient is conscious and speaking without difficulty, you may assume that the airway is patent. This assumption should not preclude you from questioning the patient further about her airway status or from suctioning if necessary. However, routine suctioning or maneuvers to open the airway would not be appropriate. If this patient did require airway positioning, the jaw thrust should be performed rather than the head-tilt,chin-lift maneuver due to the patient's mechanism of injury and chief complaint.

6-A. The radial pulse is preferred for adults for several reasons. First, it is most readily accessible and does not cause any discomfort for the patient. Second, it provides valuable information about the patient's distal perfusion status. If the radial pulse cannot be felt (but the carotid can), you should assume that distal perfusion may be compromised. Finally, if a radial pulse is present, you can temporarily conclude that the patient's systolic blood pressure is at least 80 millimeters of mercury (mm Hg).

7-B. In patients younger than 6 years of age, capillary refill is an excellent tool for evaluating perfusion status and is quickly performed. In patients older than 6 years of age, capillary refill is less precise due to the number of factors that affect its outcome (e.g., temperature, position, medications).

8-C. If despite your efforts, the patient continues to deteriorate or fails to improve, evaluate the option of decreasing the time necessary to transport the patient. For example, you may decide to use lights and sirens, re-route to a closer facility, or change transportation modes (e.g., use a medical helicopter). The transport changes may necessitate reestablishing contact with medical direction. Inserting an oropharyngeal airway would not be appropriate since its use is limited to unresponsive patients without a gag reflex. The EMT-Basic should never instruct a patient to breathe into a paper bag without specific orders from medical direction to do so. Changing the patient's oxygen delivery device to a nasal cannula would result in a decrease in the concentration of oxygen delivered and may cause further harm to the patient.

9-D. At a minimum, stable patients should be reassessed every 15 minutes. However, if the patient's level of distress, mental status, or response to treatment changes at any time, you should immediately reassess.

10-B. All patients should be continuously reassessed. In the case of a cardiac arrest victim, your reassessment should address the effectiveness of your interventions [cardiopulmonary resuscitation (CPR)]. One tool to assess the effectiveness of CPR is to check for the presence of pulses during chest compressions. Cooling cardiac arrest victims is not indicated. Efforts should be directed toward maintaining normal body temperature ($37°$ C or $98.6°$ F). A nasal cannula is a low-flow oxygen device for a spontaneously breathing patient and is therefore contraindicated for apneic (nonbreathing) patients.

11-D. The ongoing assessment allows for monitoring patient trends: improving status, deteriorating status, or stabilizing status. This information should be included in your written documentation and passed along during a verbal report to an appropriate health care provider at the receiving facility. If the information gained during the ongoing assessment suggests the patient's condition is deteriorating, you may need to contact medical direction or upgrade your transport decision to lights and siren; however, not all changes in patient condition necessitate such action. Ideally, the patient's condition will improve with prompt, appropriate treatment and continued assessments.

12-C. The components of the ongoing assessment are repeating initial assessment, reassessing and documenting vital signs, repeating focused assessment, and reevaluating emergency care interventions. Based on the ongoing assessment, you may find it necessary to contact medical direction; however, it is not standard or practical to contact medical direction at every stage of patient assessment.

13-B. Unstable patients should be reassessed at least every 5 minutes. However, you may have to reassess this patient sooner if the situation calls for it. By reassessing every 5 minutes, you can closely monitor the patient's progress and adapt your treatment and transportation decision accordingly.

14-A. To evaluate the effectiveness of the set flow rate when using a device with a reservoir, ensure that the reservoir remains at least partially inflated during inspiration. If the reservoir completely collapses during inspiration, the oxygen flow rate should be increased. Inserting an oropharyngeal airway would not be appropriate since this patient is conscious. While suctioning may be necessary, leaving the suction device on and in the patient's mouth would greatly reduce oxygen delivery concentrations and cause harm to the patient.

15-C. Since the patient is now unconscious, you will need to assist in the maintenance of a patent (open) airway. If a gag reflex is absent, an oropharyngeal airway may be used. If a gag reflex is still present, a nasopharyngeal airway may be better tolerated. If the respiratory rate is still rapid and shallow, assist ventilations by delivering slow (1.5 to 2 seconds per breath) ventilations every 5 seconds with a bag-valve mask connected to 100% oxygen. Decreasing or stopping the flow of oxygen would be inappropriate and may cause the patient to deteriorate further. The ongoing assessment is conducted so that you may adapt your treatment to changes in the patient's condition. Failure to adapt to the patient's changes negates the benefit of conducting the ongoing assessment.

BIBLIOGRAPHY

Crosby LA, Lewallen DG (eds): *Emergency Care and Transportation of the Sick and Injured*, 6th ed. Rosemont, IL, American Academy of Orthopaedic Surgeons, 1995.

Grant HD, Murray RH Jr, Bergeron JD: *Emergency Care*, 7th ed. Englewood Cliffs, NJ, Prentice-Hall, 1995.

Hafen BQ, Karren KJ, Mistovich JJ: *Prehospital Emergency Care*, 5th ed. Upper Saddle River, NJ, Prentice-Hall, 1996.

McSwain NE, White RD, Paturas JL, et al (eds): *The Basic EMT: Comprehensive Prehospital Patient Care*. St. Louis, Mosby-Year Book, 1996.

Stoy, WA: *Mosby's EMT-Basic Textbook*. St. Louis: Mosby-Year Book, 1996.

United States Department of Transportation, National Highway Traffic Safety Administration: *Emergency Medical Technician: Basic. National Standard Curriculum*, 1994.

14 COMMUNICATIONS

OBJECTIVES

*14-1 Describe the following components of an EMS communications system: base station, mobile two-way radio, portable radio, repeater, digital radio equipment, cellular telephone.

14-2 List the proper methods for initiating and terminating a radio call.

14-3 State legal aspects to consider in verbal communication.

14-4 State the proper sequence for delivery of patient information.

14-5 Explain the importance of effective communication of patient information in the verbal report.

14-6 Identify the essential components of the verbal report.

14-7 Describe the attributes for increasing effectiveness and efficiency of verbal communications.

14-8 Discuss the communication skills that should be used to interact with the patient.

14-9 Describe the communication skills that should be used to interact with family members, bystanders, and individuals from other agencies.

14-10 Describe the differences between skills used to interact with the patient and those used to interact with others on the scene.

MOTIVATION FOR LEARNING

The EMT-Basic must be able to communicate effectively with crew members, emergency dispatchers, medical direction, and other health care professionals; law enforcement personnel and other public safety workers; the patient; and the patient's family.

Communication with medical direction may be necessary if a patient refuses care, during difficult patient management situations, or to obtain orders to administer medications. The EMT-Basic must learn to communicate patient information to other health care professionals in a concise, organized manner. The EMT-Basic must also learn to communicate early with the receiving facility to ensure that adequate resources are mobilized to care for the patient.

14-11   Describe how to communicate effectively while providing patient care.

14-12   List the correct radio procedures in the following phases of a typical call:

    a. To the scene   d. At the facility

    b. At the scene   e. To the station

    c. To the facility   f. At the station

COMMUNICATIONS SYSTEMS

SYSTEM COMPONENTS

1. **Base Station**
   a. **Definition.** A **base station** is a transmitter/receiver at a stationary site such as a hospital, mountain top, or public safety agency.
   b. Power output of a base station is typically 45–275 watts.
2. **Mobile Two-Way Radio**
   a. **Definition.** A **mobile two-way radio** is a vehicle-mounted communication device.
   b. It usually transmits at a lower power than base stations (typically 20–50 watts).
   c. The typical transmission range is 10–15 miles over average terrain.
      (1)   Transmission over flat land or water increases range.
      (2)   Urban areas, mountains, and dense foliage decrease transmission range.
3. **Portable Radio**
   a. **Definition.** A **portable radio** is a handheld communication device.
   b. Typical power output is 1–5 watts, which limits its range.
   c. Portable radios are used for radio communication away from the emergency vehicle.
      (1)   They may have a single or multiple channels.
      (2)   They are often used in conjunction with repeaters to increase transmission range.
4. **Repeater**
   a. **Definition.** A **repeater** is a device that receives a transmission from a low-power portable or mobile radio on one frequency and then retransmits it at a higher power on another frequency so it can be received at a distant location.
   b. Repeaters can be fixed or mobile.
      (1)   For portable communications, repeaters may be located in the vehicle or on radio towers.
      (2)   Mobile communications use repeaters on radio towers.
   c. Repeater signals can be retransmitted by radio waves, microwaves, or telephone land lines.
5. **Digital radio equipment**
   a. The use of digital radio technology is increasing because of crowded frequencies for voice transmission.
   b. In some emergency medical services (EMS) systems, digital radio equipment is used to transmit patient monitoring data.
6. **Cellular telephones**
   a. Geographical areas are divided into "cells."
   b. Each cell has a base station to transmit and receive signals.
   c. Cellular communication systems can track a mobile unit's movements from cell to cell and transfer the unit's radio activity to the appropriate cell base station.
   d. Cellular communications are not secured and can be monitored by persons using scanners.

RADIO FREQUENCIES

1. **Regulation of radio frequencies**
   a. **Federal Communications Commission (FCC)**
      (1) In the United States, the Federal Communications Commission (FCC) regulates the use of nongovernment radio frequencies including AM, FM, television, aircraft, marine, and land-mobile frequency ranges.
      (2) The Interagency Radio Advisory Committee (IRAC) is responsible for co-ordinating radio use by agencies of the federal government.
   b. **Emergency Medical Radio Service**
      (1) The **Emergency Medical Radio Service** (EMRS) is a group of frequencies designated by the FCC exclusively for use by EMS providers.
      (2) EMRS includes many frequencies in the **VHF** (very high frequency) and **UHF** (ultra-high frequency) bands (a band is a group of radio frequencies close together).

2. **Radio bands designated for EMS use**
   a. Radio bands designated for EMS use include:
      (1) **VHF low band** = 30–50 megahertz (MHz)
      (2) **VHF high band** = 150–170 MHz
      (3) **UHF** = 450–470 MHz
   b. **VHF low band**
      (1) Radio waves in this range bend and follow the curvature of the earth, allowing radio transmission over long distances
      (2) These radio waves are subject to interference by atmospheric conditions including weather disturbances and electrical equipment.
      (3) These waves exhibit poor penetration of solid structures, such as buildings, making VHF low band less effective for use in metropolitan areas.
   c. **VHF high band**
      (1) Radio waves in this frequency range travel in a straight line.
      (2) Less interference occurs in this band than in VHF low band, but it is still susceptible to interference by solid structures, such as large buildings.
      (3) This band is better for use in metropolitan areas than VHF low band.
   d. **UHF**
      (1) Radio waves in the UHF frequency travel in a straight line.
      (2) This band has a shorter range than VHF high or low bands.
      (3) UHF is frequently used in metropolitan areas because these frequencies penetrate buildings well.
      (4) UHF frequently requires the use of repeaters due to its short range.
   e. **800 MHz**
      (1) The 800 MHz frequency allows clearer communication with minimal interference.
      (2) A trunking system is available that allows routing of a transmission to the first available frequency.
      (3) Many channels are available to choose from.
      (4) The 800 MHz frequency has the shortest range and requires the use of repeaters.

EQUIPMENT MAINTENANCE

Communications equipment requires preventive maintenance by a qualified technician to ensure proper operation.

PUBLIC ACCESS

1. Public access to EMS is influenced by:
   a. Local telephone company equipment capabilities
   b. Local and regional government public service budgets
   c. Politics between different jurisdictions
   d. Competition between jurisdictions over control of public access
2. EMS can be accessed from:
   a. Telephone land line (most common means of public access)

    b. Citizens band (CB) radios

    c. Cellular telephones

    d. Highway call boxes

3. **9-1-1**

    a. **9-1-1** allows rapid access to police, fire, and EMS.

    b. Calls are routed to different communication centers depending on the origin of the call.

    c. All calls arrive in a single location, known as a **public safety answering point (PSAP).** The PSAP may perform actual dispatch functions or direct calls to the appropriate agency.

    d. Many areas of the United States are still without 9-1-1 access. In these areas, a seven-digit number is used to access police, fire, and EMS.

4. **Enhanced 9-1-1**

    a. In an **enhanced 9-1-1** (E9-1-1) system, the computer displays the caller's telephone number and address.

        (1) E9-1-1 speeds up the transfer of information from the caller to the call-taker.

        (2) It helps decrease the number of false alarms.

        (3) It also assists in call-backs to obtain more complete information.

    b. The caller's telephone number and address may not be the actual street location.

        (1) Computer information displayed is based on telephone company records.

        (2) Large telephone systems (e.g., buildings with switchboards, hotels) do not allow E9-1-1 to distinguish a specific location

RADIO COMMUNICATION

GENERAL PRINCIPLES

1. **Before speaking:**

    a. Turn on the radio

    b. Select the proper frequency; use EMS frequencies only for EMS communication

    c. Make sure the volume is properly adjusted

    d. Reduce background noise as much as possible by closing the windows of the EMS vehicle

2. Listen to the frequency and ensure it is clear before beginning a transmission.

3. Press the push-to-talk (PTT) button on the radio and wait one second before speaking.

4. Speak with lips approximately 2–3 inches from the microphone.

5. Address the unit being called by its name and number, then identify the name of your unit (and number, if appropriate).

6. The unit being called will signal you to begin your transmission by saying "go ahead" or some other term standard in your area. A response of "stand by" means "wait until further notice."

7. Speak clearly and slowly, in a monotone voice.

8. Keep transmissions brief. If a transmission takes longer than 30 seconds, pause for a few seconds so emergency traffic can use the frequency if necessary.

9. Use plain English in your communications.

    a. Avoid the use of codes, especially those that are not standardized.

    b. Avoid meaningless phrases (e.g., "be advised").

    c. Do not use slang.

    d. Do not use profanity on the air (The FCC may impose substantial fines).

    e. Avoid words that are difficult to hear like "yes" and "no"; use "affirmative" and "negative."

10. Courtesy is assumed; there is no need to say "please," "thank you," and "you're welcome."

11. When transmitting a number that might be confused with another, give the number, then give the individual digits. For example, say the number, "seventeen" and then follow it with the individual digits, "one-seven."
12. Protect the patient's privacy.
    a. Do not give the patient's name over the air.
       (1) The airwaves are public and scanners are popular.
       (2) EMS transmissions may be overheard by more than just the EMS community.
    b. Do not offer a diagnosis of the patient's complaint or injury.
       (1) Remain objective and impartial in describing patients.
       (2) The EMT-Basic may be sued for slander if a person's reputation is injured due to information relayed during a radio transmission.
13. An EMT-Basic rarely acts alone; use "we" instead of "I" in radio transmissions.
14. Use the word "over" to indicate when the transmission is finished, and wait for confirmation that the message was received.

DISPATCH

1. **Overview**
   a. The EMS dispatcher is often, but not always, located at the central communications center. In areas where the EMS dispatcher is at a location remote from the PSAP, calls are routed by the central communications center to the dispatcher by telephone or computer.
   b. **Emergency Medical Dispatchers (EMD)**
      (1) Formal emergency medical dispatch protocols and training began in the 1980s. Before this time, medical dispatchers averaged less than 1 hour of medical training.
      (2) The Emergency Medical Dispatch program has been developed to certify personnel as Emergency Medical Dispatchers (EMDs).
      (3) The EMD is responsible for:
         (a) Asking questions of the caller
         (b) Radio dispatching
         (c) Logistics coordination; the EMD is knowledgeable about the geography of the area, the EMS system's capabilities, and the activities of other public service agencies
         (d) Providing prearrival instructions to the caller
      (4) EMS personnel may be dispatched by:
         (a) Radio
         (b) Pager
         (c) Telephone
         (d) Intercom
      (5) Once emergency units are en route, the EMD can provide specific information about:
         (a) Directions
         (b) Scene safety
         (c) Updates regarding the patient's condition
      (6) Conversations with the caller, police, fire, and EMS personnel are recorded in many EMS systems.
2. **When to notify dispatch.** The dispatcher should be notified when:
   a. Receiving the call
   b. Responding to the call
   c. Arriving at the scene
   d. Leaving the scene for the receiving facility
   e. Arriving at the receiving facility
   f. Leaving the hospital for the station
   g. Arriving at the station

COMMUNICATION WITH MEDICAL DIRECTION

1. **Overview**
   a. **Medical direction location**
      (1) In some systems, medical direction is at the receiving facility.
      (2) In others, medical direction is at a separate site.
   b. In either case, EMT-Basics may need to contact medical direction for consultation and obtain orders for administration of medications.
2. **General guidelines**
   a. Radio transmissions need to be organized, concise, and pertinent.
   b. Information given to the physician by the EMT-Basic must be accurate because the physician will use this information to determine whether to order medications and procedures.
   c. After receiving an order for a medication or procedure (or denial of such a request), use the "echo" procedure, i.e., repeat the order back to the physician, word for word.
   d. Question orders that are unclear or appear to be inappropriate.
3. **Standardized medical reporting format.** Use the following sequence when reporting information to medical direction:
   a. Unit name and level of service [Basic Life Support (BLS) or Advanced Life Support (ALS)]
   b. Estimated time of arrival (ETA)
   c. Patient's age and gender
   d. Patient's chief complaint
   e. Brief, pertinent history of the present illness
   f. Major past illnesses
   g. Patient's mental status
   h. Patient's baseline vital signs
   i. Pertinent physical examination findings
   j. Emergency medical care given
   k. Patient's response to emergency medical care

COMMUNICATION WITH RECEIVING FACILITY

1. **Purpose.** Communication with the receiving facility allows the facility to prepare for a patient's arrival by designating the right room and gathering the necessary equipment and personnel.
2. **Standardized medical reporting format.** Use the following sequence when reporting information to the receiving facility:
   a. Unit name and level of service (BLS or ALS)
   b. ETA
   c. Patient's age and gender
   d. Patient's chief complaint
   e. Brief, pertinent history of the present illness
   f. Major past illnesses
   g. Patient's mental status
   h. Patient's baseline vital signs
   i. Pertinent physical examination findings
   j. Emergency medical care given
   k. Patient's response to emergency medical care
3. **Verbal report at the receiving facility**
   a. Introduce the patient by name (if known).
   b. Summarize the information already provided by radio or telephone to the receiving facility:
      (1) Patient's chief complaint
      (2) Pertinent patient history that was not previously given
      (3) Emergency medical care given en route and the patient's response to the treatment given

(4) Vital signs taken en route

(5) Any additional information collected en route but not transmitted to the receiving facility

INTERPERSONAL COMMUNICATION

COMMUNICATING WITH THE PATIENT

1. **General Principles**
   a. Introduce yourself.
   b. Explain that you are there to provide assistance.
   c. Treat the patient with respect and courtesy.
      (1) Address the patient by proper name.
      (2) Ask the patient what he or she wishes to be called by first or last name.
   d. Position yourself directly in the patient's line of vision; when practical, position yourself at a level lower than the patient.
   e. Make and keep eye contact with the patient.
   f. Be honest with the patient.
   g. Use terms the patient can understand.
   h. Be aware of your own body language.
   i. Speak clearly, slowly, and distinctly.
   j. Allow the patient enough time to answer a question before asking the next one.
   k. Act and speak in a calm, confident manner.

SPECIAL SITUATIONS

1. **Hearing-impaired patient**
   a. If the patient has difficulty hearing, he or she may be able to read lips. If so, make sure to speak clearly with your lips visible as you speak.
   b. Determine if the patient's family members or bystanders know sign language to interpret for you.
   c. Written notes may also be used to communicate.
   d. Facial expressions may be used to emphasize points.

2. **Visually impaired patient**
   a. Approach the patient from the front and introduce yourself and identify any persons with you.
   b. Speak in a normal tone of voice.
      (1) Do not speak from a distance.
      (2) Do not avoid the use of words such as "see" and "blind;" these words are parts of normal speech.
   c. Speak before handing an object to the patient.
   d. When walking with a visually impaired patient:
      (1) Allow the patient to place his or her arm or hand on your arm so that the patient can sense the direction you are going.
      (2) Ensure that the pathway is free of clutter.
   e. Describe unfamiliar surroundings to the patient.

3. **Non-English-speaking patient**
   a. Communication with non-English-speaking patients may require the use of an interpreter.
      (1) Explain to the interpreter the type of questions that will be asked.
      (2) Avoid interrupting a family member (or bystander) and interpreter when they are communicating.
   b. If an interpreter is not present at the scene, contact dispatch or medical direction. Telephone companies often have interpreters who are available 24 hours a day.

4. **Elderly patient**
   a. The elderly patient may have difficulty hearing and poor vision.
      (1) Assume a position directly in the patient's line of vision and speak directly toward him or her.

      (2) Begin speaking to the patient in a normal tone of voice.

      (3) If the patient has difficulty hearing, speak a little more loudly until he or she can hear you.

   b. Address the patient by proper name.

      (1) Ask the patient what he or she wishes to be called.

      (2) Avoid the use of terms such as "dear," "honey," "sweetheart."

   c. Speak slowly, say each word clearly, and use short sentences.

      (1) Short simple sentences are more easily understood.

      (2) Be careful not to "talk down" to the patient.

   d. Ask the patient one question at a time.

      (1) Allow the patient time to respond.

      (2) If it is necessary to repeat the question, phrase it exactly as it was asked the first time.

      (3) Actively listen to the patient's response.

   e. Provide reassurance with a soothing voice and calm demeanor.

5. Children

   a. Assume a position that is eye level with the child.

   b. Speak in a calm, unhurried, and confident tone.

   c. Speak clearly using simple words and short sentences.

   d. Be honest with the child.

   e. Avoid sudden movements.

   f. Give the child a choice only when one exists.

   g. Allow the child to express his or her concerns and fears.

COMMUNICATING WITH OTHERS AT THE SCENE

1. Communicating with family members and bystanders

   a. Avoid interrupting when a family member or bystander is talking.

   b. Speak clearly and distinctly and use common words (avoid confusing medical terms).

   c. Speak at an appropriate speed or pace, not too rapidly and not too slowly.

   d. Listen attentively.

      (1) Face the person speaking.

      (2) Maintain eye contact.

      (3) Assume an attentive posture.

      (4) Clarify information that is unclear.

2. Communicating with individuals from other agencies

   a. Communications should be organized, concise, thorough, and accurate.

   b. When receiving a report from others at the scene, be professional and thank them for their efforts.

   c. Familiarity with local protocols and standing orders, available medications and equipment, and level of personnel training are essential.

COMMUNICATING WHILE PROVIDING PATIENT CARE

1. When communicating with the patient:

   a. Clearly explain what is happening, i.e., "Mrs. Jones, you appear to be having trouble breathing."

   b. Describe what needs to be done, i.e., "I would like to administer oxygen to help your breathing."

   c. Explain how you will accomplish what needs to be done, i.e., "I am going to put this oxygen on your face."

   d. Explain why it is important that you perform these actions, i.e., "I want you to breathe normally. The oxygen will help your breathing."

2. Reassure the patient frequently and, when appropriate, use compassionate touch to communicate your presence and understanding.

REVIEW QUESTIONS

> **Directions:** Each of the numbered items or incomplete statements in this section is followed by answers or by completions of the statement. Select the ONE lettered answer or completion that is BEST in each case.

1. Which of the following describes a base station?

   (A) A vehicle-mounted send and receive unit
   (B) A handheld device with low-output power
   (C) A handheld device with high-output power
   (D) A stationary send and receive unit with high-output power

2. Mobile two-way radios (vehicle mounted) typically have a transmission range of

   (A) 1–2 miles
   (B) 10–15 miles
   (C) 20–30 miles
   (D) 50–100 miles

3. Portable radios generally have a low-power transmission output. Which of the following can boost the range of such a device?

   (A) Installing a repeater
   (B) Installing a base station
   (C) Transmitting from a valley or tunnel
   (D) Speaking more loudly into the microphone

4. Which technological advancement is helping to ease the crowding of radio frequencies?

   (A) Digital technology
   (B) Analog technology
   (C) CD-ROM technology
   (D) Magnetic-tape technology

5. A drawback of cellular phone usage is

   (A) cellular phones are more expensive than portable radios
   (B) cellular phone transmission may be monitored by scanners
   (C) cellular phones do not support simultaneous two-way voice transmission
   (D) cellular phones generally require extensive hardware

6. The use of nongovernment U.S. radio frequencies is monitored by which agency?

   (A) The Department of Transportation (DOT)
   (B) The Federal Communications Commission (FCC)
   (C) The Associated Press (AP)
   (D) The Interagency Radio Advisory Committee (IRAC)

7. A group of radio frequencies close together is called a

   (A) band
   (B) station
   (C) repeater
   (D) transmitter

8. Which of the following radio bands follows the curvature of the earth, has the worst penetration of solid structures (e.g., buildings), and may be hindered by weather conditions or electrical equipment?

   (A) UHF
   (B) 800 MHz
   (C) VHF low band
   (D) VHF high band

9. Which of the following radio bands has a short range of transmission, many channels to choose from, and allows for clearer communications?

   (A) UHF
   (B) 800 MHz
   (C) VHF low band
   (D) VHF high band

10. What radio transmission band would be ideal for use in metropolitan areas where building penetration is needed?

    (A) UHF
    (B) VHF low band
    (C) VHF high band
    (D) VHF medium band

11. Preventative maintenance of all radio equipment should be performed by

    (A) EMT-Basics
    (B) EMT-Paramedics
    (C) dispatchers
    (D) qualified technicians

12. Routing all incoming emergency calls to one location provides an organized flow of information. Which of the following locations serves this function?

    (A) Dispatch Center
    (B) Alarm Room (AR)
    (C) Police Department
    (D) Public Safety Answering Point (PSAP)

13. The primary advantage of enhanced 9-1-1 (E9-1-1) over standard 9-1-1 is

    (A) E9-1-1 routes the call directly to the closest responding rescue unit
    (B) E9-1-1 displays the caller's telephone number and address for the call taker
    (C) E9-1-1 can be used effectively from hotel rooms and other buildings with switchboards
    (D) E9-1-1 does not require the caller to state the problem in order to get an appropriate response

14. When speaking into a microphone, you should

    (A) speak as loudly as possible
    (B) press the microphone against your lips
    (C) hold the microphone about 2 feet from your mouth
    (D) hold the microphone about 2–3 inches from your mouth.

15. You are assigned to work on an ambulance designated as "EMS-1." Which of the

following responses would be the appropriate method to make contact with EMT-Basic James McCoy on another ambulance, "EMS-5"?

(A) "EMS-1 to Jim, come in Jim."
(B) "Come in Jim, are you out there?"
(C) "EMS-5 to EMS-1, do you copy?"
(D) "EMS-1 to EMS-5, do you copy?"

16. When communicating via radio, you should

(A) keep your transmissions to 1-minute bursts of information
(B) be courteous, and say "Thank you" and "Please" when appropriate
(C) use the terms "affirmative" and "negative" in place of "yes" and "no"
(D) use as many codes as possible to speed transmission of information.

17. Which of the following regarding a patient's privacy is correct?

(A) Do not give the patient's name or condition over the air
(B) It is acceptable to give the patient's name over the air but not the condition
(C) Do not give the patient's name if you are describing the patient's complaint
(D) EMS radio frequencies are protected from eavesdroppers and therefore all information may be transmitted

18. Before administering any medications, EMT-Basics must contact

(A) dispatch
(B) medical direction
(C) the dispatch supervisor
(D) the patient's personal physician

19. Your rescue crew is called for a 78-year-old male patient complaining of chest pain. You are given orders by radio from the appropriate personnel to assist the patient in self-administering one of his nitroglycerin tablets. If your local protocol allows such intervention, an appropriate verbal response to this order would be

(A) "Copy, loud and clear"
(B) "I copy your orders"
(C) "Copy, we will attempt to relieve the patient's pain"
(D) "Copy, assist patient in taking one nitroglycerin tablet"

20. When communicating with a patient

(A) avoid eye contact with the patient
(B) treat all patients abruptly to maintain control
(C) do not tell the patient your name for legal reason
(D) position yourself at, or slightly lower, than the patient's line of vision

21. When dealing with hearing-impaired patients who are able to read lips, you should

(A) speak more loudly
(B) avoid using facial expressions
(C) speak clearly and directly at the patient
(D) pay particular attention to pronouncing every syllable slowly and concisely

22. When treating a visually impaired patient, always ensure that you

(A) speak to the patient from a distance
(B) avoid such terms as "blind" and "see"
(C) lead the patient around by grasping the patient's arm
(D) speak to the patient before handling, touching, and treating

23. You are questioning an 83-year-old male patient about his past medical history. Which of the following is correct regarding special communications needs with this patient?

    (A) You should assume that the patient is hearing impaired and speak more loudly
    (B) You should speak in a normal tone until you discover the need to do otherwise
    (C) You should communicate with the patient in written form
    (D) You should speak loudly, but refer to the patient as "honey" or "dear" to avoid having the patient mistake your loud tone for yelling at them

24. Your ambulance is called to the scene of a 4-year-old female patient who fell from a tabletop and is complaining of left arm pain. You note a gross deformity of the affected arm. The arm needs to be immobilized before transporting the patient. You should

    (A) tell the patient that your treatment won't hurt her
    (B) not splint the arm if it is going to cause the patient any discomfort
    (C) have someone distract the patient, then quickly move her arm into the splint
    (D) tell the patient that your treatment may hurt and allow her to express her fears and concerns

25. For effective radio communications, you should end each verbal message by stating

    (A) "Over"
    (B) "Over and out"
    (C) "How does that sound?"
    (D) "Did you hear my transmission?"

ANSWERS AND RATIONALES

1-D. Base stations are stationary sites for transmitting and receiving radio transmissions. These sites typically put out 45–275 watts transmitting power. To increase the range of transmission, base station transmitters may be located on mountains, special towers, or high-rise buildings. Vehicle-mounted devices typically put out 20–50 watts transmitting power and have much less range than base stations. Handheld devices are generally low output power (1–5 watts) and have even lesser range than vehicle-mounted devices.

2-B. These devices have an average output of 20–50 watts and can travel about 10–15 miles. This range, however, is affected by local terrain.

3-A. A repeater receives transmissions and rebroadcasts the transmission at a higher power, thus increasing the range of a handheld device. In order to be effective, a repeater must be located within the range of the handheld device. The transmitting power of the base station does not determine the transmitting power of handheld devices used to communicate with the base station. Transmitting from a valley or tunnel will greatly decrease the range of a radio transmission. Speaking more loudly into the microphone will not boost transmission power; rather, it may ultimately distort one's voice so that nothing can be understood.

4-A. Digital technology allows information to be more efficiently transmitted, thus relieving bandwidth crowding. CD-ROM and magnetic-tape technology are methods for storing and retrieving data. Analog data transmission is much less compact and organized than digital data transmission.

5-B. Patient privacy is not ensured by using a cellular phone for information transmission. Cellular phone traffic is easily monitored by radio scanning devices; therefore, do not transmit any sensitive information via cellular phone. Cellular phones are typically less expensive than portable radios, and the hardware requirements (in areas with existing cell phone service) are simple and relatively inexpensive. Unlike most portable radio equipment that require send-or-receive communications, cellular phones allow for simultaneous two-way conversation.

6-B. The Federal Communications Commission (FCC) regulates radio frequencies in the United States. All transmissions are subject to scrutiny by the FCC. Inappropriate transmissions may lead to prosecution under violation of federal laws. The Department of Transportation (DOT) is responsible for overseeing national standards for EMT-Basics. The Associated Press (AP) is a news agency. The Interagency Radio Advisory Committee (IRAC) assists in the coordination of radio use by federal government agencies.

7-A. A band is a group of radio frequencies. The radio bands used by EMS agencies are VHF low band (30–50 MHz), VHF high band (150–170 MHz), and UHF (450–470 MHz). Other bands include AM and FM for commercial radio transmission. A station can be one specific frequency on a given band. A repeater is a device that boosts transmissions. A transmitter is a device that sends out data on a given radio frequency.

8-C. Both VHF bands follow the curvature of the earth. Low-band VHF is much more susceptible to interference by structures or equipment.

9-B. While 800 MHz transmissions have a very short transmission range, they do provide for a much clearer transmission of information and offer many channels from which to choose. Due to their short range, these systems require repeaters.

10-A. UHF band transmissions offer strong penetrating power into densely populated areas. Like the 800 MHz systems, UHF systems necessitate the use of repeaters due to short transmission distances.

11-D. Qualified, certified technicians should be responsible for maintaining and repairing radio equipment. Unskilled individuals may become seriously injured working on these powered devices. Also, radio equipment can be very expensive. Attempting to fix these devices can be a very costly lesson for untrained personnel.

12-D. Routing all incoming calls for assistance through a central location refers to a Public Safety Answering Point (PSAP). A Dispatch Center, Alarm Room, or Police Department are all examples of facilities that may host the PSAP. Information coming into the PSAP may be processed at the PSAP, or the PSAP may route the call to an appropriate agency for processing.

13-B. Enhanced 9-1-1 uses telephone company records to provide additional information to the call processing agency. If the 9-1-1 call goes through a switchboard, the ability to pinpoint the origin of the call is lost. With E9-1-1, callers must still state the problem (medical emergency, fire, police situation). The ability to route a call to the closest appropriate response unit is a separate system, sometimes referred to as AVL (Automatic Vehicle Locator). AVL uses satellite technology to select response units based on geography.

14-D. For the clearest possible transmissions, hold the microphone approximately 2–3 inches from your mouth and speak clearly, slowly, and at a normal volume. Sometimes the information you transmit will be urgent in nature (e.g., "Rescue 204 to Alarm, dispatch a hazardous materials team, there is a large gas leak"). However, by composing oneself and speaking clearly, the information is delivered and received more quickly.

15-D. When attempting to contact another field unit, identify yourself and the unit you are seeking. Avoid using personal names.

16-C. The words "yes" and "no" are often difficult to understand in radio transmissions. Transmissions should be kept to 30 seconds or less to allow the listener an opportunity to interact in the transmission (e.g., "We didn't copy the pulse rate, Rescue 204, could you repeat"). Courtesy is assumed in radio transmissions. "Please," "thank you," and "you're welcome" are generally implied. Finally, use plain English in your transmissions (unless local protocol dictates otherwise). Codes may be misunderstood by the person on the other end of the radio transmission.

17-A. Scanners can monitor all EMS radio traffic. Take extra precautions to ensure the protection of your patients' privacy. Many receiving facilities will request the patient's name over the airwaves. This situation should be worked out ahead of time to avoid problems or confrontations during the incident.

18-B. EMT-Basics perform their duties as an extension of a physician's license. Before assisting in the administration of medications, EMT-Basics must contact medical direction (as per local policy). EMTs at all levels (Basic, Intermediate, and Advanced/Paramedic) cannot take direction from a physician outside of their medical direction without approval from medical direction.

19-D. Always echo the order you are given. Do not paraphrase, as in answer "C." The echo communication procedure ensures that the correct order has been given and will be carried out.

20-D. To facilitate a nonthreatening, comfortable exchange of information, position yourself where the patient can easily see you, if possible. Making eye contact with the patient is important for building trust. Do not assume that your patient will be "challenging" to deal with. Sometimes this assumption may cause an otherwise amicable (friendly) patient to assume a negative attitude.

21-C. Sometimes our ability to communicate with hearing-impaired patients is hindered by the knowledge that the patient is impaired. If a patient can read lips, speak in a normal tone, look at the patient when speaking, make sure you have the patient's attention before speaking, and avoid overpronunciation. Mild facial expression may assist in conveying your meaning.

22-D. Since the patient cannot visualize your actions, it is imperative that you describe what you are doing. Something as simple as obtaining a blood pressure should be clearly communicated with the patient. Avoid speaking from a great distance to the patient or moving around too much while communicating. These patients are aware of their impairment and generally will not be insulted if you tactfully question them about their degree of impairment. It is not necessary to avoid the words "blind" or "I see." When leading the patient, allow the patient to grasp your arm. Then communicate with the patient to help them understand your directions and any obstacles.

23-B. Do not assume elderly patients are impaired. Do not assume your patient cannot hear, see, or understand you. If, however, you find you are having difficulty communicating with a patient, take whatever steps necessary to facilitate your communications.

24-D. Honesty is the best policy. Help your patients (regardless of age) to understand the rationale behind your actions. If something may cause discomfort, be honest. If you lie once, your patient may not believe another word you say. Crying is acceptable and understandable; however, do not withhold necessary treatment.

25-A. "Over" indicates that you are finished with your current message. "Over and out" indicates that you are terminating the communication. Do not say "Over and out" when you mean "Over," as the receiver may discontinue your transmission. Often, the term "Clear" is used in place of "Over and out" to avoid such confusion ("Medic 201 is clear with XYZ General Hospital").

BIBLIOGRAPHY

Crosby LA, Lewallen DG (eds): *Emergency Care and Transportation of the Sick and Injured*, 6th ed. Rosemont, IL, American Academy of Orthopaedic Surgeons, 1995.

Dernocoeur KB: *Streetwise: Communications, Safety, and Control*, 3rd ed. Redmond, WA, Laing Research Services, 1996.

Grant HD, Murray RH Jr, Bergeron JD: *Emergency Care*, 7th ed. Englewood Cliffs, NJ, Prentice-Hall, 1995.

Hafen BQ, Karren KJ, Mistovich JJ: *Prehospital Emergency Care*, 5th ed. Upper Saddle River, NJ, Prentice-Hall, 1996.

McSwain NE, White RD, Paturas JL, et al (eds): *The Basic EMT: Comprehensive Prehospital Patient Care*. St. Louis, Mosby-Year Book, 1996.

Roush WR (ed): *Principles of EMS Systems*, 2nd ed. Dallas: American College of Emergency Physicians, 1994.

Staub AS, Hodges LC: *Essentials of Gerontological Nursing: Adaptation to the Aging Process*. Philadelphia, JB Lippincott, 1996.

Stoy WA: *Mosby's EMT-Basic Textbook*. St. Louis, Mosby-Year Book, 1996.

United States Department of Transportation, National Highway Traffic Safety Administration: *Emergency Medical Technician: Basic. National Standard Curriculum*, 1994.

Wong DL: *Essentials of Pediatric Nursing*, 4th ed. St. Louis, Mosby-Year Book, 1993.

OBJECTIVES

15-1	Explain the components of the written report and list the information that should be included in the written report.
15-2	Identify the various sections of the written report.
15-3	Describe the information that is required in each section of the prehospital care report and how it should be entered.
15-4	Describe the required documentation when a patient refuses care.
15-5	Describe the legal implications associated with the written report.
15-6	Discuss all state and/or local record and reporting requirements.

THE PREHOSPITAL CARE REPORT (PCR)—OVERVIEW

OTHER NAMES

The **prehospital care report** may also be called the:
1. Patient care report
2. Run report
3. Trip sheet
4. Incident report
5. Ambulance report form

● MOTIVATION FOR LEARNING ●

The prehospital care report is a legal record that documents the patient care delivered in the field. Health care professionals use the information in the prehospital care report to initiate appropriate treatment after the patient arrives at the receiving facility. Inaccurate, illegible, or incomplete information on the prehospital care report regarding the patient's condition, assessment, and care can therefore have grave consequences.

The EMT-Basic must learn to document accurately, legibly, and completely. Two precepts the EMT-Basic can follow regarding written documentation are: "If it is not written down, it was not done," and "If it was not done, do not write it down."

USES OF THE PREHOSPITAL CARE REPORT

1. **Medical uses**
   a. The prehospital care report helps ensure continuity of patient care.
   b. The PCR may be the only source of information for hospital personnel to refer to later for important information about:
      (1) The scene
      (2) The status of the patient on arrival at the scene
      (3) Emergency medical care provided or attempted
      (4) Changes in the patient's condition
2. **Legal document**
   a. The PCR is an official record of the care rendered by Emergency Medical Service (EMS) personnel.
   b. The PCR becomes part of the patient's hospital record.
   c. The PCR may be used in legal proceedings. In general, the person who completed the form must go to court with the form.
   d. The PCR may be the EMT-Basic's only source of reference to a patient incident.
3. **Administrative uses.** The PCR may be used for billing purposes and to compile agency or service statistics.
4. **Educational and research uses**
   a. The PCR may be used to show proper documentation and how to handle unusual or uncommon cases.
   b. Data obtained from the prehospital care report may be collected and used for research purposes.
5. **Quality improvement**
   a. The PCR may be used to determine the frequency with which an EMT-Basic performs specific patient care procedures.
   b. The PCR may be used to determine continuing education needs.
   c. PCRs should be reviewed for:
      (1) Adequacy of documentation
      (2) Compliance with local rules and regulations
      (3) Appropriateness of medical care

ELEMENTS OF THE PREHOSPITAL CARE REPORT

RUN DATA

1. Agency/service name
2. Unit number
3. Date
4. Times. Accurate recording of the following incident times is essential:
   (a) Time of call
   (b) Time of dispatch
   (c) Time of arrival at the scene
   (d) Time of departure from the scene
   (e) Time of arrival at the receiving facility (when transporting a patient)
   (f) Time back in service
5. Run or call number
6. Crew members' names, certification levels, and numbers

PATIENT DATA

1. Patient name, address, date of birth, age, gender
2. Billing and insurance information
3. Nature of the call

4. Mechanism of injury
5. Location where the patient was found
6. Interventions performed by first responders or bystanders before the EMT-Basic's arrival
7. Patient signs and symptoms
8. Baseline and repeat vital signs:
   a. Patient's mental status
   b. Pupillary response
   c. Skin color, temperature, and condition (moisture)
   d. Pulse
   e. Respiratory rate
   f. Blood pressure
9. SAMPLE history
10. Interventions performed by the EMT-Basic and the patient's response to each intervention
11. Changes in the patient's condition throughout the call

NARRATIVE

1. Document observations at the scene, including:
   a. Empty pill bottles
   b. Presence of a suicide note
   c. Weapons
2. Document assessment findings.
   a. Document pertinent positives and negatives.
   b. A **pertinent negative** is a finding expected to accompany the patient's chief complaint, but not found during the patient assessment.
3. Document emergency care delivered by EMS.
   a. Document interventions, who performed them, and the patient's response to the intervention.
   b. Document the time of each intervention and the name and certification number of the EMT-Basic who performed the skill.
4. Document medical direction advice and orders and the results of carrying out the advice or orders.

DOCUMENTATION ISSUES

GENERAL GUIDELINES

1. Do not intentionally leave spaces blank; use "N/A" if material does not apply.
2. Be familiar with commonly accepted medical abbreviations and acronyms and their correct spelling.
   a. Use abbreviations only if they are standard.
   b. Spell words correctly, particularly medical words.
   c. If you do not know how to spell a word, find out or use another word.
3. Describe, do not conclude.
4. Avoid radio codes.
5. When information of a sensitive nature is documented (e.g., communicable disease history), note the source of that information (e.g., patient, family member, bystander).
6. Documentation should not contain jargon, slang, bias, opinions, or impressions.

CONFIDENTIALITY

1. The PCR and the information on it are considered confidential.
   a. Do not show the form or discuss the information contained on it with unauthorized persons.

b. Be familiar with state laws and local protocols.

2. Local and state protocol and procedures will determine where the different copies of the form should be distributed.

PATIENT REFUSALS

1. The EMT-Basic must document specific observations that caused the EMT-Basic to decide that the patient can make a rational, informed decision regarding his or her own care.
2. Once the EMT-Basic has decided the patient is capable of refusing care, the patient must be informed of the risks of refusing care.
   a. The EMT-Basic must document that:
      (1) The patient understands that care is being offered
      (2) The EMT-Basic believes medical care is necessary
      (3) The patient has been informed of the possible consequences of refusing care, including potential death
   b. When possible, the EMT-Basic should explain (and document) the possible consequences of the refusal of care to the patient's relatives or others present who may be able to influence the patient. If the patient is a minor, explain possible consequences to the parent or legal guardian.
3. Consult medical direction as directed by local protocol; document any advice given by medical direction by telephone or radio.
4. If the patient still refuses, document any assessment findings and emergency medical care given, and then have the patient sign a refusal form.
   a. Have a family member, police officer, or bystander sign the form as a witness.
   b. It is preferable to have a disinterested third party witness the form rather than an EMS crew member.
   c. If the patient refuses to sign the refusal form, have a family member, police officer, or bystander sign the form, verifying that the patient refused to sign.
5. Offer (and document) the patient alternative methods of obtaining care.
6. Inform the patient of (and document) your willingness to return should his or her condition change or the patient change his or her mind.

FALSIFICATION

1. **Falsification** of information on the PCR may lead to suspension or revocation of the EMT-Basic's certification/license and other legal action.
2. Falsifying information may harm the patient, because false information may mislead other health care providers about the patient's condition, assessment, and care.
3. **Specific areas of difficulty**
   a. Vital signs: document only the vital signs that were actually taken.
   b. Interventions: if an intervention such as oxygen was overlooked, do not chart that the patient was given oxygen.

ERROR CORRECTION

1. If an error is discovered while the report form is being written:
   a. Draw a single horizontal line through the error, initial it, date it, and write the correct information beside it.
   b. Do not erase or try to obliterate the error; erasures may be interpreted as an attempt to cover up a mistake.
2. If an error is discovered after the report form is submitted:
   a. Preferably in a different color ink, draw a single line through the error, initial and date it, and add a note with the correct information.
   b. If information was omitted, or if additional information comes to the attention

of the EMT-Basic after writing the original report, add a supplemental narrative (addendum) on a separate report form with the correct information, the date, and the EMT-Basic's initials and attach it to the original.

SPECIAL SITUATIONS

MULTIPLE CASUALTY INCIDENTS

1. In a **multiple casualty incident** (MCI), comprehensive documentation must often wait until after the casualties are triaged and transported.
2. The EMT-Basic should know and follow local procedures for documentation of multiple casualty situations. The local MCI plan should include a means of temporarily recording patient information (e.g., triage tags) that can be used later to complete the PCR.

SPECIAL REPORTS

Special reports may be required for:
1. Infectious disease exposure
2. Body fluid exposure
3. Work-related injury
4. Reportable incidents

REVIEW QUESTIONS

Directions: Each of the numbered items or incomplete statements in this section is followed by answers or by completions of the statement. Select the ONE lettered answer or completion that is BEST in each case.

1. A prehospital care report (PCR) may be called a patient care report, incident report, run report, or trip sheet. After the patient encounter, this document

   (A) is intended to stay with the EMT-Basic
   (B) is used solely for billing purposes
   (C) is intended to become part of the patient's hospital record
   (D) is intended to stay with the EMS agency (ambulance service, fire department, etc.)

2. The PCR helps ensure the continuity of patient care. This document may be the only source for important information that hospital personnel need to appropriately assess and treat the patient. An example of such information is

   (A) the patient's past medical history
   (B) the patient's condition at the scene
   (C) the patient's condition at time of transfer of care at the receiving facility
   (D) the patient's current prescription medications and any allergies to medications

3. From a legal standpoint, the PCR

   (A) is the sole property of its author and may only be released with his or her consent

(B) is confidential and may only be reviewed by the agency providing EMS services

(C) is an official record of the care rendered and may be used in court proceedings

(D) is an official record of the care rendered but review of the form may be denied by the agency providing EMS services

4. The PCR should indicate

(A) the name and certification of the document author only

(B) the name and certification of the personnel performing assessment and interventions only

(C) the name and certification of the document author and all personnel assisting in patient care

(D) no names, for legal reasons

5. The PCR and the information contained in it are

(A) public record and may be freely discussed

(B) considered confidential and should not be discussed with unauthorized persons

(C) considered confidential and should not be shown to unauthorized persons, but may be discussed freely

(D) considered confidential and should not be discussed with persons other than the patient, the patient's family and friends, or the patient's employer

6. Falsification of the information on the PCR may harm the patient. Falsification may also lead to

(A) suspension of duties

(B) termination with present employer only

(C) suspension or revocation of certification and other legal action

(D) suspension or revocation of certification but not any other legal action

7. Your ambulance crew is called to the scene of a motor vehicle collision. While documenting, you accidentally record, "Patient was a front seat passenger without a seat belt on." After writing this, the patient informs you that he was the driver of the vehicle and was wearing his seat belt. You should

(A) scribble the error out completely and continue with the form

(B) start the entire form over since mistakes are not acceptable on PCRs

(C) draw a line through the error, date and initial it, and continue with the form

(D) leave the wrong information as is, but make another note on the form that the patient was the driver and was wearing his seat belt

8. Your rescue crew is called to the scene of an explosion at a large apartment complex. There are three obviously dead victims and at least 25 other residents seriously injured. For documentation purposes

(A) you need not fill out a PCR for the deceased victims

(B) no patient may be transported before having a comprehensive PCR completed

(C) a comprehensive PCR may have to wait until after the casualties are triaged and transported

(D) you must triage and treat the patients only; documentation is not needed for multiple casualty incidents (MCI)

9. You are returning to your quarters after transporting a 29-year-old female patient who accidentally cut herself with scissors. While in the back of the ambulance, this patient told you she was feeling dizzy and short of breath. While reviewing your documentation, you notice that you omitted this information. You should

(A) write the information at the bottom of the original PCR
(B) erase the misinformation on the original form and correct it
(C) write the information on a supplement (addendum) form and sign and date it
(D) ignore it since patient care has already been transferred to the hospital staff

Directions: Each of the numbered questions or incomplete statements in this section refers to a scenario that precedes them. The numbered questions or incomplete statements are followed by answers or by completions of the statement. Select the answer or completion of the statement that is BEST in each case.

Your rescue crew is called to the home of a 54-year-old male patient complaining of difficulty breathing. You arrive to find the patient sitting up in bed and very anxious. You are responsible for documentation of this patient encounter.

Questions 10–13

10. Your partner gives the patient supplemental oxygen by nonrebreather mask. For documentation purposes, you should

(A) document that the patient was given oxygen
(B) document that the patient was given oxygen and include the flow rate, delivery device, and time
(C) document that the patient was given oxygen and include the flow rate, delivery device, time, and your partner's name
(D) document that the patient was given oxygen and include the flow rate, delivery device, time, and your name since you are responsible for the documentation

11. After several minutes of oxygen therapy, you should

(A) document the patient's response to the intervention
(B) document the patient's response to the intervention only if his condition has changed
(C) document the patient's response to the intervention only if his condition has improved
(D) document the patient's response to the intervention only if his condition has deteriorated

12. Which of the following statements would be considered a "pertinent negative" for this patient's complaint?

(A) "Patient has a history of asthma"
(B) "Patient speaks in complete sentences without difficulty"
(C) "Lungs have wheezes throughout with diminished tidal volume"
(D) "Patient states that his difficulty breathing began four hours ago while working in the yard"

13. Which of the following statements would be considered a "pertinent positive" for this patient's complaint?

(A) "Patient denies chest pain"
(B) "Patient's skin is dry, warm, and pink"
(C) "Patient has not had any recent trauma or surgeries"
(D) "Patient uses accessory muscles throughout the chest and abdomen to assist respirations"

Your ambulance crew is called to the home of a 34-year-old female patient complaining of finger pain. She states that she accidentally slammed her index finger in a car door. Her finger shows gross deformity but no bleeding. She denies any other injury. You are responsible for documentation of this patient encounter.

Questions 14–16

14. Due to the minor, isolated nature of this patient's complaint, you decide a detailed physical examination is not necessary. Which of the following responses should you document on the PCR regarding the patient's posterior body?

(A) "N/A"
(B) "Pain only in the finger"
(C) "No trauma, pain, or deformity to palpation"
(D) "The patient's back was not assessed due to the minor nature of the complaint"

15. This patient requests transportation to the closest emergency department. While preparing to transport, the patient's husband informs you that she is HIV-positive. For documentation purposes, you should

(A) leave this information out since the patient is not bleeding
(B) document: "Patient has a communicable disease"
(C) document: "Patient has past medical history of AIDS"
(D) document: "Patient's husband states the patient is HIV-positive"

16. After transferring care of this patient in the emergency department, you notice that you only assessed and documented one set of vital signs. You should

(A) leave the document with only one set of vital signs recorded
(B) document that you did not want to take a second set of vital signs
(C) document that a second set of vital signs was taken 5 minutes after the first set
(D) document that a second set of vital signs was taken 15 minutes after the first set

Your rescue crew dispatched to a motor vehicle collision. Your patient is a 24-year-old man complaining of neck pain. When you arrive on scene, the patient is out of his vehicle standing on the sidewalk. You are responsible for documenting this patient encounter.

Questions 17–20

17. As you approach this patient, he tells you that he does not want any help. You notice he is massaging his neck and wincing in pain. Which of the following is correct regarding refusing care?

(A) Any patient may refuse care
(B) Patients with obvious injuries cannot refuse care
(C) Once the patient states he does not want care, you are not allowed to speak with him
(D) Competent, informed adults may refuse care for themselves or for a minor of their responsibility

18. Before acknowledging the patient's refusal, you must be certain the patient understands that care is being offered and that you believe care is needed. You must also

- (A) have a legal guardian assume responsibility for the patient
- (B) make sure that you document at least one set of vital signs
- (C) express the possible complications of refusing care, including potential death
- (D) express the possible complications of refusing care but do not mention death as the patient may mistake it for a threat

19. The patient fits the criteria for refusing treatment. He agrees to sign the "Refusal" form. To witness this form, which of the following persons should ideally sign the form?

- (A) Yourself
- (B) A third party
- (C) Your supervisor
- (D) Another EMT-Basic on your crew

20. Before leaving the scene, you should say to the patient

- (A) "This is your last chance for help"
- (B) "You are probably going to die"
- (C) "Feel free to call us back if you change your mind"
- (D) "You are probably going to be pretty sore from the collision. Take some aspirin when you get home"

ANSWERS AND RATIONALES

1-C. The patient care report (PCR) helps ensure the continuity of care and must be included in the patient's hospital record. Generally, PCRs are printed on carbonless-copy paper, which allows multiple forms to be generated at once. The original generally goes with the patient's records and the remaining copies may be filed with billing, a quality control officer, the EMS agency, or other agency. When generating a document, be aware that many people may ultimately read your report.

2-B. The hospital staff cannot be present at the scene. By painting a clear picture in the PCR, you help ensure that proper assessment and treatment are carried out. Some agencies, in fact, require a photograph of the scene in certain circumstances. For example, when transporting a motor vehicle collision victim, being able to show the hospital staff the mechanism of injury and the damage to the vehicles is sometimes helpful. Information about the patient's past medical history, current medications, and condition upon transfer of care can all be collected at the hospital. These things are important and should be included on the PCR; however, you must appreciate the hospital's need for scene-specific information.

3-C. The PCR is the official document recording prehospital care. It may be subpoenaed and used in court. Therefore, it is important to take documentation seriously. Remember that the general rules are:"If it is not written down, it was not done," and "If it was not done, do not write it down."

4-C. List all persons involved with the patient encounter. Protect yourself from punitive action by treating patients appropriately and documenting your encounter completely, honestly, and neatly. Including the names of all the personnel involved in the encounter may be life-saving. For example, your crew responds on a 12-year-old male patient complaining of a headache. You transport the patient to the hospital and think nothing of the brief encounter. However, if this patient tests positive for a certain type of meningitis, your crew can be at risk of developing the disease. Without complete documentation, notification of your exposure may be greatly delayed or absent.

5-B. Different agencies and different states regulate the confidentiality of the PCR differently. You should attempt to maintain the confidentiality of the report for your protection and for the protection of the patient's privacy. You will often be approached by concerned friends and coworkers who want to know how the patient is doing. Be tactful, compassionate, and nonspecific in your response (e.g., "I appreciate your concern. We are doing everything we can for Mr. Smith"). Do not discuss the patient's medical history, current medications, insurance status, your impression regarding the legitimacy of the complaint, or any similar topics.

6-C. The PCR is a legal document. Falsification of this document may result in punitive measures by your employer, medical direction, your local regulatory agency, and any local, state, or federal law that applies.

7-C. As the PCR is a legal document, use the standard method of correcting mistakes for such documents. Draw a single line through the error, initial and date the line, and write the correct information. It is not appropriate to scribble or erase mistakes, nor is it appropriate to leave a mistake in the document with a reference to the correct information somewhere else on the form. Both of these approaches could be confusing to anyone reading the document.

8-C. Preservation of life is the most important duty with which you may be charged. Documentation, however critical, takes a backseat to prompt, appropriate stabilization, interventions, and transportation. Sometimes the PCR has to wait. All victims must have some form of documentation, even morbidly injured ones.

9-C. This information is pertinent and should be documented. Because you already transferred care of the patient to the receiving facility (and gave the facility its copy of the PCR), putting the information at the bottom of the original form fails to ensure continuity of patient care. A separate form will need to be submitted. Use whatever form your agency deems appropriate and document the date and time of the supplement information, include the information you omitted, and sign the form. If you failed to verbally express the information to the receiving facility, you may need to contact them with the "new" information.

10-C. Be complete. When skills are performed, note the time, equipment used, and the person performing the skill. Do not give yourself credit for performing the skill simply because you are documenting completion of the skill.

11-A. With all interventions, you should record the patient's response regardless of whether the patient's condition has changed. If there was no change according to the patient, simply document, "No change." When documenting the patient's response to an intervention such as splinting or full spinal immobilization, it is important to list the condition of the body area treated before and after your intervention. For example, if a splint is applied to a possibly broken arm, it would be appropriate to document, "Motor, sensory, and circulation intact before and after splint application."

12-B. A pertinent negative is a finding contrary to what you may typically associate with the patient's chief complaint. It would be a significant pertinent negative that this patient, complaining of difficulty breathing, can speak in complete sentences without difficulty. The history of asthma and wheezes are pertinent positives (what you may expect from this patient based on his complaint). The time of onset is not a pertinent negative but does help to complete the picture for this patient's condition.

13-D. A pertinent positive is a finding that is consistent with the patient's chief complaint. The use of accessory muscles to assist respirations is significant and pertinent to the complaint. The denial of chest pain or recent trauma helps to narrow the origin of the complaint, and the skin condition (warm, dry, and pink) is a pertinent negative. Patients in respiratory distress often have cool, wet, pale, or cyanotic skin.

14-A. Be honest but not wordy. "N/A" for "not applicable" is widely understood and accepted. Responses "B" and "D" are wordy, and response "C" implies that you actually evaluated the patient's back.

15-D. Document your observations, not your conclusions. Observations are medically pertinent and should be included on the form regardless of whether the patient is bleeding. A person who is HIV-positive (infected with the Human Immunodeficiency Virus) may not necessarily have AIDS (Acquired Immune Deficiency Syndrome). If your information comes from someone other than the patient (and is not confirmed by the patient), include the source of the information. It may be appropriate to confirm this information with the patient tactfully and privately.

16-A. Be honest! If only one set of vital signs were assessed, then only one set should be recorded. Because this patient seems stable, a set of vital signs is recommended every 15 minutes (every 5 minutes for unstable patients). Do not falsify documents.

17-D. For a valid refusal of care, the patient must be informed that care is offered and recommended. Furthermore, you must indicate to the patient the possible complications of refusing care.

18-C. If you think a possible complication of this patient's refusal of care may be death, you have the responsibility to inform the patient. Be professional, not melodramatic. Seeking assistance from family or friends when encouraging a patient to accept care is often helpful. If an ill or injured patient is adamant about refusing care, you should contact medical direction, according to local protocol.

19-B. Having a third party sign the refusal form is best. It is beneficial to illustrate your efforts to care for the patient by having an outside party witness the patient's refusal.

20-C. While it is preferred that patients receive care initially, always give your patients the option of contacting EMS again for assistance. Do not take the patient's refusal of care as a personal issue. Be professional. If the patient does not want your assistance, direct the patient to contact his personal physician for follow-up care rather than instructing the patient to take aspirin or any other medication. Leave with the understanding that the patient may change his mind later and request your assistance.

BIBLIOGRAPHY

Crosby LA, Lewallen DG (eds): *Emergency Care and Transportation of the Sick and Injured*, 6th ed. Rosemont, IL, American Academy of Orthopaedic Surgeons, 1995.

Grant HD, Murray RH Jr, Bergeron JD: *Emergency Care*, 7th ed. Englewood Cliffs, NJ, Prentice-Hall, 1995.

Hafen BQ, Karren KJ, Mistovich JJ: *Prehospital Emergency Care*, 5th ed. Upper Saddle River, NJ, Prentice-Hall, 1996.

McSwain NE, White RD, Paturas JL, et al (eds): *The Basic EMT: Comprehensive Prehospital Patient Care*. St. Louis, Mosby-Year Book, 1996.

Roush W (ed): *Principles of EMS Systems*, 2nd ed. Dallas: American College of Emergency Physicians, 1994.

Stoy WA: *Mosby's EMT-Basic Textbook*. St. Louis: Mosby-Year Book, 1996.

United States Department of Transportation, National Highway Traffic Safety Administration: *Emergency Medical Technician: Basic. National Standard Curriculum*, 1994.

MEDICAL, BEHAVIORAL, AND OBSTETRIC AND GYNECOLOGICAL EMERGENCIES

FOUR

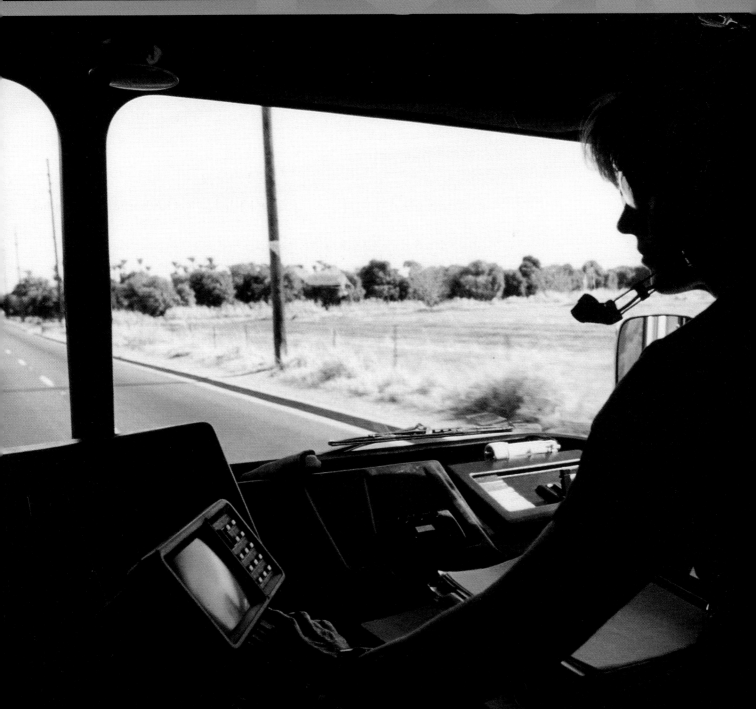

16 GENERAL PHARMACOLOGY

16

OBJECTIVES

*16-1 List four different names that may be used to identify a drug.

*16-2 List four main sources of drugs.

*16-3 List three authoritative sources for drug information.

*16-4 List two federal regulatory agencies or services.

*16-5 List examples of solid and liquid drugs.

*16-6 Differentiate between enteral and parenteral routes of drug administration.

*16-7 State two examples of enteral routes.

*16-8 State two examples of parenteral routes.

16-9 Identify the medications that may be carried on an EMS unit.

16-10 List the medications carried on the EMS unit by generic name.

16-11 Identify the medications that the EMT-Basic may help a patient self-administer.

16-12 List the generic names of the medications that the EMT-Basic can help a patient self-administer.

16-13 Discuss the forms in which the medications may be found.

*16-14 List and explain the five rights of drug administration.

● MOTIVATION FOR LEARNING ●

The EMT-Basic must be familiar with medications carried on the EMS unit and physician-prescribed medications that medical direction has authorized the EMT-Basic to assist patients in taking. Although drugs may be life saving when properly administered, they may be fatal if improperly administered. It is essential that the EMT-Basic be knowledgeable about each medication that he or she administers.

OVERVIEW

TERMINOLOGY

1. **Absorption** is the process by which a drug is transferred from its site of administration into the circulation.
2. **Administration** is the route by which a drug is given (e.g., oral, sublingual, inhalation, intravenous, intramuscular).
3. An **adverse effect** is an unintended and undesirable response to a drug.
4. An **antidote** is an agent that neutralizes or counteracts the effects of a drug or poison.
5. A **contraindication** is a condition for which a drug should not be used because it may cause harm to the patient or offer no improvement of the patient's condition or illness.
6. **Distribution** is the means by which drugs are transported by body fluids to their intended sites of action.
7. A **dose** is the amount of a drug that should be administered to a patient at one time.
8. **Dosage** refers to the frequency, size, and number of doses.
9. A **drug** is a chemical substance used in the diagnosis, treatment, or prevention of disease.
10. **Elimination** is the process by which a drug is removed from the body (e.g., urine, feces, saliva, expired air).
11. **Hypersensitivity** is an exaggerated response to a drug by an individual.
12. An **idiosyncrasy** is a reaction to a drug that is peculiar to an individual and not usually seen in the rest of the population.
13. An **indication** is a condition for which a specific drug has documented usefulness.
14. **Mechanism of action** is how a drug exerts its effect on body cells and tissues.
15. An **over-the-counter (OTC) drug** is a drug that may be purchased without a prescription.
16. **Parenteral** is administration of a drug by means other than through the gastrointestinal tract; this term is more commonly used to describe medications administered by injection.
17. **Pharmacology** is the study of drugs and their actions on the body.
18. A **prescription** is a written direction for the preparation and administration of a drug.
19. A **side effect** is an expected (and usually unavoidable) effect of a drug that usually has no consequence on the drug's intended use.

DRUG NAMES

1. The **official name** of a drug is the name under which a drug is listed in the *United States Pharmacopeia.*
2. The **chemical name** is the precise description of a drug's chemical composition and molecular structure.
3. **Generic name**
   a. The generic name is usually the name given to the drug by the company that first manufactures it.
   b. It is a simplified version of the chemical name.
   c. Generic names are printed in lowercase letters.
3. **Trade name**
   a. The trade name is also known as the brand name, proprietary name, and trademark.
   b. A trade name has the symbol "®" in the upper right-hand corner showing the drug is registered by and restricted to a manufacturer.

    c. A drug may have several different trade names if it is marketed by different manufacturers.

    d. Trade names are capitalized.

    e. Drugs may be dispensed by generic or trade name.

DRUG SOURCES

Drugs can be derived from the following sources:

1. Plants (e.g., morphine, digitalis)
2. Animals (and humans) (e.g., thyroid, insulin, vaccines)
3. Minerals or mineral products (e.g., iron, iodine, sodium chloride)
4. Synthetic sources (e.g., vitamins, narcotics, steroids). Semisynthetic drugs are naturally occurring substances that have been chemically altered (e.g., antibiotics).

DRUG REFERENCES

1. ***Physician's Desk Reference* (PDR)**
   a. Information included in this publication is a compilation of package inserts provided by drug manufacturers.
   b. Information includes the accepted use, dosages, and side effects for commercially available drugs.
   c. It only lists drugs approved by the Food and Drug Administration (FDA) for approved FDA uses.
   d. It contains a product identification guide showing actual sizes and color pictures of commonly prescribed drugs.
   e. It is published annually.
2. ***American Hospital Formulary Service* (AHFS)**
   a. This loose-leaf book is published by the American Society of Hospital Pharmacists.
   b. It is available in hospital pharmacies and most emergency departments.
   c. It contains a comprehensive evaluation of individual drugs and some investigational uses of medications.
   d. It is updated frequently.
3. ***United States Pharmacopeia* (USP)**
   a. This official publication is revised every 5 years by an elected committee of scientific personnel including pharmacists, chemists, physicians, nurses, and consumers.
   b. Supplements are printed regularly.
   c. It lists approved drugs and provides directions for their general use.
4. ***AMA Drug Evaluation***
   a. This reference is published by the American Medical Association (AMA).
   b. It provides information on drug groups, dosages, and use.
5. **Drug Inserts**
   a. Drug inserts are published by pharmaceutical firms.
   b. They are required by law.
   c. Their content is approved by the FDA.

FEDERAL REGULATORY AGENCIES AND SERVICES

1. **Drug Enforcement Agency (DEA)**
   a. The DEA is a division of the Justice Department.
   b. It became the sole legal drug enforcement agency in July 1973 and replaced the Bureau of Narcotics and Dangerous Drugs (BNDD).
2. **Food and Drug Administration (FDA)**
   a. The FDA enforces the Federal Food, Drug and Cosmetic Act by means of seizure and criminal prosecution as necessary.
   b. The FDA requires pharmaceutical firms to report adverse effects associated with new drugs at regular intervals.

3. **Public Health Service**
   a. The Public Health Service is part of the United States Department of Health and Human Services.
   b. It regulates biologic products (e.g., vaccines, antitoxins).

PHARMACOLOGY

SITES OF DRUG ACTION

1. **Local effect**
   a. The local effect of a drug usually occurs at the site of drug application.
   b. The mechanism of action of drugs with only local effects occurs only in a limited part of the body.
2. **Systemic effect.** Drugs with systemic effects are absorbed into the bloodstream and distributed throughout the body.

DRUG FORMS

1. **Solid drugs**
   a. **Capsules** are liquid, dry, or beaded drug particles enclosed in a gelatin container (e.g., Actifed®).
   b. **Pills** are powdered drugs mixed with a liquid and formed into round or oval shapes (e.g., iron).
   c. **Powders** are drugs ground into fine particles (e.g., calcium carbonate).
   d. **Suppositories** are drugs mixed in a firm base such as cocoa butter that, when placed into the rectum or vagina, melt at body temperature (e.g., glycerin).
   e. **Tablets** are powdered drugs, molded or compressed during manufacture (e.g., nitroglycerin).

LIQUID DRUGS

1. **Elixirs** are clear liquids made with alcohol, water, flavors, or sweeteners (e.g., terpin hydrate, Nyquil®)
2. **Emulsions** are mixtures of two liquids, one distributed throughout the other in small globules (e.g., cold cream).
3. **Gels** are clear or translucent semisolid substances that liquefy when applied to the skin or a mucous membrane (e.g., glucose).
4. **Liniments** are preparations in an oily, alcoholic, or soapy base that are applied to the skin.
5. **Lotions** are preparations applied to protect the skin or treat a skin disorder (e.g., Calamine® lotion).
6. **Solutions** are liquid preparations of one or more chemical substances, usually dissolved in water (e.g., 5% dextrose in water, 0.9% normal saline).
7. **Spirits** are volatile substances dissolved in alcohol (e.g., spirit of ammonia).
8. **Suspensions** are drug particles mixed with, but not dissolved in, a liquid (e.g., activated charcoal).
9. **Syrups** are drugs suspended in sugar and water (e.g., cough syrup).
10. **Tinctures** are alcohol solutions prepared from an animal or vegetable drug or chemical substance (e.g., tincture of iodine).

ROUTES OF DRUG ADMINISTRATION

OVERVIEW

1. The route of drug administration is one of the most important factors influencing the effects of a drug and the rate at which the onset of drug action occurs.
2. Although some drugs can be used both locally and systemically, most drugs are given via a single route of administration.

3. Drug routes are categorized as **enteral** or **parenteral.**
   a. **Enteral drugs**
      (1) Enteral drugs are administered through the gastrointestinal tract.
      (2) Advantages include:
         (a) Simple administration
         (b) Convenience
         (c) Relative low cost
      (3) Disadvantages include:
         (a) Slow onset of action (30–45 minutes)
         (b) Possible irritation of the gastrointestinal tract (may result in nausea, vomiting, diarrhea)
   b. **Parenteral drugs**
      (1) Parenteral drugs are those administered by means other than through the gastrointestinal tract.
      (2) This term is most commonly used to describe medications administered by injection.
      (3) Advantages include:
         (a) Rapid onset of action
         (b) Can be administered to patients who are unconscious or unable to swallow
      (4) Disadvantages include:
         (a) Need for careful selection of site and rate of injection
         (b) Need for more skill by the person administering the drug than with most enteral routes of drug administration
         (c) Possible rapid development of side effects

ROUTES OF ADMINISTRATION OF ENTERAL DRUGS

1. **Oral**
   a. The oral route of administration is used infrequently in the prehospital setting.
   b. Commonly used oral dosage forms include liquids, tablets, and capsules.
   c. **Special considerations**
      (1) Patients who are unconscious, uncooperative, have no gag reflex, or are vomiting should not be given drugs orally.
      (2) Activated charcoal may be administered by this route.
2. **Buccal**
   a. Buccal means "pertaining to the cheek."
   b. To administer a drug by this route, a drug is placed in the mouth against the mucous membranes of the cheek until the drug is dissolved.
   c. The drug may act locally on the mucous membranes of the mouth or systemically when swallowed in the saliva.
   d. Buccal drugs are rapidly absorbed into the bloodstream.
   e. Oral glucose may be administered by this route.
3. **Sublingual**
   a. Sublingual drugs are administered under the tongue and must remain under the tongue until dissolved and absorbed.
   b. The drug is absorbed rapidly into the bloodstream due to the rich blood supply under the tongue.
   c. The patient should not swallow the drug or take it with water; if swallowed, the drug may be inactivated by gastric juice.
   d. Nitroglycerin may be administered by this route.

ROUTES OF ADMINISTRATION OF PARENTERAL DRUGS

1. **Subcutaneous**
   a. These drugs are administered by a needle inserted into the connective tissue or fat immediately beneath the dermis.
   b. The onset of action of subcutaneous drugs is faster than the oral route but slower than the intramuscular route.
   c. Absorption is delayed in circulatory collapse (e.g., shock).
   d. Only a small volume of drug can be administered by this route.
2. **Intramuscular**
   a. These drugs are administered by a needle inserted into a large mass of skeletal muscle.
   b. Sites commonly used in prehospital care include:
      (1) Deltoid muscle (arm)
      (2) Vastus lateralis (midlateral thigh)
   c. Injection is usually made with a longer needle than that used with a subcutaneous injection.
   d. Larger volumes can be given by the intramuscular route than the subcutaneous route.
   e. Onset of action is faster than the subcutaneous route due to vascularity of muscle and large absorbing surface.
   f. Absorption is delayed in circulatory collapse (e.g., shock).
3. **Inhalation**
   a. Drugs administered by this route have a rapid onset of action due to the large surface area and vascularity of the lungs.
   b. To ensure that normal gas exchange of oxygen and carbon dioxide is continuous in the lungs, drugs administered by inhalation must be in the form of a gas (e.g., oxygen) or fine mist (e.g., aerosol).
   c. These drugs can be administered for their systemic effect (e.g., oxygen) or localized effect (e.g., metered dose inhaler).

DRUG ADMINISTRATION

GENERAL GUIDELINES

1. The EMT-Basic is responsible for his or her own actions when administering drugs. Although drugs may be life-saving when properly administered, they may be fatal if improperly administered.
2. Before administering any drug, the EMT-Basic must:
   a. Assess the patient's physical status
      (1) The extent of the physical examination will depend on the patient's illness or present condition.
      (2) The physical examination provides baseline information by which to evaluate the effectiveness of medications administered.
   b. Obtain a drug history from the patient including:
      (1) Prescribed medications (name, strength, daily dosage)
      (2) Over-the-counter medications
      (3) Allergies to medications
   c. Be knowledgeable about each drug that he or she administers including:
      (1) Mechanism of action (how the drug exerts its effect on body cells and tissues)
      (2) Indications [the condition(s) for which the drug has documented usefulness]
      (3) Dose (the amount of a drug that should be administered to the patient)
      (4) Route of administration (the route and form in which the drug should be administered to the patient)

(5) Contraindications [condition(s) for which a drug should not be used because it may cause harm to the patient or offer no improvement of the patient's condition or illness]

(6) Side effects [expected (and usually unavoidable) effects of the drug]

MEDICATIONS THAT CAN BE ADMINISTERED BY THE EMT-BASIC

1. The following medications can be carried on the EMS unit (*Table 16-1*):
   a. Activated charcoal
   b. Oral glucose
   c. Oxygen

2. After consulting with medical direction, these medications can be administered to patients who fit established criteria.

3. The EMT-Basic can administer, or assist a patient in administering, the following physician-prescribed medications when authorized by medical direction (*Table 16-2*):
   a. Prescribed inhaler
   b. Nitroglycerin
   c. Epinephrine

Table 16-1. Medications Carried on the EMS Unit

Generic Name	Trade Name	Drug Form	Use
Activated charcoal	SuperChar®, InstaChar®, Actidose®, LiquiChar®	Suspension	Poisoning/overdose by ingestion
Oral glucose	Insta-glucose®, Glutose®	Gel	Altered mental status with diabetic history
Oxygen	Oxygen	Gas	Hypoxia from any cause

Table 16-2. Prescribed Patient Medications that May Be Administered with Authorization from Medical Direction

Generic Name	Trade Name	Drug Form	Use
Albuterol	Proventil®, Ventolin®	Metered dose inhaler	Difficulty breathing due to asthma or chronic obstructive pulmonary disease (COPD)
Epinephrine	Adrenalin EpiPen® EpiPen Jr.®	Auto-injector	Severe allergic reaction (anaphylaxis)
Isoetharine	Bronkosol®, Bronkometer®	Metered dose inhaler	Difficulty breathing due to asthma or chronic obstructive pulmonary disease (COPD)
Metaproterenol	Metaprel®, Alupent®	Metered dose inhaler	Difficulty breathing due to asthma or chronic obstructive pulmonary disease (COPD)
Nitroglycerin	Nitrostat®, Nitrobid®, Nitrolingual spray®	Sublingual tablet, spray	Chest pain of suspected cardiac origin

DRUG ADMINISTRATION PROCEDURE

1. Consult with medical direction.
   a. The EMT-Basic can administer medications only by the order of a licensed physician.
   b. The physician's order may be:
      (1) A written protocol (standing order)
      (2) A verbal order
         (a) Relay relevant information including the patient's age, chief complaint, vital signs, signs and symptoms, allergies, current medications, and pertinent past medical history.
         (b) The physician's order will include the:
            (i) Name of the drug to be administered
            (ii) Dose of the drug to be administered
            (iii) Route of drug administration
         (c) Make sure you clearly understand the orders received from medical direction.
            (i) Repeat orders back to the physician ("echo" procedure) before administering the drug.
            (ii) Include the name of the drug, dose, and route of administration.
         (d) If an order received from medical direction is unclear or seems incorrect, ask the physician to repeat the order.
2. Use the five rights of drug administration.
   a. **Right drug**
      (1) Select the right medication.
      (2) Only use medications that are in a clearly labeled container. If the label is unclear or blurred, do not administer the drug.
      (3) Carefully read the label and check it three times before administering:
         (a) When removing the drug from the drug box
         (b) When preparing the drug for administration
         (c) Before actually administering the drug to the patient
      (4) Check the drug's expiration date.
   b. **Right patient.** If assisting a patient in taking his or her own medication, ensure that the medication is prescribed for that patient.
   c. **Right dose.** Check and recheck the dose ordered against the dose to be administered.
   d. **Right route.** The EMT-Basic must know the route(s) by which a drug can be administered.
   e. **Right time (frequency)**
      (1) Although many drugs are ordered for one-time administration, some may be repeated.
      (2) Determine from medical direction the frequency with which a drug may be administered.
3. **Reassessment strategies.** After administering a drug:
   a. Document the time of drug administration
   b. Document the patient's response to the drug
   c. Monitor the patient for possible adverse effects
   d. Reassess and record vital signs

REVIEW QUESTIONS

Directions: Each of the numbered items or incomplete statements in this section is followed by answers or by completions of the statement. Select the ONE lettered answer or completion that is BEST in each case.

1. Drug therapy may be life saving in many patient encounters. However, if improperly administered, drugs may have a harmful, even fatal, effect on the patient. Who is responsible for the actions of the EMT-Basic when he or she administers drugs?

    (A) The EMT-Basic
    (B) The receiving facility
    (C) The EMT-Basic's personal physician
    (D) The patient's personal physician

2. Which of the following medications may be carried on an EMS response unit staffed by EMT-Basics?

    (A) Albuterol
    (B) Isoetharine
    (C) Oral glucose
    (D) Nitroglycerin tablets

3. Which of the following medications may an EMT-Basic assist a patient in taking (provided the patient has a current subscription of the medication)?

    (A) Lasix®
    (B) Insulin
    (C) Epinephrine
    (D) Any prescription medication as long as the patient's name appears on the medication container

4. Drug absorption refers to

    (A) the route by which a drug is administered
    (B) the route by which a drug is removed from the body
    (C) the condition(s) for which a specific drug has documented usefulness
    (D) the process by which a drug is transferred from its site of administration into the body's circulation

5. A drug's mechanism of action refers to

    (A) the route by which a drug is administered
    (B) an exaggerated response to a drug by an individual
    (C) how a drug exerts its effect on body cells and tissues
    (D) the condition(s) for which a specific drug has documented usefulness

6. Which of the following patient statements illustrates a pharmacologic side effect?

    (A) "I am allergic to aspirin"
    (B) "My albuterol inhaler makes me feel jittery"
    (C) "The nitroglycerin tablet has completely relieved my chest pain"
    (D) "The oxygen has not helped decrease my difficulty breathing"

7. Medications are removed from the body in a number of ways. Some routes include urination, defecation, exhalation, and salivation. The process of removing medications or their by-products from the body is called

    (A) peristalsis
    (B) elimination
    (C) distribution
    (D) bowel movement

8. Which of the following patient statements would suggest medication hypersensitivity?

(A) "I am allergic to penicillin"
(B) "I take nitroglycerin for angina"
(C) "Isoetharine makes my heart beat faster"
(D) "The oxygen you are giving me is drying out my sinuses"

9. You are treating a 74-year-old male patient for difficulty breathing. He informs you that he was seen in the emergency department yesterday for the same complaint and diagnosed with a respiratory infection. The emergency department physician gave him a prescription for Augmentin®. The medication container states the patient is to take 1 pill twice daily for 10 days. These instructions refer to the drug's

(A) dosage
(B) indication
(C) distribution
(D) mechanism of action

10. Which of the following drug references is updated annually, provides color pictures of medications, and includes a compilation of the drug manufacturers' package inserts?

(A) Emergency Medical Technician: Basic. National Standard Curriculum
(B) Nursing Drug Handbook
(C) Physician's Desk Reference (PDR)
(D) Emergency Response Guide (ERG)

11. Which federal agency is solely responsible for the control of legal drugs?

(A) Drug Enforcement Agency (DEA)
(B) American Heart Association (AHA)
(C) Food and Drug Administration (FDA)
(D) Department of Health and Human Services

12. Which of the following lists the speed of medication absorption from slowest to fastest?

(A) Oral, sublingual, intramuscular
(B) Sublingual, oral, intramuscular
(C) Sublingual, intramuscular, oral
(D) Intramuscular, sublingual, oral

13. Oxygen is a drug carried by EMT-Basics. Which of the following BEST defines its indication for use?

(A) Cardiac arrest
(B) Massive blood loss
(C) Respiratory distress
(D) Hypoxia from any cause

14. Your rescue crew is called to the home of a 3-year-old male patient who may have ingested a handful of his grandmother's "heart pills." Which medication would you anticipate administering to this patient?

(A) Epinephrine
(B) Oral glucose
(C) Metaproterenol
(D) Activated charcoal

15. Your ambulance is dispatched to the nurse's office of a local high school. A 15-year-old female patient is experiencing an "asthma attack." Which medication would you anticipate assisting this patient in taking?

    (A) Ventolin®
    (B) Adrenalin
    (C) Epinephrine
    (D) Nitroglycerin

16. Your rescue crew is treating a 54-year-old male patient complaining of severe chest pain. After consulting with medical direction, you are given orders to assist this patient with taking his prescribed nitroglycerin tablets. The medical direction physician tells you that the patient can take up to 3 tablets sublingually at 5-minute intervals, provided that his systolic blood pressure remains greater than 100 millimeters of mercury (mm Hg). While preparing to administer the second nitroglycerin tablet, the patient becomes apneic and pulseless. You should immediately

    (A) reestablish contact with medical direction
    (B) begin cardiopulmonary resuscitation and rapid transport
    (C) put the tablet under the patient's tongue and reestablish contact with medical direction
    (D) put the remaining 2 nitroglycerin tablets under the patient's tongue and begin cardiopulmonary resuscitation

17. Your rescue crew is called to a local law office for a 74-year-old female patient complaining of severe, nonradiating chest pain. She states the pain is a "9" on a 1 to 10 scale (with "10" being the most severe). Her skin is cool, clammy, and ashen. A radial pulse cannot be felt, but a carotid pulse is weak and irregular at 154 beats per minute. You are unable to obtain a blood pressure. After consulting medical direction, you are ordered to assist this patient in taking her nitroglycerin tablets. You are concerned that this treatment may be harmful to the patient and should

    (A) give the medication as ordered
    (B) give the medication and begin rapid transport to the receiving facility
    (C) ask the physician to repeat the order, then give the medication as ordered
    (D) ask the physician to repeat the order, but do not give the medication as ordered if you feel it may harm the patient

18. Sublingual medications

    (A) should be chewed
    (B) are rapidly absorbed
    (C) should be swallowed
    (D) include isoetharine and albuterol

Directions: Each of the numbered items or incomplete statements in this section is negatively phrased, as indicated by a capitalized word such as NOT, LEAST, or EXCEPT. Select the ONE lettered answer or completion that is BEST in each case.

19. Which of the following is NOT an advantage of enteral drug administration?

    (A) Simple administration
    (B) Convenience
    (C) Irritation of the gastrointestinal tract
    (D) Relative low cost

Directions: Each of the numbered questions or incomplete statements in this section refers to a scenario that precedes them. The numbered questions or incomplete statements are followed by answers or by completions of the statement. Select the answer or completion of the statement that is BEST in each case.

You are called to the home of a 69-year-old male patient complaining of chest pain. Your patient is conscious and alert and complains of dull, substernal chest pain radiating to his jaw and left arm. The pain is a "10" on a 1 to 10 scale (with 10 being most severe). The patient states the pain came on about 20 minutes before your arrival while he was at rest.

Questions 20–22

20. Before administering any medication, you must

(A) assess the patient's physical status
(B) obtain a drug history from the patient
(C) obtain permission to administer the medication from medical direction
(D) all of the above

21. Nitroglycerin is administered

(A) sublingually
(B) by inhalation
(C) intramuscularly
(D) subcutaneously

22. When taken, nitroglycerin generally lowers the blood pressure. This effect is

(A) local
(B) systemic
(C) hypersensitive
(D) an idiosyncrasy

Your rescue crew is called to a local park for a 23-year-old female patient complaining of severe difficulty breathing. The patient's boyfriend informs you that the patient is allergic to bee stings, and she received a sting less than 10 minutes ago. Her lips are beginning to swell and her level of distress is increasing.

Questions 23–24

23. An appropriate medication to consider for this patient is

(A) epinephrine
(B) oral glucose
(C) nitroglycerin
(D) activated charcoal

24. After following the appropriate steps to administer this medication, you reevaluate the patient's status before administration. The patient's vital signs are as follows: pulse = 132 beats/minute, weak, and regular; respirations = 24/minute and shallow; blood pressure = 94/62; pupils = equal and slow to react to light; skin condition = cool, moist, pale. Based on these findings, you expect the medication to

(A) act more rapidly because of the patient's skin condition
(B) act more slowly because of the patient's respiratory rate
(C) act more rapidly because of the patient's blood pressure
(D) act more slowly because the patient is in shock

Your ambulance crew is called to the apartment of a 19-year-old female patient. Her friend called you for assistance because "she is just not acting right." The patient has a history of diabetes. She is conscious but answers questions inappropriately with slurred speech.

Questions 25–27

25. Which medication should you consider administering to this patient?

    (A)   Insulin
    (B)   Nitroglycerin
    (C)   Oral glucose
    (D)   Activated charcoal

26. You telephone your medical direction physician to get approval to administer this medication. After the physician tells you what medication to use, the dose of the medication, and its route into the body, you should

    (A)   immediately give the medication
    (B)   reply, "10-4, copy" and give the medication
    (C)   repeat the orders back to the physician
    (D)   begin transporting the patient to the receiving facility before administering the medication

27. While you are getting the medication out of the drug box, the patient becomes unconscious. Medical direction instructed you to give the medication buccally. You should

    (A)   give the medication sublingually and prepare to suction
    (B)   quickly proceed to give the medication according to the physician's instructions
    (C)   begin rapid transport and reestablish contact with medical direction
    (D)   mix the medication with water and have the patient drink the mixture.

ANSWERS AND RATIONALES

1-A. While EMT-Basics assist in the administration of certain medications on the advice of medical direction, the EMT-Basic must be aware that he or she is held responsible when administering medications. Communication with medical direction must be clear and accurate for desired patient outcomes.

2-C. While EMT-Basics may assist in the administration of all these medications, only oral glucose can be supplied by the EMT-Basic. The other medications must be the patient's own prescription medication. The EMT-Basic may also carry oxygen and activated charcoal.

3-C. EMT-Basics may assist in the administration of epinephrine in a severe allergic reaction (anaphylaxis). Other medications that EMT-Basics may assist patients in taking are bronchodilators (albuterol, isoetharine, and metaproterenol) and nitroglycerin. These medications must be prescriptions belonging to the patient. The EMT-Basic is not authorized to administer (or assist the patient in taking) other prescription medications, even if the patient's name appears on the medication container.

4-D. Absorption is the process of by which a drug is transferred from its form at the site of administration into a form that can be transported for use throughout the body. For example, a medication taken orally enters the stomach within seconds of ingestion; however, it may take several hours for the medication to be completely absorbed into the body's circulation. Elimination is the term used for the removal of a drug or its by-products from the body, and indication is the term used for the condition for which a specific drug has documented usefulness.

5-C. The mechanism of action is the method by which a medication acts on the body. For example, albuterol is a bronchodilator used to relieve difficulty breathing. The mechanism of action for albuterol is relaxation of the smooth muscles of the respiratory tree, thus allowing a freer flow of air.

6-B. A side effect is an expected and usually unavoidable effect of a drug that generally has no consequence on the drug's intended use. A side effect of albuterol administration may be "jitters" and agitation. It is important to know and understand the side effects of the medications you may be asked to administer. For example, headache is a common side effect of taking nitroglycerin.

7-B. Elimination is the process of removing the drug or its by-products from the body regardless of the route of administration. Peristalsis is the wavelike contraction that moves food along the gastrointestinal tract. Distribution refers to the means by which a drug is transported throughout the body. A bowel movement is the final elimination of solid waste from the body's gastrointestinal tract.

8-A. Hypersensitivity is an exaggerated response to a medication. Sometimes this response may be in the form of a severe allergic reaction (anaphylactic reaction). Hypersensitivity to a particular medication is an example of a medication's contraindication. A contraindication is a condition in which a drug should not be used because of its potential to cause further harm.

9-A. Dosage refers to the frequency, size, and number of doses for prescription and non-prescription medications. A drug's indication is the condition or conditions for which the drug has a documented usefulness. Distribution is the means by which the drug is transported throughout the body. The mechanism of action refers to how the drug works in the body.

10-C. The *Physician's Desk Reference*, commonly called the "PDR," is a text published annually and contains updates on drug information, drug inserts, and color pictures of commonly prescribed medications. The *Nursing Drug Handbook* is another source of medication information, but it is not as detailed as the PDR. The *Emergency Medical Technician: Basic. National Standard Curriculum* is the basis of EMT-Basic education in the United States. The *Emergency Response Guidebook* is a publication of the Department of Transportation that lists hazardous materials and the actions necessary to protect, contain, and stabilize hazardous materials incidents.

11-A. The Drug Enforcement Agency (DEA), a division of the Justice Department, is responsible for legal drug enforcement laws. The American Heart Association (AHA) is an organization that assists with the development of medical education programs. The Food and Drug Administration (FDA) is responsible for ensuring that pharmaceutical firms report adverse effects associated with drugs. Finally, the Department of Health and Human Services regulates biologic products such as vaccines and antitoxins through its Public Health Service branch.

12-A. Oral drugs generally take the longest to be absorbed since they must pass through the tissues of the gastrointestinal tract to enter the body's circulation. Sublingual drug administration is faster than oral administration because the medication is quickly absorbed into the capillary beds of the oropharynx (mouth). Intramuscular administration is the fastest route of drug administration listed because the medication is delivered directly to a large muscle mass with an extensive blood supply. However, expect a dramatic delay in intramuscular drug absorption if the patient is in shock. In shock (hypoperfusion), the effectiveness of circulation is decreased.

13-D. Any condition that results in hypoxia should be treated with oxygen therapy. Cardiac arrest, massive blood loss, and respiratory distress are all examples of conditions that result in hypoxia. Oxygen therapy should begin early. Do not wait until the patient becomes cyanotic (blue) or complains of respiratory difficulty before administering oxygen.

14-D. Activated charcoal is indicated for poisonings or overdoses by ingestion. Activated charcoal is an "adsorbent." Its microscopic pores adsorb many poisons and medications. The poisons or medications then pass through the gastrointestinal tract bound to the activated charcoal.

15-A. Ventolin® and Proventil® are trade names for albuterol. Albuterol, like isoetharine and metaproterenol, is a bronchodilator. Bronchodilators are inhaled and absorbed deep in the respiratory tree where they "relax" constricted airway passages. EMT-Basics may assist in the administration of albuterol, isoetharine, and metaproterenol to ease difficulty breathing associated with asthma or chronic obstructive pulmonary disease (COPD). It is important to note that these medications are absorbed deep in the respiratory tree. Patients must be instructed to inhale the atomized medication as deeply as possible for maximum benefit. If the patient's tidal volume (amount of air moved in and out of the lungs) is severely low, he or she may not benefit from inhaling a bronchodilator because the drug will not reach the terminal air sacs (alveoli) where it is absorbed.

16-B. If your patient's condition changes between the time you are given an order by medical direction and the time you prepare to carry out the order, reassess the patient. In this scenario, you should IMMEDIATELY begin cardiopulmonary resuscitation and rapid transportation. If possible (or per local protocol), re-contact medical direction to inform the physician and receiving facility of the change in the patient's condition.

17-D. Hypoperfusion is a common adverse effect of nitroglycerin administration. Therefore, it is important to assess a patient's blood pressure before each dose of nitroglycerin. Nitroglycerin should not be administered if the patient's systolic blood pressure is less than 100 millimeters of mercury (mm Hg). Although the medical direction physician has a high level of training, education, and responsibility, you should never blindly follow any order. Tactfully help the medical direction physician understand your thoughts and concerns about the intervention. If you fail to come to a mutual conclusion and you are concerned about possible adverse effects of the ordered intervention for the patient, inform the medical direction physician that you will begin rapid transportation of the patient without initiating the intervention until the physician has the opportunity to evaluate the patient firsthand. Be sure to follow up with medical direction and your employer or agency.

18-B. Sublingual medications, such as nitroglycerin, are administered under the tongue and are designed to be absorbed into the capillary beds of the mouth. These medications are rapidly absorbed within 1 to 2 minutes and should not be chewed or swallowed. Bronchodilators such as isoetharine and albuterol are inhaled medications.

19-C. Enteral drug routes include oral, buccal, and sublingual. Enteral drugs are generally simple and convenient to administer, and relatively inexpensive. Disadvantages of enteral drug administration include a slower onset of action than parenteral drugs and possible irritation of the gastrointestinal tract, resulting in nausea, vomiting, and diarrhea.

20-D. Assessing the patient's physical status is essential to ensuring that a correct treatment plan is developed. You must be knowledgeable about each drug you may administer. Obtaining a patient's drug history should include prescription medications, over-the-counter medications, and medication allergies. Finally, as an EMT-Basic, you must gain approval from medical direction before administering a medication. Approval may be in the form of on-line medical direction (speaking with the physician via phone or radio) or off-line medical direction (through standing orders).

21-A. Nitroglycerin is administered under the tongue (either in tablet or spray form). The medication is dissolved and quickly absorbed into the rich capillary beds of the mouth. Patients should be instructed not to chew or swallow nitroglycerin tablets. Furthermore, they should be informed that headache is a common side effect of nitroglycerin.

22-B. Lowering blood pressure is a systemic effect of nitroglycerin. Systemic effects are those that can be observed throughout the body, whereas local effects are those that can be observed in a specific area. Burning under the tongue is a common and acceptable localized side effect of nitroglycerin administration. An example of a hypersensitive response would be an undetectable blood pressure after administration of one nitroglycerin tablet. Before administering nitroglycerin, the patient's systolic blood pressure should be above 100 millimeters of mercury (mm Hg). An example of an idiosyncratic response would be an increase in the patient's blood pressure because of nitroglycerin therapy.

23-A. Epinephrine is indicated for severe allergic reactions, also known as anaphylaxis. Before administering this medication, you must assess the patient, obtain a medication history, get approval from medical direction, and ensure that the epinephrine has been prescribed for this patient. Oral glucose would be indicated if the patient were a known diabetic and was having a diabetic-related emergency. Nitroglycerin is used for the relief of chest pain of suspected cardiac origin. Activated charcoal is indicated for ingested poisonings or overdoses.

24-D. The rate of absorption of injected medications depends on the effectiveness of the circulatory system. This patient's blood pressure is relatively low, her skin is pale (indicating poor perfusion), and the pulse is weak. Considering these factors, you should expect a longer than normal absorption rate.

25-C. Oral glucose is indicated for patients showing signs of altered mental status with a history of diabetes. If possible, you should attempt to obtain a blood glucose reading to make sure that the patient is "sugar deficient" rather than "insulin deficient." A normal blood sugar reading is 80–120 milligrams per deciliter (mg/dL). A low reading would suggest the need for oral glucose administration. Be extremely cautious when administering oral medications to patients with an altered mental status. If the patient becomes unconscious with the medication in her mouth, the patient will require aggressive airway maintenance. EMT-Basics are not authorized to assist patients with insulin administration.

26-C. Always echo (repeat back) the orders you are given. Echoing ensures that you received the instructions correctly. Additionally, echoing allows medical direction the opportunity to hear his or her orders a second time, thus ensuring the orders are correct.

27-C. As a rule of thumb, if the patient's condition drastically changes, contact medical direction. In this case, medical direction instructed you to administer an oral medication to a conscious patient; however, by the time you were prepared to administer the medication, the patient became unconscious. The circumstances under which the physician ordered the medication to be administered have changed. Since the patient's presentation is worsening, begin immediate and rapid transport and reestablish contact with medical direction.

BIBLIOGRAPHY

Abrams AC: *Clinical Drug Therapy*, 4th ed. Philadelphia, JB Lippincott, 1995.

Beck RK: *Pharmacology for Prehospital Emergency Care*, 2nd ed. Philadelphia, FA Davis, 1994.

Bledsoe BE, Clayden DE, Papa FJ: *Prehospital Emergency Pharmacology*, 4th ed. Upper Saddle River, New Jersey, Prentice-Hall, 1996.

Crosby LA, Lewallen DG (eds): *Emergency Care and Transportation of the Sick and Injured*, 6th ed. Rosemont, IL, American Academy of Orthopaedic Surgeons, 1995.

Grant HD, Murray RH Jr, Bergeron JD: *Emergency Care*, 7th ed. Englewood Cliffs, NJ, Prentice-Hall, 1995.

Hafen BQ, Karren KJ, Mistovich JJ: *Prehospital Emergency Care*, 5th ed. Upper Saddle River, NJ, Prentice-Hall, 1996.

Kozier B, Erb G, Blais K, et al: *Fundamentals of Nursing: Concepts, Process, and Practice*, 5th ed. Redwood City, CA, Addison-Wesley, 1995.

Malseed RG, Goldstein FG, Balkon N: *Pharmacology: Drug Therapy and Nursing Considerations*, 4th ed. Philadelphia, JB Lippincott, 1995.

McKenry LM, Salerno E: *Mosby's Pharmacology in Nursing*, 18th ed. St. Louis, Mosby-Year Book, 1992.

McSwain NE, White RD, Paturas JL, et al (eds): *The Basic EMT: Comprehensive Prehospital Patient Care*. St. Louis, Mosby-Year Book, 1996.

Stoy WA: *Mosby's EMT-Basic Textbook*. St. Louis, Mosby-Year Book, 1996.

United States Department of Transportation, National Highway Traffic Safety Administration: *Emergency Medical Technician: Basic. National Standard Curriculum*, 1994.

17 RESPIRATORY EMERGENCIES

OBJECTIVES

17-1 Describe the structure and function of the respiratory system.

*17-2 Given a diagram, trace the flow of air in the respiratory system from the nose to the alveolus.

*17-3 Explain the basic mechanics of breathing.

*17-4 Define diffusion.

*17-5 Define tidal volume.

*17-6 Define minute volume.

*17-7 Explain how oxygen is transported to the tissues and how carbon dioxide is transported from the tissues.

*17-8 Explain how respiration is regulated in the human body.

*17-9 Define dyspnea.

17-10 State the signs and symptoms of a patient with breathing difficulty.

*17-11 Explain why the physical finding of quiet breathing is not always a good sign.

*17-12 Describe the following types of noisy breathing:

a. Stridor
b. Wheezing
c. Gurgling
d. Grunting

MOTIVATION FOR LEARNING

The EMT-Basic will frequently encounter patients with respiratory emergencies. The EMT-Basic must recognize the signs of breathing difficulty, determine if the patient's breathing is adequate or inadequate, and deliver appropriate patient care based on these findings.

When authorized by medical direction, the EMT-Basic may assist a patient in taking a prescribed inhaler. Before assisting with the administration of any medication, the EMT-Basic must know the generic and trade names, medication forms, dose, administration, action, indications, and contraindications for the medication to ensure patient safety.

267

*17-13 Define pleuritic chest pain.

*17-14 Describe the following abnormal breath sounds:

    a. Crackles (rales)

    b. Rhonchi

    c. Wheezes

17-15 Describe the emergency medical care of the patient with breathing difficulty.

17-16 Establish the relationship between airway management and the patient with breathing difficulty.

17-17 Explain why medical direction is needed to assist in the emergency medical care of the patient with breathing difficulty.

17-18 Describe the emergency medical care of the patient with adequate breathing.

17-19 Describe the emergency medical care of the patient with inadequate breathing.

*17-20 Describe the signs of adequate artificial ventilation.

*17-21 Describe the signs of inadequate artificial ventilation.

17-22 State the generic name, medication forms, dose, administration, mechanisms of action, indications and contraindications for a prescribed inhaler.

17-23 Distinguish among the emergency medical care of the infant, child, and adult patient with breathing difficulty.

*17-24 List eight nontraumatic causes of dyspnea.

*17-25 Differentiate between upper airway obstruction and lower airway disease in the infant and child patient.

*17-26 Explain the pathophysiology of the following respiratory conditions:

    a. Croup

    b. Epiglottitis

    c. Asthma

    d. Chronic bronchitis

    e. Emphysema

    f. Pneumonia

    g. Pulmonary embolism

    h. Acute pulmonary edema

*17-27 List the signs and symptoms of the following respiratory conditions:

    a. Croup

    b. Epiglottitis

    c. Asthma

    d. Chronic bronchitis

    e. Emphysema

    f. Pneumonia

    g. Pulmonary embolism

    h. Acute pulmonary edema

*17-28 State the emergency care for the following respiratory conditions:

    a. Croup

    b. Epiglottitis

    c. Asthma

    d. Chronic bronchitis

    e. Emphysema

    f. Pneumonia

    g. Pulmonary embolism

    h. Acute pulmonary edema

ANATOMY AND PHYSIOLOGY REVIEW

FUNCTION

The major functions of the respiratory system are to:
1. Supply oxygen from the atmosphere to body cells.
2. Transport carbon dioxide produced by body cells to the atmosphere.

DIVISIONS OF THE RESPIRATORY SYSTEM

1. **Upper respiratory tract**
   a. The upper respiratory tract consists of parts outside the chest cavity—nose, pharynx, and larynx.
   b. **Function.** The upper respiratory tract filters, warms, and humidifies the air, protecting the surfaces of the lower respiratory tract.
2. **Lower respiratory tract**
   a. The lower respiratory tract consists of parts found almost entirely within the chest cavity—trachea and lungs (including the bronchial tree and alveoli).
      (1) The lungs are enclosed and protected by a pleural membrane that consists of two layers.
         (a) The visceral pleura covers the lungs themselves.
         (b) The parietal pleura lines the chest wall.
      (2) The pleural cavity is a small potential space between the visceral and parietal pleura. The pleural cavity contains a lubricating fluid that minimizes friction between the membranes and allows them to move easily during breathing.
   b. **Function.** The lower respiratory tract conducts air to the alveoli where gas exchange occurs.
      (1) Alveoli are considered the functional units of the lungs because gas exchange occurs across them.
      (2) Each alveolus is surrounded by a network of pulmonary capillaries.
      (3) The wall of an alveolus consists of a single layer of cells.
      (4) A thin film of surfactant coats each alveolus; surfactant prevents the alveoli from collapsing.

MECHANICS OF BREATHING

1. **Definitions**
   a. **Breathing** (pulmonary ventilation) is the mechanical process of moving air into and out of the lungs.
   b. **Inspiration** (inhalation) is the process of breathing in and moving air into the lungs.
   c. **Expiration** (exhalation) is the process of breathing out and moving air out of the lungs.
   d. **Respiration** is the exchange of gases between a living organism and its environment.
2. **Breathing**
   a. The breathing process consists of four phases:
      (1) The movement of room air into and out of the lungs (pulmonary ventilation)
      (2) The diffusion of oxygen and carbon dioxide in the alveoli (external respiration). **Diffusion** is the movement of gases or particles from an area of higher concentration to an area of lower concentration.
      (3) The transport of oxygen to the cells and carbon dioxide away from the cells (internal respiration).
      (4) The regulation of ventilation

   b. The mechanics of breathing can be compared with a bellows.
- **(1)** When the bellows (lungs) is open, air enters.
- **(2)** As it closes, air is forced out.

   c. Normal breathing involves two primary muscles:
- **(1)** Diaphragm
- **(2)** External intercostal muscles between the ribs

   d. In an adult, a normal breath is approximately 500 milliliters (mL) of air. This amount is called the tidal volume.

   e. Minute volume is the total amount of air breathed in and out in one minute. Minute volume = tidal volume × respiratory rate.

3. Inspiration

   a. Inspiration is an active process (requires muscle contraction).

   b. The diaphragm and external intercostal muscles contract.

   c. The chest cavity enlarges and fills with air.

   d. Inspiration continues until the pressure between the lungs and atmosphere equalizes.

4. Expiration

   a. Expiration is normally a passive process.

   b. The diaphragm and external intercostal muscles relax.

   c. The chest cavity becomes smaller, compressing the lungs.

   d. Air is forced out of the lungs and into the atmosphere.

5. Accessory muscles

   a. The accessory muscles of breathing are used during periods of respiratory distress. This use is particularly common in patients with chronic obstructive pulmonary disease (COPD) and in infants and children.

   b. The muscles of the diaphragm and neck are used to assist in inspiration.

   c. The muscles of the abdomen and the internal intercostals are used to assist expiration.

6. Gas exchange

   a. Overview
- **(1)** The tissues of the body depend on a continuous supply of oxygen to maintain metabolism.
- **(2)** Interruption of the body's oxygen supply and/or removal of carbon dioxide can lead to shock and death.

   b. Alveolar/capillary exchange
- **(1)** Oxygen-rich air enters the alveoli during each inspiration.
- **(2)** Oxygen-poor blood in the capillaries passes into the alveoli.
- **(3)** Oxygen enters the capillaries as carbon dioxide enters the alveoli.

   c. Capillary/cellular exchange
- **(1)** Cells give up carbon dioxide to the capillaries.
- **(2)** Carbon dioxide is released during cellular metabolism.
- **(3)** Capillaries give up oxygen to the cells.

7. Control of respiration

   a. Respiration is controlled by nerve, reflex, and chemical responses in different parts of the body.

   b. The medulla of the brain stem generates impulses that travel along nerves to the respiratory muscles; the respiratory muscles are stimulated to contract, resulting in inspiration.

   c. The walls of the bronchi and bronchioles contain stretch receptors.
- **(1)** As the lungs inflate, the stretch receptors detect the stretching and generate impulses to depress the medulla.
- **(2)** Depression of the medulla limits the extent of inspiration, preventing overinflation of the lungs.

   d. The main stimulus for breathing is the level of carbon dioxide in the blood.
- **(1)** An accumulation of carbon dioxide in the blood causes an increase in the rate and depth of ventilation.

(2) An unusually low level of carbon dioxide in the blood results in a decrease in the rate and depth of ventilation.

e. Chronic respiratory diseases may alter the normal respiratory drive over time.

(1) Instead of an increase in carbon dioxide levels stimulating breathing, low levels of oxygen in the blood become the breathing stimulus; this kind of breathing stimulus is called hypoxic drive.

(2) In these patients, prolonged periods of high-concentration oxygen administration depress respirations and may result in respiratory arrest.

ASSESSING THE PATIENT WITH BREATHING DIFFICULTY

OVERVIEW

1. Shortness of breath or difficulty breathing is called **dyspnea.**
2. Dyspnea is a common chief complaint encountered by the EMT-Basic, requiring prompt assessment and treatment.

SCENE SIZE-UP

1. Determine if the patient's breathing difficulty is due to trauma or a medical condition.
   a. **Trauma.** Determine the mechanism of injury from the patient, family members, or bystanders and inspection of the scene.
   b. **Medical.** Determine the nature of the illness from the patient, family members, or bystanders.
2. Observe the patient's environment for clues to the cause of the patient's breathing difficulty.

INITIAL ASSESSMENT

1. Maintain spinal immobilization if trauma is suspected.
2. Assess the patient's mental status.
   a. As the amount of oxygen in the blood decreases, the patient may become anxious, restless, confused, and combative.
   b. As the amount of carbon dioxide in the blood increases, the patient may become increasingly difficult to arouse.
3. Observe the patient's position.
   a. Patients with dyspnea frequently sit or stand to aid their chest muscles in the process of inhaling and exhaling.
      (1) **Orthopnea** is breathlessness when lying flat that is relieved when the patient sits or stands.
      (2) **Paroxysmal nocturnal dyspnea** is a sudden onset of difficulty breathing that occurs at night; it occurs because of an accumulation of fluid in the alveoli or pooling of secretions during sleep.
   b. The patient with dyspnea may assume a "tripod" position (seated upright, leaning forward with the head hyperextended) in an effort to inhale adequate air.
4. Observe how many words the patient can speak before requiring a breath.
   a. Can the patient answer questions in full sentences?
   b. Or can he or she speak only a few words before requiring a breath?
5. Assess the airway.
   a. Assess for complete or partial airway obstruction.
   b. Signs and symptoms of complete or partial airway obstruction include:
      (1) Inability to speak, cry, cough, or make any other sound
      (2) Cyanosis
      (3) Hoarseness
      (4) Restlessness, anxiety

      (5) Difficult/labored breathing

      (6) Decreased or no air movement

      (7) Noisy breathing (e.g., snoring, crowing, gurgling, wheezing)

6. Assess breathing.

  a. Note the rise and fall of the chest.

  b. Estimate the respiratory rate.

    (1) The patient with breathing difficulty often has a respiratory rate outside the normal limits for his or her age.

    (2) An increase in the respiratory rate is an early sign of respiratory distress.

    (3) Agonal (slow, gasping) respirations may be observed just before death. The patient with agonal respirations requires immediate positive-pressure ventilation with 100% oxygen.

  c. Note the depth/equality of breathing.

    (1) The patient with difficulty breathing often has inadequate or shallow respirations. Shallow respirations, even in the presence of an increased respiratory rate, may be inadequate to ventilate the patient.

    (2) The patient with inadequate breathing requires immediate positive-pressure ventilation with 100% oxygen.

  d. Note the rhythm of respirations. Conditions that may cause irregular breathing include a head injury, drug overdose, and diabetic emergency.

  e. Note any signs of increased work of breathing (respiratory effort) including:

    (1) Nasal flaring

    (2) Pursed-lip breathing

    (3) Use of accessory muscles

    (4) Leaning forward to inhale

    (5) Presence of "seesaw" breathing in infants

    (6) **Retractions** [indentations of the skin above the clavicles (supraclavicular), between the ribs (intercostal), and/or below the rib cage (subcostal)]

    (7) Note the presence of any wounds, open or closed.

  f. Listen for air movement.

    (1) Note if respirations are quiet, absent, or noisy.

      (a) Normal breathing is quiet.

      (b) However, quiet breathing is not always a good sign.

        (i) Breathing becomes quiet when a partial airway obstruction becomes a complete obstruction.

        (ii) Quiet breathing in a patient with asthma may indicate a decrease in air movement.

      (c) Noisy breathing is indicated by stridor, wheezing, gurgling, or grunting.

        (i) **Stridor** is a harsh, high-pitched sound associated with upper airway obstruction. It is most often heard during inspiration and is frequently described as a high-pitched crowing or "seal-bark" sound.

        (ii) Wheezing is high-pitched "whistling" sounds produced by air moving through narrowed airway passages. Wheezing may be heard with or without a stethoscope throughout the lungs or, in the case of a foreign body obstruction, it may be localized.

        (iii) Gurgling is a liquid sound heard during breathing associated with fluid collection in the patient's airway.

        (iv) Grunting is heard most frequently in infants and is the sound created when forcefully exhaling against a closed glottis (which traps air and keeps the alveoli open).

    (2) Feel for air movement against your hand or cheek.

7. Assess circulation.

  a. Assess the pulse.

  b. Estimate the heart rate and assess its regularity and strength.

   c. Assess perfusion.
      (1) Note the color, temperature, and condition (moisture) of the patient's skin; the skin may be pale or cyanotic (blue), cool, clammy.
      (2) Observe the nailbeds, earlobes or tops of the ears, lips, base of the tongue, and the area around the mouth for pallor or cyanosis.
      (3) In infants and children younger than 6 years of age, assess capillary refill.
      (4) If appropriate, evaluate for possible major bleeding.

8. Establish patient priorities.
   a. Priority patients include:
      (1) Those in whom a patent airway cannot be established or maintained
      (2) Those who are experiencing difficulty breathing or who exhibit signs of respiratory distress
      (3) Those with absent or inadequate breathing and who require continuous positive-pressure ventilation
   b. Advanced-life-support (ALS) assistance should be requested as soon as possible.
   c. If ALS personnel are not available, the patient should be transported promptly to the closest appropriate facility.

FOCUSED HISTORY AND PHYSICAL EXAMINATION

1. The focused history and physical examination:
   a. Focuses on the patient's chief complaint, whether it is a medical or trauma condition
   b. Identifies other conditions that could be life-threatening if not attended to promptly
   c. Determines the severity of the condition without unnecessarily delaying transportation

2. If the patient is unresponsive:
   a. Perform a rapid physical examination
   b. Follow with evaluation of baseline vital signs and gathering of the patient's medical history

3. If the patient is responsive:
   a. Gather information about the patient's medical history before performing the physical examination
      (1) The patient should be the primary source of information.
      (2) Additional sources of information include the scene, family members, friends, and bystanders.
   b. Obtain a SAMPLE history using the OPQRST acronym to recall the pertinent questions to ask when obtaining the history of the present illness or event.
      (1) **Signs and symptoms.** Signs and symptoms of breathing difficulty (*Box 17-1*) (*Figure 17-1*) include:
         (a) Restlessness, anxiety
         (b) Altered mental status
         (c) Coughing
         (d) Hoarseness
         (e) Diaphoresis (moist skin)
         (f) Pallor, cyanosis
         (g) Sputum production
         (h) Shortness of breath (dyspnea)
         (i) Abnormal respiratory sounds (e.g., stridor, gurgling, wheezing)
         (j) Nasal flaring
         (k) Pursed-lip breathing
         (l) Use of accessory muscles
         (m) Abdominal breathing
         (n) Retractions
         (o) Hemoptysis (coughing up blood)

Box 17-1. Signs and Symptoms of Breathing Difficulty

Shortness of breath
Restlessness, anxiety
Increased or decreased pulse rate
Increased or decreased respiratory rate
Skin color changes (pallor, cyanosis)
Use of accessory muscles
Coughing
Retractions
Irregular breathing rhythm
Nasal flaring
Unusual anatomy (barrel chest)
Abdominal breathing (diaphragm only)
Inability to speak due to breathing efforts
Seesaw breathing (infants and children)
Hemoptysis
Pleuritic chest pain
Altered mental status (with fatigue or obstruction)
Noisy breathing (e.g., stridor, snoring, crowing, gurgling, audible wheezing)

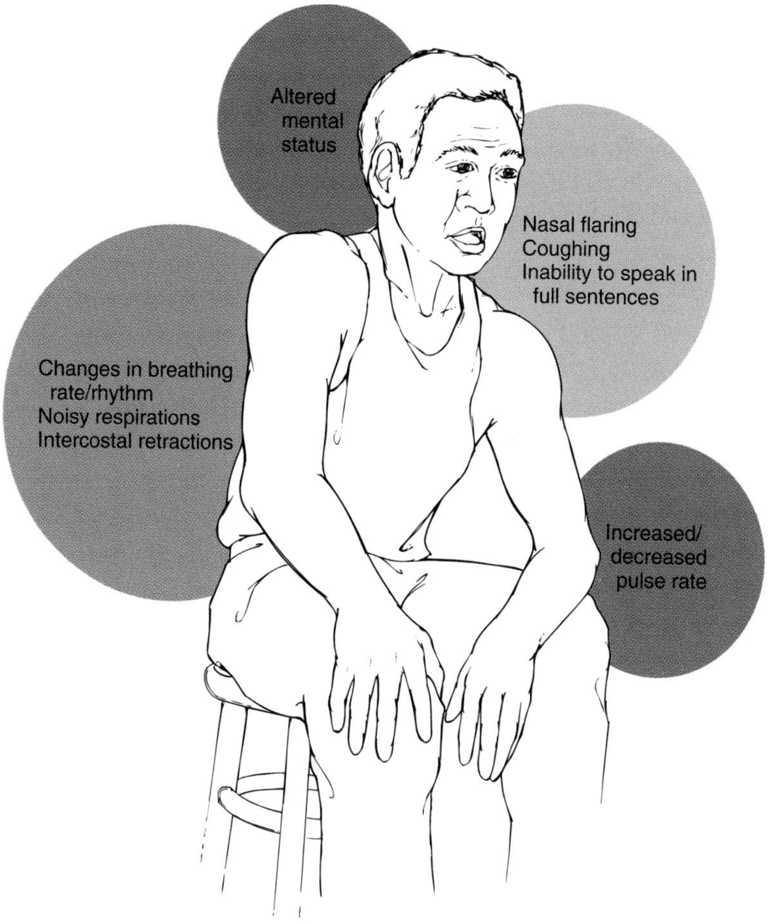

Altered mental status

Nasal flaring
Coughing
Inability to speak in full sentences

Changes in breathing rate/rhythm
Noisy respirations
Intercostal retractions

Increased/decreased pulse rate

Fig. 17-1. Signs and symptoms of difficulty breathing.

    (p) Pleuritic chest pain
      (i) Pleuritic chest pain is chest pain associated with movement of the chest wall.
      (ii) It may result from irritation of the pleura or chest wall muscles.
      (iii) It is described as sharp and stabbing and worse on deep breathing and coughing.
    (q) Barrel chest
      (i) A barrel chest occurs as a result of incomplete exhalation, which causes air to become trapped in the lungs.
      (ii) It is associated with respiratory disorders present for many years.

(2) <u>A</u>llergies
    (a) Determine if the patient has any allergies to medications and other substances or materials.
    (b) Difficulty breathing may be caused by an allergic reaction.

(3) **Medications.** Determine if the patient is taking any medications (prescription and over-the-counter) (*Table 17-1*).
    (a) Determine if the patient takes his or her medications regularly and his or her response to them. Patients with asthma or chronic obstructive pulmonary disease are frequently prescribed theophylline, steroids, or inhalers.
    (b) Determine if there has been any recent change in medications (additions, deletions, or change in dosages).
    (c) Provide all information obtained to the receiving facility.

(4) **Pertinent past medical history**
    (a) Determine if the patient has a history of asthma, allergies, tuberculosis, bronchitis, pneumonia, heart disease, diabetes, or high blood pressure.
    (b) Determine if the patient has had any chest surgery.
    (c) Determine if the patient has a family history of tuberculosis, heart disease, lung cancer.
    (d) Determine the patient's exposure to pollutants.
      (i) Determine if the patient smokes and, if so, how much.
      (ii) Determine the patient's exposure to dust, fumes, asbestos, and chemicals.

(5) <u>L</u>ast oral intake. Determine the patient's last oral intake.
(6) <u>E</u>vent. Ascertain the <u>e</u>vents leading up to this incident.

Table 17-1. Medications Commonly Prescribed for Patients with Respiratory Problems

	Generic Name	Trade Name(s)
Bronchodilators	Albuterol	Ventolin®, Proventil®
	Isoetharine	Bronkosol®, Bronkometer®
	Metaproterenol	Metaprel®, Alupent®
	Theophylline	Marax®, Quibron®, Slo-Phyllin®, Tedral®, Theo-Dur®, Slo-Bid®, Somophyllin®, Choledyl®
	Ipratropium bromide	Atrovent®
Steroids	Beclomethasone	Vanceril®, Beclovent®

  c. OPQRST
   (1) **Onset.** Determine if the onset of the patient's breathing difficulty was gradual or sudden.
    (a) What was the patient doing when the breathing difficulty began?
    (b) How long has the breathing difficulty been present?
   (2) **Provocation.** Determine what (if anything) provoked this episode of breathing difficulty.
    (a) Ascertain if the patient has noticed any changes in his or her breathing pattern, such as:
     (i) Need to sit or stand to breathe
     (ii) Difficulty breathing at night
    (b) Determine if the patient has taken any medications to relieve the problem before your arrival.
   (3) **Quality.** Determine if the patient experiences pain with breathing or activity. If pain is present, determine its location.
    (a) Ask the patient to describe the pain.
    (b) Determine if the pain occurs when the patient breathes in or out.
    (c) Ask what the patient has done to relieve the pain.
   (4) **Radiation.** If pain is present, determine if it radiates to any area.
   (5) **Severity.** Determine the patient's perception of the severity of his or her breathing difficulty. Ask, "On a scale of 1 to 10, with 1 being no shortness of breath and 10 being shortness of breath as bad as it can be, how would you rate your breathing difficulty?"
   (6) **Time.** Ascertain how long the patient's breathing difficulty has been present (e.g., seconds, minutes, hours, days).
 4. Assess baseline vital signs.
 5. Perform a focused physical examination.
  a. Look
   (1) Inspect the face for nasal flaring.
   (2) Inspect the neck for jugular venous distention (JVD).
   (3) Inspect the chest for:
    (a) Use of accessory muscles
    (b) Retractions
    (c) Equal rise and fall
    (d) Seesaw breathing (in infants and children)
   (4) Observe the patient's position.
   (5) Observe the patient's skin color.
  b. Listen
   (1) Assess breath sounds.
    (a) Auscultate breath sounds over the apex and base of each lung and on the lateral aspects of the chest in the midaxillary line.
    (b) Normal breath sounds are heard on both sides of the chest, in all areas.
    (c) Determine if breath sounds are:
     (i) Present, diminished, or absent; absent breath sounds indicate the patient is not moving enough air to adequately ventilate his or her lungs.
     (ii) Equal or unequal
     (iii) Clear or noisy
    (d) Abnormal breath sounds include:
     (i) **Crackles (rales),** which are intermittent high-pitched "popping" sounds produced by the passage of air through moisture. The sound produced by rolling strands of hair back and forth between the fingers resembles that of fine crackles. Coarse crackles sound like a Velcro fastener being opened.

> **(ii)** **Rhonchi,** which are harsh, low-pitched sounds that are usually the result of narrowing of the larger airways (bronchi) due to mucus or fluid. They frequently clear after coughing.
>
> **(iii)** **Wheezes,** which were described previously.

(2) Listen for noisy breathing, including stridor, wheezing, gurgling, and grunting.

(3) If the patient can speak, note if he or she can speak in full sentences.

(4) Note if the patient has a cough.

    (a) If a cough is present, determine if it is dry or productive of sputum.

    (b) If the cough is productive, note the color and odor of the sputum.

        (i) Pink, frothy sputum is associated with pulmonary edema.

        (ii) Thick yellow or green sputum suggests the presence of a lung infection.

(5) Note the ratio of inhalation to exhalation.

    (a) Normally, inspiration is about twice as long as expiration.

    (b) Prolonged inspiration suggests upper airway obstruction.

    (c) Prolonged expiration suggests lower airway obstruction.

c. Feel

(1) Feel for the presence of subcutaneous emphysema, which suggests the presence of an air leak from the lungs into the subcutaneous tissue.

(2) Assess for tenderness or crepitus on palpation of the chest wall.

(3) Palpate the position of the trachea.

    (a) Place one thumb on either side of the trachea above the sternal notch.

    (b) The trachea is normally in a midline position.

    (c) The position of the trachea may shift from its normal position (tracheal deviation) in conditions such as tension pneumothorax.

EMERGENCY MEDICAL CARE

FOREIGN-BODY AIRWAY OBSTRUCTION

1. Conscious adult or child

  a. If the patient is more than 1 year of age, deliver abdominal thrusts (Heimlich maneuver).

  b. Chest thrusts should be performed for patients who are very large or in the late stages of pregnancy.

  c. Repeat thrusts until effective or the patient becomes unconscious.

2. Conscious infant

  a. Perform 5 back blows and 5 chest thrusts to clear the obstruction.

  b. Repeat until effective or the patient becomes unconscious.

3. Unconscious patient

  a. Take body substance isolation precautions.

  b. Establish unresponsiveness.

  c. Open the airway. If the object can be visualized, remove it with a finger sweep.

  d. Assess breathing.

    (1) If the patient is breathing, maintain an open airway.

    (2) If the patient is not breathing, attempt to ventilate.

  e. If the chest rises, continue rescue breathing.

  f. If the chest does not rise, reposition the head and attempt to ventilate again.

  g. If the airway remains obstructed, perform manual thrusts.

    (1) In the adult and child, perform abdominal thrusts.

    (2) In the infant, administer back blows and chest thrusts.

  h. When the obstruction is removed, assess breathing.

    (1) If the patient is breathing, continue to assess breathing and pulse while maintaining an open airway.

     (a) Position the patient on his or her side.

     (b) Assist ventilations as necessary.

(2) If breathing is absent but a pulse is present:

     (a) **Adult**

          (i) Administer 100% oxygen

          (ii) Deliver 1 breath every 5 seconds (12 breaths per minute)

     (b) Child and infant

          (i) Administer 100% oxygen

          (ii) Deliver 1 breath every 3 seconds (20 breaths per minute)

(c) Continue to monitor the pulse.

ADEQUATE BREATHING

If breathing is adequate:

1. Administer oxygen by nonrebreather mask at 15 liters per minute (LPM). If the patient is breathing adequately, a nasal cannula should only be used if the patient cannot tolerate a mask.
2. Allow the patient to assume a position of comfort.
3. Assess vital signs.
4. Determine if the patient has a prescribed inhaler (metered dose inhaler).
   a. If the patient does have a prescribed inhaler:
      (1) Contact medical direction
      (2) If instructed to do so, assist the patient with its use
      (3) Continue with the focused assessment
   b. If the patient does not have a prescribed inhaler, continue the focused assessment.
5. Perform ongoing assessments until patient care is turned over to ALS personnel or medical personnel at the receiving facility.

INADEQUATE BREATHING

If the patient exhibits signs of inadequate breathing:

1. Establish and maintain an open airway.
2. Provide positive-pressure ventilation with 100% oxygen.
   a. Assess the adequacy of the ventilations delivered.
   b. Signs of adequate artificial ventilation include:
      (1) The chest rises and falls with each artificial ventilation.
      (2) The rate is sufficient.
         (a) For adults, the rate should be approximately 12 ventilations per minute.
         (b) For children and infants, the rate should be approximately 20 ventilations per minute.
      (3) The heart rate returns to normal.
   c. Signs of inadequate artificial ventilation include:
      (1) The chest does not rise and fall with artificial ventilation.
         (a) Reassess head position.
         (b) Insert an oropharyngeal or nasopharyngeal airway as necessary.
         (c) Suction as necessary.
         (d) Reassess the seal between the patient's face and mask.
      (2) The rate of ventilation is too slow or too fast. Adjust rate to deliver approximately 12 breaths per minute for an adult; approximately 20 breaths per minute for infants and children.
      (3) The heart rate does not return to normal.
3. Transport promptly to the closest appropriate medical facility.

ASSISTING THE PATIENT WITH A PRESCRIBED INHALER

1. **Prescribed inhalers**
   a. Prescribed inhalers are also called metered dose inhalers.
   b. Metered dose inhalers are aerosol cans containing medication that is released in a specific dose with each spray.
   c. **Generic name (trade names)**
      (1) Albuterol (Proventil®, Ventolin®)
      (2) Isoetharine (Bronkosol®, Bronkometer®)
      (3) Metaproterenol (Metaprel®, Alupent®)
2. **Mechanism of action.** Beta-agonist bronchodilators dilate bronchial smooth muscle, reducing airway resistance.
3. **Indications.** The EMT-Basic can assist patients in using a prescribed inhaler only if ALL of the following criteria are met:
   a. The patient exhibits signs and symptoms of breathing difficulty
   b. The patient has a physician-prescribed handheld inhaler
   c. The EMT-Basic has obtained specific authorization from medical direction (off-line or on-line)
4. **Contraindications**
   a. The patient is unable to use the device (the patient must be alert enough to use the inhaler).
   b. The inhaler is not prescribed for the patient.
   c. Medical direction does not give permission.
   d. The patient has already taken the maximum recommended dose before arrival of the EMT-Basic.
5. **Medication form.** Inhaled beta-agonists are delivered in aerosol form by a handheld metered dose inhaler.
6. **Dosage.** The total number of times the medication can be administered is determined by medical direction.
7. **Administration**
   a. Confirm that the patient is having breathing difficulty.
   b. Confirm that the patient has a physician-prescribed handheld inhaler.
      (1) Ensure that the inhaler is prescribed for the patient.
      (2) Ensure that the inhaler is not expired.
   c. Determine if the patient is alert enough to use the inhaler.
   d. Determine if the patient has already taken any doses.
   e. Obtain an order from medical direction (either on-line or off-line) to assist the patient in taking the medication.
   f. Assure right medication, right patient, right route.
   g. Assure that the inhaler is at room temperature or warmer.
   h. Shake the inhaler vigorously several times.
   i. Remove the oxygen mask from the patient.
   j. Have the patient exhale deeply.
   k. Have the patient put his or her lips around the opening of the inhaler.
   l. Have the patient depress the handheld inhaler as he or she begins to inhale deeply.
   m. Instruct the patient to hold his or her breath for as long as comfortably possible so that the medication can be absorbed.
   n. Replace the oxygen mask on the patient.
   o. Allow the patient to breathe a few times and repeat second dose per medical direction.
   p. If the patient has a spacer device for use with his inhaler, it should be used. A spacer device is an attachment between the inhaler and the patient that allows for more effective use of medication.
   q. Document the patient's name, drug name and dose administered, time of administration, and the patient's response to the drug.

r. If an on-line order was received by medical direction, document the name of the physician giving the order.

8. **Side effects.** Side effects include:
   a. Increased pulse rate
   b. Tremors
   c. Nervousness

9. **Reassessment**
   a. Reassess vital signs.
   b. Perform a focused reassessment.
      (1) Note any changes in the patient's condition.
      (2) If the patient's condition deteriorates, provide positive-pressure ventilation as necessary.

INFANT AND CHILD CONSIDERATIONS

1. Use of handheld inhalers is very common in children.
2. Retractions are more commonly seen in children than adults.
3. Cyanosis is a late finding in children.
4. Very frequent coughing may be present rather than wheezing in some children.
5. Emergency care for assisting a child with using a handheld inhaler is the same as for an adult if the indications for usage of inhalers are met by the ill child.

ENRICHMENT: COMMON RESPIRATORY DISORDERS

DYSPNEA

1. **Definition.** Dyspnea is a sensation of shortness of breath.
2. The patient may express his or her breathing difficulty in different ways (e.g., "short of breath;" "short-winded;" "can't get my breath").
3. Causes include:
   a. Trauma (see Chapter 29)
   b. Medical conditions such as:
      (1) Croup
      (2) Epiglottitis
      (3) Asthma or allergic reactions
      (4) Chronic obstructive pulmonary disease (COPD)
      (5) Chronic bronchitis
      (6) Emphysema
      (7) Pneumonia
      (8) Acute pulmonary embolism
      (9) Acute pulmonary edema

CROUP

1. **Pathophysiology**
   a. Croup is a viral infection that causes inflammation and swelling beneath the larynx and glottis.
   b. It most commonly occurs in children between the ages of 3 months and 3 years, although it can occur in older children.
   c. It is most prevalent in the fall and winter.
2. Signs and symptoms include:
   a. Stridor
   b. Barking cough
   c. Hoarse voice
   d. Low-grade fever
   e. Gradual onset, usually over 1 to 2 days

3. **Emergency care**
   a. Allow the child to assume a position of comfort.
   b. Allow the caregiver to hold the child while administering supplemental oxygen. If the mask is not well tolerated, administer oxygen by "blow-by."
   c. Transport to the hospital for further evaluation.

EPIGLOTTITIS

1. **Pathophysiology**
   a. Epiglottitis is a bacterial infection of the epiglottis most commonly occurring in children between 3 and 7 years of age, although it may also occur in adults.
   b. The onset of symptoms is usually sudden, developing over a few hours.
   c. Respiratory arrest may occur as a result of complete airway obstruction or a combination of partial airway obstruction and fatigue.
2. Signs and symptoms include:
   a. Restlessness
   b. High fever
   c. Sore throat
   d. Drooling
   e. Dyspnea
   f. Stridor
   g. Tripod position, unwilling to lie down
3. **Emergency care**
   a. Closely observe the child at all times.
   b. Allow the child to assume a position of comfort.
   c. Avoid upsetting the child.
      (1) Allow the caregiver to hold the child while administering supplemental oxygen.
      (2) If the mask is not well tolerated, administer oxygen by "blow-by."
   c. Do not attempt to visualize the airway.
   d. If respiratory arrest occurs, deliver positive-pressure ventilations with 100% oxygen.
   e. Rapidly transport the child to the closest appropriate medical facility.

ASTHMA OR ALLERGIC REACTIONS

1. **Pathophysiology**
   a. Asthma is widespread, reversible narrowing of the bronchioles that results in airflow obstruction.
   b. Asthma may be caused by many factors ("triggers") including:
      (1) Environmental irritants (e.g., smoke, smog, dust, fumes)
      (2) Weather factors (e.g., extremes of heat, cold, humidity; dusty or moldy environment)
      (3) Certain medications
      (4) Exercise
      (5) Infection
      (6) Emotional stress
   c. After exposure to the trigger:
      (1) The smooth muscles surrounding the bronchioles spasmodically contract (bronchospasm) and swell and mucus secretion increases; the mucus secreted is abnormally thick.
      (2) Airway passages are narrowed due to smooth muscle contraction, excessive mucus secretion, or a combination of both and results in the trapping of air in the bronchioles.
      (3) Exhalation becomes prolonged as the patient tries to exhale the trapped air.
2. Signs and symptoms include:

  a. Dyspnea
  b. Coughing (dry or productive)
  c. Wheezing; however, in the asthmatic patient, an absence of wheezing is an ominous sign that suggests that airflow is so diminished that wheezing is not produced.
  d. Restlessness
  e. Increased respiratory rate
  f. Increased heart rate
  g. Use of accessory muscles
3. **Emergency care**
  a. Allow the patient to assume a position of comfort.
  b. Administer 100% oxygen, preferably humidified oxygen by nonrebreather mask.
  c. Provide calm reassurance to help reduce the patient's anxiety.
  d. Encourage the patient to cough and breathe deeply to assist in the removal of secretions.
  e. If instructed to do so by medical direction, assist the patient in using his or her prescribed inhaler.
  f. Transport to the closest appropriate medical facility for further evaluation.

CHRONIC BRONCHITIS

1. **Pathophysiology** (*Figure 17-2*)
  a. Chronic bronchitis is defined as sputum production for 3 months of a year for at least 2 consecutive years.
  b. The primary cause of chronic bronchitis is cigarette smoking.
  c. Respiratory irritants, such as smoke, irritate the airways and cause an increase in mucus production.
  d. Prolonged exposure to respiratory irritants eventually causes distortion and scarring of the bronchial wall, decreasing the size of the airway opening.
  e. Excessive mucus production in the bronchi causes a chronic or recurrent productive cough.
  f. Because the size of the airway opening is decreased, some secretions are trapped in the alveoli and smaller air passages.
  g. Some individuals with chronic bronchitis retain carbon dioxide.
    (1) In healthy persons, the main stimulus to increase ventilation is an increase in carbon dioxide.
    (2) Over time, the patient with chronic bronchitis adapts to the retention of carbon dioxide and their main stimulus to breathe becomes a decrease in oxygen (hypoxic drive).
    (3) The term "blue bloater" has been used to describe these individuals because the patient is often obese with a cyanotic complexion.
2. Signs and symptoms (depend on severity of the disease and whether or not there are other problems in addition to the chronic bronchitis) include:
  a. Productive cough
  b. Cyanosis
  c. Labored breathing
  d. Use of accessory muscles
  e. Increased respiratory rate
  f. Peripheral edema
  g. Inability to speak in complete sentences without pausing for a breath
3. **Emergency care**
  a. Allow the patient to assume a position of comfort.
  b. If signs of breathing difficulty are present, administer oxygen by nonrebreather mask at 15 LPM or as ordered by medical direction.
  c. If no signs of respiratory distress are evident, administer oxygen by nasal cannula at 2 LPM or as ordered by medical direction.

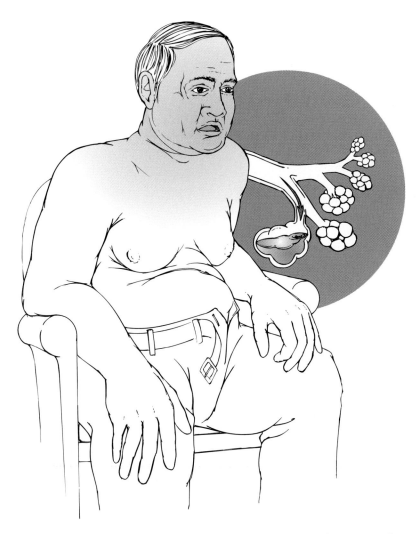

Fig. 17-2. In chronic bronchitis, respiratory irritants, such as smoke, irritate the airways and cause an increase in mucus production. Prolonged exposure to respiratory irritants eventually causes distortion and scarring of the bronchial wall, decreasing the size of the airway opening.

   d. Monitor the patient closely, reassessing every 5 minutes, and be prepared to assist ventilations as necessary.
   e. Provide calm reassurance to help reduce the patient's anxiety.
   f. Encourage the patient to cough and breathe deeply to assist in the removal of secretions.
   g. If instructed to do so by medical direction, assist the patient in using his or her prescribed inhaler.
   h. Transport to the closest appropriate medical facility for further evaluation .

EMPHYSEMA

1. **Pathophysiology**
   a. Emphysema is an irreversible enlargement of the air spaces distal to the terminal bronchioles that leads to the destruction of the walls of the alveoli, distention of the alveolar sacs, and a loss of lung elasticity.
   b. In emphysema, the lungs inflate easily but, due to the lack of elastic recoil, air becomes trapped in the lungs.
   (1)   The volume of air in the chest increases, giving the patient a barrel-chest appearance.

      (2)   The loss of elasticity causes exhalation to become an active (rather than passive) process, increasing the work of breathing.

    c. The patient with emphysema may be called a "pink puffer" because he or she can often increase his or her respiratory rate to maintain a relatively normal amount of oxygen (pink color), although his or her work of breathing is increased during exhalation (puffer) (*Figure 17-3*).

    d. Carbon dioxide levels are often normal in patients with emphysema because they hyperventilate to maintain normal oxygen levels.

2. Signs and symptoms include:

    a. Barrel chest

    b. Use of accessory muscles

    c. Pursed-lip breathing

    d. Chronic cough

    e. Prolonged exhalation

    f. Increased respiratory rate

    g. Dyspnea with exertion

3. Emergency care

    a. If signs of breathing difficulty are present, administer oxygen by nonrebreather mask at 15 LPM or as ordered by medical direction.

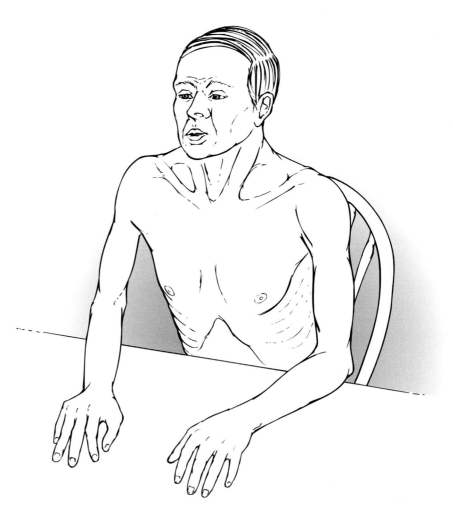

Fig. 17-3. Patients with emphysema may be called "pink puffers" because they can often increase their respiratory rate to maintain a relatively normal amount of oxygen, although their work of breathing is increased during exhalation.

   b. If no signs of respiratory distress are evident, administer oxygen by nasal cannula at 2 LPM or as ordered by medical direction.

   c. Monitor the patient closely, reassessing every 5 minutes, and be prepared to assist ventilations as necessary.

   d. Provide calm reassurance to help reduce the patient's anxiety.

   e. Encourage the patient to cough and breathe deeply to assist in the removal of secretions.

   f. If instructed to do so by medical direction, assist the patient in using his or her prescribed inhaler.

   g. Transport to the closest appropriate medical facility for further evaluation.

PNEUMONIA

1. **Pathophysiology**
   a. Pneumonia is an infection that often impairs gas exchange in the lung. It may involve the distal airways and alveoli, part of a lobe, or an entire lobe of the lung.
   b. Pneumonia is most frequently caused by bacteria and viruses, although it may also be caused by fungi and parasites.
      (1) Bacterial pneumonia can occur in any part of the lung and usually causes inflammation and swelling of the alveoli.
      (2) Viral pneumonia often begins in the bronchioles and then spreads to the alveoli. Respiratory syncytial virus (RSV) is most common in infants and children.
      (3) The alveoli fill with blood and fluid, limiting their ability to effectively exchange oxygen and carbon dioxide.
2. Signs and symptoms include:
   a. Fever
   b. Chills
   c. Increased respiratory rate
   d. Increased heart rate
   e. Possible cough
   f. Possible pleuritic chest pain
3. **Emergency care**
   a. Allow the patient to assume a position of comfort.
   b. Administer oxygen by nonrebreather mask at 15 LPM.
   c. Transport to the hospital for further evaluation and treatment.

PULMONARY EMBOLISM

1. **Pathophysiology**
   a. A pulmonary embolus is usually a clot originating from the deep veins in the leg that travels through the veins to the heart and then to the pulmonary circulation.
   b. The clot becomes trapped in the smaller branches of the pulmonary arteries, causing partial or complete blood flow obstruction.
   c. As a result, a portion of the lung is ventilated but not perfused. To compensate, the patient's respiratory rate increases.
   d. If the area involved is large, respiratory failure will occur.
   e. Factors that increase the risk for pulmonary embolism include:
      (1) Obesity
      (2) Prolonged bed rest or immobilization
      (3) Recent surgery, particularly of the legs, pelvis, abdomen, or chest
      (4) Leg or pelvic fractures or injuries
      (5) Use of high-estrogen oral contraceptives
      (6) Pregnancy

       (7) Chronic atrial fibrillation (a heart rhythm disorder)

  f. Signs and symptoms depend on the:

       (1) Size and location of the embolus

       (2) Number of emboli

       (3) Presence or absence of underlying cardiac and pulmonary disease

2. Signs and symptoms include:

  a. Sudden onset of dyspnea

  b. Apprehension, restlessness

  c. Possible pleuritic (sharp, stabbing) chest pain

  d. Possible cough

  e. Increased respiratory rate

  f. Increased heart rate

  g. Possible blood-tinged sputum

  h. Possible hypotension

3. **Emergency care**

  a. Allow the patient to assume a position of comfort unless hypotension is present.

  b. If the patient is alert but exhibiting signs of breathing difficulty, administer oxygen by nonrebreather mask at 15 LPM and provide positive-pressure ventilation with 100% oxygen as necessary.

  c. Reassess the patient frequently.

  d. Transport promptly to the closest appropriate medical facility.

ACUTE PULMONARY EDEMA

1. **Pathophysiology**

  a. Pulmonary edema is most commonly due to failure of the left ventricle of the heart, although other (noncardiac) conditions can result in pulmonary edema including:

       (1) Near-drowning

       (2) Narcotic overdose

       (3) Trauma

       (4) High altitude

  b. When the left ventricle fails, fluid is forced into the lung tissue as the right ventricle continues to pump blood into the pulmonary circulation.

  c. The alveoli fill with fluid, limiting their ability to effectively exchange oxygen and carbon dioxide.

2. Signs and symptoms include:

  a. Restlessness, anxiety

  b. Dyspnea on exertion

  c. Orthopnea (difficulty breathing when lying flat)

  d. Increased respiratory rate

  e. Frothy, blood-tinged sputum

  f. Cool, moist skin

  g. Use of accessory muscles

  h. Wheezing

  i. Crackles

  j. Increased heart rate

  k. Increased or decreased blood pressure depending on severity of edema

3. **Emergency care**

  a. Sit patient up (unless hypotension is present) to promote lung expansion.

  b. If breathing is adequate, administer oxygen by nonrebreather mask at 15 LPM.

  c. If breathing is inadequate, provide positive-pressure ventilation with 100% oxygen.

  d. Reassess frequently, monitoring vital signs at least every 5 minutes.

  e. Transport promptly to the closest appropriate medical facility.

REVIEW QUESTIONS

Directions: Each of the numbered items or incomplete statements in this section is followed by answers or by completions of the statement. Select the ONE lettered answer or completion that is BEST in each case.

1. A chief function of the upper respiratory tract is

   (A) the absorption of oxygen
   (B) the warming and humidifying of inspired air
   (C) the filtering and dehumidification of expired air
   (D) the protection of the lower airway against choking (foreign body airway obstruction)

2. The lower respiratory tract consists of the trachea, bronchi, bronchioles, and

   (A) medulla
   (B) alveoli
   (C) epiglottis
   (D) esophagus

3. The primary muscles of breathing are the

   (A) lungs and diaphragm
   (B) lungs and abdominal muscles
   (C) diaphragm and intercostal muscles
   (D) diaphragm and abdominal muscles

4. Inhalation is an active process involving muscular contraction of the primary breathing muscles. Exhalation is normally

   (A) an active process involving contraction of the abdominal muscles
   (B) a passive process involving contraction of the abdominal muscles
   (C) an active process involving contraction of the accessory muscles
   (D) a passive process involving relaxation of the primary breathing muscles

5. The exchange of cellular gases occurs in the capillary beds. In the lungs, _____ is absorbed across the lung tissue into the bloodstream of the capillary beds, and _____ is allowed to leave the bloodstream and enter the air space of the lungs.

   (A) oxygen, hemoglobin
   (B) oxygen, carbon dioxide
   (C) oxygen, carbon monoxide
   (D) hemoglobin, carbon monoxide

6. The respiratory centers of the body are found

   (A) in the alveoli
   (B) in the brain stem
   (C) in the diaphragm
   (D) between the third, fourth, and fifth cervical vertebrae

7. For most patients, the main stimulus for breathing is derived from the level of _____ in the bloodstream. However, chronic respiratory disease may change the stimulus for breathing to the level of _____ in the bloodstream.

   (A) carbon dioxide, oxygen
   (B) oxygen, carbon dioxide
   (C) oxygen, carbon monoxide
   (D) carbon dioxide, hemoglobin

8. "Difficulty breathing" is often called

   (A) dyspnea
   (B) diaphoresis
   (C) tachycardia
   (D) minute volume

9. During your initial assessment of a patient complaining of difficulty breathing, you should note the position the patient assumed before your arrival. Often this position may indicate the level of the patient's distress. Conscious, alert patients in severe distress will often be found

   (A) lying in a fetal position
   (B) sitting or standing bolt upright
   (C) lying flat on their back (supine)
   (D) lying flat on their stomach (prone)

10. An early sign of nontraumatic respiratory distress is

   (A) facial droop
   (B) unresponsiveness
   (C) agonal respirations
   (D) increased respiratory rate

11. During normal breathing, the inspiratory phase (inhalation) takes about twice as long as the expiratory phase (exhalation). Prolonged inspiration may suggest _____, and prolonged expiration may suggest _____.

   (A) upper airway obstruction, lower airway obstruction
   (B) lower airway obstruction, upper airway obstruction
   (C) partial airway obstruction, complete airway obstruction
   (D) complete airway obstruction, partial airway obstruction

12. Your ambulance responds to the home of a 34-year-old male patient complaining of difficulty breathing and chest pain. He states that his chest pain worsens with deep inspiration and coughing. He denies any recent trauma and denies any past medical history. The term given this complaint is

   (A) hemothorax
   (B) flail segment
   (C) tracheal deviation
   (D) pleuritic chest pain

13. Before assisting in the administration of a metered dose inhaler, you must ensure that

   (A) the patient is apneic and has a history of chronic bronchitis
   (B) the patient is unconscious, has a history of asthma, and has a prescribed inhaler
   (C) the patient is having difficulty breathing and has access to his brother's metered dose inhaler

(D) the patient is having difficulty breathing and has a prescribed inhaler and you have authorization from medical direction

14. You are called to a local park for a 17-year-old female patient complaining of a sudden onset of difficulty breathing. She tells you that her allergies have been bothering her lately and her distress greatly increased after playing soccer today. Her respiratory rate is 30 respirations per minute and she has wheezes throughout her lungs. Her skin is cool and moist. She speaks in five- to eight-word sentences. If this patient has not been prescribed a metered dose inhaler, you should

(A) immediately transport without further treatment
(B) insert an oropharyngeal airway and assist ventilations with a bag-valve mask
(C) continue your focused history and physical examination and treat her distress with oxygen therapy
(D) attempt to locate someone with a metered dose inhaler and treat the patient with the "loaned" inhaler

15. Anticipated side effects of metered dose inhalers include

(A) slurred speech and altered mental status
(B) seizures and unconsciousness
(C) chest pain and pulmonary edema
(D) increased pulse rate, tremors, and nervousness

16. Which of the following would be proper instructions for informing a patient how to use a metered dose inhaler?

(A) "Point the inhaler under your tongue and depress the button one time"
(B) "Spray the medication into a plastic bag several times, then breathe from the bag until you feel relief"
(C) "Exhale deeply, put the inhaler in your mouth, and depress the button several successive times while panting rapidly"
(D) "Exhale deeply, put the inhaler in your mouth, and depress the button while inhaling. Then attempt to hold your breath as long as you comfortably can"

17. Your rescue crew responds to the home of a 22-month-old male patient with difficulty breathing and a nonproductive cough. His father tells you that he has had a fever for the last several days. While assessing the patient, you observe a harsh, barklike cough and stridor. He is conscious and responds appropriately for his age. These findings are consistent with _____ . Appropriate emergency care for this patient should consist of _____.

(A) Croup; blow-by oxygen therapy, position of comfort, and transport to the hospital for further evaluation
(B) Croup; blow-by oxygen therapy, insertion of a nasopharyngeal airway, and transport in the recovery position to the hospital for further evaluation
(C) Epiglottitis; blow-by oxygen therapy, close inspection of the mouth and throat, and transport to hospital for further evaluation
(D) Epiglottitis; oxygen by nonrebreather mask, position of comfort, and transport for further evaluation

18. Asthma causes difficulty breathing due to

(A) Dilation of the bronchioles, which causes wheezing
(B) Constriction of the bronchioles, which causes wheezing
(C) Alveolar collapse, which causes diminished tidal volume
(D) Infection of the lower respiratory tract, which causes rhonchi

19. A pulmonary embolus is a clot in the bloodstream that travels to the lungs where it becomes lodged. The lung sounds of a patient with a pulmonary embolus are

(A) absent in all lobes of the lung
(B) absent in the lobes affected by the clot
(C) absent in the lobes not affected by the clot
(D) clear throughout but with a possibly diminished tidal volume due to an increased respiratory rate

20. Your ambulance is called to the home of a 7-year-old male patient complaining of difficulty breathing. His mother tells you he has been having a hard time breathing for the last 5 hours. The child appears very tired and he is using accessory muscles to assist with breathing. The child has asthma and has a prescription for metered dose albuterol. Medical direction authorizes you to assist the patient with his albuterol. Which of the following indicates that the patient is responding well to this intervention?

(A) The patient's wheezing stops and his agitation increases
(B) The patient's tidal volume decreases
(C) The patient appears to have fallen asleep
(D) The patient's level of consciousness and activity improves

21. When treating patients with a history of emphysema or chronic bronchitis, a guideline for oxygen therapy for these patients is

(A) always provide low-flow oxygen
(B) always provide high-flow oxygen
(C) do not provide oxygen therapy unless the patient is in cardiac arrest
(D) if there is respiratory distress, provide high-flow oxygen; if there is no distress, provide low-flow oxygen

Directions: Each of the numbered items or incomplete statements in this section is negatively phrased, as indicated by a capitalized word such as NOT, LEAST, or EXCEPT. Select the ONE lettered answer or completion that is BEST in each case.

22. Which of the following are NOT signs of difficulty breathing?

(A) Nasal flaring and grunting
(B) Altered mental status and cyanosis
(C) High blood pressure and slow pulse rate
(D) Use of accessory muscles and coughing

23. Many patients diagnosed with respiratory complications will be prescribed metered dose inhalers. These medications attempt to decrease difficulty breathing by dilating the smooth muscles of the respiratory tract, thus decreasing airway resistance. Which of the following is NOT a bronchodilator that EMT-Basics may assist in administering?

(A) Lasix®
(B) Alupent®
(C) Proventil®
(D) Bronkosol®

24. Your ambulance is called to an adult-care facility for a 78-year-old female patient complaining of difficulty breathing that has worsened over the past 2 days. Which of the following comments by the patient would NOT be consistent with the typical signs and symptoms of pneumonia?

(A) "My chest hurts when I take a deep breath"
(B) "My feet are much more swollen than normal"
(C) "I have had fever and the chills for the past week"
(D) "I keep coughing up yellow stuff from my lungs"

Directions: Each of the numbered questions or incomplete statements in this section refers to a scenario that precedes them. The numbered questions or incomplete statements are followed by answers or by completions of the statement. Select the answer or completion of the statement that is BEST in each case.

Your rescue crew is called to the home of a 76-year-old male patient complaining of difficulty breathing. It is 4:00 a.m. The patient is conscious and appears to be in severe respiratory distress.

Questions 25–30

25. While observing this patient, you note the skin above his collarbones (clavicles) is sucked in with each breath. This finding is called

(A) stridor
(B) tenting
(C) retractions
(D) subcutaneous emphysema

26. Upon completing the scene size-up and initial assessment, you form an impression that this patient is acutely unstable. You should immediately

(A) insert an oropharyngeal airway
(B) give the patient a bronchodilator
(C) call for advanced-life-support assistance
(D) give the patient a sublingual nitroglycerin tablet

27. The patient states he has woken up the last several nights due to an increase in his level of distress. He tells you, "Last night it was so bad that I had to sleep sitting up so I could breathe." The medical term for this specific condition is

(A) hypoxia
(B) retractions
(C) pedal edema
(D) paroxysmal nocturnal dyspnea

28. The patient says he has had a productive cough for the last 3 days. Of the following characteristics of sputum, which would indicate that this patient may have pulmonary edema (fluid in the lungs)?

(A) A thick green sputum
(B) Frothy, pink-tinged sputum
(C) A brownish-yellow sputum
(D) Copious bright red blood in the sputum

29. When listening to this patient's breath sounds, you detect a high-pitched "popping" sound in the lower lobes of his lungs. The sound is similar to the sound of Velcro tearing apart. The correct term for this abnormal breath sound is

    (A)   stridor
    (B)   grunting
    (C)   wheezes
    (D)   crackles (rales)

30. The patient's skin condition is cool, moist, and pale. He is breathing at a rate of 20 respirations per minute. His tidal volume is adequate. Appropriate oxygen therapy for this patient would be

    (A)   nasal cannula at 2 liters per minute (LPM)
    (B)   nasal cannula at 15 LPM
    (C)   nonrebreather mask at 15 LPM
    (D)   bag-valve-mask assisted ventilations at 30 respirations per minute

Your rescue crew is called to an elementary school cafeteria for a 9-year-old female patient complaining of difficulty breathing. You find the patient sitting upright in severe respiratory distress. She is crying and can only say a few words before coughing. Her skin is cool and pale. Her friend tells you the patient was tossing grapes up in the air and catching them in her mouth when her symptoms began.

Questions 31–33

31. After assessing the scene, you should immediately

    (A)   check for a pulse
    (B)   perform an initial assessment
    (C)   perform a rapid trauma assessment
    (D)   begin oxygen therapy with a nasal cannula at 6 liters per minute

32. Upon auscultation (listening), you note a harsh, high-pitched sound during inspiration that appears to be coming from the patient's throat. The term given this sound is

    (A)   stridor
    (B)   grunting
    (C)   crackling
    (D)   wheezing

33. After assessing the patient's airway and breathing status, you conclude that her airway is obstructed, possibly from a lodged grape. Her condition is deteriorating. She is now unable to talk and has a weak, ineffective cough. To clear her airway, you must

    (A)   perform back blows only
    (B)   perform back blows and chest thrusts
    (C)   perform abdominal thrusts (Heimlich maneuver)
    (D)   instruct the patient to raise both arms over her head and cough

Your ambulance crew is called to the scene of a 3-month-old infant with difficulty breathing. You arrive to find the infant in his mother's arms. She has her finger in the baby's mouth and tells you her son swallowed a small toy.

Questions 34–35

34. You assess the infant and find he is not breathing due to an obstructed airway. You should

    (A)   allow the mother to continue her efforts
    (B)   attempt to clear the airway with deep tracheal suctioning
    (C)   attempt to clear the airway with back blows and chest thrusts

(D)   attempt to clear the airway by performing abdominal thrusts (Heimlich maneuver)

35. After repeated attempts, the child coughs up the toy. The airway is now clear but the child is still not breathing. You should immediately

(A)   repeat attempts to clear the airway
(B)   begin oxygen therapy with a nonrebreather mask at 15 liters per minute
(C)   assist ventilations with a bag-valve mask and supplemental oxygen at a rate of 1 respiration every 3 seconds
(D)   assist ventilations with a bag-valve mask and supplemental oxygen at a rate of 1 respiration every 5 seconds

You are called to an office complex for a 23-year-old male patient complaining of chest pain and difficulty breathing. You arrive to find your patient sitting upright, breathing 36 times per minute. His skin is pale, sweaty, and cool. He complains of a sudden onset of sharp chest pain. He tells you that other than a skiing accident 2 weeks ago, he has no pertinent medical history.

Questions 36–38

36. Appropriate treatment for this patient may include

(A)   having the patient breathe into a paper bag to slow his respiratory rate
(B)   providing oxygen therapy by nonrebreather mask at 15 liters per minute (LPM)
(C)   administering sublingual nitroglycerin and oxygen therapy by nonrebreather mask at 15 LPM.
(D)   administering a metered dose inhaler and oxygen therapy by nonrebreather mask at 15 LPM

37. Which of the following comments by the patient would be consistent with a pulmonary embolism?

(A)   "I cannot move my legs"
(B)   "My feet are more swollen than normal"
(C)   "I have a sharp, stabbing sensation in my chest"
(D)   "This is the fifth time this has happened to me in the last month"

38. Appropriate interventions and transportation for this patient would include

(A)   immediately begin rapid transportation of this patient to a hospital
(B)   have the patient schedule an appointment with his personal physician
(C)   immediately begin rapid transportation of this patient to a doctor's office
(D)   transport the patient only after performing a detailed physical examination on the scene

ANSWERS AND RATIONALES

1-B. The upper respiratory tract consists of the nose, mouth, pharynx, and larynx. By the time air reaches the sacs of the lower respiratory tract, it must be free of contaminants and humidified. The mucous membranes and hair of the upper respiratory tract do most of this work. Oxygen is not absorbed into the bloodstream until it reaches the alveoli. Moisture is lost (not recovered) during exhalation, which is evident in cold weather situations when you "can see your breath." The epiglottis is the structure that protects the lower airway from aspiration of food or liquid.

2-B. The alveoli are the terminal air sacs of the lungs. It is at the alveolar-capillary membrane that the exchange of gases takes place between the respiratory and cardiovascular systems. The medulla is the part of the brain stem that generates impulses that travel along nerves to the respiratory muscles. The epiglottis, located just above the trachea, protects the lower airway from aspiration. The esophagus is the collapsible tube that runs behind the trachea. It is the passageway for food and drink from the mouth to the stomach.

3-C. The diaphragm and intercostal muscles are the primary muscles of respiration. To facilitate inhalation, the diaphragm contracts downward while the intercostal muscles pull the rib cage out. These movements increase the area of the chest, thus lowering pressure and attracting atmospheric air. The abdominal muscles may be used (as an accessory muscle) to assist in breathing during respiratory distress.

4-D. Normal exhalation is a passive event (it does not require muscle force). When the diaphragm and intercostal muscles relax, the chest returns to its resting position. The area of the chest decreases, causing the pressure of the air in the lungs to increase. This increase in pressure pushes the air out.

5-B. The two main gases exchanged during respiration are oxygen and carbon dioxide. Oxygen, required by all living cells, is absorbed from atmospheric air. Carbon dioxide, a cellular waste product, returns to the lungs by means of the blood and is exhaled. Hemoglobin allows the oxygen to bind to the red blood cell for transport throughout the body. Carbon monoxide is an odorless, colorless, tasteless, toxic gas.

6-B. The brain stem houses the respiratory centers. The impulse to breathe begins in the brain stem. This impulse is sent along nerves to the respiratory muscles. Damage to the spinal cord at or above the fifth cervical vertebra may impair breathing.

7-A. Normally, the primary stimulus for breathing is carbon dioxide levels (high carbon dioxide stimulates breathing). However, a backup system exists that monitors oxygen levels (low oxygen stimulates breathing). In some patients with chronically high levels of carbon dioxide (chronic bronchitis patients, for example), the carbon dioxide stimulus may be "turned off" and the oxygen stimulus "activated."

8-A. Dyspnea is difficulty breathing ("dys" = difficulty; "pnea" = breathing). Diaphoresis is another term for a moist or sweaty condition of the skin. Tachycardia means fast heart rate. Minute volume is the volume of air moved in and out of the lungs during 1 minute of breathing.

9-B. Conscious patients in respiratory distress are generally found sitting upright. This position is sometimes called the "tripod position" if the patient is sitting upright and leaning forward onto an outstretched arm. Patients assume this position to allow for maximum chest wall and diaphragm expansion.

10-D. When in distress (respiratory or otherwise), one of the body's first lines of defense is to increase the respiratory rate to increase oxygen content in the blood. A facial droop is most commonly associated with a patient who has experienced a cerebrovascular accident (stroke). Unconsciousness, if caused by respiratory distress, is a very late sign of disease progression. Patients in respiratory distress generally progress from anxious and agitated, to confused, to a sleepy or tired appearance, to unconsciousness. Agonal respirations are slow, gasping respirations associated with a critical patient who is about to become completely apneic. These patients must be quickly and aggressively managed with a bag-valve mask and supplemental oxygen.

11-A. Prolonged inspiration is generally associated with upper airway obstruction disorders such as croup or epiglottitis. Prolonged expiration is commonly associated with lower airway obstruction, such as asthma or bronchitis. A partial airway obstruction is generally associated with an upper airway foreign body obstruction and may produce prolonged inspiration. A complete airway obstruction is characterized by no air movement in or out of the respiratory tree.

12-D. Chest pain may be described as "pleuritic" if the pain increases with movement, palpation, or deep inspiration. True pleuritic chest pain is caused by an infection of the pleura (the double-walled sac that surrounds the lungs). Hemothorax (blood in the pleural space) and a flail segment (multiple rib fractures creating a free-floating section of the chest wall) may also present with this type of chest pain. Tracheal deviation, discovered on palpation of the trachea, is a late sign of a tension pneumothorax.

13-D. The following criteria must be met in order to assist a patient with a metered dose inhaler: the patient exhibits the signs and symptoms of breathing difficulty, the patient has a prescribed handheld inhaler (prescribed to this patient), and medical direction has authorized assisting the patient.

14-C. Not all wheezing patients have metered dose inhalers. For this patient, you should continue your assessment and provide appropriate interventions (oxygen therapy). Do not use someone else's metered dose inhaler.

15-D. Bronchodilators may stimulate the heart as well as the lungs. Heart stimulation can cause an increase in heart rate. Patients may also appear jumpy or agitated after taking bronchodilator medications. Slurred speech, an altered mental status, seizures, unconsciousness, chest pain, and pulmonary edema should be considered, assessed, and appropriate interventions given as these signs and symptoms are not typical side effects of bronchodilator administration.

16-D. These medications are absorbed at the alveoli; therefore, for maximum benefit from inhaled medications, most of the medication must reach the alveoli. The key is to have the patient inhale the medication as deeply as possible and momentarily hold the breath to allow the medication to settle in the alveoli. Any other method would be less effective. The plastic bag option may harm the patient.

17-A. The gradual onset, the age of the patient, the presence of stridor, and the harsh barking cough are signs and symptoms suggestive of croup. Interventions should focus on keeping the patient calm and providing supplemental oxygen. Epiglottitis generally has a more rapid onset, affects older children (age 3 to 7 years), and presents with difficulty swallowing, talking, and breathing. Epiglottitis may progress to the extent where the swollen epiglottis completely blocks the airway. These patients should be treated carefully and rapidly. Make sure the patient is comfortable (generally sitting up and next to a parent), give high-flow oxygen (blow-by if a nonrebreather mask agitates the child), and transport as quickly and safely as possible to a hospital.

18-B. Constriction of the bronchioles and an increased production of mucus associated with asthma leads to wheezing. Wheezing occurs as air is forced out of the alveoli through the narrowed air passages. The air whistles, and the accumulation of thousands of tiny whistles produces the wheeze. Remember that it takes a certain amount of air going through a whistle to create sound. The absence of wheezing in an unstable asthmatic patient may indicate that the patient is not moving sufficient air to wheeze, which is an ominous sign.

19-D. Pulmonary emboli affect the flow of blood to the lungs, not the flow of air through the lungs. Air will still be drawn into the affected area, but without perfused alveoli, gas exchange will not take place.

20-D. As this patient's hypoxia (lack of oxygen in the blood) decreases, you should note changes (possibly subtle) in the patient's interaction with his surroundings. These changes are due to increased oxygen delivery to the brain and muscle groups. If the patient's wheezing subsides but his distress is the same or worse, the patient's condition may be deteriorating. Be prepared to provide assisted ventilations. Ideally, the patient's tidal volume (amount of air moved in and out of the lungs with each breath) would increase due to dilation of the bronchioles. This patient's mother tells you that her son has been distressed for several hours. If this patient appears to have fallen asleep, this, too, could be an ominous sign that the patient's condition is deteriorating. He may need ventilatory support with a bag-valve mask and supplemental oxygen.

21-D. Since these patients typically have chronic high levels of carbon dioxide in their blood, their bodies may have switched the stimulus for breathing (refer to the answer for question 7). If these patients are operating on hypoxic drive, providing too much oxygen may knock out their stimulus to breathe. However, this does not mean that you should withhold oxygen from these patients if they need it! Be aware that some of these patients may respond adversely to oxygen therapy. Close monitoring and continuous assessments should prevent complications.

22-C. Patients in respiratory distress will most likely exhibit a normal or slightly lowered blood pressure and a rapid pulse rate. The pulse rate increases to compensate for the insult to the respiratory system. Imagine that red blood cells are the box cars of a train. They carry oxygen to all cells of the body and return with the by-products of cell life (i.e., carbon dioxide). The heart is the steam engine that pulls (pushes) the box cars. If the box cars are only capable of delivering half their normal oxygen load [either due to a problem with the engine (heart), a problem or decrease in the number of the available box cars (red blood cells), or a problem with the availability of the oxygen (respiratory compromise)], the engineer of the train (the brain) will attempt to run the train at twice its normal speed to please its customers (the cells of the body). When you provide oxygen therapy to a patient, you are, in essence, increasing the amount of oxygen each box car (red blood cell) carries.

23-A. Lasix® is a medication that helps eliminate excess fluid from the body. Patients taking Lasix® will generally have this medication in pill or tablet form. The bronchodilators you may assist in administering (if the correct criteria have been met) are: albuterol (Proventil®, Ventolin®); isoetharine (Bronkosol®, Bronkometer®); and metaproterenol (Metaprel®, Alupent®).

24-B. Pedal edema (pooling of fluid in the lower extremities) is not commonly associated with pneumonia. It is more commonly associated with congestive heart failure. Pleuritic chest pain, fever and chills, and a productive cough with yellow or green sputum are commonly associated with pneumonia. Other signs and symptoms may include an increased respiratory rate, increased heart rate, and abnormal lung sounds in the area of the lung affected by the infection.

25-C. Retractions are evident when the skin above and between accessory muscles and other structures (e.g., bones) is drawn in during the work of inspiration. Retractions are generally most notable at the clavicles, the notch above the sternum, and at the bottom of the rib cage. Stridor is a harsh high-pitched sound made during inspiration due to upper airway obstruction. Tenting of the skin generally occurs because of dehydration. To evaluate tenting, the skin is pinched to see how long it takes for it to assume its original position. Subcutaneous emphysema is the presence of air in the tissues outside the respiratory system. Found most commonly in the tissues of the chest, neck, and face, subcutaneous emphysema suggests a break in the integrity of the respiratory tree (usually following a traumatic event).

26-C. In systems where advanced-life-support (ALS) level care is available, ALS assistance should be called to assist with all unstable patients. Inserting an oropharyngeal airway would cause this conscious patient to vomit. Administering a bronchodilator may be appropriate; however, there are strict criteria you must follow first. Nitroglycerin is indicated for patients experiencing chest pain of suspected cardiac origin.

27-D. Paroxysmal nocturnal dyspnea occurs due to the pooling of fluid in the lungs. By sitting or standing up, gravity helps in moving the excess fluid down, thus increasing tidal volume. Hypoxia is the term for low oxygen content in the blood. Patients experiencing paroxysmal nocturnal dyspnea may also be hypoxic due to impaired gas exchange. Pedal edema is the pooling of fluid in the lower extremities (legs) due to impaired pumping ability of the heart.

28-B. The sputum associated with this patient's condition (pulmonary edema) would be frothy and possibly blood-tinged. The sputum is frothy from being forced through the small air passages and is pink from a small amount of blood leaking into the lungs with the fluid. Thick green or brownish yellow sputum is generally associated with a respiratory infection. Copious bright red blood is indicative of hemorrhage, rather than pulmonary edema.

29-D. Rales (crackles) are the abnormal lung sound created by fluid in the alveoli and bronchioles. The sound has been compared with the sound of opening a Velcro fastener or gentle rolling of the hair back and forth between the fingers. Grunting, most commonly associated with respiratory distress in infants, is a noise (a grunt) heard during exhalation. This grunt forms a small amount of back pressure in the lungs to help keep the alveoli from collapsing during exhalation. Stridor is a harsh, high-pitched sound associated with upper airway obstruction. Wheezes occur because of air whistling through narrowed bronchioles (as with asthma).

30-C. High-flow oxygen is important for this patient. The correct device for high-flow oxygen administration is the nonrebreather mask. The nasal cannula becomes very uncomfortable at flow rates greater than 6 liters per minute. Since this patient is breathing at an acceptable rate with good tidal volume, assisting ventilations with a bag-valve mask is not yet necessary. However, anticipate that this patient may deteriorate. Have a bag-valve mask, suction equipment, oropharyngeal airways, nasopharyngeal airways, and an automated external defibrillator readily available.

31-B. Following scene size-up, the initial assessment is your priority. An initial assessment should include an assessment of the patient's mental status, airway, breathing, circulation, and a formation of a general impression about the patient's condition. Checking a pulse is part of the initial assessment, but it is not the first step in an initial assessment. A rapid trauma assessment would be performed after the initial assessment if the patient's mental status was impaired to the point that you could not obtain a history of present illness and physical examination (i.e., the patient is unconscious). Oxygen therapy should be initiated on this patient; however, given the patient's presentation, high-flow oxygen by nonbreather mask should be administered rather than a nasal cannula.

32-A. Stridor is a harsh, high-pitched sound heard during inspiration. It is most commonly associated with an upper airway obstruction. Grunting, crackling (rales), and wheezing have been discussed in previous questions and answers.

33-C. Conscious patients older than 1 year of age should have abdominal thrusts performed to clear an obstructed airway. Back blows and chest thrusts are performed on patients younger than 1 year of age. Having the patient raise both arms over her head and coughing will only delay definitive care for this patient.

34-C. To clear an obstructed airway in an infant (younger than 1 year of age), a series of back blows and chest thrusts should be delivered. After confirming an obstructed airway, 5 back blows should be delivered followed by 5 chest thrusts. The back blows are delivered with the bottom of the palm of the hand and should strike the patient across the scapulae (shoulder blades), rather than along the length of the spine. Chest thrusts should be performed with two fingers positioned one finger-width below an imaginary line drawn between the nipples. Compression depth for chest thrusts is 0.5–1 inch. If the patient is conscious, continue to perform a series of back blows and chest thrusts until the airway is clear or the child becomes unconscious. Once the infant is unconscious, you must evaluate the airway between the series of back blows and chest thrusts.

35-C. An apneic (nonbreathing) infant with a patent (clear) airway should be managed with bag-valve-mask ventilations every 3 seconds or 20 ventilations per minute. Remember to check for a pulse once you have cleared the airway and begun ventilatory support. If the patient has a pulse but is not breathing, you should continue rescue breathing and continuously reassess the patient en route to the hospital.

36-B. Since this patient does not have a history of medical problems that would require the prescription of nitroglycerin or bronchodilators, he should not be considered for field use of these medications by EMT-Basics. This patient is clearly in distress and needs high-flow oxygen by nonrebreather mask. Never have a patient breathe into a paper bag. If you suspect the cause of the patient's distress is hyperventilation, you should provide appropriate assessment, treatment, and attempt to slow the breathing by calmly talking with the patient. Patients who hyperventilate due to emotional distress will often present with sharp chest pain and shortness of breath. This presentation is also common in patients with a pulmonary embolus. Having a patient with a pulmonary embolus breathe into a paper bag could have serious negative consequences.

37-C. The signs and symptoms of a pulmonary embolism may include sharp, stabbing chest pain, difficulty breathing (sudden onset), restlessness, a cough with blood-tinged sputum, increased respiratory rate, increased heart rate, and possible hypotension (lowered blood pressure). An inability to move or feel the extremities may be due to spinal damage. If spinal damage were present, you would need to provide full spinal immobilization. Swelling of the feet (pedal edema) combined with difficulty breathing is most commonly associated with congestive heart failure. Since pulmonary emboli may require surgical intervention, it is extremely unlikely that this patient has had four previous pulmonary emboli yet denies any past medical history.

38-A. Because a pulmonary embolism may require surgical intervention, the patient should be transported to the closest appropriate facility. Contacting medical direction may assist you in correctly triaging this patient and would also help the facility prepare for the arrival of this patient.

BIBLIOGRAPHY

Campbell JE (ed): *Basic Trauma Life Support for Paramedics and Advanced EMS Providers*, 3rd ed. Englewood Cliffs, NJ, Prentice-Hall, 1995.

Caroline NL: *Emergency Care in the Streets*, 5th ed. Boston: Little, Brown, 1995.

Crosby LA, Lewallen DG (eds): *Emergency Care and Transportation of the Sick and Injured*, 6th ed. Rosemont, IL, American Academy of Orthopaedic Surgeons, 1995.

Grant HD, Murray RH Jr, Bergeron JD: *Emergency Care*, 7th ed. Englewood Cliffs, NJ, Prentice-Hall, 1995.

Hafen BQ, Karren KJ, Mistovich JJ: *Prehospital Emergency Care*, 5th ed. Upper Saddle River, NJ, Prentice-Hall, 1996.

Henry MC, Stapleton ER, Judd RL: *EMT: Prehospital Care*. Philadelphia, WB Saunders, 1992.

Kitt S, Selfridge-Thomas J, Proehl JA, et al: *Emergency Nursing: A Physiologic and Clinical Perspective*, 2nd ed. Philadelphia, WB Saunders, 1995.

McSwain NE, White RD, Paturas JL, et al (eds): *The Basic EMT: Comprehensive Prehospital Patient Care*. St. Louis, Mosby-Year Book, 1996.

Miller RH, Wilson JK: *Manual of Prehospital Emergency Medicine*. St. Louis, Mosby-Year Book, 1992.

Stoy WA: *Mosby's EMT-Basic Textbook*. St. Louis: Mosby-Year Book, 1996.

United States Department of Transportation, National Highway Traffic Safety Administration: *Emergency Medical Technician: Basic. National Standard Curriculum*, 1994.

18-1 Describe the structure and function of the cardiovascular system.

18-2 Describe the emergency medical care of the patient experiencing chest pain or discomfort.

18-3 Discuss the position of comfort for patients with various cardiac emergencies.

18-4 Establish the relationship between airway management and the patient with cardiovascular compromise.

18-5 Discuss the need for on-line or off-line medical direction to assist in the emergency medical care of the patient with chest pain.

18-6 Predict the relationship between the patient experiencing cardiovascular compromise and basic life support.

18-7 List the indications for nitroglycerin.

18-8 State the contraindications and side effects for nitroglycerin.

18-9 Explain why not all chest pain patients become cardiac arrest patients and do not need to be attached to an automated external defibrillator.

18-10 Define the role of the EMT-Basic in the emergency cardiac care system.

18-11 Explain the importance of prehospital advanced-cardiac-life-support intervention if it is available.

18-12 Explain the importance of urgent transport to a facility with advanced cardiac life support if it is not available in the prehospital setting.

MOTIVATION FOR LEARNING

Cardiac emergencies are the most common type of medical emergency in the United States today. The EMT-Basic must learn the signs and symptoms of cardiac compromise and deliver appropriate patient care based on these findings. When authorized by medical direction, the EMT-Basic may assist a patient in taking prescribed nitroglycerin.

The EMT-Basic and the automated external defibrillator are important links in the successful resuscitation of a patient in cardiac arrest outside the hospital.

18-13 Discuss the principle of early defibrillation.

18-14 Explain the rationale for early defibrillation.

18-15 Discuss the various types of automated external defibrillators.

18-16 Differentiate between the fully automated and the semiautomated defibrillator.

18-17 Discuss the circumstances that may result in inappropriate shocks.

18-18 State the reasons for assuring that the patient is pulseless and apneic when using the automated external defibrillator.

18-19 Explain the considerations for interruption of cardiopulmonary resuscitation when using the automated external defibrillator.

18-20 Discuss the advantages and disadvantages of automated external defibrillators.

18-21 Summarize the speed of operation of automated external defibrillation.

18-22 Discuss the use of remote defibrillation through adhesive pads.

18-23 Discuss the special considerations for rhythm monitoring.

18-24 List the indications for automated external defibrillation.

18-25 List the contraindications for automated external defibrillation.

18-26 List the steps in the operation of the automated external defibrillator.

18-27 Discuss the procedures that must be taken into consideration for standard operation of the various types of automated external defibrillators.

18-28 Explain the guidelines regarding automated external defibrillator use in infants and children.

18-29 Discuss the standard of care that should be used to provide care to a patient with persistent ventricular fibrillation and no available advanced cardiac life support.

18-30 Differentiate between the single rescuer and multirescuer care with an automated external defibrillator.

18-31 Explain the reason for pulses not being checked between shocks with an automated external defibrillator.

18-32 Discuss the importance of coordinating advanced-cardiac-life-support providers with personnel using automated external defibrillators.

18-33 Discuss the importance of postresuscitation care.

18-34 List the components of postresuscitation care.

18-35 Discuss the standard of care that should be used to provide care to a patient with recurrent ventricular fibrillation and no available advanced cardiac life support.

18-36 Discuss the need to complete the Automated Defibrillator: Operator's Shift Checklist.

18-37 Discuss the role of the American Heart Association in the use of automated external defibrillation.

18-38 Explain the importance of frequent practice with the automated external defibrillator.

18-39 Explain the role medical direction plays in the use of automated external defibrillation.

18-40 State the reasons why a case review should be completed following the use of the automated external defibrillator.

18-41 Discuss the components that should be included in a case review.

18-42 Discuss the goal of quality improvement in automated external defibrillation.

18-43 Define the function of all controls on an automated external defibrillator and describe event documentation and battery defibrillator maintenance.

ANATOMY AND PHYSIOLOGY REVIEW

CIRCULATORY SYSTEM

1. **Components**
   a. The circulatory system consists of the cardiovascular and lymphatic systems.
      (1) The cardiovascular system consists of the heart, blood vessels, and blood.
      (2) The lymphatic system consists of lymph, lymph nodes, lymph vessels, tonsils, spleen, and thymus gland.
   b. Organs that form and store blood are also associated with the circulatory system. These organs include:
      (1) Spleen
      (2) Liver
      (3) Bone marrow
2. **Function**
   a. **Transport**
      (1) Blood carries oxygen, food, hormones, minerals, and other essential substances to all parts of the body.
      (2) Blood carries carbon dioxide and other waste material from the body's cells to the lungs, kidneys, or skin for elimination.
   b. **Maintenance of body temperature.** Blood vessels constrict and dilate as needed to retain or dissipate heat at the skin's surface.
   c. **Protection.** The blood and lymphatic system protect the body against invasion by foreign microorganisms through the immune (defense) system.

THE CARDIOVASCULAR SYSTEM

1. **Heart**
   a. The heart lies in the thoracic cavity (mediastinum) behind the sternum and between the lungs. Approximately two-thirds of the heart's mass lies to the left of the body's midline.
   b. The heart is attached to the thorax through the great vessels (pulmonary arteries and veins, aorta, and superior and inferior vena cavae).
   c. The heart is divided into four chambers (*Figure 18-1*).
      (1) The two upper chambers are the right and left atria.
         (a) The atria are thin-walled chambers that receive blood from the systemic circulation and lungs.
         (b) The superior and inferior vena cavae deliver oxygen-poor blood from the body to the right atrium.
            (i) The right atrium pumps oxygen-poor blood through the tricuspid valve to the right ventricle.
            (ii) The left atrium receives oxygen-rich blood from the pulmonary veins (lungs) and pumps the blood to the left ventricle.
      (2) The two lower chambers are the right and left ventricles.
         (a) The ventricles pump blood to the lungs and systemic circulation (body).
            (i) The right ventricle pumps blood to the lungs.
            (ii) The left ventricle pumps blood to the body.
         (b) The ventricles are larger and have thicker walls than the atria.
      (3) Heart valves prevent the backflow of blood and keep blood moving in one direction.
         (a) **Atrioventricular (AV) valves**
            (i) The **tricuspid valve** is located between the right atrium and right ventricle.
            (ii) The **mitral (bicuspid) valve** is located between the left atrium and left ventricle.

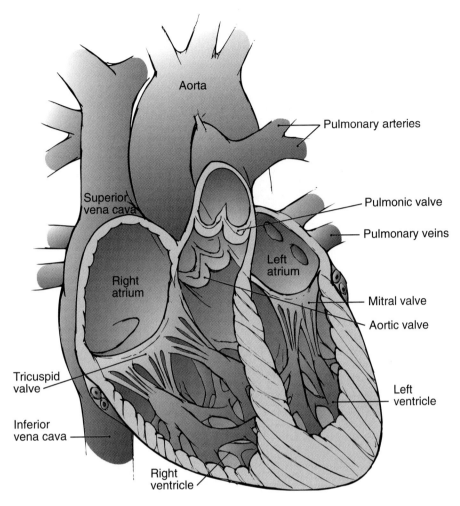

Fig. 18-1. Heart chambers, valves, and major vessels.

    (b) **Semilunar valves**
      (i) The **pulmonic valve** is located at the junction of the right ventricle and pulmonary artery.
      (ii) The **aortic valve** is located at the junction of the left ventricle and aorta.
  d. Cardiac conduction system
    (1) The heart is more than a muscle.
      (a) The heart contains specialized contractile and conductive tissue that allows the generation of electrical impulses.
      (b) Unlike other cells of the body, specialized electrical (pacemaker) cells in the heart can generate an electrical impulse without being stimulated by another source, such as a nerve. This property is called automaticity.
    (2) The electrical (pacemaker) cells in the heart are arranged in a system of pathways called the conduction system (*Figure 18-2*).
    (3) Normal pathway for electrical impulse: sinoatrial (SA) node → atrioventricular (AV) node (located between the atria and ventricles) → bundle of His → right and left bundle branches → Purkinje fibers.
    (4) Electrical stimulation normally results in contraction of the heart's muscle fibers.
    (5) Blood is then pumped to the lungs and through the aorta to the body.
2. Blood vessels

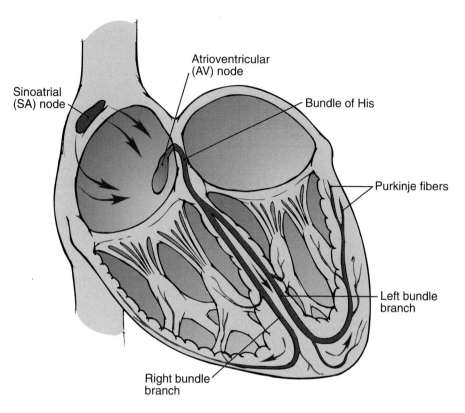

Fig. 18-2. Specialized cells in the heart are arranged in a system of pathways called the conduction system.

a. Arteries
   (1) Function
      (a) Arteries carry blood away from the heart to the rest of the body.
      (b) They are high-pressure vessels.
      (c) All arteries, except the pulmonary arteries, carry oxygen-rich blood.
      (d) Arteries help maintain blood pressure.
   (2) Major arteries
      (a) Aorta
         (i) The aorta is the major artery originating from the heart.
         (ii) It lies in front of the spine in the thoracic and abdominal cavities.
         (iii) It divides at the level of the navel into the iliac arteries.
      (b) Coronary arteries supply the heart with blood.
      (c) Carotid artery
         (i) The carotid artery is the major artery of the neck.
         (ii) It supplies the head with blood.
         (iii) Its pulsation can be palpated on either side of the neck.
         (iv) The right and left carotid arteries should never be palpated at the same time because doing so can cause severe lowering of the heart rate.
      (d) Femoral artery
         (i) The femoral artery is the major artery of the thigh.
         (ii) It supplies the lower extremity with blood.
         (iii) Pulsation can be palpated in the groin area (the crease between the abdomen and thigh).
      (e) The pulsation of the **posterior tibial artery** can be palpated on the posterior surface of the medial malleolus.
      (f) Dorsalis pedis artery

          (i)   The dorsalis pedis artery is the artery in the foot.

          (ii)   Pulsation can be palpated on the superior surface of the foot.

    (g) **Brachial artery**

          (i)   The brachial artery is the artery of the upper arm.

          (ii)   Pulsation can be palpated on the inside of the arm between the elbow and shoulder.

          (iii)   This artery is used when determining a blood pressure (BP) using a blood pressure cuff and stethoscope.

    (h) **Radial artery**

          (i)   The radial artery is the major artery of the lower arm.

          (ii)   Pulsation can be palpated at the wrist, thumb side.

    (i) **Pulmonary arteries**

          (i)   Pulmonary arteries originate at the right ventricle of the heart.

          (ii)   They carry oxygen-poor blood from the right ventricle to the lungs.

b. Arterioles are the smallest branches of arteries leading to the capillaries.

c. Capillaries

  (1) Capillaries are microscopic vessels that are one cell thick.

  (2) They serve as vessels for exchange of wastes, fluids, and nutrients between the blood and tissues.

  (3) They connect arterioles and venules.

  (4) All tissues except cartilage, hair, nails, and the cornea of the eye contain capillaries.

d. Venules are the smallest branches of veins leading to the capillaries.

e. Veins

  (1) **Function**

    (a) Veins collect blood for transport back to the heart.

    (b) They are low-pressure vessels.

    (c) They contain valves to prevent backflow of blood.

    (d) All veins, except the pulmonary veins, carry deoxygenated (oxygen-poor) blood.

  (2) **Major veins**

    (a) Pulmonary veins carry oxygen-rich blood from the lungs to the left atrium.

    (b) Venae cavae return blood to the right atrium.

        (i)   The superior vena cava carries blood from the head and upper extremities.

        (ii)   The inferior vena cava carries blood from the torso and lower extremities.

3. Blood

a. Composition of blood

  (1) Formed elements of the blood are the cellular components and include:

    (a) Red blood cells (erythrocytes)

    (b) White blood cells (leukocytes)

    (c) Platelets (thrombocytes)

  (2) Plasma is the liquid component of blood.

b. Red blood cells

  (1) Red blood cells transport oxygen to body cells.

    (a) Each red blood cell contains hemoglobin, an iron-containing protein.

    (b) Hemoglobin carries oxygen from the lungs to the tissues.

    (c) Hemoglobin gives blood its red color.

  (2) Red blood cells also transport carbon dioxide away from body cells.

c. White blood cells defend the body from microorganisms, such as bacteria and viruses, that have invaded the bloodstream or tissues of the body.

d. Platelets

    (1)   Platelets are essential for the formation of blood clots.

    (2)   They function to stop bleeding and repair ruptured blood vessels.

e. Plasma

    (1)   Plasma is the clear, straw-colored liquid component of blood (blood minus its formed elements).

    (2)   Plasma carries nutrients to the cells and waste products from the cells.

PHYSIOLOGY OF CIRCULATION

1. Pulse

    a. When the left ventricle contracts, a wave of blood is sent through the arteries, causing them to expand and recoil.

    b. A pulse is the regular expansion and recoil of an artery caused by the movement of blood from the heart as it contracts.

    c. A pulse can be felt anywhere an artery simultaneously passes near the skin surface and over a bone.

    d. Central pulses are located close to the heart and include the **carotid** and **femoral pulses** (*Figure 18-3*).

    e. Peripheral pulses are located farther from the heart and include the **radial**, **brachial**, **posterior tibial**, and **dorsalis pedis pulses.**

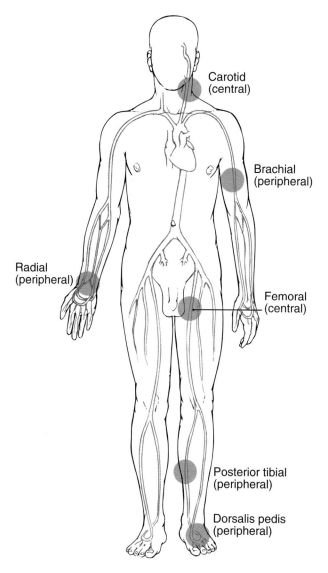

Fig. 18-3. Central and peripheral pulses.

2. **Blood pressure**
   a. Blood pressure is the force exerted by the blood on the inner walls of the heart and blood vessels.
   b. Systolic blood pressure is the pressure exerted against the walls of the arteries when the left ventricle contracts.
   c. Diastolic blood pressure is the pressure exerted against the walls of the arteries when the left ventricle is at rest.
3. **Perfusion**
   a. Perfusion is the circulation of blood through an organ or a part of the body.
   b. **Hypoperfusion** is inadequate circulation of blood through an organ or a part of the body; a state of profound depression of the vital processes of the body.
   c. Signs and symptoms of hypoperfusion include:
      (1) Pale, cyanotic, cool, clammy skin
      (2) Rapid, weak pulse
      (3) Rapid, shallow breathing
      (4) Restlessness, anxiety, or mental dullness
      (5) Nausea and vomiting
      (6) Reduction in total blood volume
      (7) Low or decreasing blood pressure
      (8) Subnormal temperature

CARDIAC COMPROMISE

CORONARY ARTERY DISEASE

1. **Coronary artery disease** is a term used for diseases that reduce or stop blood flow through the coronary arteries.
2. The heart depends on two coronary arteries and their branches for its supply of oxygen-rich blood.
   a. During relaxation (diastole) of the left ventricle, blood flows into the coronary arteries, supplying oxygen and nutrients to the heart.
   b. During times of stress, the heart requires more oxygen and depends on widening (dilation) of the arteries to increase blood flow through the coronary arteries.
3. When a coronary artery becomes blocked, the portion of the heart muscle it supplies is deprived of oxygen and nutrients (becomes ischemic).
   a. **Ischemia** is a reduction in blood flow to an organ or tissue.
   b. Ischemia can result from narrowing or blockage of an artery or spasm of an artery.
4. Body cells that lack oxygen (are ischemic) produce lactic acid.
   a. Lactic acid irritates nerve endings in the affected area, causing pain.
   b. Pain is a common symptom associated with cardiac compromise.
5. **Angina pectoris** (literally, "choking in the chest") is a symptom of coronary artery disease that occurs when the heart's need for oxygen exceeds its supply.
   a. The heart muscle lacks oxygen (becomes ischemic).
   b. Lactic acid and carbon dioxide accumulate, typically resulting in chest pain.
6. An **acute myocardial infarction** (AMI; "heart attack") occurs when the affected portion of the heart muscle is deprived of oxygen long enough so that the area dies (necrosis). If too much of the heart muscle dies, shock and sudden death will result.
7. In **congestive heart failure** (CHF), one or both sides of the heart fail to pump efficiently.
   a. When the left ventricle fails as a pump, blood backs up into the lungs (**pulmonary edema**).
   b. When the right ventricle fails, blood returning to the heart backs up causing congestion in the organs and tissues of the body.

(1) Swelling of the feet and ankles is often one of the first visible signs of CHF in patients who can walk. In patients confined to bed, swelling is observed around the lower back.

(2) Distention of the veins of the neck [jugular venous distention (JVD)] may also be observed.

ASSESSING THE PATIENT WITH CARDIAC COMPROMISE

1. **Scene size-up.** Determine if the patient's complaint is due to trauma or a medical condition.
   a. **Trauma.** Determine the mechanism of injury from the patient, family members, or bystanders and inspection of the scene.
   b. **Medical.** Determine the nature of the illness from the patient, family members, or bystanders.
2. **Initial assessment**
   a. Maintain spinal immobilization if trauma is suspected.
   b. Assess mental status.
   c. Assess the airway.
   d. Assess breathing.
      (1) Observe the rise and fall of the chest.
      (2) Estimate the respiratory rate.
      (3) Note the depth and equality of breathing.
      (4) Note the rhythm of respirations.
      (5) Note any signs of increased work of breathing (respiratory effort).
      (6) Listen for air movement and note if respirations are quiet, absent, or noisy.
      (7) Feel for air movement against your hand or cheek.
   c. Assess circulation.
      (1) Assess the pulse.
         (a) If pulseless, begin cardiopulmonary resuscitation (CPR).
         (b) If a pulse is present, estimate the heart rate and assess pulse regularity and strength.
      (2) Assess perfusion.
         (a) Note the color, temperature, and condition (moisture) of the patient's skin. The skin may be pale or cyanotic (blue), cool, clammy.
         (b) In infants and children younger than 6 years of age, assess capillary refill.
         (c) If appropriate, evaluate for possible major bleeding.
   d. Establish patient priorities.
      (1) Priority patients include:
         (a) Those with severe chest pain with a systolic blood pressure of less than 100 millimeters of mercury (mm Hg).
         (b) Pulseless patients
      (2) Advanced-life-support (ALS) assistance should be requested as soon as possible for priority patients.
      (3) If ALS personnel are not available, the patient should be transported promptly to the closest appropriate facility.

FOCUSED HISTORY AND PHYSICAL EXAMINATION

1. If the patient is unresponsive with no breathing or pulse:
   a. If the patient is older than 8 years old, start CPR and apply the automated external defibrillator (AED).
   b. If the patient is younger than 8 years old, start CPR.
2. If the patient is responsive:

a. Gather information about the patient's medical history before performing the physical examination

b. Obtain a SAMPLE history

(1) **Signs and symptoms.** Signs and symptoms of cardiac compromise may include one or all of the following (*Box 18-1*):

   (a) Chest pain or discomfort

      (i) The patient may describe symptoms of discomfort (rather than pain) such as "pressing," "tight," "squeezing," "viselike," "aching," "heaviness," "dull," "burning," or "crushing," "smothering," or indigestion-type symptoms.

      (ii) The patient usually describes chest pain located under the breastbone (substernal), but may be present across the chest or in the upper abdomen (epigastric pain).

      (iii) The pain may radiate to the jaw (the patient may complain of a toothache), neck, down the arms, and back between the shoulder blades.

   (b) Sudden onset of sweating (may be a significant finding by itself)

   (c) Difficulty breathing (dyspnea)

   (d) Anxiety, irritability

   (e) Feeling of impending doom

   (f) Abnormal or irregular pulse rate

   (g) Abnormal blood pressure

   (h) Nausea and/or vomiting

   (i) Weakness

   (j) Fatigue

   (k) Fainting (syncope). Fainting is a sudden, temporary loss of consciousness that occurs when one or both sides of the heart do not pump out a sufficient amount of blood, resulting in inadequate blood flow to the brain.

   (l) Palpitations

      (i) Palpitations are an abnormal awareness of one's heartbeat.

      (ii) Patients may describe palpitations as, "My heart is racing" or "My heart skipped a beat."

(2) **Allergies.** Determine if the patient has any allergies to medications and other substances or materials.

(3) **Medications.** Determine if the patient is taking any medications (prescription and over the counter).

   (a) Patients with primary cardiac problems are frequently prescribed medications.

      (i) Diuretics ("water pills"), such as furosemide (Lasix®), may be prescribed for high blood pressure or CHF.

Box 18-1. Signs and Symptoms of Cardiac Compromise

Abnormal or irregular pulse rate
Abnormal blood pressure
Anxiety, irritability
Chest pain or discomfort
Difficulty breathing (dyspnea)
Fatigue
Feeling of impending doom
Nausea and/or vomiting
Sudden onset of sweating
Weakness
Fainting (syncope)
Palpitations

          (ii) Medications that widen (dilate) blood vessels, such as nitroglycerin (Nitrostat®), may be prescribed to relieve chest pain and reduce the heart's workload.

          (iii) Antidysrhythmics ("heart pills")may be prescribed to control abnormal heart rates or rhythms. These drugs include propranolol (Inderal®); digoxin (Lanoxin®); procainamide (Procan®, Pronestyl®); and verapamil (Calan®, Isoptin®, Verelan®).

    (b) Determine if the patient takes his or her medications regularly and his or her response to them.

    (c) Determine if there has been any recent change in medications (additions, deletions, or change in dosages).

    (d) Provide all information obtained to the receiving facility.

  (4) **Pertinent past medical history**

    (a) Does the patient smoke? Patients who smoke are at an increased risk for diseases of the heart and blood vessels.

    (b) Does the patient have a history of high blood pressure or heart disease (e.g., history of a heart attack, angina, congestive heart failure, heart surgery)?

        (i) Patients with uncontrolled high blood pressure are at increased risk for a heart attack.

        (ii) Patients with a family history of heart or blood vessel disease are at increased risk for developing these conditions.

    (c) Does the patient have a history of diabetes, lung, liver or kidney disease, or other medical condition?

  (5) **Last oral intake.** Determine the patient's last oral intake.

  (6) **Event.** Determine the events leading up to this incident.

c. OPQRST

  (1) **Onset.** Determine the onset of the patient's symptoms.

    (a) When did the pain or discomfort begin?

    (b) Was the onset sudden or gradual?

  (2) **Provocation.** Determine what (if anything) provoked this episode of chest pain.

    (a) What was the patient doing when the symptoms began (e.g., resting, sleeping, physical activity)?

    (b) What has the patient done to relieve the pain or discomfort?

        (i) Does the discomfort disappear with rest?

        (ii) Has the patient taken any medications (such as nitroglycerin) to relieve the problem before your arrival?

  (3) **Quality.** If pain or discomfort is present, determine its quality.

    (a) Ask the patient to describe the pain or discomfort in his or her own words, e.g., dull, sharp, tearing, pressure, crushing, heavy, burning, constricting, suffocating.

    (b) Is the patient's pain or discomfort accompanied by other symptoms (e.g., sweating, shortness of breath, nausea)?

  (4) **Radiation.** If pain or discomfort is present, determine if it radiates to any area.

    (a) Chest pain may radiate to the neck, jaw, teeth, back, shoulders, arms, elbows, wrists, and, occasionally, to the back between the shoulder blades.

    (b) Pain usually radiates down the left side of the body.

  (5) **Severity.** Determine the patient's perception of the severity of his or her chest pain by asking, "On a scale of 1 to 10, with 1 being the least and 10 being the worst pain you have ever experienced, how would you rate your pain?"

  (6) **Time.** Determine how long the patient's pain or discomfort has been present (e.g., seconds, minutes, hours, days).

      (a)   Ask the patient if he has ever had this pain or discomfort before. If so, how does this episode compare with previous ones?

      (b)   Does the pain come and go (intermittent) or is it continuous?

3. Obtain baseline vital signs

  a. Respiratory rate. The patient's respiratory rate may be increased due to anxiety, pain, or CHF.

  b. Pulse

    (1)   An increased heart rate may suggest anxiety, pain, CHF, or an abnormal heart rhythm.

    (2)   A decreased heart rate may suggest an abnormal heart rhythm or the effect of some heart medications.

    (3)   A weak pulse may indicate a decrease in the amount of blood pumped out by the left ventricle due to a heart attack or CHF.

    (4)   An absent pulse in an extremity may indicate blockage of an artery in the extremity or that the patient's blood pressure is severely low.

  c. Blood pressure

    (1)   An elevated blood pressure may be the result of anxiety, emotional stress, or pain or may indicate preexisting high blood pressure.

    (2)   A fall in blood pressure may indicate shock or the effect of some heart medications.

  d. Skin color, temperature, and condition

    (1)   Cool extremities may occur from blood vessel narrowing (constriction).

    (2)   Sweating may indicate pain, anxiety, or shock.

    (3)   Pale or cyanotic skin may indicate a decrease in the amount of blood pumped out by the left ventricle due to a heart attack.

4. **Perform a focused physical examination**

  a. Look

    (1)   Observe the face for signs of distress.

    (2)   Inspect the neck for JVD.

    (3)   Inspect the chest for:

      (a)   Use of accessory muscles

      (b)   Retractions

      (c)   Equal rise and fall

    (4)   Note the presence of secretions from the mouth and nose. If present, note if the secretions are blood tinged and/or foamy suggesting advanced pulmonary edema.

    (5)   Observe the patient's position.

      (a)   The patient may place a clenched fist against his or her chest to indicate the location of the pain.

      (b)   The patient with CHF often sits upright with the legs in a dependent position, laboring to breathe.

    (6)   Observe the patient's skin color.

    (7)   Inspect the extremities for swelling.

  b. Listen

    (1)   Auscultate breath sounds. Wheezes or crackles may indicate failure of the left ventricle.

    (2)   Listen for noisy breathing (e.g., gurgling).

    (3)   If the patient can speak, note if the patient can speak in full sentences.

  c. Feel. Assess equality of pulses.

EMERGENCY MEDICAL CARE

ABSENT PULSE

1. For a medical patient older than 8 years old, CPR with AED
2. For a medical patient younger than 8 years old, CPR.

RESPONSIVE PATIENT WITH A KNOWN CARDIAC HISTORY AND SIGNS OF CARDIAC COMPROMISE

1. ALS assistance should be requested as soon as possible for patients with signs of cardiac compromise.
2. If ALS personnel are not available, the patient should be transported promptly to the closest appropriate medical facility.
3. Place the patient in a position of comfort.
   a. Most patients will prefer a semi-Fowler's position.
   b. Do not allow the patient to perform any activity (e.g., walking to the stretcher).
4. Administer oxygen.
   a. If the patient's breathing is adequate, apply oxygen by nonrebreather mask at 15 liters per minute (LPM) if not already done.
   b. If the patient's breathing is inadequate, provide positive-pressure ventilation with 100% oxygen.
   c. Assess the adequacy of the ventilations delivered.
5. Determine if the patient has been prescribed nitroglycerin.
   a. If the patient does have prescribed nitroglycerin:
      (1) Determine if the medication is with the patient
      (2) Determine when the last dose was taken
      (3) Contact medical direction
      (4) If instructed to do so, assist the patient with its use
      (5) Continue with the focused assessment
   b. If the patient does not have prescribed nitroglycerin, continue the focused assessment.
5. Transport promptly if:
   a. The patient has signs of cardiac compromise and no prior history of cardiac problems
   b. The patient has a history of cardiac problems but does not have nitroglycerin
   c. The patient has a systolic blood pressure of less than 100 mm Hg
6. Perform ongoing assessments until patient care is turned over to ALS personnel or medical personnel at the receiving facility.

MEDICATIONS: ASSISTING THE PATIENT WITH PRESCRIBED NITROGLYCERIN

1. **Medication name**
   a. The generic name is nitroglycerin.
   b. Trade names include Nitrostat®, Nitrobid®, and Nitrolingual Spray®.
2. **Mechanism of action**
   a. Nitroglycerin causes relaxation (dilation) of the smooth muscle of blood vessel walls. The effects of nitroglycerin are most pronounced on venous blood vessels, less pronounced on arterial blood vessels.
   b. Relaxation of the veins results in pooling of blood in the dependent portions of the body, due to gravity. This effect reduces the amount of blood returning to the heart, decreasing the heart's workload.
   c. Nitroglycerin causes some relaxation of the coronary arteries, improving blood flow and the delivery of oxygen to the heart.
3. **Indications.** The EMT-Basic can assist patients in using prescribed nitroglycerin only if ALL of the following criteria are met:
   a. The patient is exhibiting signs and symptoms of chest pain
   b. The patient has physician prescribed nitroglycerin
   c. The EMT-Basic has obtained specific authorization from medical direction (off line or on line)
4. **Contraindications**
   a. The patient has hypotension or blood pressure below 100 mm Hg systolic.
   b. The patient has a head injury.
   c. The patient is an infant or child.

      d. The patient has already taken the maximum recommended dose before arrival of the EMT-Basic.

      e. Medical direction does not give permission.

5. Medication forms. Nitroglycerin can be in tablet or sublingual spray forms.

6. Dosage

      a. Dosage is 1 tablet or 1 spray under the tongue.

      b. This dose may be repeated in 3 to 5 minutes (maximum of three doses) if:

         (1) The patient experiences no relief,

         (2) The patient's systolic blood pressure remains above 100 mm Hg systolic, and

         (3) The EMT-Basic is authorized by medical direction to administer another dose of the medication.

7. Administration

      a. Confirm that the patient is exhibiting signs or symptoms of chest pain.

      b. Confirm that the patient has physician prescribed nitroglycerin.

         (1) Ensure that the nitroglycerin is prescribed for the patient.

         (2) Ensure that the nitroglycerin is not expired.

         (3) Ensure that the patient is alert.

      b. Determine if the patient has already taken any doses and, if so:

         (1) The time of the last dose

         (2) The effects of the medication

      c. Assess vital signs to ensure that the patient's systolic blood pressure is greater than 100 mm Hg.

      d. Obtain an order from medical direction (either on line or off line) to assist the patient in taking the medication.

      e. Assure right medication, right patient, right route.

      f. Apply clean gloves, as the nitroglycerin can be absorbed through the EMT-Basic's skin if gloves are not worn.

      g. Remove the oxygen mask from the patient.

      h. Tablet administration

         (1) Ask the patient to raise his or her tongue

         (2) Pour 1 nitroglycerin tablet into the bottle cap

         (3) Hand the medication to the patient for self-administration or place the tablet under the patient's tongue

      i. Spray administration

         (1) Ask the patient to raise his or her tongue

         (2) Hand the medication to the patient for self-administration or spray the medication under the patient's tongue

         (3) Instruct the patient to keep his or her mouth closed and not swallow until the medication is dissolved and absorbed

      j. Replace the oxygen mask on the patient.

      k. Reassess the patient's blood pressure within 2 minutes.

      l. Document the patient's name, drug name and dose administered, time of administration, and the patient's response to the drug.

      m. If an on-line order was received by medical direction, document the name of the physician giving the order.

8. Side effects. Side effects include:

      a. Headache

      b. Hypotension

      c. Pulse rate changes

      d. Dizziness

9. Special considerations

      a. Nitroglycerin is rapid acting; relief of chest pain or discomfort may occur within 1 to 2 minutes of administration.

      b. Nitroglycerin must be protected from light, air, and heat to prevent deterioration.

       (1) Nitroglycerin deteriorates rapidly once the bottle is opened.

       (2) Patients should obtain a fresh supply every 4 to 6 months.

10. Reassessment

    a. Monitor the patient's blood pressure closely before and after administration.

    b. Question the patient about the effect of the medication on pain relief.

    c. Consult with medical direction before readministration of the medication.

    d. Document the time, dose, medication, vital signs, and patient's response to the medication.

BASIC LIFE SUPPORT (BLS)

1. Not all chest pain patients become cardiac arrest patients.

2. One-rescuer CPR

    a. EMT-Basics rarely perform one-rescuer CPR while on duty.

    b. Situations in which one-rescuer CPR may be performed include:

       (1) While the EMT-Basic's partner is preparing equipment

       (2) While the EMT-Basic's partner is driving to a receiving facility

3. Two-rescuer CPR is an essential part of the EMT-Basic's education.

4. EMT-Basics must also learn:

    a. Use of automated external defibrillation

    b. To request available ALS backup when appropriate

    c. Use of bag-valve-mask devices with oxygen attached

    d. Use of flow-restricted, oxygen-powered ventilation devices

    e. Techniques of lifting and moving patients

    f. Suctioning the airway

    g. Use of airway adjuncts

    h. Use of body substance isolation precautions for infections when necessary

    i. Techniques for interviewing bystanders and family members to obtain facts related to cardiac arrest events

CARDIAC ARREST

SUDDEN CARDIAC DEATH

1. Sudden cardiac death is the unexpected loss of life occurring either immediately or within one hour of onset of cardiac symptoms.

2. Approximately two-thirds of sudden cardiac deaths take place outside the hospital.

3. Most patients who suffer sudden cardiac death have no warning symptoms immediately before collapse.

4. It is possible that many of these deaths can be prevented by rapid entry into the emergency medical services (EMS) system, prompt CPR, and early defibrillation.

CHAIN OF SURVIVAL

1. Cardiac arrest occurs when the contraction of the heart stops and is confirmed by unresponsiveness, absent breathing, and absent pulses.

2. The most common heart rhythm seen in out-of-hospital cardiac arrest is **ventricular fibrillation** (VF).

    a. VF is an abnormal heart rhythm in which the heart muscle quivers instead of contracting normally.

    b. In VF, effective contraction of the heart and pulse are absent.

3. Survival of cardiac arrest depends on a series of critical actions that the American Heart Association (AHA) has termed the **"chain of survival."**

4. The chain has four links:

    a. Early access

(1) The public must be educated to recognize the early warning signs of a heart attack.

    (a) Many patients do nothing and hope their symptoms will go away.

    (b) The average time between the onset of symptoms and admission to a medical facility is about 3 hours.

    (c) Some patients may delay seeking help for more than 24 hours.

(2) A patient's collapse must be identified by a person who can activate the EMS system.

(3) EMS personnel must arrive rapidly at the scene with all necessary equipment.

b. Early CPR

    (1) Bystander CPR is the best treatment the patient can receive until arrival of a defibrillator and advanced-cardiac-life-support (ACLS) personnel.

    (2) CPR training teaches citizens how to contact the EMS system, decreasing the time to defibrillation.

c. Early defibrillation

    (1) Defibrillation is the delivery of a controlled electrical shock to a patient's heart to end an abnormal heart rhythm, such as VF.

    (2) Early defibrillation is the link in the chain of survival most likely to improve survival from cardiac arrest.

d. Early ACLS

    (1) Early ACLS provided by paramedics at the scene is the final critical link in the management of cardiac arrest.

    (2) ALS units combine rapid defibrillation by first-responding units with rapid intubation and intravenous medications by the ALS units.

    (3) If ACLS units are not available, thr patient should be transported rapidly to a facility for definitive ACLS care.

5. If any one link in the chain is weak or missing, the result will be poor survival, despite excellence in the rest of the chain.

AUTOMATED EXTERNAL DEFIBRILLATION

IMPORTANCE OF AUTOMATED EXTERNAL DEFIBRILLATION TO THE EMT-BASIC

1. Principle of early defibrillation. All BLS personnel must be trained to operate, equipped with, and permitted to operate a defibrillator if, in their professional activities, they are expected to respond to people in cardiac arrest.

2. Rationale for early defibrillation

    a. The most frequent rhythm seen in sudden cardiac death is VF.

    b. The most effective treatment for VF is electrical defibrillation.

    c. The likelihood of successful defibrillation decreases rapidly over time.

    d. Many EMS systems have demonstrated increased survival of cardiac arrest patients experiencing ventricular fibrillation. This increased survival was after early defibrillation programs were started and all of the links in the chain of survival were present.

TYPES OF DEFIBRILLATORS

1. A **defibrillator** is a device that delivers a controlled electrical shock to a patient to stop an abnormal heart rhythm, and defibrillation is the technique of administering the electrical shock.

2. Manual defibrillator (*Figure 18-4*)

    a. A manual defibrillator requires the rescuer to analyze and interpret the patient's cardiac rhythm.

b. If the rhythm requires defibrillation, the rescuer applies paddles or adhesive pads to the patient's chest to deliver the shock.

3. **Implantable defibrillator**
   a. An implantable defibrillator is a device that is electronically programmed to identify and stop life-threatening heart rhythms in patients at high risk for sudden cardiac death.
   b. These devices typically weigh about a half pound and are placed below the skin surface in the patient's chest wall or abdomen.
   c. Because these devices are in direct contact with the heart muscle by using wires, much less energy is needed for defibrillation than when using an external defibrillator.

4. **Automated external defibrillator (AED)**
   a. An AED is a machine that analyzes a patient's heart rhythm and, if indicated, delivers an electrical shock.
   b. AEDs are attached to the patient by means of connecting cables and two disposable adhesive pads.
   c. The adhesive pads have a thin metal pad covered by a thick layer of adhesive gel.
   d. The adhesive pads record the heart rhythm and, if appropriate, deliver a shock.

TYPES OF AEDS

1. **Fully automated external defibrillator**
   a. The adhesive pads must be attached to the patient and the power turned on.
   b. The machine analyzes the patient's heart rhythm.
   c. If ventricular fibrillation (or **ventricular tachycardia** above a preset rate) [*Figure 18-5*] is present, the machine charges and delivers a shock.
   d. Ventricular tachycardia (VT) [*Figure 18-6*] is a fast heart rhythm (rate more than 100 beats per minute) that originates in the ventricles.

2. **Semiautomated external defibrillator (SAED)** [*Figure 18-7*]
   a. The SAED is also called a shock-advisory defibrillator.
   b. The adhesive pads must be attached to the patient, the power turned on, and the operator must press an "analyze" control to begin rhythm analysis.
   c. The SAED "advises" the EMT-Basic the steps to take based on its analysis of the patient's cardiac rhythm by means of a computer synthesized voice, visual alarm, or printed message.

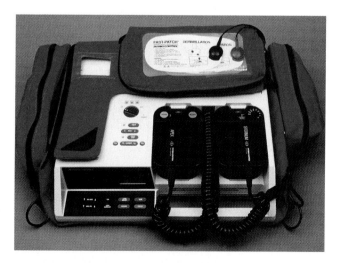

Fig. 18-4. A manual defibrillator requires the rescuer to analyze and interpret the patient's cardiac rhythm.

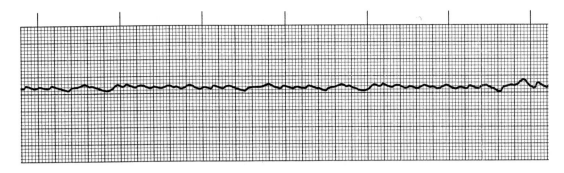

Fig. 18-5. Ventricular fibrillation.

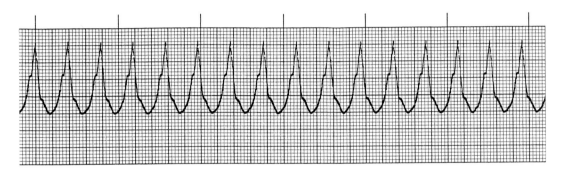

Fig. 18-6. Ventricular tachycardia.

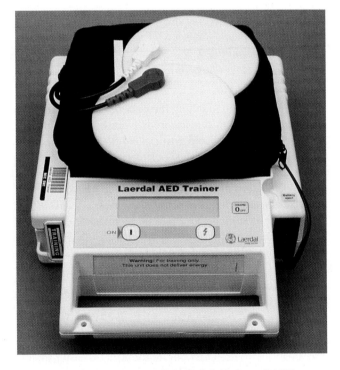

Fig. 18-7. Semiautomated external defibrillator (SAED).

AED ANALYSIS OF CARDIAC RHYTHMS

1. A defibrillator computer microprocessor evaluates the patient's rhythm and confirms the presence of a rhythm for which a shock is indicated.
2. The accuracy of AEDs in rhythm analysis has been high both in detecting rhythms needing shocks and rhythms that do not need shocks.
3. Accurate rhythm analysis is dependent on:
   a. Properly charged defibrillator batteries
   b. Proper defibrillator maintenance
4. The SAED should be placed in the "analyze" mode ONLY when:
   a. Full cardiac arrest has been confirmed (e.g., the patient is unresponsive, not breathing, and pulseless)
   b. All movement, particularly the movement of patient transport, has stopped
5. Avoid using radio transmitters during rhythm analysis. Signal "noise" may interfere with the AED's analysis of the patient's cardiac rhythm.

INAPPROPRIATE DELIVERY OF SHOCKS

1. **Human error.** Failure to follow the manufacturer's instructions in the use of the fully automated AED has, in rare instances, resulted in the delivery of inappropriate shocks.
   a. AED is inappropriately used on a patient with a pulse.
   b. AED is activated in a moving vehicle.
2. Mechanical error, such as low batteries, can cause inappropriate delivery of shocks, as accurate rhythm analysis is dependent on properly charged defibrillator batteries.

VENTRICULAR TACHYCARDIA

1. The AED should be attached only to unresponsive, nonbreathing, pulseless patients to avoid delivering inappropriate shocks.
2. The AED advises shocks for VT when the rate exceeds a certain value (e.g., above 180 beats per minute).

INTERRUPTION OF CPR

1. No one should be touching the patient when the patient's cardiac rhythm is being analyzed and when shocks are delivered.
2. Chest compressions and artificial ventilations must be stopped when the rhythm is being analyzed and when shocks are delivered. This stoppage:
   a. Allows accurate rhythm analysis, as movements caused by CPR can cause the AED to stop its analysis of the patient's rhythm
   b. Prevents accidental shocks to rescuers
3. CPR may be stopped for up to 90 seconds for diagnosing VF and delivering three shocks. Defibrillation is more effective than CPR, so stopping CPR to use the AED is more beneficial to patient outcome.
4. Resume CPR after the first three shocks are delivered or when the AED advises that no shock is indicated.

ADVANTAGES AND DISADVANTAGES OF AEDS

1. **Initial training and continuing education**
   a. Learning to use and operate the AED is easier than learning CPR.
   b. During training, the EMT-Basic:
      (1) Learns to recognize a cardiac arrest (unresponsive, nonbreathing, pulseless patient)
      (2) Learns how to properly attach the AED to the patient
      (3) Memorizes the treatment sequence
   c. The EMS delivery system should have:

    (1) Necessary links in the chain of survival

    (2) Medical direction

    (3) EMS system with audit and/or quality improvement program in place

    (4) Mandatory continuing education with skill competency review for EMS providers

  d. EMT-Basics should undergo a continuing competency skill review every three months.

2. **Speed of operation.** Studies comparing the use of manual defibrillators and AEDs have shown that the first shock can be delivered an average of 1 minute sooner with the AED than with personnel using manual defibrillators.

3. **Remote defibrillation through adhesive pads**

  a. The AED uses adhesive pads attached to the patient by connecting cables.

  b. This technique allows remote ("hands-off") defibrillation.

    (1) It is safer for the operator of the AED.

    (2) Adhesive pads cover a larger surface area than the paddles of manual defibrillators, delivering more effective shocks.

4. **Rhythm monitoring**

  a. Some AEDs have a screen for rhythm monitoring.

  b. The screen display of some AEDs may not be comparable to the bright display of manual defibrillators.

OPERATION OF THE AED

1. **Scene size-up**

  a. Ensure that the scene is safe before entering.

  b. Take body substance isolation precautions (should be done en route to the scene).

2. **Initial assessment**

  a. If CPR is in progress on arrival of the EMT-Basic, ask rescuers to stop CPR briefly.

  b. Verify that the patient is not breathing (apneic) and pulseless.

    (1) If the patient is older than 8 years of age, unresponsive, not breathing and pulseless:

      (a) Have partner resume CPR

      (b) Attach AED

    (2) If the patient is younger than 8 years of age, unresponsive, not breathing and pulseless:

      (a) Resume CPR

      (b) Transport promptly to the closest appropriate medical facility

  c. Attach AED.

    (1) Attach the AED connecting cables to the adhesive pads (*Figure 18-8*).

    (2) Attach adhesive pads to the patient's bare chest.

      (a) The sternum (negative) pad should be placed to the right of the patient's sternum with the top edge of the pad just below the right clavicle.

      (b) The apex (positive) pad should be placed over the patient's left lower ribs with the center in the midaxillary line.

  d. Turn on the AED power.

  e. If the AED is equipped with a tape recorder, begin narrative.

    (1) Identify self and EMS unit.

    (2) State location and time.

    (3) Provide a brief description of the situation.

    (4) Describe actions and patient's response throughout the resuscitation effort.

  f. Prepare to analyze the rhythm.

    (1) Stop CPR.

    (2) Clear everyone away from the patient.

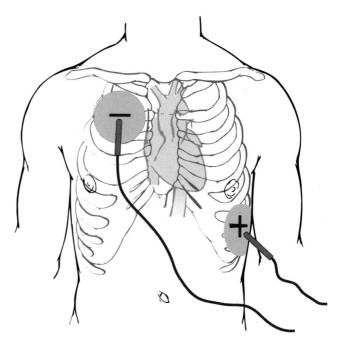

Fig. 18-8. Attach adhesive pads of the automated external defibrillator (AED) to the patient's bare chest. The sternum (negative) pad should be placed to the right of the patient's sternum with the top edge of the pad just below the right clavicle. The apex (positive) pad should be placed over the patient's lower ribs with the center in the midaxillary line.

        (a)   During rhythm analysis, there must be no movement or contact with the patient.

        (b)   Do not use radio transmitters when the AED is in analysis mode.

    (3)   Press the analyze control.

  g. If the machine advises a shock is indicated:

    (1)   Clear everyone from the patient by saying, "I'm clear, you're clear, we're all clear"

    (2)   Deliver shock. The first shock delivered by the AED is at 200 joules.

    (3)   Reanalyze the rhythm

    (4)   If the machine advises a shock, deliver a second shock. The second shock delivered by the AED is at 200 to 300 joules.

    (5)   Reanalyze the rhythm

    (6)   If the machine advises shock, deliver a third shock. The third shock delivered by the AED is at 360 joules.

    (7)   Check the patient's pulse

        (a)   If a pulse is present, check breathing.

            (i)   If the patient is breathing adequately, apply oxygen by nonrebreather mask at 15 LPM and transport.

            (ii)   If the patient is not breathing adequately, provide positive-pressure ventilation with 100% oxygen and transport.

            (iii)   Assess vital signs every 5 minutes.

        (b)   If there is no pulse:

            (i)   Resume CPR for 1 minute

            (ii)   Check pulse. If absent, reanalyze the rhythm and if indicated, deliver a second set of stacked shocks (defibrillating up to three times).

            (iii)   Transport

  h. If, after any rhythm analysis, the machine advises no shock, check the patient's pulse.

    (1)   A "no shock indicated" message may occur:

        (a) When the patient has a pulse

        (b) When the patient does not have a pulse, but the rhythm is one the AED has been programmed not to shock

    (2) If a pulse is present, check the patient's breathing.

        (a) If the patient is breathing adequately, apply oxygen by nonrebreather mask at 15 LPM and transport

        (b) If the patient is not breathing adequately, provide positive-pressure ventilation with 100% oxygen and transport

    (3) If no pulse is present:

        (a) Resume CPR for 1 minute

        (b) Check pulse; if absent, reanalyze the rhythm

        (c) If a shock is advised, deliver if necessary up to two sets of three stacked shocks separated by 1 minute of CPR

        (d) If no shock is advised and the patient is pulseless, resume CPR for 1 minute

            (i) Reanalyze the rhythm for a third time.

           (ii) If a shock is advised, deliver up to two sets of three stacked shocks separated by 1 minute of CPR if needed.

         (iii) If no shock is advised, resume CPR and transport.

3. Standard operational procedures

  a. If ALS is not on the scene, the patient should be transported when one of the following occurs:

  (1) The patient regains a pulse

  (2) A total of six shocks have been delivered

  (3) The machine gives three consecutive messages (separated by 1 minute of CPR) that no shock is advised

  b. One EMT-Basic should operate the AED while the other performs CPR.

  c. Defibrillation comes first. No other activity (e.g., setting up oxygen equipment or suction equipment) should delay analysis of the patient's rhythm or defibrillation.

  d. The EMT-Basic must be familiar with the AED used in his or her EMS setting.

  e. All contact with patient must be avoided during rhythm analysis.

  f. State "clear the patient" before delivering shocks.

  g. No defibrillator can work properly without properly functioning batteries.

    (1) Check batteries at beginning of every shift.

    (2) Carry extra batteries.

INFANT AND CHILD GUIDELINES

1. Cardiac arrest in an adult is usually cardiac in origin.

2. Cardiac arrest in infants and children is most often the result of respiratory compromise. VF is seldom the cause of cardiac arrest in infants and children.

3. In infants and children, defibrillation should not take priority over clearing the airway and providing artificial ventilation.

4. AEDs are not recommended for use in infants and children younger than 8 years of age. Currently available AEDs are not capable of the lower energy settings necessary for defibrillation of this age group.

5. For children older than 8 years of age, follow standard AED operating procedures.

PERSISTENT VENTRICULAR FIBRILLATION AND NO AVAILABLE ALS BACKUP

1. Prepare for transport after six shocks on the scene:

  a. Three initial stacked shocks

  b. Three shocks after 1 minute of CPR

2. Additional shocks may be delivered at the scene or en route by approval of local medical direction.

3. Transport considerations

    a. Perform CPR throughout transport as indicated.

    b. The AED can be left attached to the patient during transport but should never be placed in analysis mode when the vehicle is in motion.

      (1) The vehicle's movement can interfere with the AED's analysis of the patient's rhythm.

      (2) If medical direction orders additional shocks, the vehicle must be brought to a complete stop to analyze the patient's rhythm.

SINGLE RESCUER WITH AN AED

1. Perform an initial assessment.
   a. Verify unresponsiveness.
   b. Open the airway.
   c. Assess breathing. If the patient is not breathing, give two respirations.
   d. Assess the patient's pulse. If no pulse, attach the AED.
2. Turn on the AED power.
3. Begin analysis of the rhythm.
4. Deliver shock(s) as indicated.
5. Defibrillation is the first step.
   a. CPR should not be performed before rhythm analysis.
   b. EMS system activation should not occur until:
      (1) The AED advises "no shock indicated"
      (2) The patient's pulse returns
      (3) Three shocks are delivered
      (4) Help arrives on the scene

NO PULSE CHECKS BETWEEN SHOCKS

1. Pulse checks should not occur during rhythm analysis.
2. Typically, the pulse will not be checked between stacked shocks 1 and 2 and stacked shocks 4 and 5.
   a. AEDs have sensors to detect loose electrodes and regular rhythms associated with the return of a pulse.
   b. When using an AED, a pulse check between shocks:
      (1) Delays rapid identification of persistent VF
      (2) Interferes with the AED's ability to analyze the patient's rhythm
      (3) Increases the likelihood of human error

COORDINATION OF ACLS PERSONNEL WITH EMT-BASICS USING AEDS

1. Use of the AED by EMT-Basics does not require ALS personnel on the scene.
2. ACLS personnel and medical direction should be notified of arrest events as soon as possible.
3. The decision to remain on scene for ACLS, transport and rendezvous with ACLS, or transport directly to a medical facility depends on local protocol, transport time, and medical direction.

POSTRESUSCITATION CARE

1. After the AED protocol is completed, determine if the patient:
   a. Has pulses
   b. Has a pulse but the AED advises "no shock indicated"
   c. Has no pulse and the AED advises a shock is indicated
2. If pulses return:
   a. Assess the patient's airway
      (1) If breathing is adequate, administer oxygen by nonrebreather mask at 15 LPM
      (2) If breathing is inadequate, provide positive-pressure ventilation with 100% oxygen

b. Secure the patient to a stretcher and, using proper lifting and moving techniques, transfer the patient to the ambulance.

c. If appropriate, consider waiting for ALS backup.

d. Keep the AED attached to the patient during transport.

e. Perform a focused assessment.

f. Perform ongoing assessments every 5 minutes en route.

RECURRENT VF AND NO AVAILABLE ACLS

1. **Transporting the unconscious patient with a pulse**
   a. Check the patient's pulse every 30 seconds
   b. If the patient becomes pulseless:
      (1) Stop the vehicle
      (2) Start CPR if the AED is not immediately ready
      (3) Analyze the rhythm as soon as the AED is ready
      (4) Deliver up to three stacked shocks, if indicated
      (5) Check the patient's pulse; if no pulse, resume CPR for 1 minute
      (6) Continue resuscitation according to protocol
      (7) Continue transport

2. **Transporting the conscious patient who becomes unconscious**
   a. When transporting a conscious patient having chest pain who becomes unconscious, pulseless, and apneic:
      (1) Stop the vehicle
      (2) Start CPR if the AED is not immediately ready
      (3) Analyze rhythm as soon as the AED is ready
      (4) Deliver up to three stacked shocks, if indicated
      (5) Check the patient's pulse; if no pulse, resume CPR for 1 minute
      (6) Continue resuscitation according to protocol
   b. If "no shock" message is delivered and no pulse is present:
      (1) Start or resume CPR
      (2) Analyze the rhythm until:
         (a) Three consecutive "no shock" messages are given,
         (b) Six shocks are given, or
         (c) The patient regains a pulse
      (3) Continue transport

SAFETY CONSIDERATIONS

1. Before using the AED, make certain all personnel are clear of the patient, stretcher, and defibrillator.
2. Do not use the AED when the patient or rescuers are in contact with water or metal.

AED MAINTENANCE

1. Regular AED maintenance is essential.
2. An Operator's Shift Checklist for Automated Defibrillators must be completed daily by the EMT-Basic.
3. Defibrillator failure is most frequently related to improper device maintenance, commonly battery failure. EMT-Basics must ensure proper battery maintenance and battery replacement schedules.

TRAINING AND SOURCES OF INFORMATION

The American Heart Association publishes a variety of materials regarding automated external defibrillation.

MAINTENANCE OF SKILLS

1. Most EMS systems permit a maximum of 90 days between practice drills to reassess competency in AED usage; many systems practice skills as often as once a month.
2. The most successful long-term skill maintenance occurs when individuals voluntarily perform equipment checks on a frequent and regular basis that include:
   a. Visual inspection of AED components and controls
   b. Mental review of procedural steps in a cardiac arrest situation

MEDICAL DIRECTION AND QUALITY IMPROVEMENT

1. Successful completion of AED training in an EMT-Basic course does not permit usage of the device without approval by state laws/rules and local medical direction authority.
2. The medical director (or designated representative) must review every event in which an AED is used.
3. Every incident in which CPR is performed must be medically reviewed to decide whether the patient was treated according to professional standards and local standing orders.
4. Other areas that may be evaluated include:
   a. Scene command
   b. Safety
   c. Efficiency
   d. Speed
   e. Professionalism
   f. Ability to troubleshoot
   g. Completeness of patient care
   h. Interactions with other professionals and bystanders
5. Reviews of events using AEDs may be accomplished by:
   a. Written report
   b. Review of voice-ECG tape recorders attached to the AED (if so equipped)
   c. Solid-state memory modules and magnetic tape recordings stored in the AED (if so equipped)
6. Quality improvement involves:
   a. The performance of individuals using AEDs
   b. The effectiveness of the EMS system in which the AEDs are used
   c. Data collection and review:
      (1) Can identify systemwide problems
      (2) Allows evaluation of each link in the chain of survival

REVIEW QUESTIONS

Directions: Each of the numbered items or incomplete statements in this section is followed by answers or by completions of the statement. Select the ONE lettered answer or completion that is BEST in each case.

1. Blood normally flows in a coordinated fashion through the heart. To prevent the blood from flowing in the wrong direction, the heart is equipped with

   (A) two valves

    (B)   four valves
    (C)   two aortic arches
    (D)   two thoracic ducts

2. To assist in lowering body temperature, blood vessels may

    (A)   dilate, thus giving the patient a red or flushed appearance
    (B)   dilate, thus giving the patient a pale or cyanotic appearance
    (C)   constrict, thus giving the patient a red or flushed appearance
    (D)   constrict, thus giving the patient a pale or cyanotic appearance

3. The human heart is divided into chambers. By pumping blood out of these chambers in one direction, the heart effectively perfuses the body with an adequate blood supply. The upper chambers of the heart are called

    (A)   atria
    (B)   valves
    (C)   septa
    (D)   ventricles

4. The lower chambers of the heart are larger than the upper chambers and do the bulk of the work of pumping blood. These chambers are called the

    (A)   atria
    (B)   valves
    (C)   septa
    (D)   ventricles

5. Blood is carried away from the heart by high-pressure vessels that dilate and constrict to maintain blood pressure. The vessels that carry blood away from the heart are called

    (A)   aortas
    (B)   veins
    (C)   arteries
    (D)   capillaries

6. The exchange of gases (primarily oxygen and carbon dioxide) takes place in the

    (A)   aorta
    (B)   veins
    (C)   arteries
    (D)   capillaries

7. Blood is carried back to the heart in vessels of relative low pressure. Many of these vessels contain valves to prevent the backflow of blood as it returns to the heart. These vessels are called

    (A)   aortas
    (B)   veins
    (C)   arteries
    (D)   capillaries

8. The heart muscle (myocardium) requires a constant supply of fresh blood for proper functioning. The arteries that supply the heart with blood are the

    (A)   carotid arteries
    (B)   femoral arteries
    (C)   coronary arteries
    (D)   pulmonary arteries

9. Blood pressure is the force exerted by the blood on the inner walls of the heart and blood vessels. A blood pressure reading of 144/88 millimeters of mercury (mm Hg) indicates

   (A) there is 56 mm Hg of pressure when the heart is at rest
   (B) there is 144 mm Hg of pressure when the heart is at rest
   (C) there is 56 mm Hg of pressure exerted when the heart contracts
   (D) there is 144 mm Hg of pressure exerted when the heart contracts

10. Signs and symptoms of shock include

    (A) rapid pulse, warm skin, and intense thirst
    (B) rapid pulse, shallow breathing, and anxiety/restlessness
    (C) slow pulse; high blood pressure; and rapid, deep respirations
    (D) rapid pulse; dry skin; and rapid, deep respirations with a fruity breath odor

11. The term given to the death (necrosis) of heart cells is

    (A) angina pectoris
    (B) cardiac tamponade
    (C) acute myocardial infarction (AMI)
    (D) congestive heart failure (CHF)

12. The most common symptom associated with cardiac compromise and the lack of oxygenation of the heart is

    (A) nausea
    (B) pulmonary edema
    (C) chest pain or discomfort
    (D) swelling of the feet or lower back

13. Which of the following is most commonly associated with failure of or damage to the left ventricle?

    (A) Pulmonary edema
    (B) Swelling in the feet
    (C) Swelling in the lower back
    (D) Jugular venous distention (JVD)

14. Evaluating a patient's chief complaint is an important part of the focused history and physical examination. Which of the following acronyms may assist rescuers in organizing their line of questioning regarding the type and location of the patient's chief complaint?

    (A) OPQRST
    (B) SAMPLE
    (C) AEIOUTIPS
    (D) CHEST-PAIN

15. The most common cardiac rhythm prehospital cardiac arrest is ventricular fibrillation (VF). The most effective treatment for this situation is

    (A) rapid transport
    (B) early defibrillation
    (C) rapid hyperventilation
    (D) early nitroglycerin therapy

16. When performing a focused history and physical examination on a patient with chest pain, your physical examination

(A) should precede the initial assessment
(B) should be limited to a rapid assessment of the chest
(C) should be limited to a thorough assessment of the upper torso
(D) should evaluate all areas of the body that may be affected by cardiac compromise

17. EMT-Basics may, with approval from medical direction, assist a patient in taking nitroglycerin tablets or spray. This medication is

(A) to be swallowed with water
(B) to be chewed and swallowed
(C) to be given only after a full meal
(D) to be placed and dissolved under the tongue

18. Nitroglycerin may relieve chest pain associated with coronary artery disease. It does so by

(A) numbing the heart muscle
(B) constricting the coronary arteries, thus increasing blood pressure and perfusion
(C) dilating the coronary arteries, thus increasing blood flow to the heart
(D) constricting the veins of the body, thus increasing blood pressure and blood flow to the heart

19. Which of the following is a contraindication for nitroglycerin?

(A) Nausea
(B) Hypotension (low blood pressure)
(C) Hypertension (high blood pressure)
(D) Severe chest pain accompanied by a heart rate greater than 100 beats per minute

20. Your rescue crew is at the home of a 58-year-old female patient complaining of chest pain. After evaluation of the patient, medical direction instructs you to assist the patient in taking her nitroglycerin, up to a maximum of three sublingual tablets. Which of the following absolutely must be reassessed before giving the patient a nitroglycerin tablet?

(A) Pulse rate
(B) Capillary refill
(C) Blood pressure
(D) Respiratory rate

21. Common side effects of nitroglycerin administration include

(A) tremors or seizures
(B) slurred speech and partial paralysis
(C) headache, dizziness, and hypotension
(D) increase in the intensity of the chest pain and difficulty breathing

22. Semiautomated external defibrillators (SAEDs) should be applied to patients and put in the "analyze" mode

(A) if the patient is complaining of severe chest pain
(B) if the patient has chest pain accompanied by difficulty breathing
(C) if the patient is in full cardiopulmonary arrest and all movement around the patient can be stopped
(D) each time a patient complaining of chest pain is being transported to the emergency department

23. To deliver successful electrical therapy (shocks), the semiautomated external defibrillator (SAED) requires the rescuer to

(A) only apply the device
(B) only apply the device and turn on the power
(C) apply the device, turn on the power, and push the "analyze" (or similar) button
(D) apply the device, turn on the power, push the "analyze" (or similar) button, and follow commands to deliver the shock

24. To ensure an accurate reading, no one should be allowed to touch a patient once the "analyze" button has been depressed. Cardiopulmonary resuscitation (CPR) may be interrupted for up to _____ seconds to allow the automated external defibrillator to analyze the patient's cardiac rhythm and deliver three successive shocks.

(A) 10
(B) 30
(C) 60
(D) 90

Directions: Each of the numbered items or incomplete statements in this section is negatively phrased, as indicated by a capitalized word such as NOT, LEAST, or EXCEPT. Select the ONE lettered answer or completion that is BEST in each case.

25. The circulatory system is comprised of the cardiovascular system and the lymphatic system. Which of the following is NOT one of the functions of the circulatory system?

(A) Maintenance of body temperature
(B) Elimination of excess salt and fluids from the body
(C) Protection against invasion by foreign microorganisms
(D) Transport of oxygen, blood, hormones, minerals, and other substances throughout the body

26. Which of the following does NOT have to be in place for nitroglycerin administration?

(A) Patient experiencing chest pain
(B) Patient with a history of previous heart attacks
(C) Patient has physician-prescribed nitroglycerin
(D) EMT-Basic has obtained specific authorization by medical direction to assist in nitroglycerin therapy

Directions: Each of the numbered questions or incomplete statements in this section refers to a scenario that precedes them. The numbered questions or incomplete statements are followed by answers or by completions of the statement. Select the answer or completion of the statement that is BEST in each case.

Your ambulance is called to an adult care facility for a 79-year-old female patient complaining of chest pain. The patient has taken three nitroglycerin tablets before calling for assistance. Dispatch information states the patient has received no relief from the nitro-glycerin. You arrive to find the patient sitting upright in bed in a moderate-to-severe level of distress. She appears conscious.

Questions 27–30

27. Following the scene size-up, you should turn your attention to

   (A) performing an initial assessment
   (B) quickly assessing if the patient has a pulse
   (C) applying the automated external defibrillator (AED)
   (D) putting the patient on high-flow oxygen by nasal cannula

28. During the focused history and physical examination, which of the following acronyms would assist you in gathering information about the patient's medical history?

   (A) R-U-OK
   (B) SAMPLE
   (C) OPQRST
   (D) CHEST-PAIN

29. While assessing the patient's baseline vital signs, you note her blood pressure is 88/54 and her pulse is 48 beats per minute. These signs may suggest the patient

   (A) is dehydrated
   (B) is very anxious
   (C) has a normal, healthy heart
   (D) has an abnormal heart rhythm with cardiac compromise

30. Which of the following treatment plans would be most appropriate for this patient?

   (A) Provide oxygen by nasal cannula and transport to an appropriate facility
   (B) Provide oxygen by nonrebreather mask and transport to an appropriate facility
   (C) Provide oxygen by nonrebreather mask, call for advanced-life-support (ALS) assistance, and transport to an appropriate facility
   (D) Provide oxygen by nonrebreather mask, give nitroglycerin until the patient's pain in relieved, call for ALS assistance, and transport to an appropriate facility

Your rescue crew is called to an apartment complex for a 69-year-old male patient complaining of a sudden onset of "dull chest pressure." Your patient weighs 225 pounds and lives on the third flood of the complex.

Questions 31–32

31. The ideal method for getting this patient to the ambulance would be to

   (A) have the patient walk down the stairs rapidly to speed transport
   (B) have the patient walk down the stairs slowly, resting between flights
   (C) have the patient walk down the stairs slowly, only if it does not worsen his complaint
   (D) bring the stretcher to the patient and position the patient on the stretcher before going down the stairs

32. Once at the ambulance, you may place this patient in a position most comfortable for him. For conscious patients with chest pain, this is generally

(A)   sitting up at an angle
(B)   lying flat on the back
(C)   lying flat on the stomach
(D)   lying flat on the back with the feet slightly elevated

Your rescue crew is called to the scene for an unconscious 52-year-old male patient. You find the patient in his backyard in a lounge chair. He is apneic (not breathing) and pulseless. A neighbor began cardiopulmonary resuscitation (CPR) before your arrival.

Questions 33–35

33. After confirming the patient is apneic and pulseless, you apply the semiautomated external defibrillator (SAED) and push the analyze button. Three successive ("stacked") shocks are indicated and delivered. After the third shock, you should

   (A)   begin oxygen therapy by nonrebreather mask at 15 liters per minute (LPM)
   (B)   remove the SAED to avoid getting shocked when touching the patient
   (C)   check airway, breathing, and circulation status and begin cardiopulmonary resuscitation (CPR) if the patient is still in cardiopulmonary arrest
   (D)   check airway, breathing, and circulation status and press "analyze" again if the patient is still in cardiopulmonary arrest

34. After appropriately treating the patient, you press the "analyze" button again. The patient is still in cardiopulmonary arrest. The SAED informs you no shock is indicated. You should

   (A)   terminate resuscitation efforts
   (B)   continue cardiopulmonary resuscitation (CPR) and transport the patient
   (C)   administer sublingual nitroglycerin and continue cardiopulmonary resuscitation (CPR) en route to the emergency department
   (D)   deliver a shock if you are certain that the patient is still in cardiopulmonary arrest

35. Before delivering a shock by means of an external defibrillator, you must ensure that

   (A)   the patient is wearing rubber-soled shoes
   (B)   no one is touching the patient or the stretcher
   (C)   oxygen bottles are at least 20 feet from the patient
   (D)   anyone touching the patient is wearing rubber-soled shoes

ANSWERS AND RATIONALES

1-B. There are four valves in the heart that prevent the backflow of blood. These valves are the tricuspid valve (between the right atrium and right ventricle), pulmonic valve (between the right ventricle and the pulmonary artery), mitral (bicuspid) valve (between the left atrium and left ventricle), and the aortic valve (between the left ventricle and aorta).

2-A. By dilating the peripheral vessels, the circulatory system sends more blood to the surface of the body. This blood is cooled and returns to the body's core. Imagine yourself playing basketball on a hot day. Your skin may become red or flushed due to increased blood flow to the skin. Sweating allows the skin to cool down. This cooler temperature is transmitted to the blood supply. Some medications may interfere with this process.

3-A. The atria (left and right) are the upper chambers of the heart. The right atrium receives deoxygenated blood from the vena cavae. The left atrium receives freshly reoxygenated blood from the pulmonary veins as it returns from the lungs.

4-D. The lower chambers of the heart are the right and left ventricles. The ventricles receive blood from the atria. The left ventricle pumps reoxygenated blood through the aorta to the cells of the body. The right ventricle pumps deoxygenated blood through the pulmonary artery to the lungs for reoxygenation.

5-C. Arteries always carry blood away from the heart. However, all arteries do not always carry oxygenated blood. Deoxygenated blood pumped away from the right side of the heart travels through the pulmonary artery, which divides into the right and left pulmonary arteries, one to each lung. The left ventricle pumps blood into the aorta, the largest artery of the body.

6-D. Capillaries are microscopic, single-cell width vessels. Oxygen is delivered to body cells through the thin wall of the capillary. With very few exceptions, all cells of the body are no more than one cell-width away from a capillary bed. Oxygen is also absorbed into the bloodstream in the capillary beds that line the small air sacs (alveoli) of the lungs.

7-B. Veins always carry blood toward the heart. Deoxygenated blood returns from the capillary beds of the body through veins to the heart. Reoxygenated blood returns from the capillary beds through the two pulmonary veins from each lung to the left atrium.

8-C. The right and left coronary arteries are the first arteries that branch off the aorta as blood flows from the left ventricle. The carotid arteries are located in the neck just lateral to the trachea (windpipe). The femoral arteries are located in the crease between the abdomen and the thigh. The pulmonary arteries are responsible for delivering deoxygenated blood from the right ventricle to the lungs.

9-D. Blood pressure is measured in millimeters of mercury (mm Hg) and recorded as the systolic pressure over the diastolic pressure. Systole refers to contraction and diastole refers to relaxation. A blood pressure reading of 144/88 indicates that 144 mm Hg of pressure is exerted when the heart contracts. This reading further indicates that 88 mm Hg of residual pressure is exerted in the system during relaxation of the heart (between heart beats).

10-B. Perfusion is the circulation of blood through an organ or a part of the body. Perfusion is necessary for the proper functioning of all body systems. Hypoperfusion, also called shock, occurs when organs are not provided with an adequate blood supply. Other common signs and symptoms of shock include a rapid, weak pulse; rapid, shallow breathing; altered mental status; cool, pale, moist skin; nausea; and a low or falling blood pressure (a late sign). A rapid pulse with warm skin and intense thirst may be associated with hyperglycemia (a diabetic emergency). A slow pulse accompanied by high blood pressure and rapid, deep respirations may suggest a head injury with increased intracranial pressure. A rapid pulse with dry skin and rapid, deep respirations (Kussmaul respirations) with a fruity breath odor is also associated with hyperglycemia.

11-C. Coronary artery disease results in the reduced flow of blood through the coronary arteries. If the flow of blood to the heart is reduced too much, heart muscle cells will die. Infarction refers to death. Myocardium is the medical term for the heart muscle; therefore, an acute myocardial infarction (AMI) is a heart attack. While a heart attack and angina pectoris both present in much the same way and both may be attributed to coronary artery disease, a heart attack differs from angina pectoris. In angina, death of heart cells does not occur. Since EMT-Basics are not physicians, patients presenting with cardiac-type chest pain should be assumed to be having an acute myocardial infarction. Cardiac tamponade is a traumatic injury to the heart in which blood leaks into the sac surrounding the heart (pericardium), and the accumulating blood impedes the heart's ability to pump blood. Congestive heart failure (CHF) is a condition most commonly associated with patients who have suffered a heart attack. Due to decreased pumping ability of the damaged heart, blood begins to back up in the vessels. Common findings in CHF include difficulty breathing, pulmonary edema (fluid accumulation in the lungs), jugular venous distention (JVD), and swelling in the extremities or lower back.

12-C. When the heart is deprived of oxygen, the result is chest pain or discomfort. Any patient complaining of chest pain or discomfort should be immediately treated with high-flow oxygen by nonrebreather mask. The pain associated with cardiac compromise may be described in many ways: a dull ache, indigestion, a heavy weight on the chest, or a sharp pain that radiates to another body area. Pulmonary edema, nausea, and pedal or sacral edema (swelling of the feet or lower back) may accompany chest pain; however, chest pain is the most common complaint.

13-A. Because the left ventricle pumps oxygenated blood away from the lungs toward the body, a backup of this flow would result in an increase in the amount of blood in the lungs. More blood in the lungs causes the capillary beds to leak fluid into the lung's air sacs (alveoli). Fluid in the lungs is called pulmonary edema. If the right ventricle were to fail, deoxygenated blood would back up as it returns from the body to the heart. This backup may result in jugular venous distention (JVD) and swelling in the feet and lower back.

14-A. OPQRST stands for: **o**nset of pain ("What were you doing when the pain began?"), **p**rovoking/alleviating factors ("Is there anything that makes this pain better or worse?"), **q**uality of pain ("Describe how the pain feels"), **s**everity of the pain ("On a scale of 1 to 10 with 10 being the worst pain you have ever felt, how would you rate this pain?") and **t**ime of pain ("How long ago did this pain begin?"). SAMPLE is an acronym used to evaluate a patient's medical history. It stands for **s**igns and **s**ymptoms, **a**llergies, **m**edications, **l**ast oral intake, and **e**vents leading to the injury or illness. AEIOUTIPS is an acronym to help you remember some causes of unconsciousness. It stands for: **a**lcohol intoxication and **a**cidosis, **e**pilepsy, **i**nsulin (diabetic problems), **o**verdose, **u**remia (kidney failure), **t**rauma or **t**umor, **i**nfection, **p**sychosis, and **s**troke.

15-B. The most effective treatment for the reversal of this heart rhythm is rapid defibrillation. The 1994 EMT-Basic curriculum emphasizes the use of automated external defibrillators (AEDs). Transportation and appropriate airway management and oxygenation are important, but these efforts will not reverse ventricular fibrillation (VF). Nitroglycerin should never be given to a patient in cardiopulmonary arrest.

16-D. Do not be confused by the term "focused" history and physical examination. The emphasis of the physical examination is determined by the conscious patient's chief complaint. However, the physical findings for a particular complaint may be seen in body regions away from the area of distress. For example, a patient complaining of chest pain may have swelling of the feet (pedal edema) from failure of the right ventricle. This sign is an important and pertinent finding. Do not merely examine the area of discomfort or you may miss additional signs relevant to the patient's distress.

17-D. Nitroglycerin, whether in the tablet or spray form, is administered sublingually (absorbed under the tongue). Make sure you have on a clean pair of medical gloves before administering nitroglycerin as you may absorb the medication through your skin.

18-C. Nitroglycerin dilates the coronary arteries, thus improving blood flow to the heart muscle that was previously deprived of oxygen (ischemia). Relief of ischemia reduces chest pain. Nitroglycerin also dilates the veins of the body, decreasing the amount of blood returning to the heart. The decrease in the amount of blood returning to the heart, in turn, reduces the heart's workload and decreases its demand for oxygen.

19-B. Because nitroglycerin causes the blood pressure to drop, it should not be used in patients with a systolic blood pressure below 100 millimeters of mercury (mmHg). Nausea, hypertension, and heart rates greater than 100 are commonly found in patients who are candidates for nitroglycerin therapy.

20-C. Remember that nitroglycerin is a potent blood pressure lowering agent. The interval for repeating doses of nitroglycerin is 3–5 minutes, with a maximum total dose of three tablets. The blood pressure changes from nitroglycerin can generally be seen after approximately 2 minutes. Although reassessment of the patient's pulse rate, capillary refill, and respiratory rate is important, reassessing the patient's blood pressure before administering the first and subsequent tablets is absolutely essential.

21-C. Nitroglycerin also dilates the arteries in the brain and can thus cause headache and possible dizziness. A lower blood pressure is commonly observed after nitroglycerin administration. Tremors, seizures, slurred speech, and partial paralysis are not common side effects. If these events occur, it is more likely that the patient has suffered a cerebrovascular accident (stroke) than a reaction to the nitroglycerin.

22-C. The semiautomated external defibrillator (SAED) should be applied to all patients older than than 8 years of age (or per local protocol) in cardiac arrest. Before analyzing the rhythm, ensure all movement around the patient stops, all radio communications halt, transportation is stopped, and the area is safe (no metal or water contact).

23-D. Unlike the fully automated external defibrillator, which requires less training, the semiautomated external defibrillator (SAED) requires the rescuer to be knowledgeable about the application of the electrodes, powering-up the unit, activating the "analyze" mode, and delivering the shocks as instructed by readout or audible instruction.

24-D. It may take up to 90 seconds for the SAED to analyze and deliver (with your assistance) the three stacked shocks. If shocks are indicated, you should immediately deliver the shock. This may be repeated for a total of three consecutive shocks without cardiopulmonary resuscitation (CPR) or other interventions between shocks. After the third shock or a "shock is not indicated" message, reassess the patient and perform CPR if necessary. The SAED should be activated to reanalyze the patient's rhythm every 60 seconds if the pulse does not spontaneously return.

25-B. The elimination of excess salt and fluids from the body is the responsibility of the urinary system. Through the constriction and dilation of the peripheral blood vessels, the circulatory system influences body temperature. Leukocytes (white blood cells) help to combat invasion by foreign microorganisms. Finally, the circulatory system transports oxygenated blood, minerals, hormones, and other substances throughout the body.

26-B. Although many patients who have been prescribed nitroglycerin have experienced a previous heart attack, it is not necessary that the patient have such a history to be a candidate for nitroglycerin administration. The patient must, however, be experiencing chest pain, must be prescribed nitroglycerin, must have the nitroglycerin with him or her, and the EMT-Basic must receive specific authorization from medical direction to assist with nitroglycerin administration.

27-A. An initial assessment should follow the scene size-up. Evaluate the patient's level of consciousness, airway, breathing and circulatory status, and form a general impression of the patient. Although assessing a pulse is a part of the initial assessment, it is not the first step. Application of the automated external defibrillator (AED) would be indicated if the patient were apneic (not breathing) and pulseless. High-flow oxygen is indicated for this patient; however, a nasal cannula is a low-flow oxygen delivery device.

28-B. SAMPLE stands for **s**igns and **s**ymptoms, **a**llergies, **m**edications (prescribed and over the counter), **p**ertinent **p**ast medical history, **l**ast oral intake, and the **e**vents leading up to the current complaint.

29-D. A normal rate for this patient's age is 60 to 100 beats per minute. The patient's slow heart rate and low blood pressure should cause you concern. A dehydrated patient will normally have a fast heart rate and lower than normal blood pressure, as will an anxious patient. Since this patient's heart rate is lower than normal and the patient is in distress, you should not conclude that this patient has a "normal, healthy" heart.

30-C. Provide high-flow oxygen therapy. If available, advanced-life-support (ALS) assistance should be requested. If not available, begin rapid transport as soon as possible. Because nitroglycerin tends to lower a patient's blood pressure, it would not be indicated for this patient. Do not give nitroglycerin if the patient's systolic blood pressure is below 100 millimeters of mercury (mm Hg). Remember that you must obtain permission from medical direction before administering nitroglycerin.

31-D. If this patient is suffering a heart attack (which should be your assumption), the area of heart damage could be extended if this patient is required to exert himself physically. If you are going to carry the patient (either on or off a stretcher or similar device), make sure you have more than enough rescuers/helpers to control the patient's descent. Without sufficient help, the patient may become anxious. Anxiety can also result in an increase in the area of heart damage.

32-A. Generally, chest pain patients will be most comfortable sitting up at a 45° angle (semi-Fowler's position). Lying back any more may increase the patient's anxiety and worsen or cause difficulty breathing.

33-C. If indicated, defibrillation (shocks) are delivered in groups of three at 1 minute intervals. Between successive groups of analysis and defibrillation, it is imperative that you perform cardiopulmonary resuscitation (CPR) for as long as the patient remains pulseless and apneic. The semiautomated external defibrillator SAED will not (if properly maintained) shock you or the patient without being activated to do so.

34-B. Semiautomated external defibrillators (SAEDs) will not shock every apneic, pulseless patient. Lack of a shock indication does not mean that the patient is not potentially viable. It simply means that the heart rhythm that the patient is in would not benefit from electrical therapy. Continue cardiopulmonary resuscitation (CPR) and transport the patient rapidly to an appropriate facility. For your safety and the safety of the patient, you should not be able to, nor should you attempt to, "override" a resuscitation device.

35-B. Before delivering a shock with an external defibrillator, remove the patient from any contact with metal or fluid. When preparing to defibrillate, look all around (360° degrees) and be sure EVERYONE is clear of the patient. Say, "I'm clear (of any such contact), you're clear, we're all clear." You should do and say this loudly before every defibrillation. If the semiautomated external defibrillator (SAED) is applied properly and oxygen therapy is being managed properly, there should be no danger of using the SAED around oxygen equipment.

BIBLIOGRAPHY

Caroline NL: *Emergency Care in the Streets*, 4th ed. Boston, Little, Brown, 1991.

Crosby LA, Lewallen DG (eds): *Emergency Care and Transportation of the Sick and Injured*, 6th ed. Rosemont, IL, American Academy of Orthopaedic Surgeons, 1995.

Grant HD, Murray RH Jr, Bergeron JD: *Emergency Care*, 7th ed. Englewood Cliffs, NJ, Prentice-Hall, 1995.

Hafen BQ, Karren KJ, Mistovich JJ: *Prehospital Emergency Care*, 5th ed. Upper Saddle River, NJ, Prentice-Hall, 1996.

Henry MC, Stapleton ER, Judd RL: *EMT: Prehospital Care*. Philadelphia, WB Saunders, 1992.

Limmer D, Elling B, O'Keefe M: *Essentials of Emergency Care: A Refresher for the Practicing EMT-B*. Upper Saddle River, NJ, Prenctice-Hall, 1996.

McSwain NE, White RD, Paturas JL, et al (eds): *The Basic EMT: Comprehensive Prehospital Patient Care*. St. Louis, Mosby-Year Book, 1996.

Miller RH, Wilson JK: *Manual of Prehospital Emergency Medicine*. St. Louis, Mosby-Year Book, 1992.

Sloane E: *Anatomy and Physiology: An Easy Learner*. Boston, Jones and Bartlett, 1994.

Solomon EP, Phillips GA: *Understanding Human Anatomy and Physiology*. Philadelphia, WB Saunders, 1987.

Stoy WA: *Mosby's EMT-Basic Textbook*. St. Louis, Mosby-Year Book, 1996.

Thibodeau GA, Patton KT: *The Human Body in Health and Disease*. St. Louis, Mosby-Year Book, 1992.

United States Department of Transportation, National Highway Traffic Safety Administration: *Emergency Medical Technician: Basic. National Standard Curriculum*, 1994.

Yvorra JG (ed): *Mosby's Emergency Dictionary Quick Reference for Emergency Responders*. St. Louis, Mosby-Year Book, 1989.

19 ALTERED MENTAL STATUS, DIABETIC EMERGENCIES, AND SEIZURES

OBJECTIVES

*19-1 List the possible causes of altered mental status.

*19-2 Describe the general emergency care for a patient with an altered mental status.

19-3 Identify the patient taking diabetic medications with altered mental status and the implications of a diabetes history.

19-4 State the steps in the emergency medical care of the patient taking diabetic medicine with an altered mental status and a history of diabetes.

19-5 Establish the relationship between airway management and the patient with altered mental status.

19-6 State the generic and trade names, medication forms, dose, administration, mechanism of action, and contraindications for oral glucose.

19-7 Evaluate the need for medical direction in the emergency medical care of the diabetic patient.

19-8 List the common causes of seizures.

19-9 Describe the signs and symptoms of a tonic-clonic (grand mal) seizure.

19-10 Describe the emergency care for the patient experiencing a tonic-clonic seizure.

*19-11 Define the terms stroke and transient ischemic attack.

*19-12 Discuss the two main forms of stroke.

*19-13 Discuss the two types of ischemic stroke.

*19-14 Identify the risk factors for stroke.

*19-15 List the warning signs of stroke.

*19-16 Describe the emergency medical care for a patient experiencing a stroke.

MOTIVATION FOR LEARNING

The patient with an altered mental status presents a challenge for the EMT-Basic. A careful history obtained from the patient, family, or others is often useful in identifying the underlying cause of the patient's altered mental status. Regardless of cause, emergency care of the patient with an altered mental status focuses on the patient's airway, breathing, and circulation.

ALTERED MENTAL STATUS

COMMON CAUSES (BOX 19-1)

The common causes of altered mental status can be remembered by using the acronym AEIOU-TIPS.

1. **A**lcohol, **a**cidosis, **a**pnea
2. **E**pilepsy (seizures), **e**nvironmental conditions
3. **I**nfection, **i**schemia
4. **O**verdose (or underdose)
5. **U**remia (kidney failure)
6. **T**rauma, **t**emperature (hypothermia or hyperthermia), **t**umors
7. **I**nsulin (too much or too little)
8. **P**sychiatric, **p**oisoning
9. **S**troke (cerebrovascular accident), **s**hock

EMERGENCY MEDICAL CARE

1. Maintain spinal immobilization if trauma is suspected.
2. Establish and maintain an open airway.
   a. Insert an oropharyngeal or nasopharyngeal airway as needed.
   b. Suction as necessary.
3. Administer oxygen.
   a. If the patient's breathing is adequate, apply oxygen by nonrebreather mask at 15 liters per minute (LPM) if not already done.
   b. If the patient's breathing is inadequate, provide positive-pressure ventilation with 100% oxygen and assess the adequacy of the ventilations delivered.
4. Position the patient.
   a. If the patient is sitting or standing, help him or her to the floor.
   b. If there is no possibility of cervical spine trauma, place the patient in a lateral recumbent (recovery) position.
   c. If the patient is immobilized due to suspected trauma and vomits, the patient and backboard should be turned as a unit and the patient's airway cleared with suctioning.
5. Remove or loosen tight clothing.
6. Maintain body temperature.
7. Transport.

ALTERED MENTAL STATUS WITH A HISTORY OF DIABETES

PATHOPHYSIOLOGY OF DIABETES

1. Glucose, a sugar, is the basic fuel for body cells.
   a. The brain must constantly be supplied with glucose because it cannot store it.

Box 19-1. Causes of Altered Mental Status

A = Alcohol, acidosis, apnea
E = Epilepsy (seizures), environmental conditions
I = Infection, ischemia
O = Overdose (or underdose)
U = Uremia (kidney failure)
T = Trauma, temperature, tumors
I = Insulin (too much or too little)
P = Psychiatric, poisoning
S = Stroke, shock

    b. The level of sugar in the blood (the "blood sugar") must remain fairly constant to ensure proper functioning of the brain and body cells.

2. Insulin is a hormone secreted by the pancreas.

    a. Because glucose is a large molecule, insulin helps glucose enter the body's cells to be used for energy.

    b. For cells to use sugar properly, there must be an adequate supply of insulin.

3. Diabetes mellitus is a disease involving the pancreas.

    a. The pancreas either produces too little insulin or stops producing it completely.

    b. Sugar builds up in the blood.

    c. The body's cells do not have enough sugar for energy and do not perform properly.

4. There are two major types of diabetes mellitus (Table 19-1).

    a. Type I (insulin-dependent diabetes mellitus)

       (1) Type I diabetes mellitus usually begins during childhood (juvenile diabetes).

       (2) In this type of diabetes:

          (a) Little or no insulin is produced by the pancreas.

          (b) Without insulin, glucose is unable to enter most body cells.

       (3) Type I diabetes mellitus requires treatment with insulin.

    b. Type II (non-insulin–dependent diabetes mellitus)

       (1) Type II diabetes mellitus usually affects people older than 40 years of age, especially those who are overweight.

       (2) In this type of diabetes:

          (a) The amount of insulin produced by the pancreas may be adequate or may be insufficient to meet the body's needs

          (b) The body's cells are resistant to the effects of insulin

       (3) Type II diabetes mellitus can often be managed by diet, exercise, and oral medications that lower blood sugar levels. Some people require insulin.

    c. If diabetes is not controlled, complications can occur including:

       (1) Changes in the retina that can lead to blindness

       (2) Kidney damage

       (3) Nerve damage that can lead to loss of sensation, numbness and pain

       (4) Circulatory disorders (e.g., heart attack, stroke, blood vessel damage, slow wound healing)

5. **Hypoglycemia**

    a. Hypoglycemia is the most common diabetic emergency.

    b. Hypoglycemia is defined as a lower-than-normal blood sugar level.

Table 19-1. Characteristics of Type I and Type II Diabetes

	Type I	Type II
Synonyms	Insulin-dependent-diabetes mellitus (IDDM) Juvenile diabetes Brittle diabetes	Non-insulin–dependent-diabetes mellitus (NIDDM) Adult-onset diabetes Maturity-onset diabetes Stable diabetes
Age at onset	Childhood, but can begin at any age	Usually 40 years of age and older, but can begin at any age
Characteristics	Thin Diabetes often difficult to control Affects 1 in every 10 diabetics	Usually obese, but may be of normal weight Diabetes often controlled with diet, exercise, and oral medications Most common type of diabetes mellitus
Insulin	Required	Required for less than half

c. The blood sugar level may become too low if the diabetic patient:
  (1) Has taken too much insulin
  (2) Has not eaten enough food
  (3) Has overexercised and burned off sugar faster than normal
  (4) Experiences significant physical (e.g., infection) or emotional stress
d. Prolonged hypoglycemia can lead to irreversible brain damage.
e. Onset of hypoglycemia symptoms is sudden (minutes to hours).
f. Signs and symptoms of hypoglycemia include:
  (1) Altered mental status
    (a) Inability to concentrate
    (b) Irritability, combativeness
    (c) Bizarre behavior
    (d) Nervousness
    (e) Confusion
    (f) Seizures or coma
  (2) Early signs
    (a) Headache
    (b) Hunger
    (c) Nausea
    (d) Weakness
  (3) Later signs
    (a) Cool, pale, clammy skin
    (b) Increased heart rate
    (c) Tremors
6. Hyperglycemia
  a. Hyperglycemia is defined as a higher-than-normal blood sugar level.
    (1) The level of insulin in the body becomes too low.
    (2) Sugar is present in the blood but, without insulin, it cannot be transported into the body's cells.
      (a) Body cells become starved for sugar.
      (b) The body begins breaking down fats to provide energy.
    (3) The breakdown of fats produces waste products, including acids.
  b. The blood sugar level may become too high when the diabetic patient:
    (1) Has not taken his or her insulin
    (2) Has eaten too much food that contains or produces sugar
    (3) Experiences physical (e.g., pregnancy, infection, surgery) or emotional stress
  c. The onset of hyperglycemia symptoms is gradual (hours to days).
  d. Signs and symptoms of hyperglycemia include:
    (1) Altered mental status (varies from drowsiness to coma)
    (2) Rapid, deep breathing (Kussmaul respirations)
      (a) Sweet or fruity (acetone) breath odor
      (b) Loss of appetite
      (c) Thirst
      (d) Dry skin
      (e) Abdominal pain
      (f) Nausea and/or vomiting
      (g) Increased heart rate
      (h) Normal or slightly decreased blood pressure
      (i) Weakness

ASSESSMENT OF THE PATIENT WITH AN ALTERED MENTAL STATUS AND A HISTORY OF DIABETES CONTROLLED BY MEDICATION

1. Scene size-up
  a. Determine if the patient's altered mental status is due to trauma or a medical condition.

      (1) **Trauma.** Determine the mechanism of injury from the patient, family members, or bystanders and inspection of the scene.

      (2) **Medical.** Determine the nature of the illness from the patient, family members, or bystanders.

  b. Observe the patient's environment for clues to the cause of the patient's altered mental status.

      (1) Look for medical identification indicating:

        (a) History of diabetes

        (b) Current use of insulin or oral diabetic medication

      (2) If in a private residence, look in the refrigerator for insulin.

2. Perform an initial assessment.

  a. Maintain spinal immobilization if needed.

  b. Assess the patient's mental status.

  c. Assess the patient's airway.

  d. Assess breathing.

  e. Assess circulation.

  f. Identify any life-threatening conditions and provide care based on those findings.

  g. Establish patient priorities.

      (1) Priority patients include:

        (a) Patients who give a poor general impression

        (b) Unresponsive patients with no gag reflex or cough

        (c) Responsive patients who are unable to follow commands

      (2) Advanced-life-support (ALS) assistance should be requested as soon as possible.

      (3) If ALS personnel are not available, the patient should be transported promptly to the closest appropriate facility.

3. Perform a focused history and physical examination.

  a. If the patient is unresponsive:

      (1) Perform a rapid physical examination

      (2) Follow with evaluation of baseline vital signs and gathering of the patient's medical history

  b. If the patient is responsive, gather information about the patient's medical history before performing the physical examination.

  c. SAMPLE history

      (1) <u>**S**</u>**igns and <u>s</u>ymptoms.** Signs and symptoms of diabetic emergencies include (Table 19-2):

        (a) Intoxicated appearance, anxious, combative progressing to unresponsiveness

        (b) Uncharacteristic behavior

        (c) Slurred speech

        (d) Staggering walk

        (e) Increased heart rate

        (f) Cold, clammy skin

        (g) Hunger

        (h) Seizures

      (2) <u>**A**</u>**llergies.** Determine if the patient has any allergies to medications and other substances or materials.

      (3) <u>**M**</u>**edications.** Determine if the patient is taking any medications (prescription and over the counter) [Table 19-3].

        (a) Determine if the patient takes his or her medications regularly and his or her response to them.

          (i) When did the patient last take his or her medications?

          (ii) For patients taking insulin, ask whether they have taken their insulin today and how much insulin was taken.

        (b) Determine if there has been any recent change in medications (addi-

Table 19-2. Signs and Symptoms of Diabetic Emergencies

	Hypoglycemia (Low Blood Sugar)	Hyperglycemia (High Blood Sugar)
Symptom onset	Rapid (minutes to hours)	Gradual (hours to days)
Medical history	Occurs in patients with or without diabetes mellitus	Usually occurs in patients with known Type I diabetes
Precipitating factors	Insufficient food intake Excessive insulin dosage Excessive physical activity Infection, emotional stress	Excessive food intake containing sugar Insufficient insulin dosage Infection, surgery, pregnancy, emotional stress Undiagnosed diabetes
Mental status	Initially: Irritability, inability to concentrate, nervousness, confusion Late: Seizures, coma	Initially: Confusion, lack of interest in surroundings, drowsiness Coma
Breathing	Initially: Normal or rapid Late: Slow	Deep or rapid (Kussmaul breathing)
Breath odor	Normal	Fruity, acetone
Pulse	Normal or increased	Mildly increased
Blood pressure	Normal or above normal	Normal or below normal (due to dehydration)
Skin	Cool, pale, clammy	Warm, flushed, dry (due to dehydration and/or infection)

Table 19-3. Medications Commonly Prescribed for Patients with Diabetes

Type of Medication	Trade Name(s)
Oral Diabetic Agents	Diabinese® Orinase® Micronase®, DiaBeta®, Glynase® Tolinase® Glucotrol®
Insulin (injection)	Humulin®

tions, deletions, or change in dosages), e.g., has the patient's insulin dosage changed recently?

    (c) Provide all information obtained to the receiving facility.

(4) **Pertinent past medical history.** Ascertain whether the patient has the following conditions:

    (a) Diabetes (confirm with patient, family)

    (b) Heart disease

    (c) High blood pressure

    (d) Chronic obstructive pulmonary disease

(5) **Last oral intake.** Determine the patient's last oral intake.

    (a) When was the patient's last meal or snack?

    (b) How much did the patient eat (or drink)?

    (c) Did the patient vomit after eating?

    (d) Has the patient skipped any meals?

    (e) Has the patient consumed any alcohol?

(6) **Events.** Determine the events leading to the present situation.

    (a) Has the patient performed an unusual exercise or physical activity today?

(**b**) Has the patient had a recent infection?
(**c**) Has the patient suffered any psychological stress?
(**d**) What was the patient's blood sugar level the last time it was measured?

    d. Assess baseline vital signs.
    e. Perform a focused physical examination.

EMERGENCY MEDICAL CARE

1. Because a lack of glucose can cause permanent brain damage, any diabetic patient with an altered mental status should be considered to have hypoglycemia until proven otherwise.
2. Maintain spinal immobilization if trauma is suspected.
3. Establish and maintain an open airway.
    a. Insert an oropharyngeal or nasopharyngeal airway as needed.
    b. Suction as necessary.
4. Administer oxygen.
    a. If the patient's breathing is adequate, apply oxygen by nonrebreather mask at 15 LPM if not already done.
    b. If the patient's breathing is inadequate, provide positive-pressure ventilation with 100% oxygen and assess the adequacy of the ventilations delivered.
4. Position the patient.
    a. If there is no possibility of cervical spine trauma, place the patient in a lateral recumbent (recovery) position to aid drainage of secretions.
    b. If the patient is immobilized due to suspected trauma and vomits, the patient and backboard should be turned as a unit and the patient's airway cleared with suctioning.
5. Remove or loosen tight clothing.
6. Maintain body temperature.
7. If the patient is responsive:
    a. Determine if the patient is alert enough to swallow
    b. Administer oral glucose according to local or state medical direction or protocol
8. Transport. Perform ongoing assessments until patient care is turned over to ALS personnel or medical personnel at the receiving facility.

ORAL GLUCOSE

1. **Medication name**
    a. Generic name is oral glucose.
    b. Trade names are Glutose®, Insta-glucose®.
2. **Mechanism of action.** Oral glucose increases the blood sugar level.
3. **Indications.** Patients with all of the following are candidates for oral glucose:
    a. Altered mental status
    b. History of diabetes controlled by medication
    c. Ability to swallow
4. **Contraindications**
    a. The patient is unresponsive.
    b. The patient is unable to swallow.
    c. Medical direction does not give permission.
5. **Medication form.** Oral glucose is a gel and is packaged in a toothpaste-type tube.
6. **Dosage.** Dosage is one tube.
7. **Administration**
    a. Confirm that the patient:
        (**1**) Has an altered mental status
        (**2**) Has a history of diabetes controlled by medication
        (**3**) Is able to swallow and protect his or her airway

b. Obtain an order from medical direction (either on line or off line) to administer oral glucose.

c. Administer glucose.

  (1) Squeeze oral glucose on a tongue depressor and place it between the patient's cheek and gum.

  (2) Remove the tongue depressor from the patient's mouth once the gel is dissolved, or if the patient loses consciousness or seizes.

d. Document the patient's name, drug name and dose administered, time of administration, and the patient's response to the drug. If an on-line order was received by medical direction, document the name of the physician giving the order.

e. Perform ongoing assessments.

8. Side effects

a. Oral glucose causes no side effects when given properly.

b. It may be aspirated by the patient without a gag reflex.

9. Reassessment

a. If the patient loses consciousness or seizes, remove the tongue depressor from his or her mouth.

b. Perform ongoing assessments every 5 minutes, continuously monitoring the patient's airway and breathing.

SEIZURES

OVERVIEW

1. A **seizure** is a sudden period of abnormal electrical activity in the brain that causes distinctive changes in behavior and body function.

  a. A seizure is a symptom (not a disease) of an underlying problem within the central nervous system.

  b. Common causes of seizures include: (Box 19-2)

    (1) Unknown cause

    (2) Failure to take antiseizure medication (most common cause of adult seizures)

    (3) High fever (febrile seizure) [most common cause of seizures in infants and children 6 months to 3 years of age]

    (4) Infection

    (5) Head trauma

    (6) Brain tumor

    (7) Stroke

    (8) Low blood sugar level (hypoglycemia)

    (9) Electrolyte disturbances

    (10) Decreased oxygen level (hypoxia)

    (11) Alcohol or drug withdrawal

    (12) Eclampsia (seizures associated with pregnancy)

2. Epilepsy is a condition of recurrent seizures in which the cause is usually irreversible.

3. Types of seizures

  a. Tonic-clonic (grand mal)

    (1) Tonic-clonic seizures are also called a generalized motor seizures.

    (2) A tonic-clonic seizure typically consists of four phases:

      (a) Aura

        (i) An **aura** is a peculiar sensation that precedes a seizure.

        (ii) However, not all seizures are preceded by an aura.

        (iii) Typical auras include an unusual taste, a dreamy feeling, a visual disturbance (e.g., flashing light, floating light), an unpleasant odor, or a rising or sinking feeling in the stomach.

           (iv) The aura is followed by a loss of consciousness.
     (b) During the tonic phase, the body's muscles stiffen.
     (c) During the clonic phase, alternating jerking and relaxation of the body occur.
     (d) Postictal phase is the period of gradual awakening following a seizure characterized by confusion, disorientation, and fatigue.

  b. Absence (petit mal)
    (1) These seizures usually occur in children between 4 and 12 years of age, but they can occur in adults.
    (2) The patient may have a blank stare and repeat behaviors such as lip-smacking.
    (3) The seizure typically lasts from 1 to 10 seconds.

4. Status epilepticus is continuous seizures or recurrent seizures that occur at a frequency that prevents the patient from recovering from one seizure before having another one.

  a. Status epilepticus is a medical emergency that, if not treated quickly, may result in respiratory failure and death.
  b. Complications associated with status epilepticus include:
    (1) Aspiration of vomitus and blood
    (2) Long bone and spine fractures
    (3) Dehydration
    (4) Brain damage due to lack of oxygen

ASSESSMENT OF THE PATIENT WITH SEIZURES

1. Scene size-up
  a. Determine if the patient's altered mental status is due to trauma or a medical condition.
    (1) Trauma. Determine the mechanism of injury from the patient, family members, or bystanders and inspection of the scene.
    (2) Medical. Determine the nature of the illness from the patient, family members, or bystanders.
  b. Observe the patient's environment for clues to the cause of the patient's altered mental status. Look for medical identification indicating a history of epilepsy.

2. Perform an initial assessment.

3. Perform a focused history and physical examination.
  a. If the patient is unresponsive:
    (1) Perform a rapid physical examination

Box 19-2. Common Causes of Seizures

Unknown cause
Failure to take antiseizure medication (Most common cause of adult seizures)
High fever (febrile seizure) [Most common cause of seizures in infants and children 6 months to 3 years of age]
Infection
Head trauma
Stroke
Brain tumor
Low blood sugar (hypoglycemia)
Electrolyte disturbances
Decreased oxygen level (hypoxia)
Alcohol or drug withdrawal
Eclampsia (seizures associated with pregnancy)

(2) Follow with evaluation of baseline vital signs and gathering of the patient's medical history

b. If the patient is responsive, gather information about the patient's medical history before performing the physical examination.

c. SAMPLE history

(1) <u>Signs</u> and <u>symptoms</u>. Signs and symptoms of a tonic-clonic seizure include (Box 19-3):

(a) Loss of consciousness

(b) Tonic phase

(i) Stiffening of the body

(ii) Possible cyanosis

(c) Clonic phase

(i) Alternating jerking and relaxation of the body

(ii) Increased heart rate

(iii) Increased blood pressure

(iv) Warm, flushed, moist skin

(v) Possible loss of bowel and bladder control

(vi) Possible bleeding due to biting of the cheek or tongue

(d) Postictal phase

(i) Confusion

(ii) Headache

(iii) Muscle soreness

(2) <u>Allergies</u>. Determine if the patient has any allergies to medications and other substances or materials.

(3) <u>Medications</u>. Determine if the patient is taking any medications (prescription and over the counter) [Table 19-4].

(a) Determine if the patient takes his or her medications regularly and his or her response to them. When did the patient last take his or her medications?

(b) Determine if there has been any recent change in medications (additions, deletions, or change in dosages).

(c) Provide all information obtained to the receiving facility.

(4) <u>Pertinent past medical history</u>

(a) Does the patient have a history of seizures? If so, how often do the seizures usually occur?

Box 19-3. **Signs and Symptoms of a Tonic-Clonic (Grand Mal) Seizure**

Loss of consciousness

Tonic phase
- Stiffening of the body
- Loud moan or cry as air rushes from the lungs through the vocal cords
- Possible cyanosis

Clonic phase
- Alternating jerking and relaxation of the body
- Increased heart rate
- Increased blood pressure
- Possible loss of bowel and bladder control
- Possible bleeding due to biting of the cheek or tongue

Postictal phase
- Confusion
- Headache
- Muscle soreness

Table 19-4. Medications Commonly Prescribed for Patients with Epilepsy

Generic Name	Trade Name(s)
Phenytoin	Dilantin®
Carbamazepine	Tegretol®
Phenobarbital	Luminal®
Valproic acid	Depakote®, Depakene®
Clonazepam	Klonopin®

      (b) Does the patient have a history of stroke, diabetes (low blood sugar can cause seizures), or heart disease (an irregular heart rhythm can cause hypoxia, leading to seizures)?

      (c) Does the patient use or abuse alcohol or drugs? (Alcohol or drug withdrawal can result in seizures.)

  (5) <u>L</u>ast oral intake

      (a) When did the patient last eat or drink?

      (b) Has the patient consumed any alcohol?

  (6) <u>E</u>vents. Determine the events leading to the present situation.

      (a) What was the patient doing at the time of the seizure?

      (b) Did the patient cry out or attract your attention in any way?

      (c) What did the seizure look like?

      (d) When did the seizure start?

      (e) How long did the seizure last?

      (f) Did the seizure begin in one area of the body and progress to others?

      (g) Did the patient lose bowel or bladder control?

      (h) When the patient awoke, was there any change in speech or ability to move his or her extremities?

      (i) Did the patient hit his head or fall?

      (j) Has the patient recently had a fever, headache, or complained of a stiff neck?

d. Assess baseline vital signs.

e. Perform a focused physical examination.

  (1) Note any signs of injury.

      (a) Bleeding may be present from biting the cheek or tongue.

      (b) Abrasions of the head, face, or extremities may occur as a result of the seizure.

      (c) Fractures of the skull or extremities may occur as a result of the seizure.

  (2) Note any signs of alcohol or drug abuse.

  (3) Note the presence of an irregular heart beat.

EMERGENCY MEDICAL CARE

1. Position the patient.

  a. If the patient is sitting or standing, help him or her to the floor.

  b. After the tonic-clonic phase of the seizure, and if there is no possibility of cervical spine trauma, place the patient in the recovery (lateral recumbent) position to aid drainage of secretions.

2. Protect the patient from injury by moving furniture and other objects away from the patient as necessary.

3. Maintain an open airway.

  a. If the patient is actively seizing, do not insert your fingers, an oropharyngeal airway, a padded tongue blade, or bite block into the patient's mouth.

b. If the patient is immobilized due to suspected trauma and vomits, the patient and backboard should be turned as a unit and the patient's airway cleared with suctioning.

4. Administer oxygen.

  a. If the patient's breathing is adequate, apply oxygen by nonrebreather mask at 15 LPM if not already done.

  b. If the seizure is prolonged or if the patient's breathing is inadequate, provide positive-pressure ventilation with 100% oxygen and assess the adequacy of the ventilations delivered.

5. Remove or loosen tight clothing.

6. Remove eyeglasses.

7. Do not try to restrain body movements during the seizure.

8. Maintain body temperature.

9. Transport.

ENRICHMENT: CEREBROVASCULAR ACCIDENT (STROKE)

PATHOPHYSIOLOGY

1. A **cerebrovascular accident (stroke)** is caused by the blockage or rupture of an artery supplying the brain.

  a. Approximately 550,000 Americans suffer a stroke or "brain attack" each year.

  b. Strokes cause brain injury because the blood supply to the brain is reduced or cut off. The brain is deprived of necessary oxygen and nutrients, resulting in injury to the brain cells.

  c. There are two main forms of stroke: ischemic and hemorrhagic.

2. **Ischemic stroke**

  a. Ischemic strokes are caused by a blood clot that decreases blood flow to the brain.

   (1) Eighty percent of all strokes are ischemic strokes.

   (2) Ischemic strokes can be further classified as either thrombotic or emoblic.

    (a) In a thrombotic stroke, a blood clot (thrombus) forms in a blood vessel of, or leading to, the brain.

     (i) The blood vessel may be partially or completely blocked by the blood clot.

     (ii) Symptom onset is gradual.

     (iii) Thrombotic stroke is the most common cause of stroke in persons over 50 years of age.

    (b) In an embolic stroke, a blood clot breaks up and travels through the circulatory system. The blood clot is now called an embolus.

     (i) A cerebral embolus results from blockage of a vessel within the brain by a fragment of a foreign substance originating from outside the central nervous system, usually the heart or a carotid artery.

     (ii) Other types of emboli include tumor fragments, an air embolus (from injury to the chest), or fat embolus (from an injury to a long bone).

     (iii) An embolism can occur in persons of any age, but it is commonly seen in young or middle-aged adults and in persons with preexisting diseases.

     (iv) Onset of symptoms is usually sudden.

3. **Hemorrhagic stroke**

  a. Hemorrhagic strokes (also called cerebral hemorrhage) are caused by bleeding into the brain.

  b. They account for the remaining 20% of all strokes.

    c. There are two forms of hemorrhagic stroke.
      (1) Subarachnoid hemorrhage is caused by a ruptured blood vessel in the subarachnoid space, usually due to an aneurysm (an abnormal bulging of a blood vessel).
      (2) Intracerebral hemorrhage is caused by a ruptured blood vessel within the brain itself (usually due to chronic high blood pressure).

4. Transient ischemic attack (TIA)
    a. A TIA, sometimes called a "mini-stroke," is a temporary interruption of the blood supply to the brain.
    b. The patient's signs and symptoms resemble those of a stroke but are transient, lasting from a few minutes to several hours. Signs and symptoms completely resolve within 24 hours with no permanent damage.
    c. While the patient is exhibiting symptoms, it is not possible to distunguish a TIA from a stroke.
    d. Patients who experience a TIA may be at increased risk for eventual stroke.

RISK FACTORS

Risk factors for stroke include:
1. Hypertension
2. Cigarette smoking
3. Cardiovascular diseases
    a. Atheroclerosis
    b. Myocardial infarction (heart attack)
    c. Heart rhythm disorders (e.g., atrial fibrillation)
4. Diabetes mellitus
5. TIA

SIGNS AND SYMPTOMS

1. The patient's signs and symptoms are related to the artery affected and the portion of the brain deprived of oxygen, glucose, and other nutrients.
2. A stroke occurring on the right side of the brain will produce symptoms on the left side of the body.
3. A stroke occurring on the left side of the brain will affect the right side of the body.
4. Warning signs of a stroke include:
    a. Sudden weakness or numbness of the face, arm, or leg on one side of the body
    b. Sudden dimness or loss of vision, particularly in one eye
    c. Loss of speech or trouble talking or understanding speech
    d. Sudden, severe headache with no known cause
    e. Unexplained dizziness, unsteadiness, or sudden falls, especially with any of the previous symptoms
    f. Confusion, agitation
    g. Seizures
    h. Inappropriate behavior (e.g., excessive laughing or crying)

EMERGENCY MEDICAL CARE

1. Maintain spinal immobilization if trauma is suspected.
2. Establish and maintain an open airway.
    a. Remove dentures, if present.
    b. Insert an oropharyngeal or nasopharyngeal airway as needed.
    c. Have suction equipment readily available and suction as necessary.
3. Administer oxygen.
    a. If the patient's breathing is adequate, apply oxygen by nonrebreather mask at 15 LPM if not already done.
    b. If the patient's breathing is inadequate, provide positive-pressure ventilation with 100% oxygen and assess the adequacy of the ventilations delivered.

4. Position the patient.
   a. If the patient is unconscious and there is no possibility of cervical spine trauma, place the patient in the recovery (lateral recumbent) position to aid drainage of secretions.
   b. If the patient is conscious, there is no possibility of cervical spine trauma, and the patient's blood pressure is normal or elevated, transport the patient in a supine position with the head elevated 15°.
   c. If the patient is immobilized due to suspected trauma and vomits, the patient and backboard should be turned as a unit and the patient's airway cleared with suctioning.
5. Protect paralyzed extremities from injury.
6. Explain procedures to the patient. Although the patient may be unconscious, or be conscious but unable to speak, he or she may still be able to hear and understand.
7. Monitor mental status, blood pressure, pulse, and respirations frequently and document findings.
8. Do not give the patient anything to eat or drink.
9. Attempt to determine from the patient, family members, friends, or bystanders:
   a. If the patient sustained trauma to the head or neck
   b. If the patient is taking any medications, including prescription, over-the-counter (such as aspirin), and illicit drugs
   c. Time of symptom onset
   d. Whether onset of symptoms was gradual or sudden
   e. Whether the patient had any seizure activity
   f. Past pertinent medical history (e.g., previous stroke, TIA, diabetes mellitus, angina, myocardial infarction, heart rhythm disorders, smoking, high blood pressure

REVIEW QUESTIONS

Directions: Each of the numbered items or incomplete statements in this section is followed by answers or by completions of the statement. Select the ONE lettered answer or completion that is BEST in each case.

1. When dealing with patients with an altered mental status, which of the following must be done if trauma is suspected?

   (A) Maintain spinal immobilization
   (B) Insert an oropharyngeal airway
   (C) Immediately place the patient in the recovery position
   (D) Provide oxygen at 4 liters per minute (LPM) by nonrebreather mask

2. Diabetes mellitus is a disease that affects sugar metabolism. Which organ is not functioning properly in diabetes mellitus?

   (A) Liver
   (B) Spleen
   (C) Pancreas
   (D) Gallbladder

3. A lack of glucose can cause irreversible brain damage. Therefore, any diabetic patient with an altered mental status should be considered to have

   (A) hyperglycemia and should be treated with insulin therapy as per medical direction

(B)   hypoglycemia and should be treated with oral glucose therapy as per medical direction

(C)   hypoglycemia and should be treated with insulin therapy as per medical direction

(D)   hyperglycemia and should be treated with oral glucose therapy as per medical direction

4. The onset of hyperglycemia

(A)   is rapid (minutes)
(B)   is slow (hours to days)
(C)   is chronic (weeks to years)
(D)   follows no consistent time frame

5. The most common diabetic emergency is

(A)   bradycardia
(B)   hypoglycemia
(C)   hyperglycemia
(D)   hyperventilation

6. Rapid, deep, sighing respirations with a sweet or fruity breath odor may be associated with

(A)   epilepsy
(B)   hypoglycemia
(C)   hyperglycemia
(D)   non-insulin–dependent diabetes

7. Which of the following patient profiles fits the Type I diabetic?

(A)   Onset of disease after 40 years of age and manages his or her diabetes with a strict diet
(B)   Onset of disease after 40 years of age and manages his or her diabetes with insulin therapy
(C)   Onset of disease during childhood and manages his or her disease with insulin therapy
(D)   Onset of disease during childhood and manages his or her diabetes with diet, exercise, and oral medications

8. Which of the following patient profiles fits the Type II diabetic?

(A)   Onset of disease after 40 years of age and manages his or her diabetes with a strict diet
(B)   Onset of disease after 40 years of age and manages his or her diabetes with insulin therapy
(C)   Onset of disease during childhood and manages his or her disease with insulin therapy
(D)   Onset of disease during childhood and manages his or her diabetes with diet, exercise, and oral medications

9. What role does insulin play in the metabolism of sugar?

(A)   Insulin helps sugar molecules enter the cells of the body
(B)   Insulin is used inside the cells of the body to assist in "burning" the sugar for energy
(C)   Insulin works in the small intestine to "pull" the sugar out of the intestine and into the bloodstream
(D)   Insulin works in the stomach and small intestine to break down food into sugars that can be used by the cells

10. Which of the following regarding glucose (a sugar) and the brain is true?

(A) The brain has a rich store of excess glucose
(B) The brain must be constantly supplied with glucose to function
(C) The brain is the only organ in the body that does not require glucose
(D) In the absence of glucose in the bloodstream, the brain is capable of producing its own glucose

11. Which of the following regarding diabetes and diabetic patients is correct?

(A) Diabetes can generally be reversed
(B) All diabetics must take at least some insulin to manage their blood sugar level
(C) Diabetics always wear medical identification to identify themselves as such
(D) Diabetes may lead to other complications such as blindness, kidney damage, nerve damage, and circulatory disorders

12. Oral glucose is given to patients to increase their blood sugar level. Which of the following lists the indications for oral glucose administration?

(A) Patients with an altered mental status and smell of alcohol
(B) Patients with a history of diabetes who are unconscious
(C) Patients with a history of diabetes who have difficulty breathing
(D) Patients with a history of diabetes who have an altered mental status and are able to swallow

13. Seizures bring about distinctive changes in behavior and body function due to episodes of abnormal, chaotic electrical activity in the brain. The most common cause of seizures in adults is

(A) infection
(B) head trauma
(C) hypoglycemia
(D) failure to take antiseizure medication

14. Seizures in children are not uncommon. In children 6 months to 3 years old, the most common cause of seizures is

(A) fever
(B) hypoxia
(C) electrolyte imbalance
(D) failure to take antiseizure medication

15. Generalized motor seizures may be referred to as full-body seizures, tonic-clonic seizures, or grand mal seizures. Some patients experience a sensation immediately before the seizure. This sensation may be in the form of a strange taste, odor, sound, or visual disturbance. This sensation is referred to as

(A) an aura
(B) the tonic phase
(C) the clonic phase
(D) the postictal phase

16. Following a tonic-clonic seizure, the patient usually experiences a period of gradual awakening. This period is called

(A) the clonic phase
(B) status epilepticus
(C) an absence attack
(D) the postictal phase

17. Not all seizures involve exaggerated full-body convulsions. Some seizures may only involve a specific area of the body, while others may begin in one part of the body and progress to involve the entire body. In yet another type of seizure, the patient appears to be staring blankly. These seizures are called

    (A) status epilepticus
    (B) aura-only seizures
    (C) tonic-clonic seizures
    (D) petit mal seizures or absence attacks

18. Your rescue crew is called to a local manufacturing plant for a 43-year-old female patient feeling dizzy. When you arrive, the supervisor on the scene informs you the patient fell to the floor and "shook violently for about 2 minutes." The patient is lying on the floor with her eyes closed. She appears unconscious. Following the scene size-up, you should immediately

    (A) perform an initial assessment
    (B) perform a rapid physical examination
    (C) begin questioning other workers about the events leading up to the seizure
    (D) look through the patient's purse to gather information about her past medical history

Your rescue crew is called to the home of a 54-year-old female patient. A neighbor called 9-1-1 when he found the patient wandering around the neighborhood confused and disoriented.

Questions 19–21

19. Upon arrival, you find the patient standing on the sidewalk about two blocks from her home. She looks dazed and weak. You find no evidence of trauma. You should

    (A) leave the patient in a standing position
    (B) have the patient lean against a tree if necessary
    (C) instruct the patient to walk home and lie on the couch
    (D) assist the patient to the ground or gurney to assume the recovery position

20. During the focused history and physical examination, you note the patient is confused, complains of weakness and hunger, and has cool, clammy skin. These findings are consistent with

    (A) epilepsy
    (B) hypoglycemia
    (C) hyperglycemia
    (D) diabetic ketoacidosis

21. During questioning, the patient informs you she is an insulin-dependent diabetic. Which of the following statements by the patient would be consistent with your findings?

    (A) "I ate too much food today"
    (B) "I have exercised too much today"
    (C) "I have not taken my insulin in 2 days"
    (D) "I have a history of lower back problems"

Your ambulance crew is called to an adult care facility for a 76-year-old male patient with an altered mental status. The health care worker at the facility states the patient was found supine in bed shortly after she came on duty. She has never seen this patient before and leaves the room to retrieve his medical record.

Questions 22–25

22. Which of the following should be done first?

   (A) Perform an initial assessment
   (B) Insert an oropharyngeal airway (OPA)
   (C) Perform a focused history and physical examination
   (D) Leave with the health care worker to assist in retrieving the medical record

23. Following your initial assessment, your general impression about this patient's condition is poor. You should

   (A) assess baseline vital signs
   (B) begin cardiopulmonary resuscitation (CPR)
   (C) request advanced-life-support (ALS) assistance
   (D) immediately begin looking for the facility health care worker

24. While examining the patient, you find his mouth appears to be dry, and he has a faint odor, somewhat like alcohol, on his breath. His vital signs are as follows: pulse 120 beats per minute (weak and regular), blood pressure 96/64, respirations 24 per minute. His skin is warm, dry, and pink and his pupils are unequal and nonreactive (apparently from past eye surgeries). He complains of nausea. These findings are consistent with

   (A) hypoglycemia
   (B) hyperglycemia
   (C) epileptic seizure
   (D) status epilepticus

25. The patient is wearing medical identification indicating he is a diabetic and has high blood pressure. Appropriate treatment for this patient would include

   (A) placing the patient in the recovery position and administering oxygen
   (B) immobilizing the patient on a long backboard and administering oxygen
   (C) immobilizing the patient on a long backboard and administering oxygen and insulin therapy per medical direction
   (D) placing the patient in the recovery position and administering oxygen and oral glucose per medical direction

Your rescue crew is called to a local grocery store for a 27-year-old male patient experiencing a seizure. You arrive to find the patient on the ground at the checkout counter having an active, full-body seizure.

Questions 26–29

26. Which of the following would be an appropriate action?

   (A) Lie on top of the patient to control the patient
   (B) Leave the patient alone until the seizure stops
   (C) Restrain the patient by strapping him to a long backboard
   (D) Move objects away from the patient to prevent injury

27. During the seizure, the patient repeatedly strikes his head on the tile floor. After the seizure has subsided, which of the following would be indicated?

   (A) Administer oral glucose
   (B) Fully immobilize the patient's spine

(C)   Begin cooling the patient's body with ice water
(D)   Position the patient in the recovery position to help clear the airway

28. For about 2 minutes following the active seizure, this patient is slow to respond and confused. Suddenly, he begins seizing again. This condition is called:

(A)   a febrile seizure
(B)   status epilepticus
(C)   severe head trauma
(D)   Braxton-Hicks contractions

29. Following the second seizure, the patient is slow to respond. His vital signs are: pulse 112 beats per minute, blood pressure 118/90, and respiration 6 breaths per minute with diminished tidal volume. His skin is warm, moist, and pale. The patient responds to painful stimuli by moaning and pushing the stimuli away. To manage this patient's airway and breathing, you should

(A)   Provide continuous suctioning and deliver oxygen by nasal cannula at 4 to 6 liters per minute (LPM)
(B)   Insert an oropharyngeal airway (OPA) and deliver oxygen by nasal cannula at 10 to 15 LPM
(C)   Insert an OPA and deliver oxygen by nonrebreather mask at 15 LPM
(D)   Insert a nasopharyngeal airway (NPA) and assist ventilations at a rate of 12 to 20 per minute with a bag-valve mask connected to oxygen at 15 LPM

ANSWERS AND RATIONALES

1-A. Remember to immobilize the spine as soon as possible for patients with an altered mental status if trauma is suspected. Spinal immobilization should be initiated during the first stage of the initial assessment. Inserting an oropharyngeal airway (OPA) would be indicated if the patient were unconscious without a gag reflex. The recovery position (lateral recumbent) is used for patients with an altered mental status of nontraumatic origin. Finally, the use of a nonrebreather mask for these patients is indicated; however, the delivery device must flow at a higher rate [generally 10–15 liters per minute (LPM)].

2-C. Diabetes is a disease in which the pancreas does not produce sufficient insulin for cellular sugar metabolism. Diabetes may be due to a congenital disorder, poor health, trauma to the pancreas, or pregnancy. A specific region of the pancreas, known as the islets of Langerhans, is responsible for the production of insulin. Insulin, a hormone of the endocrine system, is transported throughout the body by the cardiovascular system.

3-B. Diabetic patients with an altered mental status should be considered hypoglycemic. If you administer oral glucose and the patient is ultimately diagnosed as hyperglycemic rather than hypoglycemic, the extra sugar given will not adversely affect the patient. EMT-Basics are not authorized to assist in the administration of insulin.

4-B. While hyperglycemia may take hours or days to develop, hypoglycemia has a rapid onset. For this reason, it is important to be thorough when obtaining information pertaining to the history surrounding the patient's present illness.

5-B. Because the onset of hypoglycemia is abrupt (within minutes), patients are more likely to be overcome due to this condition rather than hyperglycemia (which may take hours to days to develop).

6-C. Rapid, deep, sighing respirations, often called Kussmaul respirations, are a classic sign of hyperglycemia. To understand why hyperglycemia causes rapid, deep, sighing respirations and a fruity breath odor, it is important to understand the metabolic consequences of hyperglycemia. Without insulin, sugar cannot be used by body cells. The body, seeking energy, begins to burn fat stores. A by-product of fat metabolism is the production of fatty acids. Patients with hyperglycemia (diabetic ketoacidosis) breathe deeply and rapidly in an attempt to "blow off" some of the acids with the expired air. The somewhat fruity breath smell is the result of this acidotic condition.

7-C. Type I diabetes mellitus is sometimes called "juvenile diabetes" because its onset is usually during childhood. The pancreas of the type I diabetic does not produce sufficient insulin. Type 1 diabetes is managed with insulin therapy.

8-A. Type II diabetes generally affects individuals over 40 years of age. It is commonly associated with poor health and excessive weight. Often, type II diabetes can be managed through diet, exercise, and oral medications.

9-A. Insulin aids the transport of sugar from the bloodstream into the cell. Without insulin, sugar cannot enter the cells of the body to be used for energy.

10-B. The brain is incapable of storing glucose. Without a constant supply of glucose, the brain's ability to coordinate and control the body's systems will rapidly decrease.

11-D. While diabetes can generally be controlled, it is not generally reversible. Patients who do not closely manage their disease may suffer a number of serious consequences including blindness, kidney damage, nerve damage, and circulatory disorders. Not all diabetics must take insulin; most type II diabetics manage their disease through diet, exercise, and oral medications that lower blood glucose levels.

12-D. Patients with a history of diabetes and an altered mental status should be considered candidates for oral glucose administration if they are able to swallow. Glucose is not intended for routine administration for all patients with an altered mental status. If a patient complaining of difficulty breathing has a history of diabetes, you should only give oral glucose if the patient's mental status is altered. Diabetic patients should not be routinely treated with oral glucose unless their mental status is altered. Do not use oral glucose if the patient is incapable of maintaining her or his own airway.

13-D. The most common cause of seizures in adults is the failure to take prescribed seizure medications. Other causes include head trauma (recent or past), brain tumor, hypoglycemia, electrolyte imbalances, hypoxia (low oxygen level in the blood), drug or alcohol withdrawal, and high fever. Some seizures occur for unknown reasons.

14-A. The most common cause of seizures in young children is high fever. These seizures, called febrile seizures, occur when children "spike" a temperature. When treating a patient experiencing febrile seizures, it is appropriate to attempt to lower the patient's body temperature. However, attempts to lower the patient's temperature should not cause a shivering response because shivering is the body's defense against cold and results in increased heat production. To gently cool a febrile seizure patient, remove most of the patient's clothing and sponge the patient's skin with tepid water. It is not the temperature of the water that lowers temperature; it is the evaporation of water that draws the heat from the patient.

15-A. While not all seizures are preceded by an aura, the presence of an aura should suggest to the rescuers to position the patient in a safe place for an impending seizure. Have the patient lie down in an area free of obstructions that may cause further harm to the patient. The tonic phase of a tonic-clonic seizure is characterized by the stiffening of the body's muscles. The clonic phase is characterized by alternating jerking and relaxation of the body. Patients in the postictal phase will appear sleepy and confused.

16-D. The postictal period that follows a tonic-clonic seizure may last up to 30 minutes. As the patient slowly regains consciousness, your efforts should be focused on maintaining the patient's airway (secretions may accumulate in the mouth during seizures, so suctioning may be necessary), providing oxygen by nonrebreather mask, and completing a focused history and physical examination.

17-D. Absence attacks are seizures characterized by a blank stare and repetitive behaviors such as lip smacking. These seizures generally affect children four to twelve years of age and last less than 10 seconds.

18-A. Immediately after performing the scene size-up, turn your attention to evaluating and treating the patient's mental status, airway, breathing, circulation, and life-threatening conditions.

19-D. Assist the patient to the ground or stretcher and place her in the recovery position. Do not allow a patient with an altered mental status to remain standing, to walk unassisted, or to sit on an object from which she may fall.

20-B. Early signs and symptoms of hypoglycemia (low blood sugar level) include headache, hunger, nausea, and weakness. As this condition progresses, the patient may experience tremors and tachycardia (increased heart rate) and the skin will be cool and pale. Epilepsy is a disease associated with seizures. The signs and symptoms of hyperglycemia (high blood sugar level) are discussed in the answer to question 6. Diabetic ketoacidosis (DKA) is another term for hyperglycemia.

21-B. This patient has signs and symptoms of hypoglycemia. A patient response consistent with hypoglycemia would be "I have exercised too much today." By overexerting herself, the patient burned off most of her sugar, resulting in hypoglycemia. Overeating and a failure to take prescribed insulin would lead to hyperglycemia. Lower back pain would not be a factor.

22-A. Immediately after performing the scene size-up, begin the initial assessment. The initial assessment should include evaluation of the patient's mental status, airway, breathing, circulation, and the identification and treatment of life-threatening conditions. Assessing the patient's mental status must precede the insertion of an oropharyngeal airway (OPA) since the device should only be used in unconscious patients without a gag reflex. The focused history and physical examination follow the initial assessment. Leaving the patient to retrieve medical records is not an option unless your crew is staffed with adequate personnel to assess and treat the patient and retrieve the records. While past medical records may be important in the long-term care of this patient, stabilizing the patient is the priority.

23-C. In systems where advanced life support (ALS) is available, such assistance should be sought when dealing with critical or unstable patients. Systems that incorporate basic life support (BLS) and ALS are often called tiered systems. If ALS care is unavailable or delayed, immediate transport of critical or unstable patients should be initiated.

24-B. This patient's rapid pulse and respirations; unusual breath odor; warm, dry skin; nausea; and altered mental status are consistent with hyperglycemia. Due to the unusual odor on the breath, hyperglycemic patients may be mistaken for being under the influence of alcohol. Other signs and symptoms of hyperglycemia include loss of appetite, vomiting, and weakness.

25-D. All diabetic patients with an altered mental status should be considered hypoglycemic until proven otherwise. With approval from medical direction, this patient would be a candidate for oral glucose administration. If you have the necessary equipment, you should assess the patient's blood sugar level to further assist your patient assessment. If it is ultimately determined that the patient is hyperglycemic, the additional sugar given will not be detrimental to the patient.

26-D. While a patient is experiencing a seizure, attempt to limit the amount of harm the patient may do to himself. Move objects out of the patient's path and put padding between the patient's head and the ground. Do not attempt to physically restrain the patient; restraining the patient may cause harm to you or the patient.

27-B. This medical condition (tonic-clonic seizure) now has a trauma element to it. Because the patient struck his head, protect his spine from further injury. Patients with an altered mental status should be placed in the recovery position only if trauma is not suspected.

28-B. Status epilepticus is characterized by either continuous seizing or repeat seizures before recovering from the initial seizure. Febrile seizures are due to a rapid rise in body temperature. Severe head trauma is also a cause of seizures. Braxton-Hicks contractions is the medical term for false labor pains associated with pregnancy.

29-D. This patient is breathing well below his normal range (12 to 20 respirations per minute) and, with the patient's diminished tidal volume (the amount of air moved in and out of the lungs with each breath) and pale skin condition, aggressive airway support is needed. A nasopharyngeal airway (NPA) may be tolerated by this patient. An oropharyngeal airway (OPA) would not be tolerated and may induce vomiting. The patient's ventilations should be assisted with a bag-valve mask until his respiratory rate and tidal volume return to a normal range.

BIBLIOGRAPHY

Caroline NL: *Emergency Care in the Streets*, 4th ed. Boston, Little, Brown, 1991.

Crosby LA, Lewallen DG (eds): *Emergency Care and Transportation of the Sick and Injured*, 6th ed. Rosemont, IL, American Academy of Orthopaedic Surgeons, 1995.

Grant HD, Murray RH Jr, Bergeron JD: *Emergency Care*, 7th ed. Englewood Cliffs, NJ, Prentice-Hall, 1995.

Hafen BQ, Karren KJ, Mistovich JJ: *Prehospital Emergency Care*, 5th ed. Upper Saddle River, NJ, Prentice-Hall, 1996.

Henry MC, Stapleton ER, Judd RL: *EMT: Prehospital Care*. Philadelphia, WB Saunders, 1992.

Kitt S, Selfridge-Thomas J, Proehl JA, et al: *Emergency Nursing: A Physiologic and Clinical Perspective*, 2nd ed. Philadelphia, WB Saunders, 1995.

McSwain NE, White RD, Paturas JL, et al (eds): *The Basic EMT: Comprehensive Prehospital Patient Care*. St. Louis, Mosby-Year Book, 1996.

Miller RH, Wilson JK: *Manual of Prehospital Emergency Medicine*. St. Louis, Mosby-Year Book, 1992.

Stoy WA: *Mosby's EMT-Basic Textbook*. St. Louis: Mosby-Year Book, Inc., 1996.

United States Department of Transportation, National Highway Traffic Safety Administration: *Emergency Medical Technician: Basic. National Standard Curriculum*, 1994.

20 ALLERGIC REACTIONS

OBJECTIVES

*20-1 Define the terms antigen, antibody, allergen, allergic reaction, and anaphylaxis.

*20-2 List five possible causes of an allergic reaction.

20-3 Recognize the patient experiencing an allergic reaction.

20-4 Describe the emergency medical care of the patient with an allergic reaction.

20-5 Differentiate between those patients having an allergic reaction and those patients having an allergic reaction who require immediate medical care, including immediate use of an epinephrine auto-injector.

20-6 Establish the relationship between the patient with an allergic reaction and airway management.

20-7 Describe the mechanisms of allergic response and the implications for airway management.

20-8 State the generic and trade names, medication forms, dose, administration, action, and contraindications for the epinephrine auto-injector.

20-9 Evaluate the need for medical direction in the emergency medical care of the patient with an allergic reaction.

ALLERGIC REACTIONS

TERMINOLOGY

1. An **antigen** is any substance that is foreign to an individual and causes antibody production.
2. An **antibody** is a protein substance produced by the body to defend it against bacteria, viruses, or other antigens.

MOTIVATION FOR LEARNING

Allergic reactions can range from a mild rash to life-threatening anaphylaxis. The EMT-Basic must recognize the signs and symptoms of these conditions and provide appropriate patient care. The EMT-Basic's ability to recognize and manage anaphylaxis may be lifesaving.

3. An **allergen** is any substance that causes signs and symptoms of an allergic response.
4. An **allergic reaction** is an abnormal response by the immune system to a foreign substance. Allergic reactions can range from hay fever to anaphylaxis.
5. **Anaphylaxis** is an unusual or exaggerated allergic reaction to a foreign substance. It may be life threatening due to possible airway obstruction and circulatory collapse.

CAUSES OF ALLERGIC REACTIONS

Allergic reactions can be caused by:
1. Insect bites and stings (e.g., bees, wasps, yellow jackets, hornets, fire ants, snakes)
2. Food (e.g., nuts, milk products, strawberries, eggs, shellfish, chocolate, peanuts)
3. Plants (e.g., ragweed)
4. Medications (e.g., aspirin, ibuprofen, insulin, antibiotics such as penicillin)
5. Others (e.g., glue, latex, animal dander)

ASSESSING THE PATIENT WITH AN ALLERGIC REACTION

1. **Scene size-up**
   a. Determine the nature of the illness from the patient, family members, or bystanders and inspection of the scene.
   b. Observe the patient's environment for clues to the cause of the patient's altered mental status. Determine if the patient is wearing medical identification that indicates that the patient has an allergy.
2. **Perform an initial assessment.**
   a. Maintain spinal immobilization if needed.
   b. Assess the patient's mental status and note decreasing mental status.
   c. Assess the patient's airway and note if the following are present:
      (1) Stridor
      (2) Hoarseness
      (3) Difficulty swallowing
      (4) Swelling of the tongue
      (5) Airway obstruction
   d. Assess breathing and note if the following are present:
      (1) Coughing
      (2) Wheezing
      (3) Increased respiratory rate
      (4) Difficulty breathing
      (5) Feeling of chest tightness
   e. Assess circulation and note if the following are present:
      (1) Lightheadedness
      (2) Weakness
      (3) Increased heart rate
      (4) Low blood pressure
      (5) Irregular heart rhythm
   f. Identify any life-threatening conditions and provide care based on those findings.
   g. Establish patient priorities.
      (1) Priority patients include:
         (a) Patients who give a poor general impression
         (b) Patients experiencing difficulty breathing
         (c) Patients with signs and symptoms of shock
         (d) Unresponsive patients with no gag reflex or cough
         (e) Responsive patients who are unable to follow commands
      (2) Advanced-life-support (ALS) assistance should be requested as soon as possible.

(3) If ALS personnel are not available, the patient should be transported promptly to the closest appropriate facility.

3. Perform a focused history and physical examination.

    a. If the patient is unresponsive:

        (1) Perform a rapid physical examination

        (2) Follow with evaluation of baseline vital signs and gathering of the patient's medical history

    b. If the patient is responsive, gather information about the patient's medical history before performing the physical examination.

    c. SAMPLE history

        (1) Signs and symptoms. Signs and symptoms of an allergic reaction (Box 20-1)(Figure 20-1) include (not all are present in every case):

            (a) Skin

                (i) Warm tingling feeling in the face, mouth, chest, feet and hands

                (ii) Itching

                (iii) Hives (urticaria)

                (iv) Red skin (flushing)

                (v) Swelling of the face, neck, hands, feet and/or tongue

            (b) Respiratory system

                (i) Tightness in the throat ("lump in the throat") or chest

                (ii) Coughing

                (iii) Rapid breathing

                (iv) Labored breathing

                (v) Noisy breathing

                (vi) Hoarseness

                (vii) Stridor

                (viii) Difficulty talking

Box 20-1. Signs and Symptoms of an Allergic Reaction

Skin
- Warm tingling feeling in face, mouth, chest, feet and hands
- Itching
- Red skin (flushing)
- Swelling of face, neck, hands, feet and/or tongue
- Hives

Respiratory system
- Tightness in throat/chest
- Coughing
- Rapid breathing
- Labored breathing
- Noisy breathing
- Hoarseness (losing the voice)
- Stridor
- Wheezing (audible without a stethoscope)
- Difficulty talking

Cardiac
- Increased heart rate
- Decreased blood pressure
- Lightheadedness
- Weakness

Gastrointestinal
- Nausea
- Vomiting
- Abdominal cramps
- Diarrhea

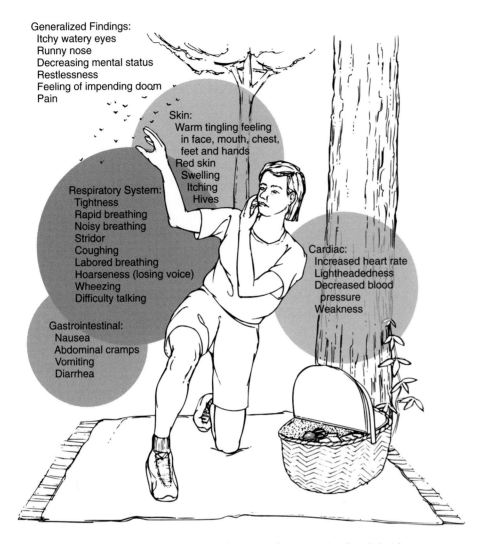

Generalized Findings:
 Itchy watery eyes
 Runny nose
 Decreasing mental status
 Restlessness
 Feeling of impending doom
 Pain

Skin:
 Warm tingling feeling
  in face, mouth, chest,
  feet and hands
 Red skin
 Swelling
 Itching
 Hives

Respiratory System:
 Tightness
 Rapid breathing
 Noisy breathing
 Stridor
 Coughing
 Labored breathing
 Hoarseness (losing voice)
 Wheezing
 Difficulty talking

Cardiac:
 Increased heart rate
 Lightheadedness
 Decreased blood
  pressure
 Weakness

Gastrointestinal:
 Nausea
 Abdominal cramps
 Vomiting
 Diarrhea

Fig. 20-1. Signs and symptoms of a severe allergic reaction (anaphylaxis).

      (ix) Wheezing (audible without a stethoscope)
    (c) Cardiac
      (i) Lightheadedness
      (ii) Weakness
      (iii) Increased heart rate
      (iv) Decreased blood pressure
    (d) Generalized findings
      (i) Restlessness
      (ii) Itchy, watery eyes
      (iii) Headache
      (iv) Fear, panic, or a feeling of impending doom
      (v) Runny nose
      (vi) Decreasing mental status
      (vii) Nausea and vomiting
      (viii) Diarrhea
  (2) **Allergies.** Determine if the patient has any allergies to medications and other substances or materials.
  (3) **Medications.** Determine if the patient is taking any medications (prescription and over the counter).
    (a) If the allergic reaction is severe, does the patient have a physician prescribed epinephrine auto-injector?

(b) Has the patient taken any medications to relieve his or her signs or symptoms before your arrival?

(c) Determine if the patient takes his or her medications regularly and his or her response to them.

(d) Determine if there has been any recent change in medications (additions, deletions, or change in dosages).

(e) Provide all information obtained to the receiving facility.

(3) **Pertinent past medical history.** Ascertain the following information:

(a) Has the patient ever experienced an allergic reaction?

(b) Is so, what was the patient exposed to that caused the reaction?

(c) How serious was the reaction?

(d) Does the patient have a history of heart disease, high blood pressure, or other illness?

(4) **Last oral intake.** Determine the patient's last oral intake.

(5) **Events.** Determine the events leading to the present situation:

(a) What was the patient doing when the symptoms began?

(b) When did the symptoms begin?

(c) How was the patient exposed?

(d) How soon after exposure did the symptoms begin?

d. Assess baseline vital signs.

e. Perform a focused physical examination.

EMERGENCY MEDICAL CARE OF ALLERGIC REACTIONS

1. If the patient has come in contact with a substance that is causing an allergic reaction without signs of respiratory distress or shock (hypoperfusion):

a. Maintain an open airway

b. Administer oxygen

c. Transport and perform ongoing assessments frequently en route

2. If the patient has come in contact with a substance that caused a past allergic reaction and complains of respiratory distress or exhibits signs and symptoms of shock (hypoperfusion):

a. Establish and maintain an open airway. The patient with an allergic reaction may initially present with airway/respiratory compromise, or airway/respiratory compromise may develop as the reaction progresses.

b. Administer oxygen

(1) If the patient's breathing is adequate, apply oxygen by nonrebreather mask at 15 liters per minute (LPM) if not already done

(2) If the patient's breathing is inadequate, provide positive-pressure ventilation with 100% oxygen and assess the adequacy of the ventilations delivered

c. Determine if the patient has prescribed preloaded epinephrine available

(1) If yes:

(a) Facilitate administration of preloaded epinephrine

(b) Contact medical direction

(c) Record and reassess in 2 minutes

(d) Record reassessment findings

(2) If no, transport immediately

d. Perform ongoing assessments every 5 minutes.

e. Transport promptly to the closest appropriate medical facility.

MEDICATIONS: EPINEPHRINE AUTO-INJECTOR

MEDICATION NAME

1. Generic name is epinephrine.

2. Trade name is Adrenalin®.

3. Trade names of the epinephrine auto-injector are Epi-Pen® and Epi-Pen Jr®.

MECHANISM OF ACTION

1. Epinephrine dilates the bronchioles.

2. It constricts blood vessels.
   a. It shrinks swollen tissues.
   b. It increases blood pressure.
      (1) It increases heart rate.
      (2) It increases the force of cardiac contractions.

INDICATIONS

Patients must meet ALL of the following criteria:

1. The patient exhibits signs and symptoms of a severe allergic reaction, including:
   (a) Respiratory distress, and/or
   (b) Signs and symptoms of shock (hypoperfusion)

2. The medication is prescribed for the patient.

3. Medical direction has authorized use for the patient.

CONTRAINDICATIONS

There are no contraindications when used in a life-threatening allergic reaction.

MEDICATION FORM

Epinephrine is a liquid administered by means of an automatic injectable needle and syringe system.

DOSAGE

1. Dosage for an adult is one adult auto-injector [(0.3 milligram (mg)].

2. Dosage for an infant or child is one infant/child auto-injector (0.15 mg).

ADMINISTRATION

1. Confirm that the patient is exhibiting signs or symptoms of a severe allergic reaction (anaphylaxis), including:
   a. Respiratory distress, and/or
   b. Shock

2. Confirm that the patient has a physician prescribed epinephrine auto-injector.

3. Confirm that the epinephrine auto-injector is prescribed for the patient.
   a. Ensure that the medication is not expired.
   b. Ensure that the medication is not discolored (if able to see).

4. Obtain an order from medical direction (either on line or off line) to administer the medication.

5. Obtain the patient's prescribed auto-injector.

6. Ensure:
   a. Right medication, right patient, right route
   b. Prescription is written for the patient experiencing allergic reactions
   c. Medication is not discolored (if able to see)

7. Remove the safety cap from the auto-injector.

8. Place the tip of the auto-injector against the lateral aspect of the patient's thigh, midway between the waist and the knee.

9. Push the injector firmly against the thigh until the injector activates.

10. Hold the injector in place until the medication is injected.

11. Dispose of the injector in a biohazard container.

12. Document the patient's name, drug name and dose administered, time of administration, and the patient's response to the drug. If an on-line order was received by medical direction, document the name of the physician giving the order.

SIDE EFFECTS

Side effects include:
1. Increased heart rate
2. Pale skin
3. Dizziness
4. Chest pain
5. Headache
6. Nausea and vomiting
7. Excitability, anxiousness

REASSESSMENT

1. Reevaluate the patient's airway, breathing, and circulatory status.
2. Observe closely for signs of worsening of the patient's condition:
   a. Decreasing mental status
   b. Increasing breathing difficulty
   c. Decreasing blood pressure
3. If the patient's condition worsens:
   a. Contact medical direction concerning administration of an additional dose of epinephrine (if a second auto-injector is available)
   b. Treat the patient for shock (hypoperfusion)
   c. Be prepared to initiate basic-life-support measures if the patient becomes pulseless [e.g., cardiopulmonary resuscitation (CPR), automated external defibrillator (AED)].
4. If the patient's condition improves, provide supportive care.
   a. Continue oxygen administration.
   b. Treat for shock if necessary.
5. Perform ongoing assessments every 5 minutes.
6. Transport promptly to the closest appropriate medical facility.

REVIEW QUESTIONS

Directions: Each of the numbered items or incomplete statements in this section is followed by answers or by completions of the statement. Select the ONE lettered answer or completion that is BEST in each case.

1. What is the appropriate site for administration of the epinephrine auto-injector?

   (A) The back of the hand
   (B) Sublingual (under the tongue)
   (C) The center of a buttock
   (D) The lateral aspect of the midthigh

2. When administering an epinephrine auto-injector, it is important to

   (A) hold the applicator at a 45° to 60° angle to the skin
   (B) hold the injector in place until all the medication has been delivered
   (C) remove the injector from the skin immediately after the needle springs forward

(D) make the needle spring forward before applying the device to the patient's skin

3. After administering an epinephrine auto-injector, you should

(A) dispose of the device in a biohazard container
(B) throw the device away in the closest available trash can
(C) tape the device to the patient's leg near the site of injection
(D) put the device in the patient's pocket so that it can be inspected by medical direction

4. When used for a severe allergic reaction, the epinephrine auto-injector helps relieve difficulty breathing by

(A) constricting the bronchi and dilating the bronchioles
(B) increasing the percentage of oxygen delivered to the alveoli
(C) constricting the blood vessels and dilating the bronchioles
(D) inhibiting the release of histamines that cause an allergic reaction

5. The generic name for the drug administered by an epinephrine auto-injector is epinephrine. A trade name for this drug is

(A) Albuterol
(B) Bronkosol®
(C) Adrenalin®
(D) Solu-Medrol®

6. Which one of the following is a contraindication for use of the epinephrine auto-injector?

(A) Do not use the epinephrine auto-injector if the patient has an altered mental status
(B) Do not use the epinephrine auto-injector if the patient is experiencing chest pain
(C) Do not use the epinephrine auto-injector in patients older than 50 years of age because it may cause a heart attack
(D) There are no contraindications for use of the epinephrine auto-injector if the patient is having a severe allergic reaction

7. Which of the following regarding the use of an epinephrine auto-injector for an infant or child is correct?

(A) An epinephrine auto-injector should not be used on patients younger than 12 years of age
(B) Epinephrine auto-injectors are prescribed for children, but generally at half the adult dose
(C) Children do not have severe allergic reactions and would derive no benefit from epinephrine auto-injector administration
(D) An epinephrine auto-injector can be used, but administration of the medication is at a different site than for adult patients

8. Common side effects from the administration of an epinephrine auto-injector may include

(A) nausea, vomiting, and unconsciousness
(B) seizures, unequal pupils, and gastric distention
(C) increased heart rate, chest pain, anxiousness, and pale skin
(D) decreased heart rate, decreased tidal volume, and increased blood pressure

9. Anaphylaxis is best described as

   (A) a normal body response to a poison
   (B) a normal body response to an antigen
   (C) an asthma attack induced by bee stings
   (D) an unusual or exaggerated allergic reaction

10. Which of the following may cause an anaphylactic reaction?

    (A) Food
    (B) Medications
    (C) Insect bites or stings
    (D) All of the above may cause an anaphylactic reaction

Directions: Each of the numbered questions or incomplete statements in this section refers to a scenario that precedes them. The numbered questions or incomplete statements are followed by answers or by completions of the statement. Select the answer or completion of the statement that is BEST in each case.

Your rescue crew is called to a local garden store for "a man stung by a bee." Upon arrival, you are met by the patient's wife who informs you that her husband is allergic to bee stings, and he was stung approximately 5 minutes ago. He has no other medical history.

Questions 11–14

11. The patient is found standing near the checkout counter. He appears very nervous and anxious. You should immediately

    (A) insert an oropharyngeal airway (OPA)
    (B) administer an epinephrine auto-injector
    (C) assist the patient to the ground or the stretcher
    (D) begin ventilating with a bag-valve mask and supplemental oxygen

12. You note the patient is in severe distress and his level of consciousness is decreasing. He is confused, dizzy, and weak. An appropriate action would be to

    (A) administer oral glucose
    (B) begin cardiopulmonary resuscitation (CPR)
    (C) call for the hazardous materials team
    (D) call for advanced-life-support (ALS) assistance.

13. As you are assessing this patient's airway and breathing status, you note an audible high-pitched whistling sound coming from the patient during exhalation. This sound is most probably

    (A) grunting
    (B) wheezing
    (C) rales (crackles)
    (D) gastric distention

14. The patient's wife hands you an epinephrine auto-injector and informs you that a doctor prescribed it for her husband. You should immediately

    (A) administer the medication without prior authority

(B)   administer the medication only if the patient stops breathing

(C)   empty the contents of the auto-injector under the patient's tongue

(D)   contact medical direction for authorization to assist with medication administration

*Your ambulance crew is called to the scene of a one-car vehicle collision. You arrive at the
scene to find a pick-up truck has hit a tree. There is only one occupant in the vehicle, and
his seat belt is still on. The damage to the vehicle is minimal. Your scene size-up indicates
that the patient's car is not leaking any fluids, and there do not appear to be any hazards
other than oncoming traffic. Local law enforcement has diverted traffic away from the
scene. You are wearing a reflective traffic vest and appropriate personal protective equipment.*

Questions 15–20

15. Following the scene size-up, you should immediately

(A)   remove the patient from the vehicle

(B)   begin an initial assessment of the patient

(C)   attempt to pry the vehicle away from the tree

(D)   provide supplemental oxygen by nonrebreather at 15 liters per minute
(LPM)

16. The patient is unconscious. His respiratory rate is 30 breaths per minute. His pulse
rate is 96 beats per minute with moderate strength at the radial pulse. Which of
the following signs would lead you to believe that this patient may be experiencing
an anaphylactic reaction?

(A)   The patient's abdomen is rigid to palpation

(B)   The patient's face is swollen and blotchy red

(C)   The patient's blood pressure is 150/84 and rising

(D)   The patient's pupils are unequal and do not react to light

17. During the detailed physical examination, you find the patient has a stinger imbedded in his neck. The area around the sting is swollen and white surrounded by a
red, rash-like appearance. While the police are attempting to gather information
about the patient, they find a note attached to several epinephrine auto-injectors
that states that the patient is allergic to bee stings. Use of an epinephrine auto-injector

(A)   is contraindicated because the patient is unconscious

(B)   is contraindicated because the patient has suffered trauma

(C)   is appropriate if authorization is given by medical direction

(D)   is appropriate regardless of authorization from medical direction because
this patient is near death

18. Assuming you administer the epinephrine auto-injector, which of the following is
true regarding the administration of subsequent (additional) epinephrine auto-injectors?

(A)   Only one may be given

(B)   Subsequent administrations may be given if approved by medical direction

(C)   Subsequent administrations may be given only if the patient stops breathing

(D)   A second may be given without consulting medical direction, if medical direction authorized the first dose

19. If the patient's breathing is adequate, which of the following regarding airway and
breathing support for this patient is correct?

(A)   The patient's airway should be maintained with an oropharyngeal airway (OPA) and oxygen should be given by nonrebreather mask at 15 liters per minute (LPM)

(B)   The patient's airway should be maintained with the head-tilt, chin-lift maneuver. Oxygen therapy should be delivered by nonrebreather mask at 15 LPM.

(C)   The patient's airway should be maintained with the head-tilt, chin-lift maneuver and an OPA. Oxygen should be delivered by nasal cannula at 4 to 6 LPM

(D)   The patient's airway should be maintained with a jaw thrust and an OPA. Oxygen should be administered by nonrebreather mask at 15 LPM

20. While en route to the hospital, you reassess the patient and find that he is breathing at a rate of 40 breaths per minute with a greatly decreased tidal volume. He is also becoming increasingly cyanotic, and his pulse is now 150 beats per minute at the brachial artery (you cannot feel the radial pulse). Which of the following would be an appropriate intervention?

(A)   Begin cardiopulmonary resuscitation (CPR)

(B)   Increase the oxygen flow to 20 liters per minute (LPM) by nonrebreather mask

(C)   Begin assisting the patient's ventilations with a bag-valve mask and supplemental oxygen at a rate of one breath every 3 seconds

(D)   Begin assisting the patient's ventilations with a bag-valve mask and supplemental oxygen at a rate of one breath every 5 seconds

ANSWERS AND RATIONALES

1-D.   Epinephrine is injected into the large muscle of the thigh. The correct placement of the auto-injector is the lateral (outside) aspect of the thigh, midway between the waist and the knee.

2-B.   When the auto-injector is pressed flush against the skin, the spring-loaded needle is released to pierce the skin. The medication is then injected. You must keep the device flush with the skin until all of the medication is delivered. If the needle is not flush (at a 90° angle) with the skin, the medication may not be delivered deep enough for proper absorption. Do not release the spring-loaded needle before applying the device to the skin. These devices are designed for use by nonmedical personnel and should be complete with instructions. When in doubt, read the instructions and consult medical direction.

3-A.   The needle has pierced the patient's skin and come in contact with the patient's body fluids. Failure to treat the device as a biohazard could lead to an exposure hazard. If medical direction wants the device retained for inspection, secure the device in an approved container (e.g., sharps container).

4-C.   By constricting the blood vessels, epinephrine increases blood pressure and shrinks swollen tissues, leading to improved perfusion. By dilating the bronchioles, epinephrine allows air to enter and exit the lungs (alveoli) more easily. Tidal volume is thus increased and oxygenation is improved. The percent of oxygen delivered can be accomplished by supplementing the patient's oxygen [e.g., by nonrebreather mask at 15 liters per minute (LPM)]. Epinephrine increases the amount of oxygen delivered to the alveoli but does not change the *percentage* of oxygen in inspired air. A medication does exist that inhibits the release of histamines. This medication (diphenhydramine or Benadryl®) is not authorized for administration by EMT-Basics. Advanced-life-support (ALS) personnel may be authorized to administer this medication.

5-C. Adrenalin® is a trade name for epinephrine. Albuterol (generic name) and Bronkosol® (trade name) are metered dose bronchodilators. Solu-Medrol® is a trade name for a steroid medication that may be given to the patient by advanced life support (ALS) or hospital personnel. Solu-Medrol® helps to decrease inflammation and can be useful in treating patients with allergic reactions.

6-D. If the patient is having a severe allergic reaction, there is no contraindication for use of the epinephrine auto-injector. Although no contraindications exist, the medical direction physician may instruct you NOT to use this device. The lack of a contraindication means that there is no preexisting medical indication that precludes the use of an epinephrine auto-injector. Since epinephrine increases the work of the heart, it should be used with caution in patients with certain preexisting medical conditions.

7-B. Children are susceptible to anaphylactic reactions just like adults. The dose of the injector is generally half the adult dose. You should not be concerned with changing the dose of an injector to match the patient's size. If the injector is prescribed for the specific patient, the dose should be considered correct.

8-C. Side effects of epinephrine administration include an increased heart rate which may lead to chest pain, dizziness, pale skin, headache, nausea, vomiting, and anxiousness. Any other signs or symptoms should be assessed and treated as individual findings. This information should be communicated to medical direction and the receiving facility.

9-D. Anaphylaxis is not a "normal" response just as a heart attack is not a "normal" event. Anaphylaxis is an allergic reaction out of control. While some signs and symptoms of an anaphylactic reaction are similar to the signs and symptoms of asthma, the two processes are not identical.

10-D. Any substance that causes an abnormal response by the immune system can cause an anaphylactic reaction. These substances include insect bites and stings, food (e.g., shellfish, peanuts, milk, strawberries), plants, and medications (most commonly penicillin). Other substances such as glue, latex, and animal dander may also cause anaphylaxis.

11-C. The patient should not be left standing since his altered mental status may lead to a ground-level fall. Insertion of an oropharyngeal airway (OPA) is only appropriate for unconscious patients with no gag reflex. Administration of an epinephrine auto-injector may be considered, but strict criteria must be met before its administration. Ventilating the patient may also be considered if the patient's breathing is not adequate; however, you must first assist the patient to a safe position and carefully evaluate his airway and breathing status.

12-D. These findings should assist you in forming a "poor" impression about this patient's condition. If available, advanced-life-support (ALS) personnel should be called for assistance with all unstable patients. If ALS personnel are not available (or greatly delayed), immediate and rapid transport should be considered. Oral glucose would be administered only if the patient were a known diabetic, exhibited the signs and symptoms of a diabetic emergency, and medical direction authorized its use. A hazardous materials team would be called (if available) for incidents involving dangerous chemicals. While a beesting is dangerous for this patient, it possesses no threat to the public at large.

13-B. Wheezes are the whistling sounds created as air exits the alveoli (air sacs) through narrowed bronchioles. This abnormal lung sound is common in asthmatics and patients experiencing anaphylaxis. Grunting is an abnormal sound created during exhalation and is generally associated with infants. Grunting is a sound made by the patient during exhalation to help keep the alveoli from collapsing. Rales (crackles) are the fine bubbling noises of air as it passes through fluid. Rales sound somewhat like the sound created when Velcro is released. Gastric distention is the accumulation of air in the stomach. Gastric distention may occur during assisted ventilations if ventilations are delivered too quickly and forcefully.

14-D. The sooner you get the medication "on board" (in the patient), the sooner you will begin to reverse the process that is compromising this patient's airway, breathing, and circulatory status. However, you must follow proper protocol, which includes gaining authorization from medical direction. Authorization may be on line or off line. If medical direction has authorized off-line administration of epinephrine auto-injectors, you may immediately give the medication if the patient is symptomatic for a severe allergic reaction and has his auto-injector with him. If you do not have off-line authority (prior authority), you must contact medical direction before administering this medication.

15-B. The scene size-up indicates the patient is in no danger in his current position; therefore, you should turn your attention to an initial assessment of the patient's mental status, airway, breathing, circulation, and life-threatening conditions. Freeing the vehicle from the tree does not appear to be at all necessary and may only result in disturbing the patient's spinal alignment. Any such actions should only be carried out by properly trained personnel when access to the patient is denied due to obstruction. The method of maintaining the patient's airway and delivering oxygen should be decided upon after evaluating the mechanism of injury, the patient's presentation, status, and past medical history.

16-B. Red, swollen skin with hives suggests an allergic reaction. A rigid abdomen should lead you to suspect that the patient has damaged an abdominal organ and may be bleeding internally. Generally, in anaphylactic reactions, the patient's blood pressure will decrease. An increasing blood pressure in a trauma patient may indicate closed head trauma. Deviation from normal pupil response may also suggest closed head injury.

17-C. As with all medications that EMT-Basics are trained to assist in administering, specific criteria must be met before administration of the drug. First, the patient must be exhibiting the signs and symptoms associated with the indication of giving the medication. Second, the patient must have been prescribed an epinephrine auto-injector and must have the epinephrine auto-injector with him or her. Finally, the EMT-Basic must have specific authorization from medical direction to administer this medication (either on-line or off-line medical direction).

18-B. In severe cases, several epinephrine auto-injectors may be used. If you know that the patient has several epinephrine auto-injectors, when you consult with medical direction for permission to use the device, you may ask about the possibility and time frame for repeat doses. Asking up front may save you time if the patient fails to improve after the first dose and subsequent doses are needed.

19-D. You are dealing with a patient with two main problems. First, he has been involved in a vehicle collision, and second, he is possibly having a severe allergic reaction. Both problems must be addressed. Opening and maintaining the patient's airway must be accomplished with the modified jaw thrust and the patient's spine must be fully immobilized. If the patient has no gag reflex, either an oropharyngeal (OPA) or nasopharyngeal airway (NPA) may be used. However, if the patient is semiconscious, an NPA may be tolerated whereas an OPA will not be tolerated. High-flow oxygen should be administered by nonrebreather mask because the patient's breathing is adequate but his condition is unstable.

20-D. The patient's breathing status is now inadequate as evidenced by the increased respiratory rate (twice the normal adult rate of 12 to 20 breaths per minute), increased cyanosis, and decreased peripheral perfusion (lack of a radial pulse). Assisting ventilations in an apneic adult is accomplished at a rate of one breath every 5 seconds (12 breaths per minute) with high-flow oxygen connected to the bag-valve mask. Cardiopulmonary resuscitation (CPR) should be initiated only if the patient were apneic and had no palpable pulse (radial, brachial, or carotid). This patient has a brachial (upper arm) pulse.

BIBLIOGRAPHY

Crosby LA, Lewallen DG (eds): *Emergency Care and Transportation of the Sick and Injured,* 6th ed. Rosemont, IL, American Academy of Orthopaedic Surgeons, 1995.

Grant HD, Murray RH Jr, Bergeron JD: *Emergency Care,* 7th ed. Englewood Cliffs, NJ, Prentice-Hall, 1995.

Hafen BQ, Karren KJ, Mistovich JJ: *Prehospital Emergency Care,* 5th ed. Upper Saddle River, NJ, Prentice-Hall, 1996.

Henry MC, Stapleton ER, Judd RL: *EMT: Prehospital Care.* Philadelphia, WB Saunders, 1992.

Kitt S, Selfridge-Thomas J, Proehl JA, et al: *Emergency Nursing: A Physiologic and Clinical Perspective,* 2nd ed. Philadelphia, WB Saunders, 1995.

McSwain NE, White RD, Paturas JL, et al (eds): *The Basic EMT: Comprehensive Prehospital Patient Care.* St. Louis, Mosby-Year Book, 1996.

Stoy WA. *Mosby's EMT-Basic Textbook.* St. Louis, Mosby-Year Book, 1996.

United States Department of Transportation, National Highway Traffic Safety Administration: *Emergency Medical Technician: Basic. National Standard Curriculum,* 1994.

21 POISONING AND SUBSTANCE ABUSE

POISONING

TERMINOLOGY

1. An **antidote** is a substance that neutralizes a poison.
2. A **poison** is any substance taken into the body that interferes with normal body function.
3. **Poisoning** is exposure to a substance that is harmful in any dosage.
4. A **toxin** is a poisonous substance of plant or animal origin.

MOTIVATION FOR LEARNING

Poisoning and substance abuse calls are common emergencies. It is essential to understand the routes by which poisons may enter the body, the signs and symptoms associated with poisoning and overdose, and the emergency medical care for these patients.

ROUTES OF ENTRY OF POISONS INTO THE BODY (*FIGURE 21-1*)

1. **Ingestion.** Poisons that can be ingested include:
   a. Medications
   b. Foods
   c. Poisonous plants
   d. Pesticides
   e. Cosmetics/toiletries
   f. Cleaning products
   g. Petroleum-based products (e.g., gasoline, lighter fluid, furniture polish)
2. **Inhalation.** Poisons that can be inhaled include:
   a. Carbon monoxide
   b. Chlorine
   c. Ammonia
   d. Propane
   e. Cyanide
   f. Freon
   g. Tear gas
3. **Injection.** Poisons that can be injected include:
   a. Bee, wasp, and ant venom
   b. Spider, tick, and scorpion venom
   c. Snake venom
   d. Drugs
4. **Absorption.** Poisons that can be absorbed through the skin or mucous membranes include:
   a. Toxins from plants, such as:
      (1) Poison ivy
      (2) Poison oak
      (3) Poison sumac
   b. Pesticides
   c. Fertilizers
   d. Cocaine

GENERAL CARE FOR POISONING

SCENE SIZE-UP

1. Observe the patient's environment for clues as to the source of the poisoning, such as:
   a. Unusual odors
   b. Smoke or flames
   c. Open medicine cabinet
   d. Open or overturned containers
   e. Syringes or other drug paraphernalia
2. Use appropriate protection or have trained rescuers remove the patient from the poisonous environment.

INITIAL ASSESSMENT

1. Maintain spinal immobilization if needed.
2. Assess the patient's mental status.
3. Assess the patient's airway.
4. Assess breathing.
5. Assess circulation.
6. Identify any life-threatening conditions and provide care based on these findings.
7. Establish patient priorities.

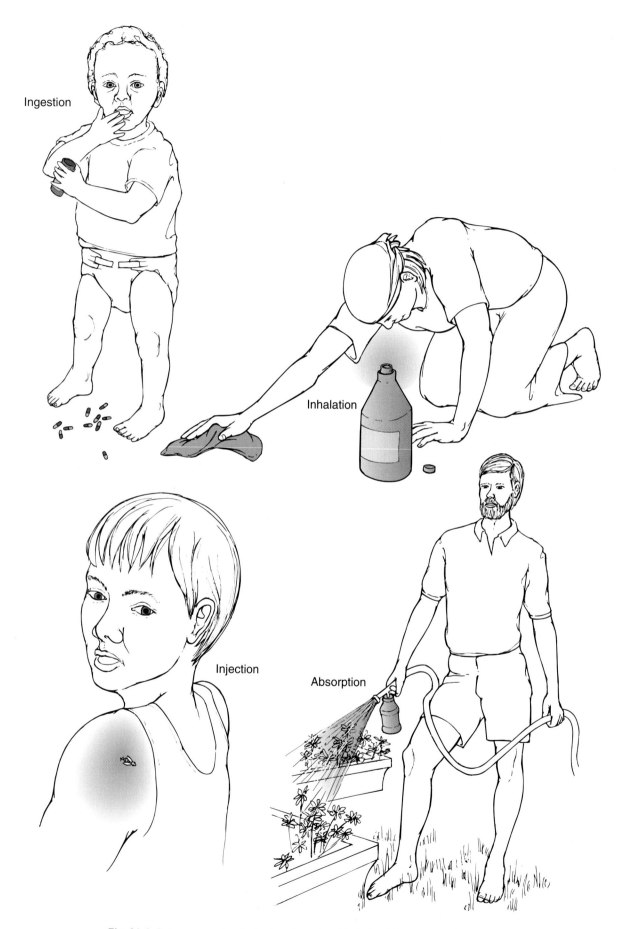

Fig. 21-1. Poisons can enter the body by ingestion, inhalation, injection, and absorption.

a. Priority patients include the following:
   (1) Patients who give a poor general impression
   (2) Patients experiencing difficulty breathing
   (3) Patients with signs and symptoms of shock
   (4) Unresponsive patients with no gag reflex or cough
   (5) Responsive patients who are unable to follow commands
b. Advanced-life-support (ALS) assistance should be requested as soon as possible.
c. If ALS personnel are not available, transport the patient promptly to the closest appropriate facility.

FOCUSED HISTORY AND PHYSICAL EXAMINATION

1. If the patient is unresponsive:
   a. Perform a rapid physical examination
   b. Follow with evaluation of baseline vital signs and gathering of the patient's medical history
2. If the patient is responsive, gather information about the patient's medical history before performing the physical examination.
3. **SAMPLE history**
   a. **Signs and symptoms.** Common signs and symptoms of poisoning include:
      (1) Altered mental status
      (2) Difficulty breathing
      (3) Headache
      (4) Nausea
      (5) Vomiting
      (6) Diarrhea
      (7) Chest or abdominal pain
      (8) Sweating
      (9) Seizures
      (10) Burns around the mouth
      (11) Burns on the skin
   b. **Allergies.** Determine if the patient has any allergies to medications and other substances or materials.
   c. **Medications.** Determine if the patient is taking any medications (prescription and over the counter).
      (1) Determine if the patient takes his or her medications regularly and his or her response to them.
      (2) Determine if there has been any recent change in medications (additions, deletions, or change in dosages).
      (3) Provide all information obtained to the receiving facility.
   d. **Pertinent past medical history.** Ascertain whether the patient has any of the following conditions:
      (1) Chronic obstructive pulmonary disease
      (2) Heart disease
      (3) High blood pressure
      (4) Kidney disease
      (5) Liver disease
      (6) Seizures
      (7) Psychiatric problems (important in determining the possibility of a suicide attempt)
   e. **Last oral intake.** Determine the patient's last oral intake.
   f. **Events.** Determine the events leading to the present situation.
      (1) What poison was involved?
      (2) How much was taken?
      (3) When was it taken (or when did the exposure occur)?
         (a) If the patient is unresponsive, obtaining the time of ingestion or exposure may be impossible unless someone witnessed the event.

(b) In such situations, an estimate of the time of ingestion or exposure can often be made by determining when the patient was last seen.

(4) Over what period was the substance ingested?

(5) Why was it taken? (Attempt to determine whether the ingestion was accidental or intentional.)

(6) What else was taken? (Many intentional ingestions involve more than one substance.)

(7) Was any seizure activity observed?

(8) What has been done to treat the poisoning?

(9) How much does the patient weigh? (In cases of ingested poisons, this information is necessary to determine the dose of activated charcoal.)

4. Assess baseline vital signs.

5. Perform a focused physical examination.

EMERGENCY MEDICAL CARE

1. Have trained rescuers remove the patient from the source of the poison.

2. Follow proper decontamination procedures, if necessary, and prepare the ambulance to receive the patient.

3. Establish and maintain an open airway.

a. Remove pills, tablets, or fragments with gloves from the patient's mouth, as needed, without injuring oneself.

b. Be alert for vomiting and have suction ready.

4. Administer oxygen.

a. If the patient's breathing is adequate, apply oxygen by nonrebreather mask at 15 liters per minute (LPM) if not already done.

b. If the patient's breathing is inadequate, provide positive-pressure ventilation with 100% oxygen and assess the adequacy of the ventilations delivered.

5. If the patient has ingested a poison (and is awake), consult medical direction regarding the administration of activated charcoal.

6. Bring all containers, bottles, labels, etc. of suspected poisons to receiving facility.

7. Anticipate complications, including:

a. Seizures

b. Vomiting

c. Shock

d. Agitation

e. Irregular heart rhythm

8. Transport promptly.

a. If the patient is stable, perform ongoing assessments every 15 minutes.

b. If the patient is unstable, perform ongoing assessments every 5 minutes.

INGESTED POISONS

SIGNS AND SYMPTOMS

Signs and symptoms of ingested poisoning include:

1. History of ingestion

2. Nausea

3. Vomiting

4. Diarrhea

5. Altered mental status

6. Abdominal pain

7. Chemical burns around the mouth

8. Different breath odors

EMERGENCY MEDICAL CARE

1. Using gloves, remove pills, tablets, or fragments from the patient's mouth, as needed, without injuring oneself.
2. Establish and maintain an open airway.
3. Administer oxygen.
    a. If the patient's breathing is adequate, apply oxygen by nonrebreather mask at 15 LPM if not already done.
    b. If the patient's breathing is inadequate, provide positive-pressure ventilation with 100% oxygen and assess the adequacy of the ventilations delivered.
4. Be alert for vomiting; have suction ready.
5. Consult medical direction regarding activated charcoal administration.
6. Bring all containers, bottles, labels, etc. of suspected poisons to receiving facility.

INHALED POISONS

SIGNS AND SYMPTOMS

Signs and symptoms of inhaled poisoning include:
1. History of inhalation of toxic substance
2. Difficulty breathing
3. Chest pain
4. Cough
5. Hoarseness
6. Dizziness
7. Headache
8. Confusion
9. Seizures
10. Altered mental status

EMERGENCY MEDICAL CARE

1. Have trained rescuers remove the patient from the poisonous environment.
2. Remove the patient's contaminated clothing.
2. Establish and maintain an open airway.
3. Administer oxygen.
    a. If the patient's breathing is adequate, apply oxygen by nonrebreather mask at 15 LPM if not already done.
    b. If the patient's breathing is inadequate, provide positive-pressure ventilation with 100% oxygen and assess the adequacy of the ventilations delivered.
5. Bring all containers, bottles, labels, etc. of suspected poisons to receiving facility.

INJECTED POISONS

SIGNS AND SYMPTOMS

Signs and symptoms of injected poisoning include:
1. Weakness
2. Dizziness
3. Chills
4. Fever
5. Nausea
6. Vomiting

EMERGENCY MEDICAL CARE

1. Remove the patient (and rescuers) from the environment if repeated stings or bites are likely.
2. Establish and maintain an open airway.
3. Be alert for vomiting; have suction ready.
4. Administer oxygen.
   a. If the patient's breathing is adequate, apply oxygen by nonrebreather mask at 15 LPM if not already done.
   b. If the patient's breathing is inadequate, provide positive-pressure ventilation with 100% oxygen and assess the adequacy of the ventilations delivered.
5. Monitor the patient closely for signs and symptoms of anaphylaxis.
6. Bring all containers, bottles, labels, etc. of suspected poisons to receiving facility.

ABSORBED POISONS

SIGNS AND SYMPTOMS

Signs and symptoms of absorbed poisoning include:
1. History of exposure
2. Liquid or powder on the patient's skin
3. Burns
4. Itching
5. Irritation
6. Redness

EMERGENCY MEDICAL CARE

1. Remove the patient from the source of the poison.
2. While wearing chemical protective clothing and gloves, remove the patient's contaminated clothing and jewelry.
3. Establish and maintain an open airway.
4. Administer oxygen.
   a. If the patient's breathing is adequate, apply oxygen by nonrebreather mask at 15 LPM if not already done.
   b. If the patient's breathing is inadequate, provide positive-pressure ventilation with 100% oxygen and assess the adequacy of the ventilations delivered.
5. **Skin**
   a. If the poison is in powder form, brush powder off patient, then continue as for other absorbed poisons.
   b. If the poison is in liquid form, irrigate the skin with clean water for at least 20 minutes (and continue en route to facility if possible). Pay particular attention to skin creases and fingernails.
6. **Eye.** Irrigate with clean water away from the affected eye for at least 20 minutes and continue en route to facility if possible.

MEDICATIONS—ACTIVATED CHARCOAL

MEDICATION NAMES

1. The generic name is activated charcoal.
2. Trade names are SuperChar®, InstaChar®, Actidose®, and LiquiChar®.

MECHANISM OF ACTION

1. Activated charcoal binds (adsorbs) certain poisons from the gastrointestinal tract and prevents them from being absorbed into the body.
2. Not all brands of activated charcoal are the same.
   a. Some brands bind more poison than others.
   b. Consult medical direction about the brand to use .

INDICATIONS

Activated charcoal is indicated in patients who have ingested poison.

CONTRAINDICATIONS

1. Patient has an altered mental status.
2. Patient has ingested acids or alkalis.
   a. Examples of acids include rust removers, phenol, and battery acid.
   b. Examples of alkalis include ammonia, household bleach, and drain cleaner.
3. Patient is unable to swallow.
4. Medical direction does not give authorization.

MEDICATION FORM

1. Activated charcoal is premixed in water, frequently available in a plastic bottle containing 12.5 grams (g) of activated charcoal.
2. The powder form should be avoided in the field.

DOSAGE

1. For adults and children, the dose is 1 g of activated charcoal per kilogram (kg) of body weight.
2. The usual adult dose is 25–50 g.
3. Usual infant/child dose is 12.5–25.0 grams.

ADMINISTRATION

1. Confirm that the patient has ingested a poison.
2. Obtain an order from medical direction (either on line or off line) to administer the medication.
3. Shake the charcoal container thoroughly.
4. Because activated charcoal looks like mud, the patient may need to be persuaded to drink it. A covered opaque container and a straw may improve patient compliance since the patient cannot see the medication this way.
5. If the patient takes a long time to drink the medication, the charcoal will settle and will need to be shaken or stirred again.
6. Document the patient's name, drug name and dose administered, time of administration, and the patient's response to the drug. If an on-line order was received by medical direction, document the name of the physician giving the order.

SIDE EFFECTS

Side effects include:
1. Black stools
2. Constipation
3. Abdominal cramping
4. Vomiting in some patients (particularly those who have ingested poisons that cause nausea); if the patient vomits, the dose should be repeated once.

SPECIAL CONSIDERATIONS

Do not administer activated charcoal with ice cream, sherbet, or milk as these products decrease charcoal's effectiveness.

REASSESSMENT

1. Reevaluate the patient's airway, breathing, and circulatory status.
2. The EMT-Basic should be prepared for the patient to vomit or further deteriorate.
3. Observe closely for signs of worsening of the patient's condition:
   a. Decreasing mental status
   b. Increasing breathing difficulty
   c. Decreasing blood pressure
4. If the patient's condition improves, provide supportive care.
5. Perform ongoing assessments every 5 minutes.
6. Transport promptly to the closest appropriate medical facility.

SUBSTANCE ABUSE

TERMINOLOGY

1. **Addiction** is a psychological and physical dependence on a substance that has gone beyond voluntary control.
2. An **overdose** is exposure to excessive amounts of a substance.
3. **Substance abuse** is the deliberate, persistent, and excessive self-administration of a substance in a way that is not medically or socially approved.
4. **Substance misuse** is the self-administration of a substance for unintended purposes, or for appropriate purposes but in improper amounts or doses.
5. **Tolerance** occurs when an individual requires progressively larger doses of a drug to achieve the desired effect.
6. **Withdrawal** is the condition produced when an individual stops using or abusing a drug to which he or she is physically or psychologically addicted.

COMMONLY MISUSED AND ABUSED SUBSTANCES

1. Commonly misused and abused substances include stimulants, depressants, hallucinogens, and designer drugs.
2. **Stimulants**
   a. Stimulants increase mental and physical activity.
   b. They include amphetamines and cocaine.
      (1) Stimulants produce feelings of alertness and well-being, loss of appetite, increased heart rate, sweating, tremors, increased blood pressure, and hallucinations.
      (2) They may produce violent behavior.
   c. Common legal stimulants include caffeine and nicotine.
   d. When the effects of the drug wear off, the user is often exhausted and sleeps.
   e. On awakening, the user may be depressed, suicidal, or incoherent.
2. **Depressants**
   a. **Barbiturates**
      (1) Barbiturates include Nembutal®, Seconal®, and phenobarbital.
      (2) These drugs relieve anxiety, promote sleep, and relax muscles.
      (3) Overdose can produce respiratory depressions, coma, and death.
      (4) Withdrawal can cause anxiety, tremors, nausea, fever, convulsions, and death.
   b. **Narcotics (opiates)**
      (1) Narcotics include morphine, codeine, and Demerol®.
      (2) These drugs are used to relieve pain and anxiety.

(3) Overdose can result in respiratory depression, shock, and death.

(4) Withdrawal can cause abdominal cramps, increased heart rate, increased body temperature, tremors, loss of appetite, diarrhea, and intense agitation.

c. Benzodiazepines

(1) Benzodiazepines include Valium®, Librium®, Klonopin®, and Ativan®.

(2) These drugs are used to control anxiety and stress and to promote sleep.

(3) Overdose can result in respiratory depression and death.

(4) Withdrawal can cause anxiety, tremors, nausea, fever, convulsions, and death.

d. Alcohol

(1) Alcohol slows mental and physical activity.

(2) It affects judgement, vision, reaction time, and coordination.

(3) In large quantities, it can cause death.

(4) When approaching the patient who has ingested alcohol, observe the scene for evidence of trauma.

(5) Signs and symptoms of alcohol misuse or abuse can mimic those of other medical conditions (e.g., diabetes, head injury, epilepsy).

    (a) Do not assume the patient is intoxicated.

    (b) Carefully evaluate the patient for the presence of other injuries or illnesses.

(6) Disulfiram (Antabuse®) is a medication prescribed for alcoholics to discourage them from drinking.

    (a) When combined with alcohol, Antabuse® produces unpleasant, and sometimes serious, reactions lasting 30 minutes to 8 hours (usually 3–4 hours). Reactions include:

        (i) Nausea, vomiting, abdominal discomfort

        (ii) Chest discomfort, palpitations

        (iii) Headache, dizziness, blurred vision

    (b) Although rare, seizures, congestive heart failure, heart attack, and cardiac arrest have occurred.

(7) Alcohol withdrawal syndrome occurs 6–48 hours after a decline in or ceasing alcohol consumption.

(8) Signs and symptoms of alcohol withdrawal include tremors, anxiety, gastrointestinal distress, hallucinations, disorientation, and seizures. In some individuals, alcohol withdrawal may cause death.

3. Hallucinogens

a. Hallucinogens include LSD, PCP (angel dust), and mescaline.

b. These drugs produce changes in mood, thought, emotion, and self-awareness.

c. They can also cause hallucinations, profound depression, and irrational and disruptive behavior that can make the user dangerous to himself or herself and others.

4. Designer drugs

a. Designer drugs are variations of federally controlled substances that have high abuse potential (e.g., narcotics, amphetamines).

b. These drugs are produced by persons ranging from amateurs to highly skilled chemists and sold on the street.

c. Designer drugs are often much stronger than the original form of the drug, thus overdose occurs frequently.

d. Fentanyl (Sublimaze®), a surgical anesthetic, is one drug used to make designer narcotics.

(1) Street names include "china white," "synthetic heroin," "Persian white," and "Mexican brown."

(2) Signs and symptoms of misuse or abuse include respiratory depression and mental status depression.

e. Designer amphetamines include "ecstasy," also called "Adam," "XTC," and "essence." Signs and symptoms of misuse or abuse include increased heart rate, sweating, agitation, erratic mood swings, and increased blood pressure.

SIGNS AND SYMPTOMS OF SUBSTANCE MISUSE OR ABUSE

1. Signs and symptoms of stimulant misuse or abuse include:
   a. Fever
   b. Headache
   c. Dizziness
   d. Increased heart rate
   e. Increased respiratory rate
   f. Increased blood pressure
   g. Moist or flushed skin
   h. Sweating
   i. Chest pain
   j. Restlessness
   k. Irritability
   l. Combativeness
   m. Nausea/vomiting
2. Signs and symptoms of depressant misuse and abuse include:
   a. Drowsiness
   b. Slurred speech
   c. Decreased heart rate
   d. Decreased respiratory rate
   e. Poor coordination
   f. Confusion
3. Signs and symptoms of hallucinogen misuse and abuse include:
   a. Flushed face
   a. Sudden mood changes
   b. Fear
   c. Anxiety
4. Signs and symptoms of designer drug misuse and abuse are unpredictable signs and depend on the drug that is being chemically altered.

EMERGENCY MEDICAL CARE FOR SUBSTANCE MISUSE OR ABUSE

1. Ensure that the scene is safe before entering and be prepared for unpredictable patient behavior.
2. Establish and maintain an open airway.
   a. Wear gloves to remove pills, tablets or fragments from the patient's mouth, as needed, without injuring oneself.
   b. Be alert for vomiting; have suction ready.
3. Administer oxygen.
   a. If the patient's breathing is adequate, apply oxygen by nonrebreather mask at 15 LPM if not already done.
   b. If the patient's breathing is inadequate, provide positive-pressure ventilation with 100% oxygen and assess the adequacy of the ventilations delivered.
4. If trauma is not suspected, place the patient in a recovery (lateral recumbent) position.
5. Obtain a SAMPLE history.
6. If the patient has ingested a drug (and is awake), consult medical direction regarding the administration of activated charcoal.
7. Bring all containers, bottles, labels, etc. to the receiving facility.
8. Transport promptly.
   a. If the patient is stable, perform ongoing assessments every 15 minutes.
   b. If the patient is unstable, perform ongoing assessments every 5 minutes.

Directions: Each of the numbered items or incomplete statements in this section is followed by answers or by completions of the statement. Select the ONE lettered answer or completion that is BEST in each case.

1. Which of the following signs and symptoms suggest a possible poisoning incident?

   (A) Headache, bruising behind the ears, and repetitive statements
   (B) Burns with an entrance and exit wound, abnormal heart rhythm, and altered mental status
   (C) Burns around the mouth, nausea, difficulty breathing, and altered mental status
   (D) Fruity breath odor, altered mental status, and extreme thirst

2. Which of the following are "depressant" substances?

   (A) LSD, PCP, and mescaline
   (B) Albuterol®, Alupent®, and Bronkosol®
   (C) Adrenaline®, epinephrine, Actidose®, and InstaChar®
   (D) Barbiturates, alcohol, narcotics, and benzodiazepines

3. Which of the following are "designer" drugs?

   (A) Mescaline and Fentanyl
   (B) Persian white and Ecstasy
   (C) Disulfiram and Antabuse®
   (D) Valium® and Demerol®

4. Which of the following correctly lists all the routes by which poisons may enter the body?

   (A) Ingestion, inhalation, and injection
   (B) Ingestion, inhalation, injection, and absorption
   (C) Ingestion, inhalation, injection, and diaphoresis
   (D) Ingestion, inhalation, injection, absorption, and diaphoresis

5. Activated charcoal may assist in limiting the effects of ingested poisons by

   (A) adsorbing the poison
   (B) neutralizing the poison
   (C) causing the patient to throw up (vomit) the poison
   (D) lining the stomach, thus not allowing the poison to be absorbed

6. Your rescue crew is called to the scene of a 2-year-old female patient who has ingested approximately 5–10 "heart pills" prescribed for her grandfather. After determining that the patient meets the appropriate criteria and obtaining permission from medical direction, you prepare to administer activated charcoal. Which of the following would be the best way to get this patient to take this medication?

   (A) Mix the medication with chocolate milk or ice cream
   (B) Shake it vigorously, put it in an opaque container with a lid, and have the patient drink it through a straw

    (C)   Do not shake the medication and have the patient drink the more liquefied solution at the top of the bottle

    (D)   Pour the entire solution into a clear glass, mix with chocolate milk, and have the patient drink the solution with a straw

7. Which of the following are common side effects of activated charcoal ingestion?

    (A)   Difficulty breathing and chest pain

    (B)   Abdominal cramping and constipation

    (C)   Unconsciousness and rapid pulse rate

    (D)   Altered mental status and difficulty breathing

8. Which of the following is true regarding medical direction and activated charcoal?

    (A)   Activated charcoal can be given without approval from medical direction because it is "charcoal"

    (B)   Authorization must be given by medical direction for the administration of activated charcoal

    (C)   Activated charcoal can only be given if the patient has already been prescribed, has a bottle(s) of activated charcoal, and medical direction approval has been obtained

    (D)   Activated charcoal can be given before approval by medical direction but the physician must be contacted after administration

9. The correct dose of activated charcoal is

    (A)   1 gram (g) of activated charcoal per kilogram (kg) of body weight

    (B)   1 g of activated charcoal per pound (lb) of body weight

    (C)   1 gram of activated charcoal per 10 lb of body weight

    (D)   25 g of activated charcoal per lb of body weight

10. The most serious potential side effect from the ingestion of large quantities of alcohol is

    (A)   death

    (B)   loss of brain cells

    (C)   impaired judgment

    (D)   damage to the liver

11. Alcohol withdrawal syndrome occurs after a decline in or cessation of alcohol consumption. The signs and symptoms associated with this syndrome include tremors, anxiety, gastrointestinal distress, hallucinations, disorientation, and seizures. These signs and symptoms generally appear within _____ after the last ingestion of alcohol.

    (A)   30 to 60 minutes

    (B)   1 to 2 hours

    (C)   6 to 48 hours

    (D)   1 to 2 weeks

Directions: Each of the numbered items or incomplete statements in this section is negatively phrased, as indicated by a capitalized word such as NOT, LEAST, or EXCEPT. Select the ONE lettered answer or completion that is BEST in each case.

12. Which of the following patients would NOT be a candidate for activated charcoal administration?

(A) A patient who has ingested "rock" cocaine and is complaining of chest pain
(B) A patient who has ingested an overdose of Valium® and is unconscious
(C) A patient who has ingested approximately 150 Tylenol® and has no complaint of illness or injury
(D) A patient who has ingested an overdose of aspirin combined with alcohol and is complaining of cramping

Directions: Each of the numbered questions or incomplete statements in this section refers to a scenario that precedes them. The numbered questions or incomplete statements are followed by answers or by completions of the statement. Select the answer or completion of the statement that is BEST in each case.

Your rescue crew responds for an "unknown" medical problem at a local apartment complex. Your scene size-up reveals a female patient found lying in bed. There are pill and alcohol bottles on the night stand. No weapons are apparent in the immediate area.

Questions 13–19

13. Before making contact with this patient, you should

(A) look for a suicide note
(B) inspect the labels of the pill bottles
(C) check the fluid level in the alcohol bottles
(D) ensure that body substance isolation precautions have been taken

14. Which of the following should be performed first?

(A) SAMPLE history
(B) Initial assessment
(C) Baseline vital signs
(D) Detailed physical examination

15. The patient is conscious and crying. She will not answer any of your questions but appears to be alert. While assessing her airway, you note there are pill fragments in her mouth. You should

(A) instruct the patient to spit out all the fragments
(B) give the patient a glass of water to rinse the fragments down
(C) probe the patient's mouth with your finger to get all the fragments
(D) leave the fragments in place for further examination at the receiving facility

16. You are successful in gaining the patient's trust, and she ultimately confides in you that she has ingested an unknown amount of the pills on the night stand. Administration of which of the following (trade name) medications may be appropriate for this patient's condition?

(A) Alupent®
(B) LiquiChar®
(C) Adrenaline®
(D) Bronkometer®

17. To administer the correct dose of this medication, you must determine the

   (A) patient's weight
   (B) number of pills ingested
   (C) presence of alcohol in the patient's stomach
   (D) patient's past medical history including past suicide attempts

18. You are preparing to transport this patient. What should you do with the pill bottles?

   (A) Bring them in a bag to the hospital for further examination
   (B) Throw them away in an approved biohazard waste container
   (C) Leave them where found for a subsequent police investigation
   (D) Leave them on the night stand, but write down the names of the medications for further examination at the hospital

19. Which of the following is true about the presence of alcohol at this scene?

   (A) It is not important since alcohol is a legal substance
   (B) It is important only if the patient is under legal drinking age
   (C) It is only important if the substance is distilled spirits rather than beer or wine
   (D) It is important because alcohol may enhance, hasten, or otherwise change the nature of the drug overdose

Your ambulance is called to a local park for a 24-year-old male patient with an altered mental status. You arrive to find your patient standing on a park bench yelling gibberish and laughing hysterically. His face is flushed and red. As you approach, he begins crying uncontrollably. He attempts to get away from you by digging a hole in the cement.

Questions 20–22

20. Which of the following substances would most commonly be associated with this reaction?

   (A) Alcohol
   (B) Barbiturates
   (C) Hallucinogens
   (D) Benzodiazepines

21. When treating this patient, you should anticipate what type of behavior?

   (A) Joyful and funny
   (B) Slow to respond and sleepy
   (C) Calm and introspective
   (D) Disruptive, possibly violent, and dangerous

22. Your physical examination of this patient fails to reveal any findings other than his altered mental status. If physically possible, this patient should be transported in what position?

   (A) Fully immobilized and restrained if appropriate (according to local protocol and patient's signs and symptoms)
   (B) Recovery position (lateral recumbent) and restrained if appropriate (according to local protocol and patient's signs and symptoms)
   (C) Prone with a backboard secured over the patient to prevent any patient movement
   (D) Supine between two secured backboards (one on top and one on the bottom) to prevent any patient movement

Your rescue crew is called to the scene of a 22-year-old male patient who has been "burned" (according to the information at time of dispatch). You arrive at an industrial complex to find your patient standing in an assembly area. Bystanders state that a container of dry chlorine powder burst open and covered the patient. The material is used for pool maintenance and is all over the patient and his immediate area. The shipping container information states that the product may cause irritation to the skin and mucous membranes. You call for a Hazardous Materials team. Their estimated time to the scene is 20 minutes. Your crew has taken body substance isolation precautions with gloves, eye and respiratory protection, and gowns.

Questions 23–28

23. You should immediately

    (A) begin an initial assessment
    (B) wait until the Hazardous Materials team arrives
    (C) remove the patient, your crew, and the bystanders from the area
    (D) begin irrigating the patient with water to remove the gross contaminants

24. As performed by trained personnel, the first step in decontaminating this patient should be

    (A) immediate removal of all dry powder
    (B) immediate irrigation with warm water
    (C) neutralization of the acid with a corresponding base (such as lye)
    (D) immediate submersion of the patient in a chemical bath of bicarbonate of soda and water

25. Which of the following is correct regarding the decontamination of this patient?

    (A) All clothing and jewelry must be removed before or during irrigation
    (B) The patient must strip down to his underwear before or during irrigation
    (C) The patient should change into clean clothes if available before or during irrigation
    (D) The patient should be decontaminated with his clothes on so the clothing becomes decontaminated as well

26. After continuous irrigation, the patient begins to complain of left eye discomfort. He states it feels like his eye is burning and itching. Appropriate treatment for this complaint would be

    (A) cover the left eye with a moistened, sterile gauze pad
    (B) lay the patient on his left side and continuously irrigate the left eye until arrival at the hospital
    (C) lay the patient on his right side and continuously irrigate the left eye until arrival at the hospital
    (D) have the patient submerse his head in a container of water and bicarbonate of soda until the discomfort is relieved

27. Which of the following would suggest that this patient may have inhaled some chlorine powder?

    (A) Abdominal cramping
    (B) Vomiting and nausea
    (C) Blisters on the chest and neck area
    (D) Difficulty breathing with rales (crackles)

28. Appropriate management of this patient en route to the hospital would be

(A) continuous irrigation and no oxygen due to an explosion hazard

(B) continuous irrigation and low-flow oxygen [nasal cannula at 4 to 6 liters per minute (LPM)]

(C) continuous irrigation and high-flow oxygen (nonrebreather mask at 15 LPM)

(D) continuous irrigation, high-flow oxygen (nonrebreather mask at 15 LPM) and application of occlusive dressing to all burned areas

ANSWERS AND RATIONALES

1-C. Signs and symptoms of poisoning include burns to the mouth and hands (from handling and ingestion), nausea, difficulty breathing, altered mental status, headache, vomiting, diarrhea, chest or abdominal pain, sweating, and seizures. Bruising behind the ears and repetitive statements are generally associated with head trauma. Burns with an entrance and exit wound combined with cardiac abnormalities and an altered mental status are generally indicative of an electrical burn. The presence of a fruity breath odor and intense thirst in a patient with an altered mental status is most closely associated with a diabetic emergency (hyperglycemia).

2-D. Barbiturates, alcohol, narcotics, and benzodiazepines are depressants and "numb" the body's ability to react appropriately to its environment. LSD, PCP, and mescaline are hallucinogens. Albuterol®, Alupent®, and Bronkosol® are bronchodilators. Adrenaline® and epinephrine are synthetic versions of a naturally occurring chemical in our body. Actidose® and InstaChar® are trade names for activated charcoal.

3-B. Designer drugs are chemical variants of federally controlled substances. Often, these extremely potent drugs are produced in contaminated, makeshift laboratories. Other examples of designer drugs are Adam, XTC, Mexican brown, China white, and Essence. There are literally hundreds of other slang and street names for these drugs. Mescaline is a plant product with hallucinogenic characteristics. Fentanyl is a surgical anesthetic after which designer drugs may be patterned. Disulfiram (Antabuse®) is used to discourage alcoholics from drinking. Valium® is a benzodiazepine (depressant), and Demerol® is a narcotic (depressant).

4-B. The four routes by which poisons may enter the body are ingestion (via the gastrointestinal tract), inhalation (via the respiratory tract), injection (by creating a break in the skin or mucous membranes), and absorption (by moving through intact skin or mucous membranes). Diaphoresis is a term for a clammy or sweaty condition of the skin.

5-A. Activated charcoal is a very porous substance. It acts by adsorbing and binding to the ingested poison. The charcoal then moves through the gastrointestinal tract without being absorbed. The poison and charcoal are then eliminated as a bowel movement.

6-B. Activated charcoal is a thick, chalky, black substance. It is generally tasteless, but its appearance is less than appetizing. The best method to administer the medication is to shake it vigorously (because the charcoal tends to settle rapidly), keep it in its container (they are generally white and not "see-through"), and have the patient drink it with a straw. Mixing the charcoal with milk products reduces its effectiveness.

7-B. Common side effects of activated charcoal administration are constipation, black stools, abdominal cramping, and possibly vomiting. Because activated charcoal is not absorbed into the bloodstream, any other complications should be attributed to the poison or the patient's underlying medical history.

8-B. The criteria for administration of activated charcoal are the same as for other EMT-Basic assisted medications: the patient must be exhibiting the signs and symptoms of the illness for which the medication is indicated (in this case, an ingested poison) and medical direction authority must be given (either on-line medical control or off-line medical direction). Activated charcoal is one of three medications that EMT-Basics may supply for the patient (oral glucose and oxygen are the other two). Metered dose inhalers, nitroglycerin, and epinephrine auto-injectors must be prescribed for the specific patient.

9-A. Activated charcoal is given in doses according to the patient's body weight. The exact dose is 1 gram (g) of activated charcoal per kilogram (kg) of the patient's body weight. An estimate of the patient's weight in kg can be made by dividing the patient's weight in pounds (lb) by 2. For example, a 200-lb patient would weigh approximately 100 kg and would receive 100 g of activated charcoal. When obtaining authorization to administer the medication from medical direction, request a dose from the physician (be prepared to give the patient's weight).

10-A. Alcohol is a poison. In large amounts, the concentration of this poison can be potentially fatal. The root word of the term "intoxicated" is "toxin." A toxin is a poisonous substance. Chronic alcohol use may also contribute to or worsen conditions (e.g., diabetes, liver disease).

11-C. Typically, the signs and symptoms associated with alcohol withdrawal syndrome will occur within 6 to 48 hours after the last ingestion of alcohol. The onset of these symptoms does not necessarily mean that all the alcohol has left the patient's body. Rather, it means that the blood alcohol level has fallen below the patient's physical dependency level. In other words, a patient may begin to exhibit the signs and symptoms of withdrawal while still legally intoxicated. These patients should be considered unstable, and advanced-life-support (ALS) care should be requested immediately.

12-B. Because activated charcoal is given orally and must be swallowed by the patient, its use is limited to patients with an intact gag reflex and alert mental status. Its effectiveness is limited or absent in patients who have ingested acids, alkalis, iron products, arsenic, or lithium.

13-D. After a rapid scene size-up, you need to turn your attention to assessing the patient. There will be adequate time later to gather specific information about the medications and the alcohol; they are potentially important "pieces of the puzzle." The most important piece is your patient's condition. You cannot (should not) address the patient's condition before taking proper body substance isolation precautions.

14-B. The initial assessment of the patient's mental status, airway, breathing, circulation status, and potentially life-threatening conditions must take precedence over any other activity. If the patient is conscious, the focused history and physical assessment should follow the initial assessment. If unconscious, a detailed physical examination should follow.

15-A. Do not stick your fingers in the mouth of a conscious patient with a possible altered mental status. The patient may follow your instructions and spit the pill fragments out. If not, you may attempt to remove the fragments with a suction catheter or other appropriate device. Do not have the patient wash the fragments down or leave the fragments in the patient's mouth. Swallowing the fragments may further complicate the incident and the patient's outcome. If the fragments are left in the patient's mouth, they will dissolve in the mouth and be ingested.

16-B. LiquiChar® is a trade name for a type of activated charcoal. Activated charcoal is indicated for ingestion poisonings. Alupent® and Bronkometer® are trade names for bronchodilator medications, and Adrenaline® is a trade name of epinephrine (given for severe allergic reactions).

17-A. Activated charcoal is given according to patient body weight. The number of pills ingested, the presence of alcohol, and the patient's past medical history are all important; however, these factors do not typically change the dose of the medication.

18-A. Whenever possible, bring the medication bottles to the hospital. The name of the medication is important but is only one part of the total picture. Bringing the bottles allows the hospital the opportunity to compare the date of purchase of the medication to the daily dose prescribed and the amount of medications in the bottle. This comparison allows the facility to better appreciate the total ingestion dose. The pill bottle labels may also contain other information valuable to the hospital.

19-D. Alcohol is a "drug" and a "toxin" (a poisonous substance). Alcohol may affect the reaction to the pill overdose. This information is important and should be passed on to the receiving facility.

20-C. While alcohol can cause erratic behavior, the presence of the irrational behavior and quick mood swings are suggestive of hallucinogens. The other choices (alcohol, barbiturates, and benzodiazepines) are depressants and are not typically associated with the behavior described in this scenario.

21-D. Use extreme caution when handling this patient. He may go from being calm to violent very quickly. Make sure that local law enforcement personnel are available to help you control this patient.

22-B. The ideal position would be the recovery position since no factors are present that indicate the need for spinal immobilization. Do NOT "sandwich" the patient between backboards or between a backboard and the stretcher. Continuous assessments and treatment are hampered by this unnecessary and unprofessional technique of controlling the patient. Patients placed in these positions have died from unwitnessed aspiration of vomitus. Contact medical direction and follow local protocol if restraints are necessary to protect you and the patient from harm.

Questions 23–28

Many of you are studying this text to become or continue as EMT-Basics, not Hazardous Materials Technicians. Do not assume that because you have some prehospital education about treating exposed patients that you are capable or expected to be able to manage hazardous materials. Once you recognize that your "medical" incident has a "hazardous materials" element, immediately return to the scene size-up mode. Ensure the safety of yourself, your crew, the patient, and all potential patients (bystanders). Call for available resources (fire department, "HazMat" team, on-site specialists, local public safety department, local public health department, etc.). Find out what your particular resources are before you encounter a hazardous materials incident.

23-C. Your scene assessment reveals that you, your crew, the patient, and the bystanders may be harmed by staying in the immediate area. In all cases where your location may put you in harm's way, you need to move as quickly as the situation warrants. Since the patient is conscious and standing, it would be appropriate for you to instruct him to follow you out of the area. Have all bystanders leave the area but direct them to a different site other than where you are directing the patient. Remember, as long as the patient is contaminated, everywhere he goes is contaminated until proven otherwise.

24-A. Since the patient is covered in a dry product, you should attempt (or instruct the patient to) sweep off the material. Immediate and continuous irrigation with water should follow. Never attempt to "correct" a product's pH to reduce an injury or burn. Do not add an acid to an alkali or vice versa. The result could be fatal. The only substance you should use to irrigate is water.

25-A. Protecting a patient's modesty and privacy is important; however, when decontaminating a patient, all clothing must be removed, including jewelry, wigs, toupees, or other body adornments. Do not be concerned with decontaminating these things as your efforts should be directed toward saving the patient. Do not transport the clothing or other effects with the patient—it is contaminated. If you are concerned about the safety of valuables, ensure that law enforcement personnel secure the entire area from nonessential personnel. Allowing the patient to wear "clean" clothing during the decontamination may only result in ineffective decontamination. If bystanders and nonessential personnel are removed from the area, you have met the privacy concerns of the patient to the best of your ability.

26-B. The correct method for treating an eye exposure is to have the patient with the affected eye lie down and continuously irrigate the eye with water or normal saline solution. The affected eye is lowered so that contaminants are not washed into the unaffected eye. If both eyes are affected, you may position the patient on either side. Laying the patient flat may cause the contaminated irrigation fluid to run down the face toward the nose and mouth.

27-D. The signs and symptoms of inhaled poisoning include difficulty breathing, rales/crackles (typically from damage to the lungs leading to leaking fluid in the lung space), chest pain, cough/hoarseness (typically from damage to the larynx), dizziness (typically from shock and inadequate oxygenation), and headache/confusion/ seizures/altered mental status (typically from inadequate oxygen delivery to the brain). Abdominal cramping, vomiting, and nausea generally accompany ingested poisoning incidents. Blisters on the chest and neck area suggest an absorbed poisoning incident.

28-C. Continuously irrigate to ensure that most of the contaminants are washed away. CAUTION: Your patient may become extremely cold during continuous irrigation. The ideal way to warm the patient without stopping irrigation is to use the heater in the transport vehicle. Monitor your patient closely for signs of hypothermia, especially if severe burns are present. Oxygen should be delivered by nonrebreather mask at 15 liters per minute (LPM).

BIBLIOGRAPHY

American Red Cross: *Emergency Response,* 2nd ed. St. Louis, Mosby-Year Book, 1996.

Crosby LA, Lewallen DG (eds): *Emergency Care and Transportation of the Sick and Injured,* 6th ed. Rosemont, IL, American Academy of Orthopaedic Surgeons, 1995.

Grant HD, Murray RH Jr, Bergeron JD: *Emergency Care,* 7th ed. Englewood Cliffs, NJ, Prentice-Hall, 1995.

Hafen BQ, Karren KJ, Mistovich JJ: *Prehospital Emergency Care,* 5th ed. Upper Saddle River, NJ, Prentice-Hall, 1996.

Henry MC, Stapleton ER, Judd RL: *EMT: Prehospital Care.* Philadelphia, WB Saunders, 1992.

Kitt S, Selfridge-Thomas J, Proehl JA, et al: *Emergency Nursing: A Physiologic and Clinical Perspective.* 2nd ed. Philadelphia, WB Saunders, 1995.

McSwain NE, White RD, Paturas JL, et al (eds): *The Basic EMT: Comprehensive Prehospital Patient Care.* St. Louis, Mosby-Year Book, 1996.

Olson, KR (ed): *Poisoning and Drug Overdose*. 2nd ed. Norwalk, Connecticut, Appleton & Lange, 1994.

Sanders, MJ. *Mosby's Paramedic Textbook*. St. Louis, Mosby-Year Book, 1994.

Stoy WA: *Mosby's EMT-Basic Textbook*. St. Louis, Mosby-Year Book, 1996.

United States Department of Transportation, National Highway Traffic Safety Administration: *Emergency Medical Technician: Basic. National Standard Curriculum*, 1994.

22 ENVIRONMENTAL EMERGENCIES

22-1 Describe the various ways that the body loses heat.

22-2 List the signs and symptoms of exposure to cold.

22-3 Explain the steps in providing emergency medical care to a patient exposed to cold.

22-4 List the signs and symptoms of exposure to heat.

22-5 Explain the steps in providing emergency care to a patient exposed to heat.

22-6 Recognize the signs and symptoms of water-related emergencies.

22-7 Describe the complications of near-drowning.

22-8 Discuss the emergency medical care of bites and stings.

BODY TEMPERATURE

OVERVIEW

1. Body temperature is the balance between the heat produced by the body and the heat lost from the body.
2. Body temperature is measured in heat units called degrees (°).
3. The body is divided into two areas for temperature control:
   a. Core temperature
   b. Peripheral (surface) temperature

CORE AND PERIPHERAL TEMPERATURES

1. **Core temperature**
   a. The body core (the deep tissues of the body) includes the contents of the skull, vertebral column, thorax, abdomen, and pelvis.

● MOTIVATION FOR LEARNING ●

Environmental emergencies include exposure to heat and cold, water-related emergencies, and bites and stings. The EMT-Basic must be aware of methods of heat loss to effectively manage patients with temperature-related emergencies. The EMT-Basic must be able to recognize the signs and symptoms of environmental emergencies in order to provide appropriate emergency care.

    b. The body core is normally maintained at a relatively constant temperature, usually within 1° of normal, unless a person develops a fever.

      (1) The average normal temperature is generally considered between 98.0° and 98.6° Fahrenheit (F) when measured orally.

      (2) The temperature measured in the armpit (axillary) or orally is about 1° F less than the rectal temperature.

      (3) In a resting adult, rectal temperature is about the same as the temperature of the liver and slightly lower than that of the brain.

    c. When the body produces excessive heat, such as through strenuous exercise, the temperature can temporarily rise to as high as 101° to 104° F.

    d. When the body is exposed to cold, the temperature can often fall to below 96° F.

2. Peripheral (surface) temperature

    a. The peripheral area of the body includes the skin, subcutaneous tissue, and fat.

    b. Unlike core body temperature, the temperature of the body's periphery rises and falls in response to the environment.

    c. At room temperature, the temperature in the peripheral areas of the body is slightly below those of the body core.

3. Body temperature remains constant if the heat produced by the body equals the heat lost.

TEMPERATURE REGULATION

1. Brain

    a. The hypothalamus (located in the brain) functions as the body's thermostat, coordinating the body's response to temperature.

    b. Receptors throughout the body detect changes in the temperature of the skin and certain mucous membranes and relay the information to the hypothalamus.

    c. When high temperatures are detected, blood vessels in the skin dilate.

    d. When low temperatures are detected, blood vessels in the skin constrict, sweating stops, and the body shivers to increase heat.

2. Cardiovascular system

    a. Blood vessels dilate and constrict in response to messages from the hypothalamus.

    b. The cardiovascular system regulates the blood flow to the skin.

3. Skin

    a. The skin plays a primary role in temperature regulation.

    b. Cold and warmth receptors detect changes in temperature and relay the information to the hypothalamus.

HEAT PRODUCTION

1. Body heat is produced primarily by the conversion of food to energy (metabolism).

    a. Most of the heat produced in the body is generated by the liver, brain, heart, and the skeletal muscles during exercise.

    b. Heat produced by skeletal muscle is important in temperature control because muscle activity can be increased to produce heat when needed.

2. When the body's cold sensors are stimulated, the body begins mechanisms to conserve heat and increase heat production (*Figure 22-1*).

    a. Production of epinephrine and other hormones is increased.

      (1) The increased production of epinephrine and other hormones increases the rate of metabolism, thus increasing heat production.

      (2) It also stimulates narrowing (constriction) of peripheral blood vessels.

    b. Peripheral blood vessels narrow.

      (1) Narrowing of these vessels decreases blood flow and heat loss through the skin.

      (2) It also keeps warm blood in the body's core.

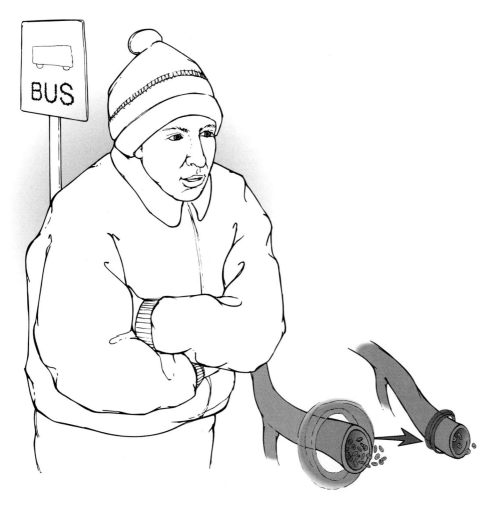

Fig. 22-1. When the body's cold sensors are stimulated, the body begins to conserve heat and increase heat production. Blood vessels near the skin constrict, decreasing blood flow and heat loss through the skin and keeping warm blood in the body's core. Increased muscle activity, such as moving about and involuntary shivering, increases heat production.

    c. Muscle activity increases. Muscle activity may be voluntary (e.g., walking, running, or moving about) or involuntary (e.g., shivering).

HEAT LOSS

1. Heat is lost from the body to the air and nearby objects through the processes of radiation, convection, conduction, evaporation, and breathing.
    a. Most heat loss is transferred from the deeper body organs and tissues to the skin where it is lost to the air and other surroundings.
    b. Some heat loss occurs through the mucous membranes of the respiratory, digestive, and urinary systems.
2. **Mechanisms of heat loss** (*Figure 22-2*)
    a. **Radiation**
        (1) Radiation is the transfer of heat, as infrared heat rays, from the surface of one object to the surface of another without contact between the two objects.
        (2) When the temperature of the body is more than the temperature of the surroundings, the body will lose heat.
        (3) More than half of the heat loss from the body occurs by radiation.
    b. **Convection**
        (1) Convection is the transfer of heat by the movement of air currents.

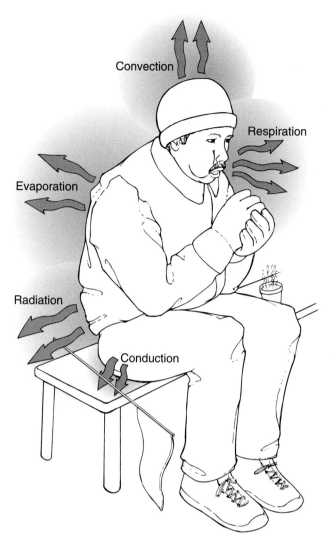

Fig. 22-2. Mechanisms of heat loss.

    (2) Wind speed affects heat loss by convection (wind chill factor).
- **c. Conduction**
  - **(1)** Conduction is the transfer of heat between objects that are in direct contact.
  - **(2)** Heat flows from warmer areas to cooler ones.
  - **(3)** The amount of heat lost from the body by conduction depends on the:
    - **(a)** Temperature difference between the body and the object
    - **(b)** Amount of time the objects are in contact
    - **(c)** Amount (surface area) of the body in contact with the object
- **d. Evaporation**
  - **(1)** Evaporation is a loss of heat by vaporization of moisture on the body surface.
  - **(2)** The body will lose heat by evaporation if the skin temperature is higher than the temperature of the surroundings.
  - **(3)** When the temperature of the surrounding air is higher than body temperature, the body gains heat.
  - **(4)** As relative humidity rises, the effectiveness of cooling of the body by evaporation decreases.
- **e. Respiration (breathing).** With normal breathing, the body continuously loses a relatively small amount of heat through the evaporation of moisture.

3. When the body's warmth sensors are stimulated, the body begins mechanisms to increase heat loss (*Figure 22-3*).

    a. Peripheral blood vessels widen (dilate).

        (1) Blood flow to the body surface increases.

        (2) Heat escapes from the skin surface by radiation and conduction.

        (3) When air currents pass across the skin, additional heat is lost by convection, cooling the body's core.

    b. Sweat gland secretion is increased.

        (1) Sweat travels to the skin surface.

        (2) When air currents pass across the skin, heat loss occurs through evaporation.

4. The EMT-Basic must be aware of methods of heat loss when treating patients with a cold-related injury to prevent further heat loss.

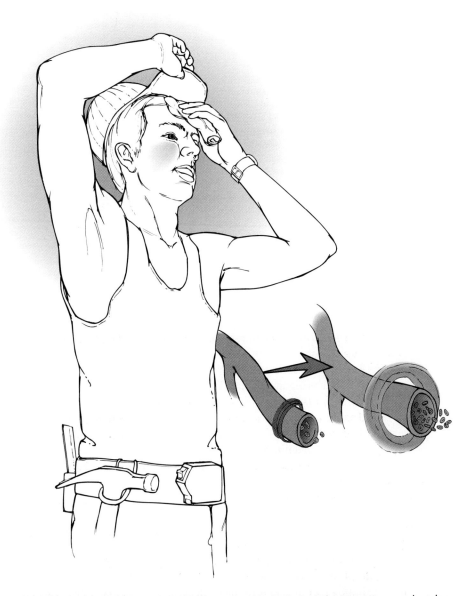

Fig. 22-3. When the body's warmth receptors are stimulated, the body begins to increase heat loss. Blood vessels near the skin surface dilate, increasing blood flow to the body surface. This increased surface blood flow allows heat to escape. Sweat travels to the skin surface. When air currents pass across the skin, heat loss occurs by evaporation.

EXPOSURE TO COLD

TYPES OF COLD EMERGENCIES

1. When the body loses more heat than it gains or produces, **hypothermia** (low body temperature) results.
2. The two primary types of cold emergencies are generalized cold emergency (generalized hypothermia) and local cold injury.
   a. Generalized cold emergency (generalized hypothermia) includes:
   (1) Mild hypothermia (body temperature of 90° to 95° F). Temperatures below 95° F are considered significant because at or below this temperature, the body typically does not generate sufficient heat to restore normal body temperature or maintain proper organ function.
   (2) Moderate hypothermia (82° to 89.9° F)
   (3) Severe hypothermia (less than 82° F)
   b. Local cold injury is damage to a specific area of the body, such as fingers or toes.

GENERALIZED HYPOTHERMIA

1. **Predisposing factors**
   a. **Cold environment**
   (1) Extremes in temperature are not necessary for hypothermia to occur.
   (2) Factors such as clothing, wind velocity, duration of exposure, illness, poor physical condition, immersion in water, and injury increase the risk of hypothermia.
   b. **Age**
   (1) Elderly individuals are at risk of hypothermia because:
   (a) Lack of heat in home
   (b) Poor diet/appetite
   (c) Loss of subcutaneous fat for body insulation
   (d) Lack of activity/mobility
   (e) Decreased efficiency of temperature control mechanisms
   (f) Delayed circulation
   (2) Young individuals are at risk of cold-related injury because:
   (a) Less subcutaneous fat for body insulation
   (b) Large surface area in relation to their overall size resulting in more rapid heat loss
   (c) Inadequate ability to shiver due to small muscle mass
   (i) Shivering mechanism is not well-developed in children.
   (ii) Infants (newborns) are unable to shiver.
   (d) Inability of infants and younger children to protect themselves from the cold
   (i) They cannot put on or take off clothes.
   (ii) They cannot move to a warm environment.
   c. **Medical conditions.** Medical conditions that predispose to generalized hypothermia include:
   (1) Shock (hypoperfusion)
   (2) Head injury
   (3) Burns
   (4) Generalized infection
   (5) Injuries to the spinal cord
   (6) Diabetic emergencies (e.g., hypoglycemia)
   d. **Alcohol, drugs, and poisons**
   (1) Some drugs and poisons interfere with the body's ability either to produce or conserve heat.

(2) Drugs or alcohol may affect judgment, preventing the individual from taking appropriate precautions (e.g., wearing more clothing, increasing room temperature, coming in from the cold).

(3) Alcohol dilates the peripheral vessels and depresses the central nervous system.

    (a) Heat loss may occur rapidly due to dilation of vessels.

    (b) Sedation from alcohol causes the sedation due to cold to go unrecognized.

2. Patient assessment

  a. Scene size-up

    (1) Observe the patient's environment for signs of exposure, including:

      (a) Obvious exposure

      (b) Subtle exposure, such as:

        (i) Ethanol ingestion

        (ii) Underlying illness

        (iii) Overdose/poisoning

        (iv) Major trauma

        (v) Outdoor recreation

        (vi) Decreased ambient temperature (e.g., home of elderly patient)

    (2) Use trained rescuers to remove the patient from the environment; cold environment requires special safety considerations due to presence of ice, snow, or wind.

  b. Initial assessment

    (1) Maintain spinal immobilization if needed.

    (2) Assess the patient's mental status.

    (3) Assess the patient's airway.

    (4) Assess breathing.

    (5) Assess circulation.

    (6) Identify any life-threatening conditions and provide care based on these findings.

    (7) Establish patient priorities.

      (a) Priority patients include:

        (i) Patients who give a poor general impression

        (ii) Patients experiencing difficulty breathing

        (iii) Patients with signs and symptoms of shock

        (iv) Unresponsive patients with no gag reflex or cough

        (v) Responsive patients who are unable to follow commands

      (b) Advanced-life-support (ALS) assistance should be requested as soon as possible.

      (c) If ALS personnel are not available, the patient should be transported promptly to the closest appropriate facility.

  c. Focused history and physical examination

    (1) The focused history and physical examination should be done in the back of a warmed ambulance.

    (2) If the patient is unresponsive:

      (a) Perform a rapid physical examination

      (b) Follow with evaluation of baseline vital signs and gathering of the patient's medical history

    (3) If the patient is responsive:

      (a) Gather information about the patient's medical history before performing the physical examination

      (b) Gather a SAMPLE history

  d. SAMPLE history

    (1) <u>S</u>igns and <u>s</u>ymptoms. Signs and symptoms of generalized hypothermia include:

      (a) Mild hypothermia:

      (i) Increased heart rate
      (ii) Increased respiratory rate
      (iii) Cool skin (to preserve core temperature)
      (iv) Shivering
      (v) Difficulty in speech and movement
      (vi) Memory lapse (amnesia), mood changes, combative
      (vii) Patient may complain of joint aches/muscle stiffness
      (viii) Altered mental status, confusion, or poor judgment (patient may actually remove clothing)

  (b) Moderate hypothermia:
      (i) Shivering that may progressively decrease and become absent; replaced with muscle rigidity
      (ii) Progressively decreasing pulse and respirations
      (iii) Irregular pulse
      (iv) Progressive loss of consciousness
      (v) Dilated pupils
      (vi) Blood pressure difficult to obtain

  (c) Severe hypothermia:
      (i) Low to absent blood pressure
      (ii) Irrational proceeding to unconsciousness
      (iii) Muscle rigidity
      (iv) Skin cold to touch; may appear cyanotic
      (v) Slow or even absent breathing
      (vi) Slowly responding pupils
      (vii) Pulse slow and barely palpable and/or irregular, or completely absent
      (viii) Cardiopulmonary arrest

(1) Allergies. Determine if the patient has any allergies to medications and other substances or materials.

(2) Medications. Determine if the patient is taking any medications (prescription and over the counter).
  (a) Some patients taking medications such as phenothiazines, cyclic antidepressants, steroids, or barbiturates may be predisposed to developing hypothermia.
  (b) Determine if the patient takes his or her medications regularly and his or her response to them.
  (c) Determine if there has been any recent change in medications (additions, deletions, or change in dosages).
  (d) Provide all information obtained to the receiving facility.

(3) Pertinent past medical history. Ascertain whether the patient has a history of any of the following conditions:
  (a) Alcohol abuse
  (b) Thyroid disorder
  (c) Diabetes
  (d) Stroke
  (e) Trauma to the head, neck, or spine

(4) Last oral intake. Determine the patient's last oral intake.

(5) Event. Determine the events leading to the present situation.
  (a) How long has the patient been exposed to the cold?
  (b) What was the source of the cold (e.g., water, snow)?
  (c) What was the patient doing at the time his or her symptoms began?

e. Assess baseline vital signs.

f. Perform a focused physical examination.
  (1) Decreasing mental status correlates with the degree of hypothermia. Patient may show the following signs:
    (a) Difficult (slow, slurred) speech
    (b) Confusion

        (c) Memory lapse

        (d) Mood changes

        (e) Combativeness

    (2) Changing vital signs correlate with the degree of hypothermia.

        (a) Breathing rate is initially increased, then slow and shallow, and finally absent.

        (b) Pulse rate is initially increased, then slow and irregular, and finally absent.

        (c) Blood pressure is low to absent.

        (d) Skin is initially red; then pale; then cyanotic; and finally gray, hard, and cold to the touch.

            (i) To assess skin temperature, the EMT-Basic should place the back of his or her hand between the patient's clothing and abdomen to assess the patient's general temperature.

            (ii) The patient experiencing a generalized cold emergency will have a cool abdominal skin temperature.

        (e) Pupils dilate and are slow to respond.

    (3) Decreasing motor and sensory functions correlate with the degree of hypothermia.

        (a) Patient may complain of joint aches or muscle stiffness.

        (b) Patient may demonstrate:

            (i) Lack of coordination

            (ii) Staggering walk

            (iii) Shivering initially, gradually decreasing until absent

            (iv) Loss of sensation

            (v) Muscle rigidity

    (4) Assess the patient for other injuries.

3. Emergency medical care for generalized hypothermia

  a. The decision to rewarm the hypothermic patient depends on local protocol, consultation with medical direction, and the degree of hypothermia.

    (1) **Passive rewarming** is the warming of the patient without the use of additional heat sources beyond the patient's own heat production. Passive rewarming includes placing the patient in a warm environment, applying blankets, and preventing drafts.

    (2) **Active rewarming** involves adding heat directly to the surface of the patient's body.

  b. Protect the patient from further heat loss.

    (1) Remove the patient from the environment.

    (2) Remove wet clothing. Cut the patient's clothing away rather than jostle the patient by tugging and pulling at his or her clothes.

    (3) Keep the patient's head covered.

    (4) Insulate the patient from the cold with available materials (e.g., blankets, sleeping bag, newspapers, plastic garbage bags). Be sure to cover the patient's head, leaving the face exposed to monitor the airway.

    (5) Place insulating material between the patient and the surface on which he or she is lying (e.g., ground, backboard, stretcher).

    (6) Protect the patient from drafts.

  c. Handle the patient gently.

    (1) Avoid rough handling.

    (2) Do not allow the patient to walk or exert himself or herself.

    (3) Rough handling or exertion may shunt cold, acidotic blood in the periphery to the body's core.

    (4) When possible, transport the hypothermic patient in a supine position.

  d. Establish and maintain an open airway.

    (1) As the body cools, the cough reflex is depressed and respiratory secretions increase.

    (2) Frequent suctioning may be necessary.

    e. Administer high-concentration oxygen, if not already done. Oxygen should be warmed and humidified, if possible.

    f. Assess pulses for 30 to 45 seconds. If pulseless, start cardiopulmonary resuscitation (CPR).

    g. If the patient is alert and responding appropriately, actively rewarm (follow local protocol).

       (1) Apply warm blankets.

       (2) Apply heat packs or hot water bottles to the groin, armpits, and back of neck.

       (3) Place a towel or dressings under a heat pack or hot water bottle before applying to the patient's skin to prevent burns.

       (4) Turn the heat up high in the patient compartment of the ambulance.

    h. If the patient is unresponsive or not responding appropriately, rewarm passively (follow local protocol).

       (1) Apply warm blankets.

       (2) Turn the heat up high in the patient compartment of the ambulance.

    i. Do not allow the patient to eat or drink stimulants (e.g., coffee, tea, chocolate) or alcohol.

    j. Do not rub or massage the extremities.

    k. Transport promptly.

       (1) If the patient is stable, perform ongoing assessments every 15 minutes.

       (2) If the patient is unstable, perform ongoing assessments every 5 minutes.

LOCAL COLD INJURY

1. Local cold injury (also called frostbite) involves tissue damage to a specific area of the body.

    a. It occurs when a part of the body (e.g., nose, ears, cheeks, chin, hands, feet) is exposed to prolonged or intense cold.

    b. Cold causes narrowing of the blood vessels in the body part, reducing circulation to the involved area.

    c. Ice crystals form, causing damage and destruction to body cells.

    d. Frostbite is often accompanied by hypothermia.

2. Predisposing factors

    a. Anxiety

    b. Exhaustion

    c. Dehydration

    d. Smoking (nicotine causes narrowing of peripheral blood vessels)

    e. Patients with a history of:

       (1) Diabetes

       (2) Substance abuse

       (3) Heart or blood vessel disease

       (4) Previous burns, frostbite, or other tissue damage

    f. Ambient temperature

    g. Wind-chill factor

    h. Length of exposure

    i. Type and number of layers of clothing worn including tight gloves, tight or tightly laced footwear

    j. Whether or not the patient was wet

    k. Whether or not the patient had direct contact with cold objects

3. Signs and symptoms of local cold injury

    a. Early or superficial injury

       (1) Exposed area first appears red and inflamed.

       (2) Area then becomes gray or white with continued cooling.

       (3) When the skin is palpated, normal color does not return (blanching).

       (4) Feeling and sensation is lost in the injured area.

       (5) Skin beneath the affected area remains soft.

(6) If rewarmed, the patient experiences tingling or burning followed by a pins-and-needles sensation as the area thaws and circulation improves.

b. Late or deep injury
   (1) Whitish skin color is followed by a waxy appearance.
   (2) When the affected area becomes frozen, it will feel stiff and hard on palpation.
   (3) Patient may complain of slight burning pain followed by a feeling of warmth, then numbness.
   (4) Swelling may be present.
   (5) Blisters may be present (usually appear in 1 to 7 days).
   (6) If the affected area has thawed or partially thawed, the skin may appear flushed with areas that are purple, pale, mottled, or cyanotic.

4. **Emergency medical care for local cold injuries**
   a. Follow local protocol.
   b. Remove the patient from the environment.
   c. Protect the affected area from further injury.
   d. Administer oxygen, if not already done.
   e. If the injury is early or superficial:
      (1) Gently remove any jewelry or wet or restrictive clothing. If clothing is frozen to the skin, leave it in place.
      (2) Splint the affected extremity and apply soft padding (avoid pressure).
      (3) Cover the affected area with dry sterile dressings or clothing.
      (4) Do not:
         (a) Rub or massage the affected area
         (b) Re-expose the affected area to the cold
   f. If the injury is late or deep:
      (1) Gently remove any jewelry or wet or restrictive clothing. If clothing is frozen to the skin, leave it in place.
      (2) Cover the affected area with dry sterile dressings or clothing.
      (3) Do not:
         (a) Break blisters
         (b) Rub or massage the affected area
         (c) Apply heat to or rewarm the affected area
         (d) Allow the patient to walk on an affected extremity
   g. When an extremely long or delayed transport is inevitable:
      (1) Contact medical direction or follow local protocol.
      (2) Do not begin rewarming if there is a risk of refreezing.
      (3) If instructed to begin active rapid rewarming:
         (a) Anticipate that the patient will complain of intense pain during thawing
         (b) Handle the affected area gently
         (c) Immerse the affected area in a warm water bath (*Figure 22-4*). Do not use dry sources of heat (e.g., heat packs) because these heat sources are more difficult to control and may burn the tissue.
         (d) Monitor the water to ensure it does not cool from the frozen part. Continuously stir the water around the affected part to keep heat evenly distributed.
         (e) Continue rewarming until the affected part is soft and color and sensation return
         (f) Gently dry the area after rewarming
         (g) Dress the area with dry sterile dressings (*Figure 22-5*)
         (h) If the affected area is a hand or foot:
         (i) Place dry sterile dressings between the fingers or toes
         (ii) Elevate the extremity to decrease swelling
         (i) Protect against refreezing of the warmed part
   h. Transport promptly.

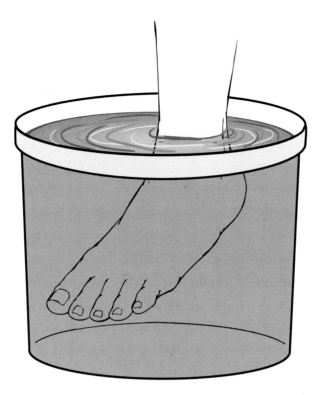

Fig. 22-4. If instructed to begin rewarming of a late or deep cold injury, immerse the affected area in a warm water bath.

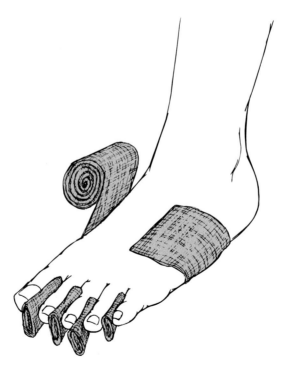

Fig. 22-5. Gently dry the area after rewarming. Dress the area with dry sterile dressings. If the affected area is a hand or foot, place dry sterile dressings between the fingers or toes.

EXPOSURE TO HEAT

TYPES OF HEAT EMERGENCIES

1. When the body gains or produces more heat than it loses, **hyperthermia** (high core body temperature) results.
2. Primary types of heat emergencies are:
   a. **Heat cramps**
   b. **Heat exhaustion**
   c. **Heat stroke**

PREDISPOSING FACTORS

1. **Climate**
   a. High ambient temperature reduces the body's ability to lose heat by radiation.
   b. High relative humidity reduces the body's ability to lose heat by the evaporation of sweat.
2. **Exercise and strenuous activity**
   a. Exercise and strenuous activity can cause the loss of more than 1 liter (L) of sweat per hour.
   b. Electrolytes (e.g., sodium, chloride) and fluid through sweat may also be lost.
3. **Age**
   a. The elderly are at higher risk for heat emergencies due to:
      (1) Medications
      (2) Lack mobility (cannot escape hot environment)
      (3) Impaired ability to maintain a normal temperature
      (4) Impaired ability to adapt to temperature changes
      (5) Impaired sense of thirst
   b. Newborns and infantsare at higher risk for heat emergencies due to:
      (1) Impaired ability to maintain a normal temperature
      (1) Inability to remove own clothing
4. **Preexisting illness and/or conditions.** The following illnesses and conditions increase the risk of a heat-related emergency:
   a. Heart disease
   b. Dehydration
   c. Obesity (increased insulation)
   d. Fever
   e. Fatigue
   f. Diabetes
   g. Thyroid disorder
   h. Parkinson's disease
   i. Previous history of a heat-related emergency
5. **Drugs/medications**
   a. Amphetamines and cocaine increase muscle activity, increasing heat production.
   b. Alcohol and phenothiazines impair the body's ability to regulate heat.
   c. Cyclic antidepressants, antihistamines, and phenothiazines impair the body's ability to lose heat.

PATIENT ASSESSMENT

1. **Scene size-up**
   a. Observe the patient's environment for signs of exposure, including:
      (1) Obvious exposure
      (2) Subtle exposure
2. **Initial assessment**
   a. Maintain spinal immobilization if needed.

b. Assess the patient's mental status.

c. Assess the patient's airway.

d. Assess breathing.

e. Assess circulation.

f. Identify any life-threatening conditions and provide care based on these findings.

g. Establish patient priorities.

    (1) Priority patients include:

        (a) Patients who give a poor general impression

        (b) Patients experiencing difficulty breathing

        (c) Patients with signs and symptoms of shock

        (d) Unresponsive patients with no gag reflex or cough

        (e) Responsive patients who are unable to follow commands

    (2) Advanced-life-support (ALS) assistance should be requested as soon as possible.

    (3) If ALS personnel are not available, the patient should be transported promptly to the closest appropriate facility.

3. Focused history and physical examination

  a. If the patient is unresponsive:

    (1) Perform a rapid physical examination

    (2) Follow with evaluation of baseline vital signs and gathering of the patient's medical history

  b. If the patient is responsive:

    (1) Gather information about the patient's medical history before performing the physical examination

    (2) Gather a SAMPLE history

4. SAMPLE history

  a. Signs and symptoms. General signs and symptoms of a heat-related emergency include:

    (1) Muscle cramps

    (2) Weakness or exhaustion

    (3) Dizziness or faintness

    (4) Moist and pale skin with normal to cool temperature. Skin that is hot and dry or moist indicates a dire emergency.

    (5) Rapid heart rate

    (6) Nausea/vomiting

    (7) Headache

    (8) Altered mental status to unresponsive

  b. Allergies. Determine if the patient has any allergies to medications and other substances or materials.

  c. Medications. Determine if the patient is taking any medications (prescription and over the counter).

    (1) Some medications may predispose the patient to a heat-related emergency.

    (2) Determine if the patient takes his or her medications regularly and his or her response to them.

    (3) Determine if there has been any recent change in medications (additions, deletions, or change in dosages).

    (4) Provide all information obtained to the receiving facility.

  d. Pertinent past medical history. Ascertain whether the patient has a history of any of the following conditions:

    (1) Thyroid disorder

    (2) Diabetes

    (3) Parkinson's disease

    (4) Heart disease

    (5) History of a heat-related emergency

    e. <u>L</u>ast oral intake. Determine the patient's last oral intake.

    f. <u>E</u>vent. Determine the events leading to the present situation.

        (1) Assess the environment and note:

            (a) High ambient temperature

            (b) High relative humidity

            (c) Enclosed area/restricted ventilation

        (2) How long was the patient exposed to the heat?

        (3) What was the patient doing at the time his or her symptoms began (exercise, exertion)?

5. Assess baseline vital signs.

6. Perform a focused physical examination.

EMERGENCY MEDICAL CARE FOR HEAT EMERGENCIES

1. Consult medical direction or follow local protocol.

2. Patient with moist, pale, normal to cool temperature skin

    a. Remove the patient from the hot environment and into a cool environment, such as the patient compartment of an air-conditioned ambulance.

    b. Administer oxygen.

        (1) If the patient's breathing is adequate, apply oxygen by nonrebreather mask at 15 liters per minute (LPM).

        (2) If the patient's breathing is inadequate, provide positive-pressure ventilation with 100% oxygen and assess the adequacy of the ventilations delivered.

    c. Remove as much of the patient's clothing as possible; loosen clothing that cannot be easily removed.

    d. Cool the patient by fanning. Do not cool the patient to the point of shivering; shivering generates heat.

    e. Place the patient in a supine position with the legs elevated 8–12 inches (shock position).

    f. If patient is responsive and is not nauseated, have the patient drink water. Consult medical direction or follow local protocol.

    g. If the patient is unresponsive or is vomiting:

        (1) Do not administer fluids

        (2) Transport to the hospital with the patient on his or her left side

    h. Perform ongoing assessments.

        (1) If the patient is stable, perform ongoing assessments every 15 minutes.

        (2) If the patient is unstable, perform ongoing assessments every 5 minutes.

2. Patient with hot and dry or moist skin

    a. Remove the patient from the hot environment into a cool environment, such as the patient compartment of an air-conditioned ambulance with the air conditioner running on high.

    b. Administer oxygen.

        (1) If the patient's breathing is adequate, apply oxygen by nonrebreather mask at 15 liters per minute (LPM).

        (2) If the patient's breathing is inadequate, provide positive-pressure ventilation with 100% oxygen and assess the adequacy of the ventilations delivered.

    c. Begin measures to cool the patient.

        (1) Do not cool the patient to the point of shivering; shivering generates heat.

        (2) Remove the patient's clothing.

        (3) Apply cool packs to the neck, armpits, and groin.

        (4) Place a towel or dressings under the cool pack before applying to the patient's skin to prevent frostbite.

        (5) Wet the patient's skin and keep it wet by applying water with a sponge or wet towels.

        (6) Fan the patient aggressively.

    d. Transport immediately.
        (1) If the patient is stable, perform ongoing assessments every 15 minutes.
        (2) If the patient is unstable, perform ongoing assessments every 5 minutes.

WATER-RELATED EMERGENCIES

NEAR-DROWNING AND DROWNING

1. **Terminology**
   a. Drowning is death that occurs within 24 hours of submersion/suffocation in fluid.
   b. Near-drowning is at least a temporary recovery (more than 24 hours) after a submersion injury.
2. Factors that influence a near-drowning victim's chances for survival:
   a. Ability to swim
   b. Age of victim
   c. Length of submersion
   d. Cleanliness of the water
   e. Temperature of the water
   f. Preexisting medical conditions
3. Predisposing factors include:
   a. Seizures
   b. Exhaustion
   c. Heart disease
   d. Hypothermia
   e. Hypoglycemia
   f. Inability to swim
   g. Suicide or homicide
   h. Alcohol or other drug use
   i. Trauma (head or spinal injury from diving)
4. Possible associated injuries include:
   a. Spinal cord injury (diving)
   b. Air embolism or the "bends"
   c. Hypothermia

PATIENT ASSESSMENT

1. **Scene size-up**
   a. Study the scene and determine if approaching the patient is safe.
   b. Evaluate the mechanism of injury and determine, if possible:
       (1) Length of submersion
       (2) Cleanliness of the water
       (3) Temperature of the water
   c. Obtain additional help before contact with the patient(s).
       (1) Call for specially trained personnel as needed to remove the patient from the environment.
       (2) A cold environment requires special safety considerations due to the presence of ice, snow, or wind.
   d. Do not enter a body of water unless you have been trained in water rescue.
   e. Do not enter fast-moving water or venture out on ice unless you have been trained in this type of rescue.
   f. Protect the patient from environmental temperature extremes.
2. **Initial assessment**
   a. Maintain spinal immobilization as needed.
       (1) Suspect neck injury:
           (a) When the mechanism of injury is unknown

        (b) Facial trauma is evident

        (c) In swimming, boating, water-skiing, and diving accidents

    (2) If the patient is in the water and spinal injury is suspected, place the patient on a long backboard before removing the patient from the water.

  b. Assess the patient's mental status.

    (1) Mental status may range from awake and alert to combative, difficult to arouse, or unresponsive.

    (2) These variations in mental status may be due to an associated injury or due to a lack of oxygen from submersion.

  c. Assess the patient's airway.

  d. Assess breathing.

  e. Assess circulation.

  f. Identify any life-threatening conditions and provide care based on these findings.

  g. Establish patient priorities.

    (1) Priority patients include:

        (a) Patients who give a poor general impression

        (b) Patients experiencing difficulty breathing

        (c) Patients with signs and symptoms of shock

        (d) Unresponsive patients with no gag reflex or cough

        (e) Responsive patients who are unable to follow commands

    (2) ALS assistance should be requested as soon as possible.

    (3) If ALS personnel are not available, the patient should be transported promptly to the closest appropriate facility.

3. Focused history and physical examination

  a. If the patient is unresponsive:

    (1) Perform a rapid physical examination

    (2) Follow with evaluation of baseline vital signs and gathering of the patient's medical history

  b. If the patient is responsive:

    (1) Gather information about the patient's medical history before performing the physical examination

    (2) Gather a SAMPLE history

4. SAMPLE history

  a. <u>S</u>igns and <u>s</u>ymptoms. Signs and symptoms of near-drowning will vary depending on the type and length of submersion and include:

    (1) Coughing, vomiting, choking, and airway obstruction

    (2) Absent or inadequate breathing

    (3) Difficulty breathing

    (4) Absent, slow, or increased heart rate

    (5) Seizures

    (6) Cool, clammy, and pale or cyanotic skin

    (7) Possible gastric distention

  b. <u>A</u>llergies. Determine if the patient has any allergies to medications and other substances or materials.

  c. <u>M</u>edications. Determine if the patient is taking any medications (prescription and over the counter).

    (1) Determine if the patient takes his or her medications regularly and his or her response to them.

    (2) Determine if there has been any recent change in medications (additions, deletions, or change in dosages).

    (3) Provide all information obtained to the receiving facility.

  d. Pertinent past medical history. Ascertain whether the patient has a history of any of the following conditions:

    (1) Heart disease

    (2) Seizures

        (3)   Alcohol or drug use

    e. <u>L</u>ast oral intake. Determine the patient's last oral intake.

    f. <u>E</u>vent. Determine the events leading to the present situation.

        (1)   When did the incident occur?

        (2)   Where did the incident occur (e.g., near rocks, pool, bathtub)?

        (3)   How did the incident occur?

        (4)   Did the patient experience any loss of consciousness?

        (5)   Was the incident witnessed? (This information is useful in determining possible head or spinal injury.)

        (6)   Look for signs of abuse or neglect in infants, children, and the elderly.

5. Assess baseline vital signs.

6. Perform a focused physical examination, carefully assessing the patient for other injuries.

EMERGENCY MEDICAL CARE FOR NEAR-DROWNING

1. Ensure the safety of all rescue personnel.

2. Remove the patient from the water as quickly and safely as possible.

3. If spinal injury is suspected and the patient is still in the water:

    a. Maintain in-line immobilization of the head and spine

    b. Move and secure the patient onto a long backboard

    c. Remove the patient from the water

4. If spine injury is not suspected, place the patient on the left side to allow water, vomitus, and secretions to drain from the upper airway.

5. Any pulseless, nonbreathing patient who has been submerged in cold water should be resuscitated.

6. Suction as needed.

7. Administer oxygen.

    a. If the patient's breathing is adequate, apply oxygen by nonrebreather mask at 15 LPM if not already done.

    b. If the patient's breathing is inadequate, provide positive-pressure ventilation with 100% oxygen.

        (1)   Assess the adequacy of the ventilations delivered.

        (2)   If gastric distention interferes with artificial ventilation:

            (a) Place the patient on the left side

            (b) With suction immediately available, the EMT-Basic should place his or her hand over the epigastric area of the patient's abdomen and apply firm pressure to relieve the distention. This procedure should be performed only if the gastric distention interferes with the ability to ventilate the patient effectively

8. Remove wet clothing and dry the patient to prevent heat loss.

9. Transport promptly.

    a. If the patient is stable, perform ongoing assessments every 15 minutes.

    b. If the patient is unstable, perform ongoing assessments every 5 minutes.

BITES AND STINGS

SIGNS AND SYMPTOMS

Signs and symptoms of bites and stings include:

1. History of bite (spider, snake) or sting (insect, scorpion, marine animal)

2. Pain

3. Redness

4. Swelling

5. Weakness

6. Dizziness

7. Chills
8. Fever
9. Nausea/vomiting
10. Bite marks
11. Stinger

EMERGENCY MEDICAL CARE FOR BITES AND STINGS

1. Establish and maintain an open airway.
2. Administer oxygen.
    a. If the patient's breathing is adequate, apply oxygen by nonrebreather mask at 15 LPM if not already done.
    b. If the patient's breathing is inadequate, provide positive-pressure ventilation with 100% oxygen and assess the adequacy of the ventilations delivered.
3. If a stinger is present, remove it (*Figure 22-6*).
    a. Gently scrape the stinger out by using the edge of a plastic card or cardboard.
    b. Avoid pinching or using tweezers or forceps, as pinching can squeeze venom from the venom sac into the wound.
4. Gently wash the area.
5. If possible, remove jewelry from the injured area before swelling begins.
6. If the injection site is on an extremity, position the extremity slightly below the level of the patient's heart.
7. Do not apply cold to snakebites.

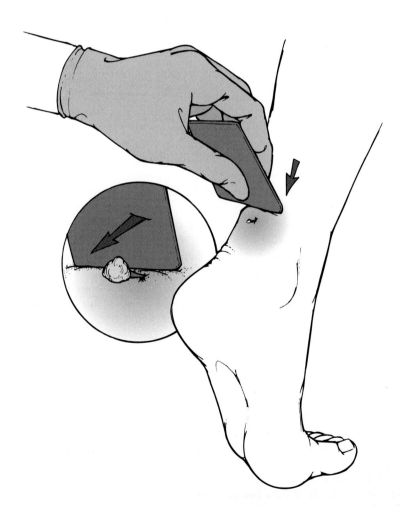

Fig. 22-6. If a stinger is present, remove it by gently scraping the stinger out with the edge of a plastic card or cardboard. Avoid pinching or using tweezers or forceps.

8. Consult medical direction regarding the use of a constricting band for snakebite.
9. Observe the patient closely for the development of signs and symptoms of an allergic reaction; treat as needed.

ENRICHMENT—DIVING EMERGENCIES

BAROTRAUMA

1. **Pathophysiology**
   a. Barotrauma is injury caused by pressure.
   b. It can occur on ascent or descent.
      (1) Barotrauma occurring on ascent is called pulmonary overpressurization syndrome (POPS) or "burst lung."
      (2) Barotrauma occurring on descent is called "lung squeeze" or "the squeeze." Air pressure in the body's air-filled cavities increases, causing damage to the tissues within the cavity (e.g., ear, sinuses, lungs, gastrointestinal tract).
2. Signs and symptoms of barotrauma include:
   a. Ear: bloody drainage from the ear, mild to severe pain in the ear, nausea, dizziness, disorientation
   b. Sinuses: mild to severe pain over the sinuses, bleeding from the nose
   c. Lungs: difficulty breathing, chest pain, cough, pulmonary edema
   d. Gastrointestinal tract: mild to severe abdominal pain
3. Emergency medical care for barotrauma
   a. Establish and maintain an open airway.
   b. Administer oxygen at 15 LPM by nonrebreather mask. Some authorities do not recommend positive-pressure ventilation because of the risk of further injury.
   c. Transport promptly.

AIR EMBOLISM

1. **Pathophysiology**
   a. Air embolism may occur when divers ascend too rapidly or hold their breath during ascent.
   b. Onset is usually rapid and dramatic, frequently occurring within minutes of surfacing.
   c. As the diver ascends, air trapped in the lungs expands.
   d. If the air is not exhaled, the alveoli rupture, damaging adjacent blood vessels.
   e. Air bubbles are forced into the circulatory system through ruptured pulmonary veins.
   f. The air bubbles become lodged in small arteries, cutting off circulation.
   g. The size and location of the bubbles determine the patient's signs and symptoms.
2. **Signs and symptoms of air embolism include:**
   a. Dizziness
   b. Confusion
   c. Shortness of breath
   d. Visual disturbances
   e. Weakness or paralysis in extremities
   f. Sudden unconsciousness after surfacing (can occur before surfacing)
   g. Pink, frothy sputum
   h. Respiratory arrest
   i. Cardiac arrest
3. **Emergency medical care for air embolism**
   a. Establish and maintain an open airway.
   b. Administer oxygen.

(1) If the patient's breathing is adequate, apply oxygen by nonrebreather mask at 15 LPM if not already done.

(2) If the patient's breathing is inadequate, provide positive-pressure ventilation with 100% oxygen and assess the adequacy of the ventilations delivered.

c. If neck or spine injury is not suspected, the patient should be placed on the left side with the head and chest tilted downward.

(1) Some authorities recommend placing the patient in a supine position due to the difficulty of maintaining the position described above.

(2) Consult medical direction or follow local protocol regarding patient positioning.

d. Maintain body temperature.

(1) Remove wet clothing.

(2) Dry the patient and cover with blankets, towels, or dry clothing.

e. If possible, obtain all relevant information regarding the patient's dive and relay to the receiving facility.

f. Consult medical direction regarding transport to a recompression facility.

DECOMPRESSION SICKNESS (BENDS)

1. **Pathophysiology**

    a. As a diver descends, nitrogen and oxygen are dissolved in the blood.

    b. If the diver ascends rapidly, there is not enough time for the nitrogen to be reabsorbed from the blood.

    c. Nitrogen bubbles form in the bloodstream, interfering with tissue perfusion.

    d. The size and location of the bubbles determine the patient's signs and symptoms.

2. Signs and symptoms of decompression sickness include:

    a. Fatigue

    b. Weakness

    c. Shortness of breath

    d. Skin rash

    e. Itch

    f. Joint soreness

    g. Dizziness

    h. Headache

    i. Paralysis

    j. Seizures

    k. Unconsciousness

3. **Emergency medical care for decompression sickness**

    a. Establish and maintain an open airway.

    b. Administer oxygen.

    (1) If the patient's breathing is adequate, apply oxygen by nonrebreather mask at 15 LPM if not already done.

    (2) If the patient's breathing is inadequate, provide positive-pressure ventilation with 100% oxygen and assess the adequacy of the ventilations delivered.

    c. If neck or spine injury is not suspected, the patient should be placed on the left side with the head and chest tilted downward.

    (1) Some authorities recommend placing the patient in a supine position due to the difficulty of maintaining the position described above.

    (2) Consult medical direction or follow local protocol regarding patient positioning.

    d. Maintain body temperature.

    (1) Remove wet clothing.

    (2) Dry the patient and cover with blankets, towels, or dry clothing.

    e. If possible, obtain all relevant information regarding the patient's dive and relay to the receiving facility.

f. Consult medical direction regarding transport to a recompression facility.

ENRICHMENT—BITES AND STINGS

SNAKEBITES

1. Venomous snakes in the United States include pit vipers and coral snakes.
   a. Pit vipers [rattlesnakes, cottonmouth (water) moccasins, and copperheads]
      (1) These snakes have the following features:
         (a) Pit (heat sensor) between eye and nostril
         (b) Catlike elliptical pupils
         (c) Triangular head
         (d) Two fangs
      (2) The bites of copperheads are rarely fatal.
   b. Coral snakes. These snakes have the following features:
      (1) Black, red, and yellow bands
         (a) "Red on yellow, kill a fellow."
         (b) "Red on black, venom lack."
      (2) Small fangs
      (3) Black head
      (4) Round, black eyes
2. **Signs and symptoms**
   a. Pit vipers
      (1) Local signs and symptoms include:
         (a) Fang marks or semicircle of teeth marks
         (b) Instant burning pain
         (c) Area becomes red and swollen
         (d) Discoloration and blisters common
      (2) Systemic signs and symptoms include:
         (a) Weakness
         (b) Sweating
         (c) Nausea and vomiting
         (d) Shock
   b. Coral snakes
      (1) Early signs and symptoms include:
         (a) Scratch marks or tiny puncture marks
         (b) Little or no pain at the site
         (c) Minimal to moderate swelling
         (d) Slurred speech
         (e) Muscle weakness
      (2) Late signs and symptoms (may be delayed for 12 hours or more) include:
         (a) Nausea/vomiting
         (b) Difficulty breathing
         (c) Seizures
         (d) Paralysis
         (e) Respiratory failure
3. **Emergency medical care for snakebites**
   a. Ensure the safety of all rescuers.
   b. Establish and maintain an open airway.
   c. Administer oxygen.
      (1) If the patient's breathing is adequate, apply oxygen by nonrebreather mask at 15 LPM if not already done.
      (2) If the patient's breathing is inadequate, provide positive-pressure ventilation with 100% oxygen and assess the adequacy of the ventilations delivered.

d. Keep the patient calm.

e. Gently wash the area.

f. If possible, remove jewelry from the injured area before swelling begins.

g. If the bite is on an extremity, position the extremity slightly below the level of the patient's heart.

    (1) Frequently reassess the presence of distal pulses in the affected extremity.

    (2) If swelling is present, note the circumference of the extremity at the site of the bite and reassess frequently to evaluate swelling progression.

h. Do not:

    (1) Apply cold

    (2) Cut the wound

    (3) Attempt to suck out the venom

i. Consult medical direction regarding the use of a constricting band.

j. Observe the patient closely for the development of signs and symptoms of an allergic reaction; treat as needed.

k. Transport promptly.

    (1) If the patient is stable, perform ongoing assessments every 15 minutes.

    (2) If the patient is unstable, perform ongoing assessments every 5 minutes.

SPIDER BITES

1. Black widow spider

  a. These spiders have shiny, black bodies with a red hourglass figure on the abdomen.

  b. The male is approximately half the size of the female, brown, and nonvenomous to humans.

  c. Signs and symptoms of a black widow spider bite include:

    (1) Vague history of sharp pinprick followed by dull, numbing pain

    (2) Tiny red marks at the point of entry of the venom

    (3) Swelling

    (4) Difficulty breathing

    (5) Severe pain beginning 15–60 minutes after bite and increasing for 12 to 48 hours

    (6) Lower extremity bite: localized pain followed by abdominal pain and rigidity

    (7) Upper extremity bite: pain and rigidity in chest, back, and shoulders

2. Brown recluse spider

  a. Brown recluse spiders are small, brown or tan in color and have a dark band shaped like a violin on the head/thorax.

  b. Signs and symptoms of a brown recluse spider bite include:

    (1) Mild stinging sensation at the site of bite

    (1) Local swelling

    (2) Fever

    (3) Weakness

    (4) Nausea/vomiting

    (5) Joint pain

    (6) Bluish ring around the bite appears within 2 to 8 hours after the bite

    (7) Redness and blister formation at site

    (8) Open sore formation at site in 7 to 14 days

3. Emergency medical care for spider bites

  a. Establish and maintain an open airway.

  b. Administer oxygen

    (1) If the patient's breathing is adequate, apply oxygen by nonrebreather mask at 15 LPM if not already done.

    (2) If the patient's breathing is inadequate, provide positive-pressure ventilation with 100% oxygen and assess the adequacy of the ventilations delivered.

c. Gently wash the area.

d. If possible, remove jewelry from the injured area before swelling begins.

e. If the bite is on an extremity, position the extremity slightly below the level of the patient's heart.

f. Observe the patient closely for the development of signs and symptoms of an allergic reaction; treat as needed.

g. Transport promptly.

  (1) If the patient is stable, perform ongoing assessments every 15 minutes.

  (2) If the patient is unstable, perform ongoing assessments every 5 minutes.

SCORPION STINGS

1. In North America, the sculptured or bark scorpion is the only species of scorpion that injects a venom that is dangerous to humans.

2. The scorpion injects venom by means of a stinger located on its tail.

3. Signs and symptoms of a scorpion sting include:

  a. Local pain at the sting site

  b. SLUDGE [salivation, lacrimation (tearing), urination, diarrhea, gastric cramping, emesis (vomiting)]

  c. Slurred speech

  d. Blurred vision

  e. Restlessness, jerking, and involuntary shaking

  f. Increased heart rate

  g. Seizures

4. **Emergency medical care for scorpion stings**

  a. Establish and maintain an open airway; excessive oral secretions may require frequent suctioning.

  b. Administer oxygen.

    (1) If the patient's breathing is adequate, apply oxygen by nonrebreather mask at 15 LPM if not already done.

    (2) If the patient's breathing is inadequate, provide positive-pressure ventilation with 100% oxygen and assess the adequacy of the ventilations delivered.

  c. Gently wash the area.

  d. If possible, remove jewelry from the injured area before swelling begins.

  e. If the bite is on an extremity, position the extremity slightly below the level of the patient's heart.

  f. Observe the patient closely for the development of signs and symptoms of an allergic reaction; treat as needed.

  g. Transport promptly.

    (1) If the patient is stable, perform ongoing assessments every 15 minutes.

    (2) If the patient is unstable, perform ongoing assessments every 5 minutes.

REVIEW QUESTIONS

Directions: Each of the numbered items or incomplete statements in this section is followed by answers or by completions of the statement. Select the ONE lettered answer or completion that is BEST in each case.

1. The body's core temperature is generally maintained within one degree of its normal temperature. When assessing and recording oral temperatures, the "normal" range is generally considered

    (A)   37–37.6° Fahrenheit (F)
    (B)   96–96.6° F
    (C)   96–98° F
    (D)   98–98.6° F

2. Oral or axillary temperature readings tend to be _____ than rectal temperature readings.

    (A)   about 1° Fahrenheit (F) lower
    (B)   about 1° F higher
    (C)   about 5° F lower
    (D)   about 5° F higher

3. Nerves throughout the body monitor changes in skin temperature and relay the information to the hypothalamus, the body's "thermostat." The hypothalamus is found

    (A)   in the neck
    (B)   in the chest
    (C)   in the brain
    (D)   in the dermal layer of the skin

4. When exposed to cold stimuli, the body attempts to preserve its core temperature. One method the body uses to preserve core temperature is

    (A)   stimulation of the sweat glands
    (B)   dilation of the peripheral blood vessels
    (C)   constriction of the peripheral blood vessels
    (D)   decreased production of epinephrine and slow metabolism

5. Which of the following is the preferred method for removing the clothes of this patient?

    (A)   The patient's clothing should be cut off in the back of the ambulance
    (B)   Removing the clothing of a patient in the prehospital setting is not necessary
    (C)   Have the patient remove her wet clothing before getting in the ambulance so water is not tracked into the ambulance
    (D)   Have the patient remove her wet clothing only after the temperature in the back of the ambulance is above 95° Fahrenheit (F)

6. Which of the following are signs and symptoms associated with moderate hypothermia?

    (A)   Cardiopulmonary arrest
    (B)   Shivering gradually replaced by muscular rigidity, decreasing pulse and respirations, decreasing level of consciousness
    (C)   Low to absent blood pressure, muscular rigidity, slow or absent breathing, slowly responding pupils
    (D)   Shivering, increased pulse and respiratory rates, difficulty in speech and movement, confusion, poor judgment

7. Which of the following is an example of a "passive warming" method for cold-exposure patients?

    (A)   Placing the patient in a drafty atmosphere
    (B)   Placing the patient in a warm environment
    (C)   Having the patient do calisthenics (e.g., jumping jacks)
    (D)   Placing warming pads in the patient's groin, armpits, and neck areas

8. Your rescue crew has been called to the scene for a 26-year-old male patient found floating in a lake. A friend of the patient states that he was "ice fishing" on the frozen lake when the patient fell in the ice. Time of submersion was approximately 3–5 minutes. The patient is cyanotic and cold to the touch. During the initial assessment, pulselessness should be assessed for _____ before beginning cardiopulmonary resuscitation (CPR).

   (A) 3–5 seconds
   (B) 5–10 seconds
   (C) 20–30 seconds
   (D) 30–45 seconds

9. Which of the following is appropriate management of a mildly hypothermic patient?

   (A) Rub or massage cold extremities to increase distal perfusion
   (B) Whenever possible, transport the patient in the prone position
   (C) Cover the patient's head with a blanket, but leave the face exposed
   (D) Encourage the patient to drink coffee or hot tea if conscious with an intact gag reflex

10. Local cold injury (frostbite) occurs when a specific area of the body is damaged due to exposure to prolonged or intense cold. These injuries are classified as either superficial or deep. Superficial cold injuries affect

   (A) all layers of the skin causing the affected area to be firm to palpation
   (B) only the fingers and toes causing the immediate formation of blisters
   (C) some layers of the skin causing numbness followed by tingling during rewarming efforts
   (D) the underlying tissues (muscles and organs) of the body causing a dull, waxy appearance of the skin

11. Your ambulance crew has been called to a local mountain range to assist in the treatment of a 34-year-old male patient who got lost while hunting. He was out overnight in freezing temperatures and was unable to get a fire started. While examining the patient, you discover that both feet appear to have suffered a deep cold injury. After consulting medical direction, you are instructed to begin active, rapid rewarming of the affected areas. This may be accomplished by

   (A) covering the bare feet with sterile gauze and a blanket
   (B) massaging the affected areas with warm compresses
   (C) submersing the patient's feet in circulating, warm water
   (D) starting a fire and putting the patient's bare feet near the fire

12. When treating a heat exposure patient with hot, dry skin and an altered mental status, your treatment should be geared toward

   (A) decreasing the patient's body temperature slowly and methodically
   (B) rapidly decreasing the patient's body temperature to induce shivering
   (C) rapidly decreasing the patient's body temperature without inducing shivering
   (D) maintaining the patient's current temperature until arrival at the emergency department

13. Which of the following is the preferred method of removing the stinger of an insect?

   (A) Suck the stinger out using your mouth
   (B) Scrape the stinger out using the edge of a plastic card
   (C) Pinch the stinger with gloved hands and pull straight out
   (D) Carefully grasp the stinger with tweezers and pull straight out

14. Your ambulance crew is called to treat a 34-year-old male patient complaining of severe abdominal cramping and difficulty breathing. He states that he was cleaning the garage about 10 hours ago when something pricked his thigh. The site is red and tender but has no discolored "rings" surrounding it. You suspect

(A) coral snake bite and treat by cleaning the site and administering high-flow oxygen
(B) black widow spider bite and treat by removing all distal jewelry, cleaning the site, and administering high-flow oxygen
(C) scorpion sting and treat by cleaning the site, applying a tourniquet, and suctioning the area en route to the hospital
(D) brown recluse spider bite and treat by making a small incision over the site and suctioning

Directions: Each of the numbered items or incomplete statements in this section is negatively phrased, as indicated by a capitalized word such as NOT, LEAST, or EXCEPT. Select the ONE lettered answer or completion that is BEST in each case.

15. Which of the following water-related scenarios would indicate that spinal immobilization would NOT be a primary concern?

(A) Suicide attempt by jumping from a 40-foot bridge
(B) A swimmer found unconscious in the water with a bloody nose
(C) An elderly swimmer experiencing chest pain while swimming in the ocean
(D) A jet skier who hit a log and is complaining of numbness in his feet and hands

16. Pit vipers and coral snakes are two types of venomous snakes found in the United States. Pit vipers include rattlesnakes, cottonmouth (water) moccasins, and copperheads. When treating a patient who has been bitten by a snake, which of the following treatments should NOT be initiated?

(A) Wash the site with soap and water
(B) Reassess the patient every 5 minutes
(C) Remove all jewelry distal to the bite
(D) Apply ice to the bite area to slow absorption of the venom

Directions: Each of the numbered questions or incomplete statements in this section refers to a scenario that precedes them. The numbered questions or incomplete statements are followed by answers or by completions of the statement. Select the answer or completion of the statement that is BEST in each case.

Your rescue crew is called to a lake recreation area for a 7-year-old female patient who had a submersion (under the water) incident. She reportedly fell out of a sailboat in the middle of the lake. According to the dispatch information, she was pulled from the water and taken to a dock. You arrive to find your patient shivering and wet sitting on a large rock. It is 68° Fahrenheit (F) outside with gusting winds.

Questions 17–20

17. While in the 58° F water, the patient lost body heat to the currents of water that swirled around her. This is an example of what type of heat loss?

(A) Radiation
(B) Convection
(C) Conduction
(D) Evaporation

18. The rock on which the patient sits is cold to the touch. The patient's loss of heat to the rock is an example of what type of heat loss?

(A) Radiation
(B) Convection
(C) Conduction
(D) Evaporation

19. The patient is wearing jeans and a long-sleeved sweater that are soaked. Heat loss through the wet clothes is an example of heat loss by

(A) Radiation
(B) Convection
(C) Conduction
(D) Evaporation

20. An assessment of the patient's oral temperature reveals that she is in moderate hypothermia. Appropriate treatment for this patient would be to

(A) wrap the patient in a sheet or blanket, provide high-flow oxygen, and transport
(B) continuously irrigate the patient with warm water, provide high-flow oxygen, and transport
(C) remove the patient's wet clothing, wrap her in a blanket, turn on the ambulance heater, provide high-flow oxygen, and transport
(D) remove the patient's wet clothing, wrap her in a blanket, vigorously massage the extremities, turn on the ambulance heater, provide high-flow oxygen, and transport

Your rescue crew has been called to a local park for a 65-year-old female patient complaining of weakness and dizziness. It is a hot, humid summer day. You arrive to find your patient sitting in the sun on a park bench. Her skin condition is cool, pale, and moist. She greets you as you approach and is in a moderate level of distress.

Questions 21–23

21. Which of the following should you do first?

(A) Assess baseline vital signs
(B) Perform a rapid trauma assessment
(C) Assist the patient to the back of your air-conditioned ambulance
(D) Begin cooling the patient with ice packs to the groin, armpits, and neck area

22. This patient is responsive and does not complain of nausea. Which of the following regarding oral intake is correct?

(A) You may allow the patient to drink water
(B) You may allow the patient to drink iced tea
(C) You may allow the patient to eat but not drink
(D) You may allow the patient to drink a cold soda

23. The preferred position in which to transport this patient is

  (A) Sitting upright at a 90° angle
  (B) Fully immobilized to a long backboard
  (C) Prone with the arms dangling off the stretcher
  (D) Supine with the legs elevated about 8 to 12 inches

You have been called to the home of a 24-year-old female patient complaining of weakness, nausea, and joint pain. She informs you she just returned from a SCUBA diving excursion. She tells you, "I think it is just the flu, but my boyfriend made me call." She denies any past medical history.

Questions 24–25

24. This patient should be transported in what position?

  (A) Fully immobilized on a long backboard
  (B) On her left side with the head and chest tilted downward
  (C) Sitting upright at a 90° angle with her legs dangling over the edge of the stretcher
  (D) Prone, with her head slightly elevated

25. En route, the patient suffers a full-body seizure and does not regain consciousness. Based on the history of present illness, you suspect

  (A) barotrauma and treat with low-flow oxygen by nasal cannula and continuous reassessment
  (B) epilepsy and treat with high-flow oxygen by nonrebreather mask and continuous reassessment
  (C) hypoglycemia and treat with oral glucose, low-flow oxygen by nasal cannula, and continuous reassessment
  (D) decompression sickness (the "bends") and treat with high-flow oxygen by nonrebreather mask and continuous reassessment intermittently en route to the hospital

ANSWERS AND RATIONALES

1-D. A "normal" oral temperature is between 98° and 98.6° Fahrenheit (F) [approximately 37° Centigrade (Celsius)]. Oral temperatures can be influenced by previous oral intake, patient compliance, and atmospheric conditions, among other factors.

2-A. Rectal temperature readings are more reliable, but more invasive than a temperature obtained orally or in the armpit (axillary). The temperature measured in the armpit or orally is about 1° Fahrenheit less than the rectal temperature.

3-C. The hypothalamus is positioned at the base of the brain (just above and behind the pituitary gland, the "master" gland of the body and the endocrine system). Receptors throughout the body send information about the body's temperature to the brain, where the hypothalamus processes and responds to this information. Hypothalamus function in elderly individuals may be impaired, thus making them more susceptible to heat or cold emergencies.

4-C. Constriction of the peripheral blood vessels decreases the amount of blood (and heat) flowing from the body's core. When stimulated by cold, the body will also increase the production and release of epinephrine and other hormones, which cause the metabolism rate to rise. [Metabolism is the body's process of "burning" sugar (glucose) in the presence of oxygen to produce energy or heat.] Stimulation of the sweat glands leads to sweat production that lowers the body temperature due to evaporation. Dilation of the peripheral blood vessels increases the amount of blood (and heat) leaving the core, hence the flushed, "beet red" appearance observed in persons working outside in moderate to high temperatures.

5-A. Hypothermic patients must be handled with extreme care because you do not want to stimulate cold, acidotic blood in the extremities to return to the core. The best way to remove clothing without much movement by the patient is to cut the clothing away. Do not be concerned with water tracked into the ambulance. If you have ample towels and blankets, you will be able to properly treat the patient regardless of the amount of water she may have on her. Do not leave the clothing on until the ambulance temperature reaches a certain level. If the patient is covered with a blanket, she will retain more heat than if she were to keep her wet clothes on.

6-B. This response lists some of the more classic signs and symptoms of moderate hypothermia. There are four main body responses (other than temperature) that may give you a good idea of the patient's changing condition: mental status, airway and breathing status, circulatory status, and motor function status. Mental status may progress (decline) from difficulty speaking, to confusion and memory lapse, to combativeness, to unconsciousness. Airway and breathing status may progress from increased respirations, to slow and shallow respirations, to apnea (absence of breathing). Circulation may progress from rapid heart rate, to irregular heart rate and low blood pressure, to slow or absent heart rate with low or absent blood pressure. Motor function may progress from lack of coordination, to shivering, to rigidity.

7-B. Heating the passenger's area of the ambulance and covering the patient with a blanket are examples of passive warming. Placing warming pads on the patient is an example of active warming. Consult medical direction and local protocol before initiating active warming measures. Placing a patient in a drafty area would result in decreased temperature due to convection (the movement of the air). Having the patient exercise is absolutely contraindicated.

8-D. Severely hypothermic patients may have a very slow heart rate. When assessing these patients, check the pulse for an extended period. If cardiopulmonary resuscitation (CPR) is indicated, it would be appropriate to reevaluate the patient for the presence of a pulse about every 2 minutes. Remember, "They are not dead until they are warm and dead."

9-C. Roughly half the patient's body heat is lost through radiant energy escaping from the head. Therefore, protecting against this form of heat loss is essential. Leave the patient's face uncovered so that you may continuously assess the patient's airway and breathing. Never rub or massage a cold emergency patient. Transporting the patient prone (on the stomach) decreases your ability to assess the airway properly. Do not allow any cold (or heat) emergency patient to drink any fluid that contains caffeine or alcohol.

10-C. Patients may be unaware of their superficial frostbite due to the numbing effect on local nerves. The skin may appear red and inflamed; however, the skin retains its supple, elastic nature. While the most commonly affected areas are the nose, cheeks, chin, ears, hands, and feet, any portion of the skin (if exposed) can be frostbitten. If all layers of the skin are affected and the area is firm to palpation and/or has a dull, white, waxy appearance, the injury is most likely a deep frostbite.

11-C. The best method for warming an affected extremity is to submerse the extremity in warm water since the temperature of water can be closely monitored. The water temperature should be consistent and uniform. Make sure that the water is not allowed to cool. Anticipate that this patient will experience extreme pain as the area warms. As with all unstable heat and cold emergency patients, advanced-life-support (ALS) level care should be requested early. Covering the patient's feet with gauze and a blanket is an example of passive warming measures. Massaging is contraindicated. Finally, the use of an open fire is not a good idea for several reasons. This patient needs to be transported to a medical facility. The heat from a fire cannot be adequately measured. You may burn the patient, causing more harm. If you are unable to begin transport and are considering starting a fire, do not attempt to warm/thaw a frostbitten area if the danger of refreezing exists. The damage will be worse than if the area were initially allowed to stay cold.

12-C. Core body temperatures can soar above 105° F. The brain and internal organs can only take this type of punishment for a short period before irreversible damage takes place. Your efforts should be directed at cooling the body as quickly as possible without activating the body's heat-generating mechanisms (e.g., shivering). Move the patient to a cool area; remove clothing; moisten the skin with cool water; and apply padded cool compresses to the armpits, back of the neck, and the groin. Never apply ice directly to the skin as you may cause a local cold emergency (frostbite), which can also result in shivering.

13-B. Care should be taken not to squeeze or pinch the venom sac of a stinger. The venom sac contains a toxin. By scraping the stinger and avoiding contact with the venom sac, you may be able to decrease the dose of the injected venom.

14-B. The location, sensation, and side effects of the bite suggest a black widow spider bite. A coral snakebite would not, in an awake and conscious patient, go unnoticed (especially on the thigh). While a scorpion sting may produce similar complaints, treatment with a tourniquet is inappropriate. Brown recluse spider bites will usually present with a "target" mark within 8 hours. A "target" mark is a bluish ring surrounding the bite area and a blister at the bite. The treatment for these bites and stings is basically the same: continue to monitor closely to ensure that the patient is not having an allergic (anaphylactic) reaction to the bite, obtain SAMPLE information, perform a focused history and physical examination, clean the site, remove distal jewelry, provide oxygen therapy, and transport.

15-C. Full spinal immobilization should be instituted for water emergencies that involve trauma or where the cause of the emergency is unknown (i.e., a patient found floating in a pool). An elderly swimmer experiencing cardiac problems need not be immobilized.

16-D. While washing the bite area is appropriate, remove distal jewelry (due to later swelling), and continuously monitor your patient. The application of ice to the bite area should be avoided because it may result in further tissue damage. Washing the site of a coral snake bite is especially important since coral snakes, unlike pit vipers, do not inject their venom. Rather, they secrete (drool) their venom over their short, stubby teeth. The venom is then absorbed through the small cuts created by the grinding action of the coral snake's bite. You may successfully wash off much of the poison by immediately washing the area with cool water and soap. Avoid using hot water, because hot water tends to open the pores of the skin.

17-B. The loss of heat by moving liquids or air is convection. Patients will lose heat in liquid much more rapidly than in air of the same temperature. Radiation is the loss of body heat as heat rays (which travel much like light rays). The warmth felt from the sun is an example of radiant heat. Conduction is the loss of heat through direct contact (e.g., touching an ice cube). Evaporation is the loss of heat due to the vaporization of a liquid. The sweating mechanism is the most common example of this form of heat loss.

18-C. The loss of heat through direct contact is conduction. Do not underestimate these factors (convection, conduction, radiation, and evaporation) in your patient's decline toward hypothermia. You need to be aware of the factors influencing your patient's status. Once this patient slipped into a hypothermic state [temperature below 95° Fahrenheit (F)], she lost the ability to sufficiently generate heat to restore a normal core temperature. The low core temperature affects the ability of the organs to function. Your swift and appropriate response may make the difference between life and death.

19-D. Evaporation is the loss of heat through the vaporization of a fluid. While the most common form of evaporation is sweating, any fluid may vaporize and reduce body temperature.

20-C. If the patient stays wet, evaporation will continue. Park your ambulance as close to the patient as possible and preheat the patient area (if you think hypothermia may be a concern based on the dispatch information and the weather). Move the patient to the back of the ambulance as soon as possible. Remove the patient's clothing including wet socks, undergarments, hats, etc. Cover the patient with a warm, dry blanket. Provide high-flow oxygen, heated and humidified if possible, and transport. Contact medical direction for further instructions regarding the care of this patient. Do not irrigate the patient with warm water. Do not rub the patient to increase warmth; rubbing may cause chilled, acidotic blood to return to the body's core.

21-C. Before obtaining your SAMPLE history and focused physical exam, you must prevent further injury to the patient. All other assessments and interventions should be conducted in a less oppressive atmosphere.

22-A. If allowed by local protocol and medical direction, this patient may take sips of water. If, however, the patient complains of nausea or has an altered mental status, you should not allow any oral intake. Never allow a heat (or cold) emergency patient to drink any caffeinated or alcoholic beverage.

23-D. The preferred position for this patient is the "shock position," supine with the legs elevated. Elevating the legs helps reduce the workload of the heart by facilitating the return of blood. This position may also assist in maintaining an acceptable blood pressure. Sitting at a 90° angle would have the opposite effect. There are no indications that spinal immobilization is necessary. Positioning the patient prone (on her stomach) complicates your ability to monitor the patient's airway. Allowing the arms to dangle below the level of the heart causes the heart to work harder.

24-B. If this patient has had a diving-related injury, the possibility exists that small bubbles of gas are floating around in her body. The best way to remember the proper positioning of such a patient is to remember that the brain and the heart are important organs, and gases tend to rise. Therefore, lower the brain and lower the heart.

25-D. Decompression sickness, also known as the "bends," occurs when divers ascend (come up) too quickly. Gases in their body expand too rapidly and bubbles are formed. The signs and symptoms associated with this are fatigue, weakness, shortness of breath, skin rash, itch, joint pain, dizziness, headache, paralysis, seizures, and unconsciousness. If the possibility exists that you will treat a diving-related injury, you should be aware of the nearest decompression chamber. When patients are put in this device, the pressure is increased so that the air bubbles "dissolve," and then the pressure is brought down in a controlled manner so bubbles do not form. Barotrauma is also an ascent injury. It occurs when divers surface too quickly. he change in atmospheric pressure changes too rapidly for the air-filled chambers of the body (e.g., sinus cavities, abdomen, lungs, ears). These cavities become damaged or rupture. The signs and symptoms are associated with the rupture of these chambers.

BIBLIOGRAPHY

Crosby LA, Lewallen DG (eds): *Emergency Care and Transportation of the Sick and Injured*, 6th ed. Rosemont, IL, American Academy of Orthopaedic Surgeons, 1995.

Grant HD, Murray RH Jr, Bergeron JD: *Emergency Care*, 7th ed. Englewood Cliffs, NJ, Prentice-Hall, 1995.

Guyton AC, Hall JE: *Textbook of Medical Physiology*, 9th ed. Philadelphia, WB Saunders, 1996.

Hafen BQ, Karren KJ, Mistovich JJ: *Prehospital Emergency Care*, 5th ed. Upper Saddle River, NJ, Prentice-Hall, 1996.

Henry MC, Stapleton ER, Judd RL: *EMT: Prehospital Care*. Philadelphia, WB Saunders, 1992.

Kitt S, Selfridge-Thomas J, Proehl JA, et al: *Emergency Nursing: A Physiologic and Clinical Perspective*, 2nd ed. Philadelphia, WB Saunders, 1995.

McSwain NE, White RD, Paturas JL, et al (eds): *The Basic EMT: Comprehensive Prehospital Patient Care*. St. Louis, Mosby-Year Book, 1996.

Sanders MJ: *Mosby's Paramedic Textbook*. St. Louis, Mosby-Year Book, 1994.

Sheehy SB, Lombardi JE: *Manual of Emergency Care*. 4th ed. St. Louis, Mosby-Year Book, 1995.

Sloane E: *Anatomy and Physiology: An Easy Learner*. Boston, Jones and Bartlett, 1994.

Stoy WA: *Mosby's EMT-Basic Textbook*. St. Louis, Mosby-Year Book, 1996.

Thibodeau GA, Patton KT: *The Human Body in Health and Disease*. St. Louis, Mosby-Year Book, 1992.

Tortora GJ, Grabowski SR: *Principles of Anatomy and Physiology*, 7th ed. New York, Harper-Collins, 1993.

United States Department of Transportation, National Highway Traffic Safety Administration: *Emergency Medical Technician: Basic. National Standard Curriculum*, 1994.

23 BEHAVIORAL EMERGENCIES

23-1 Define behavioral emergencies.

23-2 Discuss the general factors that may cause an alteration in a patient's behavior.

23-3 State the various reasons for psychological crises.

23-4 Discuss the characteristics of an individual's behavior that suggest that the patient is at risk for suicide.

23-5 Discuss the special considerations for assessing a patient with behavioral problems.

23-6 Discuss methods to calm behavioral emergency patients.

23-7 Discuss the general principles of an individual's behavior that suggest that he or she is at risk for violence.

23-8 Discuss special medical/legal considerations for managing behavioral emergencies.

BEHAVIOR

TERMINOLOGY

1. **Behavior** is the manner in which a person acts or performs. It includes any or all activities of a person, including physical and mental activity.
2. **Abnormal behavior** is a manner of acting or conducting oneself that:
   a. Is not consistent with society's norms and expectations
   b. Interferes with the individual's well-being and ability to function

MOTIVATION FOR LEARNING

Behavioral emergencies generally require long-term management. In the field, the EMT-Basic must recognize the general factors that can cause alteration in a patient's behavior and know the medical/legal considerations for management of these patients. The EMT-Basic must also ensure his or her own safety when caring for these patients.

    c. May be harmful to the individual or others

3. A **behavioral emergency** is a situation in which the patient exhibits abnormal behavior within a given situation that is unacceptable or intolerable to the patient, family members, or community. A behavioral emergency can be due to:

    a. Extremes of emotion leading to violence or other inappropriate behavior

    b. A psychological or physical condition (e.g., mental illness, lack of oxygen, low blood sugar)

BEHAVIORAL CHANGE

1. Factors that may cause a change in a patient's behavior include:

    a. Alcohol or drugs

    b. Situational stresses, such as:

        (1) Rape

        (2) Loss of a job

        (3) Career change

        (4) Death of a loved one

        (5) Marital stress or divorce

        (6) Physical or psychological abuse

        (7) Disasters, either natural (e.g., tornado, flood, earthquake, hurricane) or man-made (e.g., war, explosion)

    b. Medical illnesses, such as:

        (1) Poisoning

        (2) Central nervous system infection

        (3) Head trauma

        (4) Seizure disorder

        (5) Lack of oxygen (hypoxia)

        (6) Low blood sugar (hypoglycemia)

        (7) Inadequate blood flow to the brain

        (8) Extremes of temperature (e.g., excessive cold or heat)

    c. Psychiatric problems, such as:

        (1) Phobia

        (2) Paranoia

        (3) Depression

        (4) Schizophrenia

        (5) Suicidal acts

        (6) Homicidal acts

        (7) Bipolar disorder

        (8) Anxiety disorder

PSYCHOLOGICAL CRISES

ANXIETY/PANIC

1. Fear and anxiety are normal responses to a perceived threat.

2. Fear and anxiety bring on symptoms including worry, confusion, apprehension, helplessness, and negative thoughts.

3. **Fear.** Fear is usually triggered by a specific object or situation, such as:

    a. Fear of failing an examination

    b. Fear of being unable to pay the bills

4. **Anxiety**

    a. **Anxiety** is a state of apprehension and uneasiness, usually triggered by a vague or imagined situation. Anxiety includes:

        (1) Feeling of "losing control"

        (2) Feeling of not being able to meet another person's expectations

b. Anxiety can appear in different forms and at different levels of intensity, ranging from uneasiness to a panic attack.
   (1) Some anxiety is believed to increase awareness and the ability to perform.
   (2) As anxiety increases, it drains energy, shortens the attention span, and interferes with thinking and problem-solving.
c. Signs and symptoms of anxiety can be due to a medical cause, such as:
   (1) Asthma
   (2) Diabetes
   (3) Heart problems
   (4) Thyroid disorder
   (5) Seizure disorder
   (6) Inner ear disturbances
   (7) Premenstrual syndrome (PMS)
   (8) Withdrawal from alcohol, sedatives, tranquilizers
   (9) Reaction to cocaine, amphetamines, caffeine, aspartame or other stimulants
   (10) Environmental toxins (e.g., hydrocarbons, food additives, mercury, pesticides)
   (11) Medications (e.g., some blood pressure medications, cold medications, thyroid medications, sleeping pills, steroids, stimulants)
d. Anxiety disorder differs from normal anxiety. An anxiety disorder:
   (1) Is more intense than normal anxiety (e.g., panic attacks)
   (2) Lasts longer (e.g., lasts for months instead of going away after a stressful situation is over)
   (3) Leads to phobias that interfere with the individual's life
5. Panic attack
   a. A **panic attack** is an intense state of fear that occurs for no apparent reason.
   b. Panic attacks can build gradually over several minutes or hours or occur suddenly.
   c. Most panic attacks do not last longer than one-half hour.
   d. A panic attack is defined by the presence of four or more of the following symptoms at the same time:
      (1) Choking
      (2) Sweating
      (3) Hot flashes or chills
      (4) Trembling or shaking
      (5) Dizziness or faintness
      (6) Nausea or abdominal distress
      (7) Fear of going crazy or being out of control
      (8) Fear of becoming seriously ill or dying
      (9) Shortness of breath or a smothering sensation
      (10) Heart palpitations (rapid or irregular heartbeat)
      (11) Feeling of detachment or being out of touch with oneself
      (12) Numbness or tingling sensations (usually in the fingers, toes, or lips)
   e. A panic disorder is characterized by unexpected panic attacks that occur "out of the blue" for no apparent reason (e.g., no medical cause or external threat is present).

PHOBIAS

1. A **phobia** is an irrational and persistent fear of a specific activity, object, or situation.
2. Specific phobias are common and usually do not create a problem in life because the individual simply avoids the specific activity, object, or situation.
3. Common specific phobias include a fear of heights, darkness, elevators, flying, insects, doctors or dentists, thunder and/or lightning, blood, and animals.
4. Agoraphobia is a fear of open spaces.
   a. Individuals with panic disorder often develop agoraphobia.

b. The individual is afraid of being in a place or situation in which escaping might be difficult or where help might be unavailable if he or she were to experience a panic attack.

c. The individual with agoraphobia often:

    (1)   Avoids being outside his or her home alone

    (2)   Avoids public transportation

    (3)   Avoids restaurants, grocery stores, department stores

5. A phobic reaction may include panic, sweating, difficulty breathing and/or increased heart rate.

DEPRESSION

1. Depression is a mental state characterized by feelings of sadness, worthlessness, and discouragement.

2. Depression often occurs in response to a loss (e.g., job, independence, death of a loved one, end of a relationship).

3. Signs of depression vary with age.

  a. Children

    (1)   Depressed children may be sad, irritable, or cry frequently.

    (2)   They may express anger by acting out toward parents, teachers, or other authority figures.

    (3)   Older children may have no appetite and may experience headaches or skin disorders.

  b. Adolescents

    (1)   Depressed adolescents may behave unpredictably, run away, or change their physical and social activities.

    (2)   They may have no appetite, show no interest in their appearance, excessively use alcohol or drugs, or attempt suicide.

  c. Adults

    (1)   Depressed adults have feelings of guilt, anger, sadness, helplessness, hopelessness, loneliness, and worthlessness.

    (2)   Depression in adults is characterized by crying, sadness, or irritability.

    (3)   Depressed adults show a lack of interest in job, home, or appearance.

    (4)   They focus on negative aspects of life, past events, and failures.

    (5)   They may attempt suicide.

    (6)   Physical signs and symptoms may include loss of appetite, diarrhea or constipation, fatigue, inability to sleep, muscle aches, vague pains, weight loss, and early awakening with an inability to resume sleep.

  d. Elderly

    (1)   Depression in the elderly is often related to retirement; a loss, such as death of a spouse or other loved one; or the belief that he or she lacks control over his or her life (or present situation).

    (2)   Older adults may not label their feelings as depression but instead as "helplessness."

    (3)   The elderly individual may experience:

        (a) Feelings of uselessness or of being a "burden"

        (b) Feelings of loneliness as loved ones die or move away

    (4)   Signs and symptoms of depression in the elderly:

        (a) Are often confused with normal changes of aging

        (b) May include confusion, irritability, headaches, changes in appetite, constipation, inability to sleep, and thoughts of suicide

    (5)   It is common for depressed older adults to withdraw and not speak to anyone, confine themselves to bed, and not take care of bodily functions.

BIPOLAR DISORDER

1. Bipolar disorder is also known as manic-depressive disorder.

2. The patient has alternating episodes of mood elevation (mania) and depression.

3. When manic, the patient:
   a. Appears restless
   b. Is easily distracted
   c. Requires little sleep
   d. Develops unrealistic plans
   e. Is extremely energetic and enthusiastic
   f. Believes he or she possesses special powers and/or abilities
   g. Has racing thoughts and speech, often rambling and changing topics with little or no logical pattern
4. The patient with bipolar disorder will also usually experience periods of major depression in which he or she feels worthless and may consider suicide.

PARANOIA

1. **Paranoia** is a mental disorder characterized by excessive suspiciousness or other delusions, often of persecution or grandeur.
   a. **Delusions** are false beliefs that the patient maintains are true, despite facts to the contrary.
   b. Common delusions of paranoid patients include:
      (1) Believing that people are out to get them (persecution); being followed, harassed, plotted against
      (2) Believing that he or she possesses great power or special abilities (grandeur)
      (3) Believing that he or she is a famous person
2. Paranoid patients may experience **hallucinations.**
   a. Hallucinations are false perceptions (e.g., the patient sees things others cannot see).
   b. Hallucinations can be auditory (hearing voices), visual (worms or snakes crawling on the floor), or tactile (insects crawling on the skin).
3. Paranoid patients:
   a. Are suspicious and distrustful, often feeling they are being mistreated and misjudged
   b. Tend to carry grudges, recalling wrongs done to them years before
   c. Are excitable and unpredictable with outbursts of bizarre or aggressive behavior

SCHIZOPHRENIA

1. **Schizophrenia** is a group of mental disorders.
2. Characteristics of schizophrenia include:
   a. Confusion
   b. Combative behavior
   c. Reserved and withdrawn
   d. Delusions and hallucinations
   e. Rambling, disorganized speech
   f. Bizarre or disorganized behavior
   g. Indifferent to the feelings of others
   h. High risk for suicidal and homicidal behavior
   i. Prefers to be alone, has few, if any, close friends
   j. Disorganized and fragmented thoughts, perceptions, and emotional reactions

SUICIDE

OVERVIEW

1. **Suicide** is any willful act designed to end one's own life.
2. Most patients who commit suicide express their intentions beforehand.

3. Every suicide threat or gesture should be taken seriously and the patient transported for evaluation.
4. The EMT-Basic must recognize and take steps to prevent a patient from committing the act of suicide.

ASSESSMENT FOR SUICIDE RISK

1. SAD PERSONS is a scale that may be used as a guide to determine suicide potential (*Table 23-1*).
   a. Each portion of the scale is assigned a point value of 0 or 1; 10 possible points.
   b. 0 represents lowest risk, 10 highest risk.
2. **Sex**
   a. Men commit suicide more frequently than women, although women attempt suicide more frequently than men.
   b. Men tend to use more lethal methods than women.
      (1) Men tend to use firearms.
      (2) Women tend to use drugs.
3. **Age**
   a. Suicide is a leading cause of death in individuals 15–45 years old.
   b. Adolescents, college students, and persons over age 45 are at higher risk than the general population.
   c. Older men (more than 55 years of age) are most likely to succeed at suicide.
   d. Younger persons attempt suicide more often.
4. **Depression**
   a. Depression is a significant factor contributing to suicide.
   b. The patient with feelings of hopelessness, helplessness, or exhaustion is at increased risk.
   c. Arrest, imprisonment, or loss of job may be a source of depression.
5. **Previous suicide attempt**
   a. Risk is greatest in those who have previously attempted suicide.
   b. If there have been several attempts in a short period, risk is significantly increased.
   c. Lethality (the probability of successful suicide) may increase with successive attempts, increasing risk (e.g., patient previously ingested pills, slashed wrists on second attempt).
6. **Ethanol (alcohol) abuse**
   a. Substance abuse increases suicide risk.
   b. The alcoholic may commit suicide on impulse.
   c. Some patients become suicidal only when intoxicated.
7. **Rational thinking (impaired)**
   a. Suicide may be viewed as "the only way out" of an emotional situation.

Table 23-1. Assessment of Suicide Risk: SAD PERSONS Scale

S	Sex
A	Age
D	Depression
P	Previous suicide attempt
E	Ethanol (alcohol) abuse
R	Rational thinking (impaired)
S	Social support lacking
O	Organized plan
N	No spouse
S	Sickness

    b. Patients with delusions or hallucinations are at increased risk (e.g., schizophrenia).

8. **Social support lacking**
   a. Those who live alone or are single, separated, widowed, or divorced are at increased risk.
   b. Unemployed individuals are at increased risk.
   c. Some occupations have an increased suicide risk (e.g., law enforcement personnel, physicians, dentists).
9. **Organized plan**
   a. The more well-thought out the plan, the more serious the risk.
   b. The patient who has chosen a lethal plan of action and verbalized it to others is at increased risk.
   c. An unusual gathering of articles that could be used to commit suicide increases risk (e.g., purchase of a gun, large volumes of pills).
10. **No spouse.** Suicide risk is high in those who are widowed or divorced.
11. **Sickness**
   a. Recent diagnosis of a serious illness increases risk.
   b. Chronic, severe, or debilitating illness increases risk.

ASSESSING THE PATIENT WITH A BEHAVIORAL EMERGENCY

GENERAL PRINCIPLES

1. Be prepared to spend time at the scene.
2. Approach the patient slowly and purposefully; do not make any quick movements. If the patient is lying supine, it is safer to approach from the head.
3. Clearly identify yourself.
   a. Explain who you are and what you are trying to do for the patient.
   b. If the patient is confused, repeating this information may be necessary.
4. Maintain good eye contact with the patient.
   a. Face the patient.
   b. Sit or stand at or below the patient's level.
   c. Maintain a comfortable distance from the patient.
5. Be calm, direct, courteous, and respectful.
   a. Ask questions in a calm, reassuring voice.
   b. Do not talk down to the patient.
6. Allow the patient to tell his or her story without being judgmental.
   a. Accept the patient's right to have his or her own feelings.
   b. Avoid threatening actions, statements, and questions.
   c. Do not allow your personal feelings to obstruct your professional judgment.
   d. Be aware of your own reactions (e.g., an anxious patient may make you anxious; a hostile patient may make you angry).
   e. Show you are listening by rephrasing or repeating part of what is said.
7. Provide honest reassurance.
   a. Respond honestly to the patient's questions.
   b. Tell the truth; do not lie to the patient.
   c. Do not make promises you cannot keep.
   d. Do not "play along" with visual or auditory disturbances of the patient.
      (1) Do not tell the patient you believe his or her hallucinations or delusions in an attempt to win his or her trust.
      (2) Letting the patient know that you do not hear what he or she is hearing but are interested in knowing what it is he or she is hearing is recommended.
   e. Let the patient know what you expect and what he or she can expect from you.
8. Take a definite plan of action.

    a. Inform the patient of what you are doing.

    b. Encourage purposeful activity (e.g., help the patient gather the belongings he or she wants to take to the hospital).

    c. Remain with the patient at all times.

9. Do not threaten, challenge, or argue with disturbed patients.

10. Involve trusted family members or friends.

11. Avoid unnecessary physical contact.

    a. Respect the patient's territory; limit physical touch.

    b. If physical restraint is necessary, call additional help as needed.

12. Do not assume you cannot talk with a patient until you have tried.

SCENE SIZE-UP

1. Determine if a violent or potentially unsafe situation exists.

    a. When approaching a violent or potentially violent patient, your primary concern should always be for your own safety first.

    b. Approach the patient from the head if the patient is lying supine.

    c. Evaluate the scene for possible dangers.

        (1) Visually locate the patient.

        (2) Note the presence of drugs or alcohol.

        (3) Scan the area for possible weapons.

    d. If you suspect a dangerous situation, do not enter the scene until law enforcement personnel are present and the safety of the scene is assured.

2. **Assessment of potential violence**

    a. **History.** Check with family and bystanders to determine if the patient has a known history of aggression or combativeness.

    b. **Posture.** The following patient postures may indicate potential violence:

        (1) Patient stands or sits in a position that threatens self or others

        (2) Inability to sit still, pacing

        (3) Fists or jaw clenched

        (4) Unsafe object in hands

    c. **Speech.** The following speech patterns may indicate potential violence:

        (1) Yells, shouts

        (2) Uses abusive language

        (3) Threats of harm to self or others

        (4) Erratic speech pattern

    d. **Physical activity.** The following physical activities may indicate potential violence:

        (1) Moves toward rescuers

        (2) Carries heavy or threatening objects

        (3) Makes quick, irregular movements

    e. Other signs of potential violence include:

        (1) Has flushed face, agitation

        (2) Turns away when spoken to

        (3) Avoids eye contact

        (4) Patient in an unsafe environment (e.g., domestic violence, gang activity)

3. In the absence of obvious danger, observe the scene for information to assist with patient assessment and care, including:

    a. Signs of violence

    b. Evidence of suicide attempt

    c. Evidence of substance abuse

    d. General environmental condition

4. Do not place the patient between yourself and the exit.

INITIAL ASSESSMENT

1. Limit the number of people around patient; isolate the patient if necessary.

2. Maintain alertness to danger.

3. Assess the patient's mental status.
   a. Observe the patient's appearance, dress, hygiene.
   b. Note the patient's orientation to person, place, time, and event.
   c. Note the patient's speech (e.g., garbled, unintelligible).
   d. Observe the patient's mood (e.g., anxiety, depression, elation, agitation, angry, hostile, fearful).
   e. Note the patient's thought process (e.g., disordered, delusions, hallucinations, unusual worries, fears).
4. Assess the patient's airway.
5. Assess breathing.
6. Assess circulation.
7. Identify any life-threatening conditions and provide care based on these findings.
8. Establish patient priorities.
   a. Priority patients include:
      (1) Patients who give a poor general impression
      (2) Patients experiencing difficulty breathing
      (3) Patients with signs and symptoms of shock
      (4) Unresponsive patients with no gag reflex or cough
      (5) Responsive patients who are unable to follow commands
   b. Advanced-life-support (ALS) assistance should be requested as soon as possible.
   c. If ALS personnel are not available, the patient should be transported promptly to the closest appropriate facility.

FOCUSED HISTORY AND PHYSICAL EXAMINATION

1. Remove the patient from the crisis or disturbing situation, if not already done.
2. If the patient is unresponsive:
   a. Perform a rapid physical examination
   b. Follow with evaluation of baseline vital signs and gathering of the patient's medical history
3. If the patient is responsive:
   a. Gather information about the patient's medical history before performing the physical examination
   b. Gather a SAMPLE history
4. **SAMPLE history**
   a. **Signs and symptoms.** Determine the patient's signs and symptoms.
   b. **Allergies.** Determine if the patient has any allergies to medications and other substances or materials.
   c. **Medications.** Determine if the patient is taking any medications (prescription and over the counter).
      (1) Determine if the patient takes his or her medications regularly and his or her response to them.
      (2) Determine if there has been any recent change in medications (additions, deletions, or change in dosages).
      (3) Provide all information obtained to the receiving facility.
   d. **Pertinent past medical history.** Ascertain whether the patient has any of the following conditions:
      (1) Head trauma
      (2) Alcohol or substance abuse
      (3) Seizure disorder
      (4) Psychiatric history (e.g., diagnosis, hospitalizations, response to treatment)
   e. **Last oral intake.** Determine the patient's last oral intake.
   f. **Event.** Determine the events leading to the present situation.
      (1) Who called for help? (e.g., patient, family member)
      (2) Why is the patient (or family member) asking for help now?
      (3) Has the patient thought of harming himself or anyone else?
      (4) Is the patient hearing voices or seeing things?

5. Assess baseline vital signs.
6. Perform a focused physical examination.

EMERGENCY MEDICAL CARE FOR BEHAVIORAL EMERGENCIES

1. Ensure the safety of rescuers, the patient, and bystanders.
   a. Control violent situations.
   b. Do not leave the patient alone.
   c. Do not turn your back on a violent or potentially violent patient.
2. Assess the patient for the presence of trauma or a medical condition and treat accordingly.
3. If the patient is in imminent danger to himself or others, physical restraint may be necessary.
   a. Physical restraint should be a last resort.
   b. Consider the need for law enforcement personnel.
   c. Follow local protocol.
4. Transport the patient to an appropriate facility for further evaluation and treatment.
   a. If cases of an overdose, bring any medications or drugs found at the scene to the receiving facility.
   b. If the patient is stable, perform ongoing assessments every 15 minutes.
   c. If the patient is unstable, perform ongoing assessments every 5 minutes.

RESTRAINTS

OVERVIEW

1. Physical restraint should be avoided unless the patient is a danger to himself and/or others.
2. When using restraints:
   a. Obtain approval from medical direction
   b. Have law enforcement personnel present, if possible
   c. Follow local protocol
3. **Types of restraints**
   a. Acceptable restraints include:
      (1) Soft leather straps
      (2) Padded cloth straps
      (3) Nylon restraints
      (4) Velcro straps
      (5) Full-jacket restraint
   b. Metal handcuffs are unacceptable restraints.

RESTRAINT PROCEDURE

1. Be sure to have adequate help.
2. Plan your activities before attempting to restrain the patient.
3. Use body substance isolation precautions for protection against airborne saliva, emesis, and blood.
4. Use reasonable force (only the force necessary) for restraint.
5. Estimate the range of motion of the patient's arms and legs and stay beyond that range until you are ready to restrain the patient.
6. Once the decision has been made to restrain, act quickly.
7. One rescuer should talk to the patient throughout the restraint procedure.
8. At least four persons should approach the patient, one assigned to each of the patient's extremities ("limb assignments"). Restrain on cue to gain rapid control of the patient.

9. Secure the patient's extremities with restraints approved by medical direction.
10. Secure the patient to the stretcher with chest, waist, and thigh straps.

> **Note:** Some authorities recommend placing the patient in a prone position. Recent literature suggests this position may be associated with death due to positional asphyxia. Positioning of the restrained patient on the abdomen physically interferes with movement of the diaphragm and downward displacement of abdominal contents. It is suggested that restrained patients be placed in a lateral or supine position, rather than a prone position.
> Stratton SJ, Rogers C, Green R: Sudden death in individuals in hobble restraints during paramedic transport. *Annals of Emergency Medicine* 1995; 25:710–712.

11. If the patient is spitting, cover the patient's face with a disposable surgical mask.
12. Reassess the patient's airway, breathing, and circulation frequently.
    a. Assess the patient's airway; suction as necessary.
    b. Chest straps should not hinder the patient's breathing.
    c. Reassess distal pulses in each extremity to ensure circulation is not impaired due to restraints.
13. Document:
    a. The reason(s) for using restraints
    b. The number of personnel used to subdue the patient
    c. The type of restraint used
    d. The status of the patient's airway, breathing, and circulation before and after restraints are applied
14. Do not:
    a. Inflict unnecessary pain
    b. Use unreasonable force
    c. Leave a restrained patient unattended
    d. Remove applied restraints before arrival at the receiving facility

LEGAL CONSIDERATIONS

CONSENT AND REFUSAL OF CARE

1. Legal or potential legal problems are greatly reduced when the emotionally disturbed patient consents to care.
2. Emotionally disturbed patient will often resist treatment or refuse care.
3. To provide care against the patient's will, you must show a reasonable belief that the patient would harm himself or others.
4. If the patient is a threat to himself or others, the patient may be transported without consent after contacting medical direction. If possible, have law enforcement personnel participate in the transport of the patient.

USING REASONABLE FORCE

1. Reasonable force is the minimum force necessary to keep the patient from injuring himself or others.
2. Reasonableness is determined by looking at all circumstances involved, including:
    a. Patient's size and strength
    b. Type of abnormal behavior
    c. Gender of patient
    d. Mental state of patient
    e. Method of restraint

3. Be aware after a period of combativeness and aggression some calm patients may cause unexpected and sudden injury to self and others.
4. Avoid acts or use of physical force that may cause injury to the patient.
5. EMS personnel may use reasonable force to defend against an attack by an emotionally disturbed patient.

POLICE AND MEDICAL DIRECTION INVOLVEMENT

1. Seek medical direction when considering restraining a patient.
2. Ask for the assistance of law enforcement personnel if the patient appears or acts aggressive or combative during the scene size-up.

PROTECTION AGAINST FALSE ACCUSATIONS

1. Documentation of abnormal behavior exhibited by the patient is very important.
2. Emotionally disturbed patients may accuse rescuers of sexual misconduct.
3. When possible:
   a. Have witnesses present during patient care, especially during transport
   b. Use same-gender attendants to provide or assist with care
   c. Involve third-party witnesses

REVIEW QUESTIONS

Directions: Each of the numbered items or incomplete statements in this section is followed by answers or by completions of the statement. Select the ONE lettered answer or completion that is BEST in each case.

1. Abnormal behavior is best defined as

   (A) predictable behavior under normal circumstances
   (B) behavior defined by one individual as inappropriate
   (C) all activities of a person, including physical and mental activity
   (D) possibly harmful behavior that is not consistent with society's norms or expectations

2. A panic attack is an intense state of fear that generally does not last longer than 30 minutes. These attacks occur

   (A) for no apparent reason
   (B) because of low blood sugar
   (C) due to tumors in the brain or spine
   (D) immediately following a traumatic injury

3. Which of the following scenarios suggests a phobia?

   (A) Being chronically sad and feeling worthless
   (B) Being afraid of large open spaces like stores and theaters
   (C) Attempting to commit suicide by ingesting an overdose of pills and alcohol
   (D) Suddenly being overcome with an intense state of fear that passes with time

4. Which of the following regarding depression and patient age is correct?

 (A) Children younger than 13 years old never have true depression
 (B) Depression is often first observed following a suicide attempt
 (C) The signs and symptoms of depression differ according to the age of the patient
 (D) Depressed patients have the same signs and symptoms, regardless of age

5. Your crew has been called to the home of a 43-year-old female patient who is severely depressed. Her husband states that she ran out of her prescribed medications last week. He tells you his wife has not slept much for the last 3 days and is now very depressed. This description is consistent with

 (A) phobias
 (B) paranoia
 (C) schizophrenia
 (D) bipolar disorder

6. The acronym SAD PERSONS may be used as a guide

 (A) to determine the suicide potential of a patient
 (B) to determine when physical restraints are appropriate
 (C) to remember the different psychological illnesses commonly seen in field medicine
 (D) to conduct the physical examination of a patient who has successfully committed suicide by overdose

7. When treating a patient experiencing a behavioral emergency, you should assess, question, and treat

 (A) as quickly as possible
 (B) at a slow, comfortable rate
 (C) without making eye contact with the patient
 (D) as you would for any other patient emergency

8. When dealing with a potentially violent patient, you should position yourself

 (A) between the patient and a stairwell
 (B) between the patient and a door or window
 (C) between the patient and a police officer
 (D) out of the patient's way if he or she decides to leave the scene

9. Which of the following is correct regarding the use of physical restraints?

 (A) The use of handcuffs, rather than Velcro or nylon straps, is preferred
 (B) Once the decision to restrain a patient is made, you must act quickly and decisively
 (C) Physical restraints should be the first measure taken when attempting to control a patient
 (D) The use of body substance isolation precautions is not practical or recommended when physically restraining a patient

10. If a restrained patient is spitting, it is acceptable to cover the patient's mouth with

 (A) duct tape
 (B) medical tape
 (C) a surgical mask
 (D) a nonrebreather mask that is not connected to oxygen

11. The legal considerations for patients experiencing a behavioral emergency who refuse treatment can be confusing. Field health care professionals are often put in

the middle, with the patient adamantly denying treatment on one side and a medical facility requesting transport on the other. To provide care against a patient's will, you must be able to show a reasonable belief that the patient may harm himself or others. When operating in such a situation, your best resource for advice is

(A) the patient
(B) the patient's family
(C) local law enforcement
(D) your medical direction physician

12. Panic attacks are identified by the presence of four or more defined symptoms. Which of the following should NOT be attributed to a panic attack?

(A) Hot flashes and chills
(B) Trembling and shaking
(C) Chest pain during emotional stress
(D) Feeling of detachment or being out of touch with oneself

Directions: Each of the numbered questions or incomplete statements in this section refers to a scenario that precedes them. The numbered questions or incomplete statements are followed by answers or by completions of the statement. Select the answer or completion of the statement that is BEST in each case.

Your ambulance crew is called to the home of a 21-year-old male patient who called 9-1-1 and threatened that he was going to kill himself with an overdose of sleeping pills. You arrive to find your patient sitting in his bedroom. He is quiet but willing to answer your questions.

Questions 13–15

13. Following the scene size-up, you should turn your attention to

(A) restraining the patient
(B) making sure the scene is safe
(C) looking around for any guns or knives near the patient
(D) obtaining an initial assessment, SAMPLE history, and focused history and physical examination

14. This patient begins to relate to you that his girlfriend left him last night and he got in a fight with his roommate this morning. He tells you he feels "worthless" and just wants to "end it all." While the patient is relating his feelings to you, you should

(A) show active listening by repeating or rephrasing part of what is said
(B) ask him to only tell you things that concern his medical condition
(C) promise that he can work things out with his girlfriend and roommate
(D) show indifference by interrupting the patient and talking with your crew members

15. After deciding what needs to be done with this patient (possibly after contacting medical direction), you should

(A) not inform the patient of your plan
(B) inform the patient about the plan of action

(C) discourage the patient from physically assisting you in carrying out the plan of action

(D) assume the patient will not understand the action plan and only tell him information on a need-to-know basis

ANSWERS AND RATIONALES

1-D. Abnormal behavior is measured according to society's norms and expectations. For example, skydiving is a potentially dangerous sport; however, our society does not consider skydiving abnormal behavior, although the possibility exists that the participant may become seriously injured. Abnormal behavior is the combination of potentially harmful or disruptive behavior that is not acceptable to local norms or cultures.

2-A. True panic attacks occur for no particular reason. If a stressor is involved, then the patient is probably suffering from fear or anxiety. If an underlying medical condition is causing the panic attack, then the patient is exhibiting an altered mental status because of disease or injury, not a panic attack.

3-B. Phobias are irrational and persistent fears. They do not come and go like panic attacks and are not characterized by a chronic depressed state. Rather, a phobia is a constant fear of something (i.e., heights, open spaces, tunnels, snakes, blood, dentists, etc.). Avoiding the source of the fear allows phobic individuals to lead an otherwise normal life. When confronted with the particular fear, patients have been known to "shut down," stop all activity, and retreat inward.

4-C. Depression is not limited to adults and adolescents. Children, too, may become depressed. The signs and symptoms of depression tend to differ according to age. Reactions to depression range from crying to acting out to use of drugs and alcohol to suicide attempts. Suicide attempts are not generally the first indicator that a patient is depressed; unfortunately it may be the first time that the patient is given the help he or she needs.

5-D. Bipolar disorder is characterized by radical mood swings. One end of the spectrum (mania) may be hyperactivity, restlessness, and the perceived presence of "superhuman" powers or abilities. The other end is major depression, possibly with suicidal tendencies. Paranoia is a disorder marked by the patient's irrational and excessive suspiciousness or perception of grandeur. Schizophrenia is a term used for a group of mental disorders.

6-A. The acronym SAD PERSONS may assist you in determining the potential of a patient to carry out a suicide attempt. Each letter stands for a different factor. Positive responses to the different factors are given a point. The scale is from 0 to 10, with 10 being a very high probability of suicide attempt.

7-B. When treating behavioral emergency patients, be prepared to spend some time with them. Acting quickly may be perceived as either threatening behavior or as an indicator that you do not truly care for the patient (in an emotional sense). Your time, understanding, and professional experience may make the difference in these patients' ultimate outcome.

8-D. When dealing with potentially violent patients, never place yourself between the patient and a possible exit. Also, if local law enforcement is on the scene (which is a good idea), do not block their field of view or field of action.

9-B. Once you have carefully evaluated and exhausted all other methods to control a potentially violent or harmful patient, restraining a patient should be coordinated and carried out quickly. Make sure all personnel involved in restraining a patient have taken the appropriate level of body substance isolation precautions. Anticipate that the patient will attempt to spit. The use of "soft restraints" rather than handcuffs is essential. Patients in restraints often continue to fight even after they are restrained. Handcuffs may cause further injury.

10-C. Do not tape a patient's mouth closed. If the patient were to vomit, he could aspirate the vomitus into his lungs and die. It is acceptable to cover the patient's mouth with a disposable surgical mask because it is designed to allow adequate ventilation. If you use an oxygen delivery device, you must turn the oxygen on and flow it at an appropriate rate.

11-D. When in doubt, contact medical direction. Medical direction is your ultimate authority in treating patients and will often shed light into your gray area. Get to know your medical direction physician(s) so that when problems or gray areas arise, open lines of communications result in positive outcomes, for the patient and you.

12-C. The signs and symptoms of panic attacks include hot flashes, chills, trembling, detachment, sweating, nausea, feeling "out of control," shortness of breath, numbness and tingling, and heart palpitations. Chest pain experienced during emotional stress should be attributed to a cardiac problem. Emotional stress may increase the heart's workload and could cause a heart attack.

13-D. The goal of obtaining an initial assessment, SAMPLE history, and focused physical examination is the same in behavioral emergencies as in medical or trauma situations. However, in a behavioral emergency, the method needs to be altered to coincide with the patient's signs and symptoms. Limit the number of personnel near or around the patient. Take the time to explain your actions, especially when they involve making physical contact or approaching the patient. Once you have completed the scene size-up, you should be aware of the safety of the scene and the presence of any weapons. Be especially observant when sizing up the scene on behavior incidents. Restraining the patient does not appear to be necessary (as of yet) in this situation.

14-A. The patient needs to feel like he is getting through to you. After all, you may be the first person who has been willing to listen (nonjudgmentally) to the patient's side of what is happening in his life. Allow the patient some time to vent before trying to get him back on track with the current plan. Pay particular attention that there is no whispering or pointing by your crew. This may immediately cause the patient to mistrust you and feel threatened by you.

15-B. Be as open and honest about your plan as possible. Acknowledge and address the patient's concerns. You may need to bargain on little issues, but do not lose sight of the ultimate goal or desired outcome. Involve the patient in carrying out the plan. For example, if you are going to walk the patient out to the ambulance, have the patient put on his shoes and grab a sweater (as long as he stays in your view).

BIBLIOGRAPHY

Bourne EJ: *The Anxiety and Phobia Workbook*, 2nd ed. Oakland, California, New Harbinger, 1995.

Crosby LA, Lewallen DG (eds): *Emergency Care and Transportation of the Sick and Injured*, 6th ed. Rosemont, IL, American Academy of Orthopaedic Surgeons, 1995.

Grant HD, Murray RH Jr, Bergeron JD: *Emergency Care*, 7th ed. Englewood Cliffs, NJ, Prentice-Hall, 1995.

Hafen BQ, Karren KJ, Mistovich JJ: *Prehospital Emergency Care*, 5th ed. Upper Saddle River, NJ, Prentice-Hall, 1996.

Henry MC, Stapleton ER, Judd RL: *EMT: Prehospital Care*. Philadelphia, WB Saunders, 1992.

McSwain NE, White RD, Paturas JL, et al (eds): *The Basic EMT: Comprehensive Prehospital Patient Care*. St. Louis, Mosby-Year Book, 1996.

Peurifoy RZ: *Anxiety, Phobias, and Panic*, 2nd ed. Citrus Heights, California, Life Skills, 1992.

Sanders MJ: *Mosby's Paramedic Textbook*. St. Louis, Mosby-Year Book, 1994.

Sheehy SB, Lombardi JE: *Manual of Emergency Care*. 4th ed. St. Louis, Mosby-Year Book, 1995.

Stoy WA: Mosby's EMT-Basic Textbook. St. Louis, Mosby-Year Book, 1996.

United States Department of Transportation, National Highway Traffic Safety Administration: *Emergency Medical Technician: Basic. National Standard Curriculum*, 1994.

24-1 Identify the following structures:

   a. Amniotic sac

   b. Fetus

   c. Perineum

   d. Placenta

   e. Umbilical cord

   f. Uterus

   g. Vagina

24-2 Identify predelivery emergencies.

24-3 Differentiate the emergency medical care provided to a patient with predelivery emergencies from a normal delivery.

24-4 State indications of an imminent delivery.

24-5 State the steps in the predelivery preparation of the mother.

24-6 Identify and explain the use of the contents of an obstetrics kit.

24-7 Establish the relationship between body substance isolation and childbirth.

24-8 State the steps to assist in a delivery.

24-9 Describe care of the baby as the head appears.

24-10 Describe how and when to cut the umbilical cord.

24-11 Discuss the steps in the delivery of the placenta.

24-12 List the steps in the emergency medical care of the mother postdelivery.

24-13 Summarize neonatal resuscitation procedures.

24-14 Describe the procedures for the following abnormal deliveries: prolapsed cord, breech birth, and limb presentation.

MOTIVATION FOR LEARNING

The EMT-Basic may be called to care for a woman in labor or a woman experiencing a gynecological emergency. Knowledge of normal delivery procedures, postdelivery care of the mother, and management of a newborn is essential for appropriate emergency care. Emergency situations involving the reproductive system require professionalism and understanding by the EMT-Basic.

24-15 Describe the special considerations for multiple births.

24-16 Describe the special considerations when the delivery is complicated by meconium.

24-17 Describe special considerations for a premature baby.

24-18 Discuss the emergency medical care of a patient with a gynecological emergency.

ANATOMY AND PHYSIOLOGY REVIEW

FEMALE REPRODUCTIVE SYSTEM (FIGURE 24-1)

1. The female reproductive organs are found in the pelvic cavity.
2. **Ovaries**
   a. The **ovaries** are paired, walnut-shaped structures located on either side of the uterus in the pelvic cavity.
   b. They produce the hormones estrogen and progesterone.
   c. Each ovary contains thousands of follicles.
   d. About once a month during a woman's reproductive years, a follicle matures to release an egg (**ovulation**).
2. **Fallopian tubes**
   a. The **fallopian tubes** are also called uterine tubes or oviducts.
   b. Each fallopian tube extends from an ovary to the uterus.
   c. They receive and transport the egg to the uterus after ovulation.
   d. Fertilization normally takes place in the upper third of the fallopian tube.
3. **Uterus**
   a. The **uterus** is also called the womb.
   b. It is a pear-shaped, hollow, muscular organ located in the pelvic cavity.
   c. It prepares for pregnancy each month of a woman's reproductive life.
   d. If pregnancy does not occur, the inner lining of the uterus sloughs off and is discarded (**menstruation**).

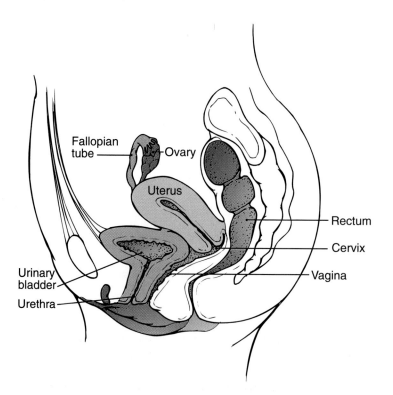

Fig. 24-1. Female reproductive organs.

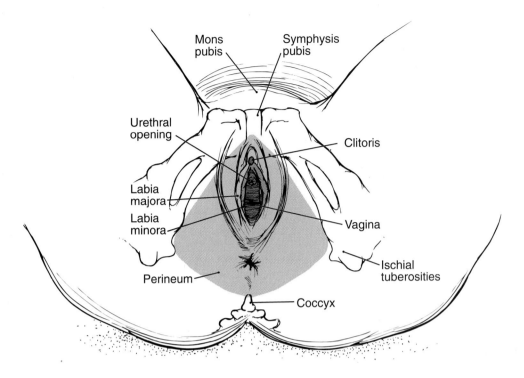

Fig. 24-2. The female external genital organs.

   e. If pregnancy does occur:
     (1)   The developing **fetus** (unborn infant) implants in the uterine wall and develops there.
     (2)   The uterus stretches throughout pregnancy to adapt to the increasing size of the fetus.
     (3)   During labor, the uterus contracts powerfully and rhythmically to expel the infant from the mother's body.
     (4)   After delivery of the infant, the uterus quickly clamps down to stop bleeding.

4. Cervix
   a. The **cervix** is the narrow opening at the distal end of the uterus.
   b. It connects the uterus to the vagina.
   c. During pregnancy, it contains a plug of mucus.
     (1)   The **mucus plug** seals the opening to the uterus, keeping bacteria from entering.
     (2)   When the cervix begins to widen during early labor, the mucus plug, sometimes mixed with blood **(bloody show),** is expelled from the vagina.

5. Vagina
   a. The **vagina** is also called the birth canal.
   b. It is a muscular tube that serves as a passageway between the uterus and the outside.
   c. It receives the penis during intercourse.
   d. It also serves as the passageway for menstrual flow and delivery of an infant.

6. Accessory organs
   a. Mammary glands (breasts) function in milk production after delivery of an infant.
   b. The external genitalia (vulva) includes the mons pubis, clitoris, urethral opening, vagina, labia minora, and labia majora (*Figure 24-2*).
   c. Perineum
     (1)   The **perineum** is the area between the vaginal opening and anus.
     (2)   It is commonly torn during childbirth.

STRUCTURES OF PREGNANCY

1. Pregnancy begins when an egg unites with a sperm cell (fertilization).
2. After approximately 3 days, the fertilized egg (ovum) passes from the fallopian tube into the uterus.
3. The ovum implants in the wall of the uterus (implantation).
   a. During the first 3 weeks after fertilization, the developing structure is called an ovum.
   b. From the third to the eighth week, the developing structure is called an embryo.
   c. From the eighth week until birth, the developing structure is called a fetus.
4. **Placenta** (*Figure 24-3*)
   a. The **placenta** is also called the afterbirth because it is expelled after the baby is born.
   b. This specialized structure of pregnancy begins to develop about 2 weeks after fertilization occurs.
   c. It attaches to the mother at the inner wall of the uterus and to the fetus by the **umbilical cord.**
   d. The placenta is responsible for:
      (1) Exchange of oxygen and carbon dioxide between the blood of the mother and fetus (the placenta serves the function of the lungs for the developing fetus)
      (2) Removal of waste products
      (3) Transport of nutrients from the mother to the fetus
      (4) Production of a special hormone of pregnancy that maintains the pregnancy and stimulates changes in the mother's breasts, cervix, and vagina in preparation for delivery
      (5) Maintaining a barrier against harmful substances
      (6) Transfer of heat from the mother to the fetus

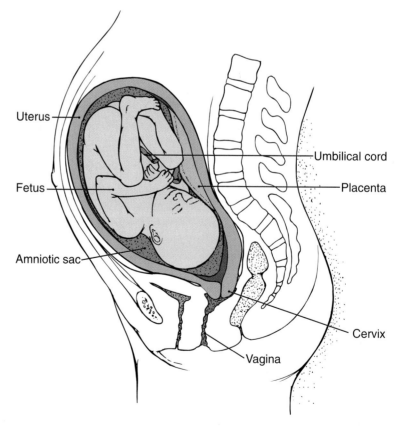

Fig. 24-3. The structures of pregnancy.

5. **Umbilical cord**
   a. The umbilical cord is the lifeline connecting the placenta to the fetus.
   b. It contains two arteries and one vein.
      (1) The umbilical arteries carry deoxygenated blood from the fetus to the placenta.
      (2) The umbilical vein carries oxygenated blood to the fetus.
   c. The umbilical cord attaches to the umbilicus (navel) of the fetus.
6. **Amniotic sac**
   a. The **amniotic sac** is also called the bag of waters.
   b. The amniotic sac is a membranous bag that surrounds the fetus inside the uterus.
   c. It contains fluid (amniotic fluid) that helps protect the baby from injury.
      (1) The amniotic fluid provides a controlled environment.
      (2) It functions much like a shock absorber.
   d. It contains about 1 liter (L) of fluid at term.

ENRICHMENT—NORMAL PREGNANCY

1. Pregnancy is divided into three 90-day intervals called trimesters.
2. **First trimester (months 1–3)**
   a. The mother stops menstruating (missed period).
   b. Breasts become swollen and tender.
   c. The mother urinates more frequently and may sleep more than usual.
   d. Nausea and vomiting are usually at their worst during the second month.
   e. The fetus is undergoing rapid development.
      (1) Cells are differentiating into tissues.
      (2) At this time, the fetus is vulnerable to effects of some drugs and certain organisms (e.g., rubella).
3. **Second trimester (months 4–6)**
   a. **Mother**
      (1) The uterus can be felt above the symphysis pubis.
      (2) The mother begins to feel fetal movement at about the fourth month.
   b. **Fetus**
      (1) Muscles become active (kicks).
      (2) Heart sounds can be heard with a stethoscope at about the fifth month.
4. **Third trimester (months 7–9)**
   a. **Mother**
      (1) The mother may complain of backache due to muscle strain.
      (2) Stretch marks may appear.
      (3) Frequent urination is due to the weight of the uterus pressing on the bladder.
   b. **Fetus**
      (1) The fetus continues to gain weight and grow in length.
      (2) Normally, the head of the fetus settles in the pelvis in preparation for delivery.

PREDELIVERY EMERGENCIES

ASSESSMENT

1. **Scene size-up**
   a. Take body substance isolation precautions. Obstetric emergencies (emergencies related to pregnancy or childbirth) are frequently associated with bleeding.
   b. Evaluate scene safety.
   c. Determine the mechanism of injury or nature of the patient's illness.
   d. Determine the total number of patients. If delivery is imminent, there is going to be an additional patient.

    e. Determine the need for additional resources.

2. **Initial assessment**

    a. Maintain spinal immobilization if needed.

    b. Assess the patient's mental status.

    c. Assess the patient's airway.

    d. Assess breathing.

    e. Assess circulation.

    f. Identify any life-threatening conditions and provide care based on these findings

    g. Establish patient priorities.

       (1) Priority patients include:

          (a) Patients who give a poor general impression

          (b) Patients experiencing difficulty breathing

          (c) Patients with signs and symptoms of shock

          (d) Unresponsive patients with no gag reflex or cough

          (e) Responsive patients who are unable to follow commands

       (2) Advanced-life-support (ALS) assistance should be requested as soon as possible.

       (3) If ALS personnel are not available, the patient should be transported promptly to the closest appropriate facility.

3. **Focused history and physical examination**

    a. If the patient is unresponsive:

       (1) Perform a rapid physical examination

       (2) Follow with evaluation of baseline vital signs and gathering of the patient's medical history

    b. If the patient is responsive:

       (1) Gather information about the patient's medical history before performing the physical examination

       (2) Gather a SAMPLE history

4. **SAMPLE history**

  a. <u>Signs and symptoms.</u> Signs and symptoms of predelivery emergencies include:

       (1) Seizures

       (2) Weakness

       (3) Dizziness

       (4) Faintness

       (5) Signs of shock

       (6) Lightheadedness

       (7) Vaginal bleeding

       (8) Altered mental status

       (9) Passage of clots or tissue

       (10) Swelling of the face and/or extremities

       (11) Abdominal cramping or pain that may be intermittent or constant

    b. <u>Allergies.</u> Determine if the patient has any allergies to medications and other substances or materials.

    c. <u>Medications.</u> Determine if the patient is taking any medications (prescription and over the counter).

       (1) Determine if the patient takes her medications regularly and her response to them, including:

          (a) Vitamins

          (b) Illegal substances (e.g., crack, heroin, methadone, cocaine, marijuana)

       (2) Determine if there has been any recent change in medications (additions, deletions, or change in dosages).

       (3) Provide all information obtained to the receiving facility.

    d. **Pertinent past medical history.** Ascertain whether the patient has had any of the following:

       (1) Surgeries

    (2)   Heart disease

    (3)   Lung disease

    (4)   Kidney disease

    (5)   High blood pressure

    (6)   Diabetes

    (7)   Smoking

    (8)   Alcohol use

    (9)   Previous pregnancies and any problems (e.g., prematurity, large babies, hemorrhage, cesarean section, miscarriage, abortion)

e. Last oral intake. Determine the patient's last oral intake.

f. Event. Determine the events leading to the present situation by asking:

    (1)   Is there a possibility that you might be pregnant?

    (2)   When was your last menstrual period?

    (3)   Was it a normal period?

    (4)   Are your periods usually regular?

    (5)   Did you have any bleeding after that period?

    (6)   Have you seen a doctor?

    (7)   If pregnant:

        (a)   Do you know your due date?

        (b)   Is this your first pregnancy?

        (c)   How many children do you have?

        (d)   Were your children delivered vaginally?

        (e)   Have you had any prenatal care?

        (f)   Have you had any problems with this pregnancy?

        (g)   Are you having any contractions?

        (h)   When did they start?

        (i)   How close are they now?

        (j)   Has your bag of waters broken? When? What color was the fluid?

        (k)   Is the baby moving the way it usually does?

        (l)   Do you feel the need to push or bear down?

    (8)   Vaginal bleeding:

        (a)   Are you having any bleeding?

        (b)   How long have you been bleeding?

        (c)   What color is it?

        (d)   How much are you bleeding? (How many pads has the patient used?)

        (e)   What is the consistency of the bleeding (e.g., thick with mucuslike bloody show or bright red, thin blood)?

5. Assess baseline vital signs.

6. Perform a focused physical examination.

PREDELIVERY EMERGENCIES—GENERAL GUIDELINES FOR EMERGENCY MEDICAL CARE

1. Take appropriate body substance isolation precautions.

2. Provide specific treatment based on the patient's signs and symptoms.

3. Establish and maintain an open airway.

4. Administer oxygen.

    a. If the patient's breathing is adequate, apply oxygen by nonrebreather mask at 15 liters per minute (LPM) if not already done.

    b. If the patient's breathing is inadequate, provide positive-pressure ventilation with 100% oxygen and assess the adequacy of the ventilations delivered.

5. Treat for shock if indicated.

    a. If trauma is not suspected, place the pregnant patient on her left side (*Figure 24-4*).

    b. When the pregnant patient is placed in a supine position, the weight of the pregnant uterus compresses the vena cava and aorta, decreasing cardiac output and blood pressure.

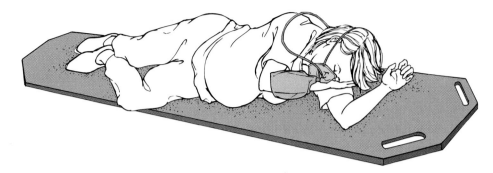

Fig. 24-4. If trauma is not suspected, place the pregnant patient on her left side.

   c. Maintain body temperature.
6. Apply external vaginal pads as necessary.
   a. As the pad becomes blood-soaked, replace it with a new one.
   b. All blood-soaked garments and pads should accompany the patient to the hospital; these items will be used to estimate the patient's blood loss.
7. Provide emotional support to the patient and family members.
8. Transport promptly.
   a. If the patient is stable, perform ongoing assessments every 15 minutes.
   b. If the patient is unstable, perform ongoing assessments every 5 minutes.

ABORTION

1. An **abortion** is the termination of pregnancy before the fetus is capable of survival outside the uterus (age of viability). Most sources define the age of viability as the 20th week of gestation (fetal growth); however, others define it as 24 or 28 weeks.
2. An **induced abortion** is an abortion performed under sterile conditions in an authorized medical setting.
   a. A therapeutic abortion is an abortion performed for medical reasons, often because the pregnancy poses a threat to the mother's health.
   b. An elective abortion is an abortion performed at the request of the mother.
3. A **criminal abortion** is an illegally performed abortion, usually in undesirable conditions by unqualified medical personnel.
4. A **spontaneous abortion** occurs naturally and is often called a miscarriage by lay people.
   a. An inevitable abortion is a spontaneous abortion that cannot be prevented.
   b. In an inevitable and spontaneous abortion, the cervix has begun to open and the patient may pass tissue or clots.
   c. The patient often experiences heavy vaginal bleeding and painful uterine contractions.
5. A **threatened abortion** is a pregnancy in which the cervix remains closed and the fetus remains in the uterus.
   a. The patient often complains of vaginal bleeding and/or pain resembling menstrual cramps.
   b. A threatened abortion may progress to a complete abortion or may subside, and the pregnancy may continue to term.
6. An **incomplete abortion** is one in which part of the products of conception have been passed, but some remain in the uterus. The cervix is open and the patient will bleed heavily until all of the products of conception are removed from the uterus.
7. **Emergency medical care**
   a. See general guidelines previously outlined in this chapter.
   b. Bring fetal tissues to the hospital.
   c. Provide emotional support for the patient and family.
   d. Transport promptly.

ECTOPIC PREGNANCY

1. An **ectopic pregnancy** occurs when the fertilized egg implants outside the uterus, usually inside the fallopian tube.
2. As the fetus grows, the fallopian tube tears and eventually ruptures.
3. Signs and symptoms include:
   a. Missed menstrual period or intermittent spotting over 6 to 8 weeks
   b. Vaginal bleeding ranging from spotting to hemorrhage
   c. Sudden onset of severe pain on one side of the lower abdomen
   d. Severe pain in the back of the shoulder
   e. Abdominal tenderness
   f. Signs of shock (e.g., cool, clammy skin; decreasing blood pressure; increased heart rate)
4. **Emergency medical care**
   a. An ectopic pregnancy is a medical emergency.
   b. See general guidelines previously outlined in this chapter.
   c. Transport promptly.

SEIZURES DURING PREGNANCY

1. Some women with no history of a seizure disorder may experience seizures during pregnancy.
2. Seizures experienced during pregnancy may be associated with high blood pressure (hypertension).
3. Hypertensive disorder of pregnancy (formerly called toxemia of pregnancy) is the name given to a group of disorders associated with high blood pressure and pregnancy.
4. **Pregnancy-induced hypertension** (PIH) is a disorder of pregnancy in which the patient has a blood pressure of 140/90 millimeters of mercury (mm Hg) or more during pregnancy but had a normal blood pressure before the pregnancy.
5. **Emergency medical care**
   a. See general guidelines previously outlined in this chapter.
   b. Closely monitor the patient's vital signs.
   c. Transport for further evaluation and treatment.

PREECLAMPSIA

1. **Preeclampsia** tends to occur in young mothers during their first pregnancies.
2. If untreated, it may progress to the next stage **(eclampsia).**
3. Signs and symptoms include:
   a. Abnormal weight gain
   b. Swelling of the face, hands, and lower back
   c. Visual disturbances
   d. Headaches
   e. Irritability
   f. Right upper quadrant abdominal pain
   g. Increased blood pressure (more than 140/90 mm Hg)
4. If the patient complains of blurred vision, nausea, a severe headache, and right upper quadrant abdominal pain, she may be very close to having a seizure.
5. **Emergency medical care**
   a. See general guidelines previously outlined in this chapter.
   b. Keep the patient calm.
   c. Dim the lights.
   d. Place the patient on her left side.
   e. Transport promptly without lights or siren.

ECLAMPSIA

1. Eclampsia is the convulsive phase of preeclampsia.
2. Eclampsia is associated with a significant risk of death of the mother and fetus.

3. Signs and symptoms include:
   a. Signs and symptoms of preeclampsia
   b. Grand mal seizure activity
4. **Emergency medical care**
   a. See general guidelines previously outlined in this chapter.
   b. Have suction readily available.
   c. Dim the lights.
   d. Place the patient on her left side.
   e. If the patient seizes, protect the patient from injury.
   f. Transport promptly without lights or siren.

VAGINAL BLEEDING IN LATE PREGNANCY

1. Vaginal bleeding may occur late in pregnancy (third trimester) and may or may not be accompanied by pain.
2. All third-trimester bleeding should be considered a life-threatening emergency.
3. Possible causes of vaginal bleeding in late pregnancy include placenta previa, abruptio placenta, and ruptured uterus.
   a. **Placenta previa** (*Figure 24-5*)
      (1) **Placenta previa** accounts for most cases of hemorrhage in the third trimester of pregnancy.
      (2) Placenta previa occurs when part or all of the placenta covers the opening of the cervix (e.g., the placenta is the presenting part).
      (3) The patient usually experiences vaginal bleeding when the cervix begins to open and thin out in preparation for delivery or when the pressure from the fetus increases.
      (4) Placenta previa tends to occur in women who have delivered more than one baby and in women older than 35 years of age.
      (5) Signs and symptoms include:
         (a) Sudden, painless, bright red vaginal bleeding
         (b) Signs of shock
      (6) **Emergency medical care**
         (a) See general guidelines previously outlined in this chapter.
         (b) Transport promptly.
   b. **Abruptio placenta** (*Figure 24-6*)

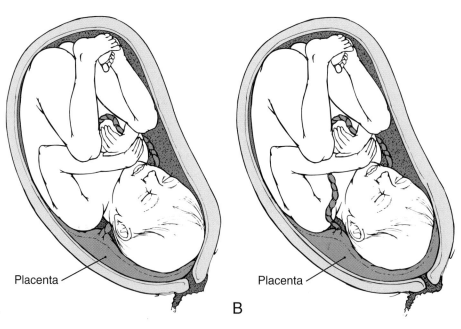

Placenta   Placenta

A   B

Fig. 24-5. Placenta previa occurs when *(A)* part or *(B)* all of the placenta covers the opening of the cervix.

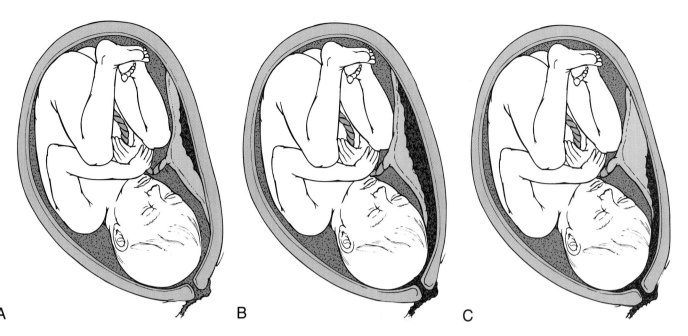

A   B   C

Fig. 24-6. Abruptio placenta occurs when a normally implanted placenta separates prematurely from the wall of the uterus during the last trimester of pregnancy. *(A)* Partial separation without visible bleeding; *(B)* partial separation with visible bleeding; *(C)* complete separation.

(1) **Abruptio placenta** occurs when a normally implanted placenta separates prematurely from the wall of the uterus during the last trimester of pregnancy.

(2) The uterus may separate partially or completely.

 (a) Partial separation may allow time for treatment of mother and fetus.

 (b) Complete separation often results in death of the fetus.

(3) Abruptio placenta is more common in patients with multiple pregnancies, high blood pressure, or significant abdominal trauma.

(4) Signs and symptoms include:

 (a) Severe abdominal pain

 (b) Decreased or absent fetal movement

 (c) Bleeding

  (i) If the placenta is partially separated, bleeding may be minimal (dark red) or absent.

  (ii) If the placenta is completely separated, severe hemorrhage can occur (bright red bleeding).

 (d) Signs of shock, which may seem out of proportion to the amount of blood loss seen

(5) **Emergency medical care**

 (a) See general guidelines previously outlined in this chapter.

 (b) Transport promptly.

c. Ruptured uterus

(1) A ruptured uterus is caused by the actual tearing (rupture) of the uterus.

(2) **Uterine rupture** can occur:

 (a) When the patient has been in strong labor for a long period (most common cause)

 (b) When the patient has sustained abdominal trauma, such as a severe fall or sudden stop in a motor vehicle collision

(3) Signs and symptoms include:

 (a) Sudden, severe abdominal pain

 (b) Tender, rigid abdomen

 (c) External bleeding may or may not be present

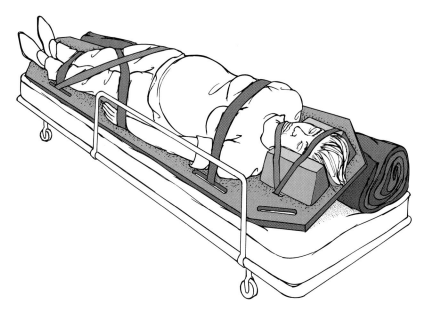

Fig. 24-7. If spine injury is suspected, the pregnant patient should be immobilized on a long backboard. The entire board can be tilted to the left by placing a rolled towel, small pillow, blanket, or other padding under the right side of the backboard.

            (d) Signs of shock
            (e) Absence of fetal movement
      (4) **Emergency medical care**
            (a) See general guidelines previously outlined in this chapter.
            (b) Transport promptly.

TRAUMA AND PREGNANCY

1. Assessment of the pregnant trauma patient is the same as that of other trauma patients.
2. **Shock in the pregnant patient**
   a. The pregnant patient may lose as much as 1500 milliliters (mL) of blood before a decrease in blood pressure and changes in other vital signs are observed.
   b. To compensate for shock in the mother, available blood are shunted to the heart and brain and away from other organs, including the uterus, thus compromising the fetus.
   c. Blood flow to the fetus may be significantly decreased before signs of shock are evident in the mother.
   d. One of the best defenses against fetal compromise is to place the pregnant patient on her left side to increase her blood pressure and increase blood flow to the uterus.
3. If spine injury is suspected, the patient should be immobilized on a long backboard (*Figure 24-7*). The entire board can be tilted to the left by placing a rolled towel, small pillow, blanket, or other padding under the right side of the backboard.

ENRICHMENT—NORMAL LABOR

TERMINOLOGY

1. **Labor** is the time and process in which the uterus repeatedly contracts to push the fetus and placenta out of the mother's body. It begins with the first uterine muscle contraction and ends with delivery of the placenta.
2. **Delivery** is the actual birth of the baby at the end of the second stage of labor.

STAGES OF LABOR

1. Before labor begins:
   a. The head of the fetus normally settles in the pelvis. The mother may feel she can "breathe easier" but she will also feel the need to urinate frequently.
   b. The cervix begins to open (dilate) and thin out (efface), and the mucus plug may be expelled (bloody show).
2. **First stage of labor**
   a. The first stage of labor begins with the first uterine contraction and ends with complete thinning out and opening of the cervix.
   b. Contractions are timed from the beginning of one cycle to the beginning of the next.
   c. Contractions usually begin as regular cramplike pains that progressively increase in intensity.
      (1) They usually last from 30 to 50 seconds.
      (2) They occur every 5–15 minutes.
   d. The amniotic sac often ruptures during this stage.
   e. This stage of labor averages:
      (1) Eight to twelve hours in a woman who has not previously borne a child
      (2) Six to eight hours in a woman who has previously given birth
2. **Second stage of labor**
   a. The second stage of labor begins with full dilation of the cervix and ends with delivery of the infant.
   b. Contractions are stronger and last longer.
      (1) They last from 45 to 60 seconds.
      (2) They occur every 2–3 minutes.
   c. The fetus begins its descent into the vagina.
      (1) The presenting part is the part of the infant/fetus that comes out of the mother first.
      (2) Normally, the head of the fetus descends into the vagina first [this is called a cephalic (head) presentation].
      (3) If the buttocks or feet descend first, it is called a **breech** presentation.
   d. Toward the end of this stage of labor, the mother experiences an urge to bear down or push with each contraction.
      (1) The presenting part will appear and disappear at the vaginal opening between contractions.
      (2) As the presenting part presses on the rectum, the mother will feel an urge to move her bowels.
      (3) Eventually, the presenting part will remain visible at the vaginal opening between contractions (crowning).
   e. This stage of labor averages:
      (1) One to two hours in a woman who has not previously borne a child
      (2) Twenty to thirty minutes in a woman who has previously given birth
4. **Third stage of labor**
   a. The third stage of labor begins with delivery of the infant and ends with delivery of the placenta.
   b. The placenta separates from the wall of the uterus, leaving tiny blood vessels exposed.
   c. The uterus normally contracts to squeeze these blood vessels shut.
   d. The placenta normally delivers within 15 to 20 minutes after the infant's birth.
   e. This stage of labor normally lasts 5–60 minutes.

NORMAL DELIVERY

PREDELIVERY CONSIDERATIONS

1. Generally, transporting a woman in labor to the hospital is best unless delivery is expected within a few minutes.

2. The EMT-Basic must determine if there is time to transport the patient to the hospital or if preparations should be made for delivery at the scene.
3. To make this decision, the EMT-Basic should ask the patient the following questions:
   a. Is this the patient's first delivery?
   b. When is the baby due?
   c. Has there been any bleeding or discharge?
      (1) If so, when?
      (2) What did the fluid look like? (bloody show, amniotic fluid)
   d. Are there any contractions or pain?
   e. What are the frequency and duration of contractions?
   f. Is crowning occurring with contractions?
   g. Does the mother feel as if she needs to move her bowels?
   h. Does the mother feel the need to push?
   i. Does the abdomen (uterus) feel hard?

SIGNS OF IMMINENT DELIVERY

1. Consider delivering at the scene when:
   a. Delivery can be expected in a few minutes
      (1) The patient feels the urge to push, bear down, or have a bowel movement.
      (2) Crowning is present.
      (3) Contractions are regular, lasting 45–60 seconds, and are 1–2 minutes apart.
   b. No suitable transportation is available
   c. The hospital cannot be reached (e.g., heavy traffic, bad weather, natural disaster)
2. If there is time to transport the patient to the hospital:
   a. Place the patient on her left side
   b. Remove any undergarments that might obstruct delivery
   c. Transport promptly

PREPARING FOR DELIVERY

1. If the decision is made to deliver on the scene, take the following precautions.
2. Use body substance isolation precautions, including gloves, mask, eye protection, and a gown. Blood and amniotic fluid are expected and may splash.
3. Do not touch the patient's vaginal area except during delivery and when your partner is present.
4. Do not let the mother go to the bathroom.
   a. The mother will feel as if she needs to move her bowels.
   b. This sensation is caused by the head of the fetus in the vagina pressing against the walls of the patient's rectum.
5. Do not hold the mother's legs together or attempt to delay or restrain delivery in any way.
6. If delivery is imminent with crowning, contact medical direction concerning the decision to commit to delivery on the scene.
7. If delivery does not occur within 10 minutes, contact medical direction for permission to transport.

CONTENTS OF A CHILDBIRTH DELIVERY KIT

A childbirth delivery kit (also called an obstetrics or OB kit) contains the following items:
1. Surgical scissors (used to cut the umbilical cord)
2. Hemostats or cord clamps (used to clamp the umbilical cord)
3. Umbilical tape or sterilized cord (used to tie the placenta side of the umbilical cord)
4. Bulb syringe (used to suction the infant's mouth and nose)
5. Towels (used to dry the infant)

6. 2 × 10 gauze sponges (used to clear secretions from the infant's mouth)
7. Sterile gloves (worn by the rescuer during delivery)
8. One baby blanket (used to warm the infant)
9. Sanitary napkins (used to absorb vaginal drainage after delivery)
10. Plastic bag (used to transport the placenta to the hospital)
11. Sterile sheet or drape paper (to create a sterile field around the vaginal opening)

DELIVERY PROCEDURE

1. Take appropriate body substance isolation precautions (e.g., gloves, mask, gown, eye protection).
2. Position the patient.
   a. Remove the patient's undergarments.
   b. Have the patient lie on her back.
   c. Place clean absorbent towels, a folded sheet, or drape under her buttocks.
   d. Make sure there is enough room in front of the mother's buttocks to provide support for the infant after delivery.
   e. Have the patient bend her knees and spread her thighs apart.
3. Organize the OB kit.
4. Create a sterile field around the vaginal opening with sheets from the OB kit, sterile towels, or paper barriers (*Figure 24-8*).
5. Prepare oxygen and blankets for the newborn infant.
6. When the infant's head appears during crowning:
   a. Place your gloved fingers on the bony part of the infant's skull
   b. Exert very gentle pressure to prevent an explosive delivery
   c. Do not apply pressure to the infant's face or **fontanelles** (soft spots on the head)
7. If the amniotic sac does not break, or has not broken, use a clamp or your gloved fingers to puncture the sac and push it away from the infant's head and mouth as they appear.
8. As the infant's head is being born, determine if the umbilical cord is around the infant's neck (sometimes called **nuchal cord**).

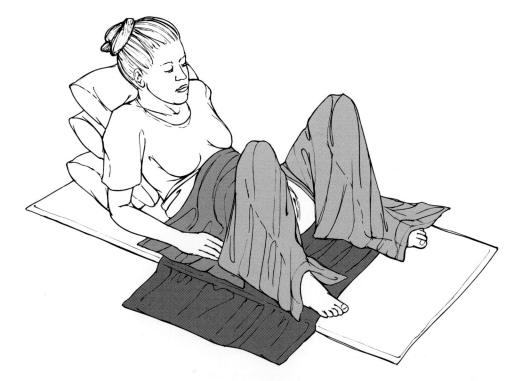

Fig. 24-8. Preparation for delivery. Place clean absorbent towels, a folded sheet, or a drape under the mother's buttocks. Create a sterile field around the vaginal opening.

     a. If the cord is around the neck, attempt to loosen the cord and slip it over the infant's shoulder.

     b. If the cord cannot be removed:

       (1) Place two umbilical clamps on the cord, approximately 3 inches apart

       (2) Carefully cut the cord between the two clamps

       (3) Remove the cord from the infant's neck

  9. When the infant's head is delivered, support the head with one hand and suction the infant's mouth and nose with a bulb syringe.

     a. Infants are primarily "nose breathers."

     b. The mouth should be suctioned first to be sure there is nothing for the infant to aspirate if he or she should gasp when the nose is suctioned.

     c. Squeeze the bulb of the bulb syringe before inserting it into the infant's mouth or nose (*Figure 24-9*).

     d. Gentle suctioning is usually adequate to remove secretions.

     e. Do not suction for more than 3–5 seconds per attempt.

     f. Be careful how far the bulb syringe is inserted. Stimulation of the back of the throat during the first few minutes after birth can cause severe slowing of the heart rate (bradycardia) and/or absence of breathing (apnea).

  10. After the head is delivered:

     a. The head will turn to line up with the shoulders

     b. Guide the head downward to deliver the top shoulder

     c. Guide the head upward to deliver the bottom shoulder

     d. Tell the mother not to push during this time

  11. As the torso and full body are born, support the infant with both hands.

  12. As the feet are born, grasp the feet.

  13. Clean the infant's mouth and nose.

     a. Wipe blood and mucus from the infant's mouth and nose with sterile gauze.

     b. Suction the mouth and nose again to stimulate breathing and crying.

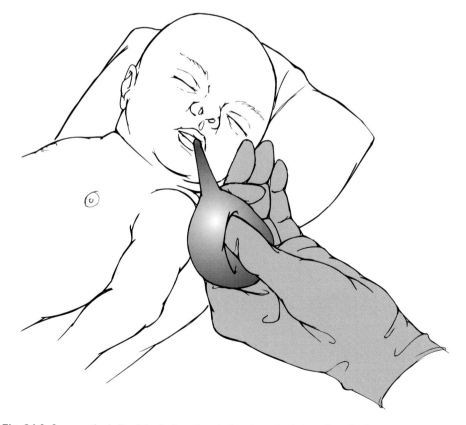

Fig. 24-9. Squeeze the bulb of the bulb syringe before inserting it into the infant's mouth or nose. The mouth should be suctioned first.

14. Dry, warm, and position the infant.

    a. Quickly dry the infant's body and head to remove amniotic fluid.

    b. Remove the wet towel or blanket from the infant.

    c. Wrap the infant in a clean, warm blanket.

    d. Cover the infant's body and head to prevent heat loss (keep the face exposed).

    e. Place the infant on his or her back or side with the neck in a neutral position.

    f. Hold the infant level with the vagina until the cord is cut. Raising the baby above or below the level of the uterus causes blood to shift from the baby to the placenta and vice versa.

15. Assign your partner to monitor and complete the initial care of the newborn.

16. Clamp, tie, and cut the umbilical cord after the cord stops pulsating (*Figure 24-10*).

    a. The umbilical cord usually stops pulsating 3–5 minutes after delivery of the infant.

    b. Place the first clamp (or tie) approximately 4 finger-widths (6 inches) from the infant.

    c. Place the second clamp (or tie) 2–3 inches distally (toward the placenta) from the first.

    d. When the clamps (or ties) are firmly in place, cut the cord between the two clamps.

    e. Periodically check the cut ends of the cord for bleeding.

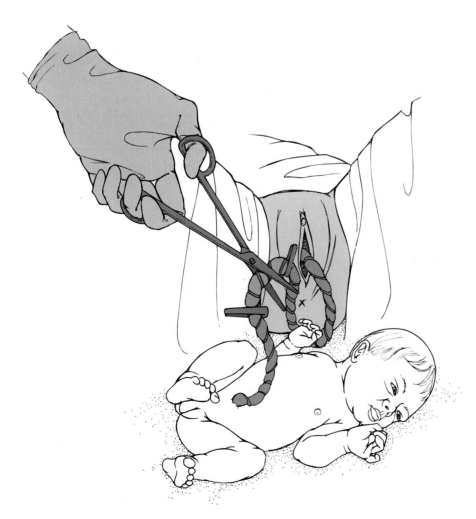

Fig. 24-10. Clamp, tie, and cut the umbilical cord after the cord stops pulsating. Place the first clamp approximately 4 finger-widths from the infant. Place the second clamp 2–3 inches distally (toward the placenta) from the first clamp. When the clamps are firmly in place, cut the placenta.

(1) If the cut end of the cord attached to the infant is bleeding, clamp (or tie) the cord proximal to the existing clamp.

(2) Do not remove the first clamp.

17. Observe for delivery of the placenta.

   a. While preparing mother and infant for transport, continue to warm and assess the infant and watch for delivery of the placenta.

   b. The placenta is usually delivered within 20 minutes of the infant.

   (1) In many areas, waiting for the placenta to deliver before transporting the mother and infant is not necessary.

   (2) Check local protocol.

   c. Signs of placental separation include:

   (1) A gush of blood

   (2) Lengthening of the umbilical cord

   (3) Contraction of the uterus

   (4) An urge to push

   d. Encourage the mother to push to help deliver the placenta.

   (1) Do not pull on the umbilical cord to deliver the placenta.

   (2) Pulling can cause the uterus to invert (turn inside out).

   e. After delivery of the placenta:

   (1) Put the infant to the mother's breast to nurse, which stimulates the uterus to contract, thus constricting blood vessels within its walls and decreasing bleeding

   (2) Wrap the placenta in a towel and put in a plastic bag

   (3) Transport the placenta to the hospital with the mother

   (a) Hospital personnel will examine the placenta for completeness.

   (b) Retained pieces of placenta in the uterus will cause persistent bleeding.

18. Examine the skin between the anus and the vagina (the perineum) for tears and apply pressure to any bleeding tears with a sanitary napkin.

19. Place a sterile pad over the vaginal opening, lower the mother's legs, and help her hold them together.

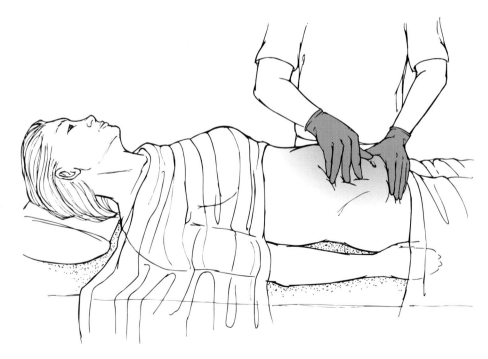

Fig. 24-11. Uterine massage. With the fingers fully extended, place one hand horizontally across the abdomen, just above the pubic bone. Cup the other hand around the uterus and, using a kneading motion, massage the uterus. Bleeding should decrease as the uterus becomes firm.

20. Record the time of delivery and transport the mother, infant, and placenta to the hospital.

VAGINAL BLEEDING FOLLOWING DELIVERY

1. Up to 500 mL of blood loss is normal after delivery.
2. If blood loss appears excessive:
  a. Administer oxygen to the mother by nonrebreather mask.
  b. Massage the uterus (*Figure 24-11*).
    (1) With the fingers fully extended, place one hand horizontally across the abdomen, just above the symphysis pubis (pubic bone) to help prevent downward displacement of the uterus during the massage.
    (2) Cup the other hand around the uterus and, using a kneading motion, massage the area.
    (3) Continue massaging until the uterus feels firm.
    (4) Bleeding should lessen as the uterus becomes firm.
  c. Reassess the patient every 5 minutes.
3. If bleeding continues to appear excessive:
  a. Reassess your massage technique
  b. Transport immediately, continuing uterine massage en route
4. Whatever the amount of blood loss, if the mother appears to be in shock (hypoperfusion), treat her for shock and transport immediately, continuing uterine massage en route.

INITIAL CARE OF THE NEWBORN

1. Dry the infant's body and head to remove amniotic fluid.
2. Remove the wet towel or blanket from the infant.
3. Wrap the infant in a clean, warm blanket.
4. Cover the infant's body and head to prevent heat loss.
5. Place the infant on his or her back or side with the neck in a neutral position.
6. Repeat suctioning of the mouth and nose as needed.
7. An Apgar score is used to assess the infant's condition after birth.
  a. The Apgar score is used to assess five specific signs (*Table 24-1*):
    (1) **A**ppearance (color)
    (2) **P**ulse (heart rate)
    (3) **G**rimace (irritability)
    (4) **A**ctivity (muscle tone)
    (5) **R**espirations
  b. Each sign is assigned a value of either 0, 1, or 2 and added for a total Apgar score.
  c. An Apgar score should be recorded at 1 and 5 minutes after birth.
  d. Apgar scores
    (1) A score of 0 to 3 indicates a newborn in severe distress.
    (2) A score of 4 to 6 indicates a newborn in moderate distress.

Table 24-1. Apgar Score

Sign	0	1	2
Appearance (color)	Blue or pale	Body pink Extremities blue	Completely pink
Pulse (heart rate)	Absent	Below 100/minute	Above 100/minute
Grimace (irritability)	No response	Grimace	Cough, sneeze, cry
Activity (muscle tone)	Limp	Some flexion of extremities	Active motion
Respirations (respiratory effort)	Absent	Slow, irregular	Good, crying

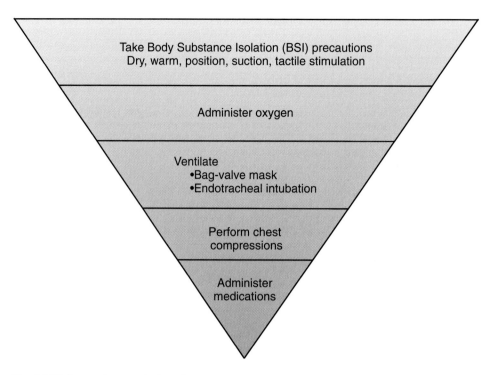

Fig. 24-12. Inverted pyramid of newborn resuscitation. The inverted pyramid shows the relative frequency of resuscitation efforts for the newborn.

    (3)   A score of 7 to 10 indicates a newborn in mild distress or with no distress.
  e. Stimulate the newborn if he or she is not breathing or is not breathing adequately.
    (1)   Flick the soles of the feet.
    (2)   Rub the infant's back.

RESUSCITATION OF THE NEWBORN

  1. Assessment of the newborn should begin immediately after birth and focus on the following areas:
    a. Respiratory rate and effort
    b. Heart rate
    c. Skin color
  2. Although the Apgar score is an important tool in assessment of the newborn, it is not recorded until 1 and 5 minutes after birth. If resuscitation of the newborn is needed, waiting until the first Apgar score is obtained could be disastrous.
  3. Newborn resuscitation follows the inverted pyramid (*Figure 24-12*).
  4. Respiratory rate and effort
    a. Assess respiratory rate and effort after the infant is dried, warm, suctioned, and stimulated.
    b. If respirations are adequate, assess heart rate.
    c. If respirations are shallow or slow:
      (1)   Stimulate the infant and administer 100% oxygen
      (2)   If there is no improvement after 5 to 10 seconds, provide positive-pressure ventilation with 100% oxygen
    d. If respirations are absent or gasping, begin positive-pressure ventilation with 100% oxygen immediately.
    e. Ventilate at a rate of 40 to 60 breaths per minute.
    f. Reassess after 30 seconds.
    g. If no improvement, continue ventilations and reassessments.
  5. Heart rate

    a. The newborn's pulse may be evaluated by:
        (1)   Palpating the brachial pulse
        (2)   Palpating the femoral pulse
        (3)   Palpating the pulse at the base of the umbilical cord
    b. If the heart rate is greater than 100 beats/minute and spontaneous respirations are present, assess skin color.
    c. If the heart rate is less than 100 beats/minute, begin positive-pressure ventilation with 100% oxygen immediately.
    d. Begin chest compressions if:
        (1)   The heart rate is less than 60 beats/minute or
        (2)   The heart rate is 60–80 beats/minute and not increasing rapidly despite positive-pressure ventilation with 100% oxygen for approximately 30 seconds
    e. Newborn CPR. To provide chest compressions for the newborn:
        (1)   Place your thumbs on the middle third of the newborn's sternum with your fingers encircling the chest and supporting the back (*Figure 24-13*)
            (a) Your thumbs should be positioned side by side on the sternum, just below the nipple line.
            (b) If the newborn is very small or your thumbs are extremely large, your thumbs may have to be placed one on top of the other.
            (c) If your hands are too small to encircle the newborn's chest, or if the newborn is very large, compress the sternum with the ring and middle fingers of one hand, just below the nipple line.
        (2)   Compress the sternum approximately ½ to ¾ inch at a rate of 120 times per minute
        (3)   Three chest compressions should be followed by a brief pause to deliver one breath

6. Color
    a. If the newborn's body is blue (cyanotic), with spontaneous breathing and an adequate heart rate, administer free-flow oxygen.
        (1)   Free-flow oxygen refers to blowing oxygen over the newborn's nose so that the newborn breathes oxygen-enriched air.

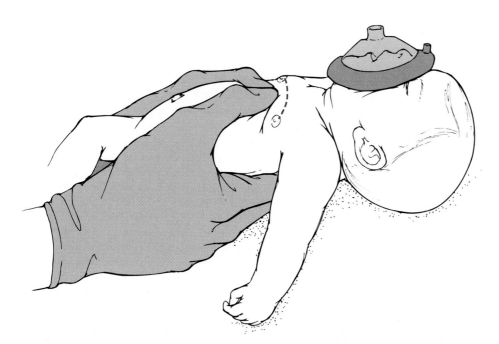

Fig. 24-13. Chest compressions in the newborn. The rescuer's thumbs should be positioned side by side on the middle third of the newborn's sternum, just below the nipple line.

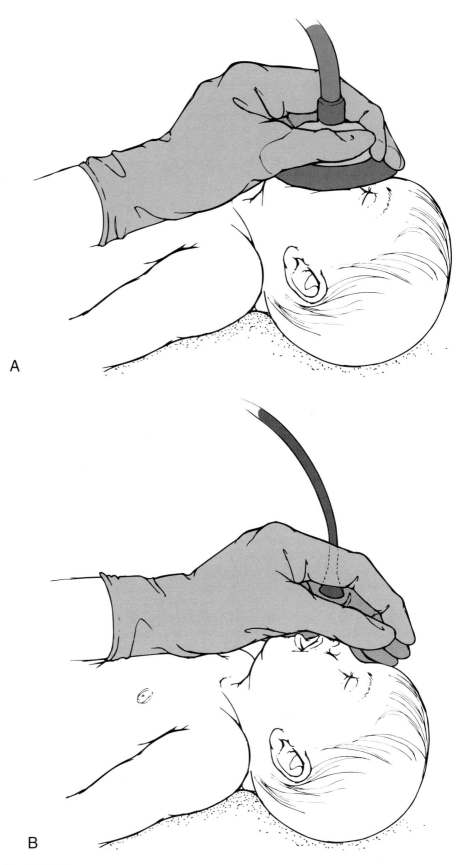

Fig. 24-14. (A) Administering free-flow oxygen to the newborn by mask. Connect the osygen mask to oxygen at 5 liters per minute (LPM) and hold the mask firmly on the newborn's face. (B) Administering free-flow oxygen to the newborn by means of oxygen tubing. Connect the oxygen tubing to oxygen set to at least 5 LPM. Cup your hand around the oxygen tubing and direct the oxygen at the baby's face.

(2) Free-flow oxygen can be administered by oxygen mask or oxygen tubing.

(3) If an oxygen mask is used (*Figure 24-14A*):

    (a) Connect the oxygen mask to oxygen at 5 LPM

    (b) Hold the mask firmly on the newborn's face

(4) If oxygen tubing is used (*Figure 24-14B*):

    (a) Connect the oxygen tubing to oxygen set to at least 5 LPM

    (b) Cup your hand around the oxygen tubing and direct the oxygen at the baby's face

(5) Oxygen is not indicated if the newborn's body is pink but the extremities are blue (acrocyanosis). This condition is common in newborns in the first few minutes of life.

ABNORMAL DELIVERIES

PROLAPSED CORD

1. **Prolapsed cord** is a serious emergency that endangers the life of the unborn fetus.

2. Prolapsed cord occurs when the umbilical cord falls down below the presenting part of the fetus and presents through the birth canal before delivery of the head (*Figure 24-15*).

    a. With each contraction of the uterus, the cord is compressed between the presenting part and the bony pelvis.

    b. Death of the fetus will occur quickly if blood cannot flow through the cord.

3. **Emergency medical care**

    a. Administer oxygen to the mother by nonrebreather mask at 15 LPM.

    b. Position the mother with her head down in a knee-chest position or raise her buttocks as high as possible to lessen pressure on the cord in the birth canal.

    c. Insert a sterile gloved hand into vagina and push the presenting part of the fetus away from the pulsating cord.

        (1) Once this has been accomplished, leave your hand in place.

        (2) Do NOT attempt to push the cord back into the vagina.

    d. With a wet gauze pad or cloth moistened with saline solution, cup the cord against the mother's body to keep it warm and moist.

    e. Transport rapidly while keeping pressure off the cord and monitoring cord pulsations.

BREECH BIRTH

1. A breech presentation occurs when the buttocks or feet are low in the uterus and are the first part of the fetus delivered (*Figure 24-16*).

    a. In a frank breech, the legs are extended on the chest.

    b. In a complete breech, the legs are flexed on the chest.

    c. In a footling breech, one or both feet are present in the vaginal opening.

2. These positions are dangerous for the fetus because of the increased likelihood of a prolapsed cord and delivery trauma.

3. A breech presentation is best managed in the hospital, therefore you should transport immediately upon recognition of a breech presentation.

    a. Administer oxygen to the mother by nonrebreather mask at 15 LPM.

    b. Place the mother in head-down position with the pelvis elevated.

4. If delivery is imminent, prepare for delivery.

    a. Use body substance isolation precautions, including gloves, mask, eye protection, and a gown.

    b. Prepare the mother in the same way as for a head-first delivery.

    c. Position the mother and prepare the OB kit.

    d. Allow the buttocks and trunk of the baby to deliver on their own.

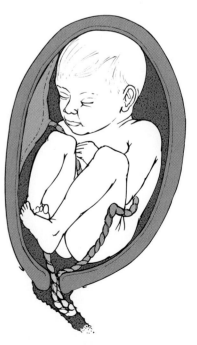

Fig. 24-15. Prolapsed cord occurs when the umbilical cord falls down below the presenting part of the fetus and presents through the birth canal before the head.

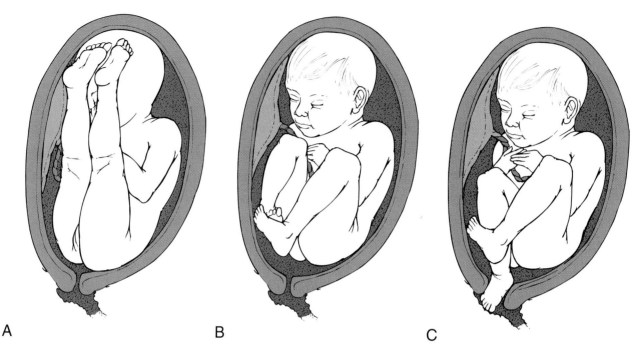

Fig. 24-16. Types of breech presentations. *(A)* Legs extended on the chest (frank breech); *(B)* legs flexed on the chest (complete breech); *(C)* one or both feet present in the vaginal opening (footling breech).

      (1) Do not pull on the infant.

      (2) Pulling may cause the cervix to clamp down tighter on the infant's head.

  e. Once the legs are clear, support the infant's legs and trunk.

  f. If the head does not deliver within 3 minutes of the time the trunk was delivered: (*Figure 24-17*)

      (1) Place a gloved hand into the vagina with the palm toward the infant's face

      (2) Form a "V" with the index and middle finger on either side of the infant's nose

      (3) Push the vaginal wall away from the infant's face

      (4) If necessary, continue this position during transport

LIMB PRESENTATION

1. A limb presentation occurs when a limb of the infant protrudes from the vagina before the head.

2. Transport immediately upon recognition of a limb presentation.

3. Administer oxygen to the mother by nonrebreather mask at 15 LPM.

4. Place the mother in a head-down position with the pelvis elevated.

MULTIPLE BIRTHS

1. Multiple birth should be anticipated if the mother's abdomen appears unusually large or if it remains large after the first infant is delivered.

2. If multiple births are expected, call for assistance and be prepared for more than one resuscitation.

MECONIUM

1. **Meconium** is material that collects in the intestines of a fetus and forms the first stools of a newborn.

  a. It is thick and sticky in consistency and usually greenish to black in color.

  b. Meconium contains swallowed amniotic fluid, mucus, fine hair, blood, and other by-products of growth.

  c. In the newborn with a properly functioning gastrointestinal tract, the color and consistency of meconium changes after 3 or 4 days of feedings of breast milk or formula.

2. The presence of meconium in the amniotic fluid is an indication of possible fetal distress.
   a. Normally, meconium is not passed from the infant's rectum until after birth.
   b. However, during birth, if there is a low oxygen supply, the fetus's anal sphincter may relax and allow the passage of meconium into the amniotic fluid. A low oxygen supply may occur from compression of the umbilical cord, abruptio placenta, or maternal shock, among other causes.

3. If inhaled, meconium may cause severe inflammation of the lungs and pneumonia in the newborn.

4. Amniotic fluid is normally colorless; amniotic fluid containing meconium may be thin and watery or thick and may be brownish-yellow or green in color.

5. If meconium is observed during delivery:
   a. The infant must be vigorously suctioned before he or she begins breathing
   b. As soon as the head is delivered, the newborn's mouth and nose should be thoroughly suctioned
   c. Suctioning must be performed before the shoulders and chest are delivered to reduce the risk of aspiration of meconium
   d. The infant should NOT be stimulated before suctioning is performed

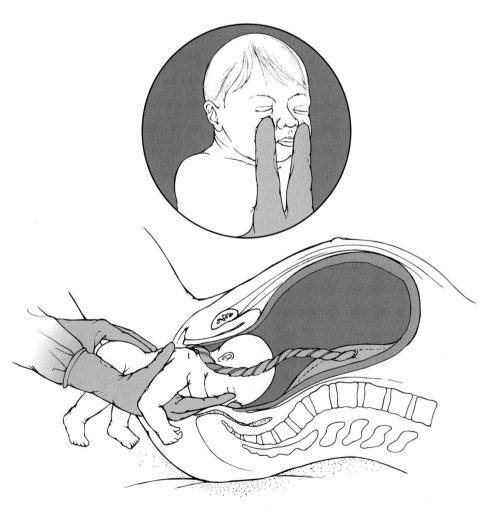

Fig. 24-17. In a breech delivery, if the head does not deliver within 3 minutes of the time the trunk was delivered, place a gloved hand into the vagina with the palm toward the baby's face. Form a "V" with the index and middle finger on either side of the infant's nose and push the vaginal wall away from the baby's face.

   e. Transport as soon as possible, maintaining the airway throughout transport

   f. Report the presence of meconium to personnel at the receiving facility

PREMATURE BIRTH

1. A premature infant is one weighing less than 5.5 pounds or an infant born before the 38th week of gestation.

2. Premature infants are at risk for hypothermia, hypoglycemia, some respiratory problems, and infection.

3. Premature infants often require resuscitation.

4. **Management of the premature infant**

   a. Keep the infant warm to reduce heat loss.

      (1) Wrap the infant in a warm blanket.

      (2) Cover the infant's body and head (keep the face exposed).

   b. Keep the mouth and nose clear of fluid and mucus.

   c. Administer oxygen.

      (1) Do not allow cold oxygen to blow directly into the infant's face.

      (2) Provide positive-pressure ventilation if breathing is inadequate.

   d. Prevent bleeding from the umbilical cord.

      (1) Frequently check the cut end of the umbilical cord to be sure it is not bleeding.

      (2) Premature infants cannot tolerate the loss of even small amounts of blood.

   e. Protect the infant from contamination.

      (1) Premature infants are highly susceptible to infection.

      (2) Do not breathe directly into the infant's face.

GYNECOLOGICAL EMERGENCIES

VAGINAL BLEEDING WITH NO HISTORY OF TRAUMA

1. While taking the patient's history, ask the following questions:

   a. When was the patient's last menstrual period? Was it normal?

   b. Is the patient sexually active?

   c. Is there any possibility of pregnancy?

   d. How long has the patient been bleeding?

   e. Is the blood dark red (like menstrual blood) or bright red?

   f. How many sanitary napkins has she used?

   g. Is the bleeding heavier or lighter than a normal menstrual period?

   h. Has the patient had these same symptoms before?

   i. Does the patient have a history of:

      (a) Urinary tract infections

      (b) Gallbladder problems

      (c) Endometriosis (a condition in which uterine tissue is located outside the uterus; causes pain and bleeding)

      (d) Kidney stones

   j. Does the patient feel dizzy when standing?

2. Assess baseline vital signs.

3. **Emergency medical care**

   a. Take appropriate body substance isolation precautions.

   b. Provide specific treatment based on the patient's signs and symptoms.

   c. Establish and maintain an open airway.

   d. Administer oxygen.

      (1) If the patient's breathing is adequate, apply oxygen by nonrebreather mask at 15 LPM if not already done.

      (2) If the patient's breathing is inadequate, provide positive-pressure ventila-

tion with 100% oxygen and assess the adequacy of the ventilations delivered.
   e. Treat for shock, if indicated.
   f. Maintain body temperature.
   g. Apply external vaginal pads as necessary.
      (1) As the pad becomes blood-soaked, replace it with a new one.
      (2) All blood-soaked garments and pads should accompany the patient to the hospital.
   h. Transport.
      (1) If the patient is stable, perform ongoing assessments every 15 minutes.
      (2) If the patient is unstable, perform ongoing assessments every 5 minutes.

VAGINAL BLEEDING WITH A HISTORY OF TRAUMA

1. Trauma to the external genitalia may occur from:
   a. Straddle injuries
   b. Blunt trauma
   c. Childbirth
   d. Sexual assault
2. **Emergency medical care**
   a. Take appropriate body substance isolation precautions.
   b. Ensure and maintain an open airway.
   c. Administer oxygen.
   d. Control bleeding with local pressure to the area using trauma dressings or sanitary napkins.
   e. Do not pack or place dressings inside the vagina.
   f. Monitor the patient's vital signs.
   g. Treat for shock if indicated.
   h. Provide additional care based on the patient's signs and symptoms.
   i. Provide reassurance and privacy.

ALLEGED SEXUAL ASSAULT

1. Criminal assault situations require initial and ongoing assessment/management and psychological care.
2. **Emergency medical care**
   a. Take appropriate body substance isolation precautions.
   b. When possible, have an EMT-Basic of the same gender assess the sexual assault victim.
   c. Ensure and maintain an open airway.
   d. Maintain a nonjudgmental attitude during the SAMPLE history and focused assessment.
   e. Protect the crime scene.
      (1) Discourage the patient from bathing, douching, voiding, or cleaning wounds until after transport and evaluation at the receiving facility.
      (2) Do not allow the patient to comb the hair or clean the fingernails.
      (3) Handle the patient's clothing as little as possible.
      (4) Bag all items separately.
      (5) Do not use plastic bags for bloodstained articles. Plastic holds in moisture, which can promote the growth of bacteria. Bacterial growth can contaminate evidence.
   f. Examine the genitalia only if profuse bleeding is present.
   g. Transport to appropriate medical facility for further evaluation and treatment.

REVIEW QUESTIONS

Directions: Each of the numbered items or incomplete statements in this section is followed by answers or by completions of the statement. Select the ONE lettered answer or completion that is BEST in each case.

1. The _____ of the female reproductive system produce(s) the hormones estrogen and progesterone and releases an egg once a month.

    (A) ovaries
    (B) fallopian tubes
    (C) uterus
    (D) cervix

2. In a normal pregnancy, the egg will travel to the uterus through the

    (A) cervix
    (B) vagina
    (C) urethra
    (D) fallopian tubes

3. Another term for the shedding of the uterine lining is

    (A) menopause
    (B) menstruation
    (C) placental delivery
    (D) the first stage of labor

4. During delivery, especially very rapid deliveries, the tissue between the mother's anus and vagina may tear. This area is called the

    (A) colon
    (B) cervix
    (C) perineum
    (D) labia majora

5. The organ responsible for the exchange of oxygen and carbon dioxide between the blood of the mother and the fetus is the

    (A) cervix
    (B) vagina
    (C) placenta
    (D) fallopian tubes

6. Your rescue crew has been called to the home of a 23-year-old female patient complaining of severe flulike symptoms. She is 7 months pregnant with her first child. She informs you that she has been vomiting for the past 2 days and has a mild fever. She requests transport to a local clinic. You should position this patient

    (A) on her left side
    (B) on her stomach (prone)
    (C) flat on her back with her legs elevated (shock position)
    (D) flat on her back with the head lower than the feet (Trendelenburg position).

7. A premature infant is an infant weighing less than 5.5 pounds or born before the

38th week of gestation. Prompt, proper care of these infants is critical to their survival. Infants are generally considered viable after what age of fetal growth?

(A) Approximately 15–20 weeks
(B) Approximately 24–28 weeks
(C) Approximately 32–36 weeks
(D) Approximately 36–38 weeks

8. Your ambulance crew has been called to a local high school for an 18-year-old female patient complaining of severe left lower abdominal pain. She is pale and sweaty with a weak radial pulse at 124 beats per minute. She denies any recent illness or trauma. She does, however, state that she is sexually active and missed her last period, but she does not think she is pregnant. This patient's pain is most likely due to

(A) eclampsia
(B) placenta previa
(C) abruptio placenta
(D) ectopic pregnancy

9. Your ambulance crew has been called to transport a 19-year-old female patient. She states she is about to deliver her first child, and her estimated delivery date is tomorrow. She has been having contractions for about the last 20 minutes. Normally, the first stage of labor for this patient will be

(A) 1–2 hours long
(B) 8–12 hours long
(C) 5–15 minutes long
(D) the last 90 days of the pregnancy

10. When delivering the placenta (afterbirth), it is important to

(A) retain the placenta for inspection at the hospital
(B) massage the uterus before delivery of the placenta
(C) gently pull on the umbilical cord to help the delivery
(D) hold the delivered placenta about 2–3 feet above the level of the infant before clamping and cutting the cord

11. Normally, the placenta will deliver

(A) just before the infant
(B) at the same time as the infant
(C) about 2–3 hours after the infant
(D) about 10–20 minutes after the infant

12. If, during delivery of an infant, the umbilical cord is wrapped around the neck and cannot be released, you should

(A) cut the cord immediately because there is no time to clamp
(B) not allow the infant to deliver and begin rapid transport
(C) clamp the cord about 3 inches apart and cut between the clamps
(D) gently pull on the cord and the infant to deliver both at the same time

13. Which of the following may indicate that the infant was in distress before delivery?

(A) Yellowish-green amniotic fluid
(B) An initial pulse rate of 160 beats per minute
(C) An initial respiratory rate of 40 to 60 breaths per minute
(D) The child has a strong cry and his or her limbs resist straightening

14. Your rescue crew is called to a restaurant for a 26-year-old female patient who states her water has broken. She is 9 months pregnant with her fourth child. Upon examination, you note that a loop of the umbilical cord is protruding from the vaginal opening. In addition to high-flow oxygen therapy and rapid transport, you should

(A) gently push the cord back into the birth canal and position the patient on her left side

(B) position the patient in a knee-chest position, clamp and cut the cord, and prepare for delivery

(C) position the patient in a knee-chest position, gently push the fetus way from the cord, and keep the cord moist

(D) gently pull on the cord to ease delivery of the infant and transport with the patient on her back with the head slightly elevated

15. Your ambulance is transporting a 31-year-old pregnant woman who is 8½ months pregnant with her first child. While en route to the hospital, the patient states she feels like she has to move her bowels. When looking at the vaginal opening, you observe one of the infant's arms dangling from the birth canal. You should

(A) stop the ambulance and prepare for a "field" delivery

(B) position the mother on her left side and rapidly transport to the hospital

(C) position the mother in a head-down position with the pelvis elevated, and rapidly transport to the hospital

(D) place the arm back in the birth canal, position the mother on her left side, and rapidly transport to the hospital

16. Your rescue crew has been dispatched to transport an assault patient from a crime scene. Local law enforcement personnel have secured the scene. Your patient is a 24-year-old woman complaining of head pain. She states she was jumped while jogging in the park and was hit in the head with a small bat. A police officer informs you the patient told her that she was raped. Appropriate interventions should include

(A) having the police officer transport the patient to the hospital to complete a "rape kit"

(B) full spinal immobilization, oxygen therapy, focused history and physical examination, and transport

(C) full spinal immobilization, oxygen therapy, focused history and physical examination to determine if a rape occurred, and transport

(D) allowing the patient to bathe quickly, full spinal immobilization, focused history and physical examination, and transport

Directions: Each of the numbered questions or incomplete statements in this section refers to a scenario that precedes them. The numbered questions or incomplete statements are followed by answers or by completions of the statement. Select the answer or completion of the statement that is BEST in each case.

Your ambulance crew is called to the home of a 32-year-old female requesting transportation to the hospital maternity ward. You arrive to find your patient lying in bed. She is conscious and alert, complaining of contractions.

Questions 17–19

17. After performing a scene size-up and initial assessment, you should turn your attention to

(A) gathering a SAMPLE history
(B) gathering baseline vital signs
(C) performing a rapid physical examination
(D) performing a focused physical examination

18. The patient informs you that her third child is due to deliver next week. She is

(A) in the third stage of labor
(B) in the first trimester of pregnancy
(C) in the third trimester of pregnancy
(D) in the fourth trimester of pregnancy

19. The patient informs you that she has been having contractions all morning, but they have increased in intensity over the last hour. Which of the following would suggest that delivery may be imminent?

(A) The patient has been urinating frequently
(B) The patient feels as though she needs to have a bowel movement
(C) The patient feels weak and dizzy when lying flat on her back
(D) The patient has been experiencing contractions that last about 30 seconds and are about 10 minutes apart

Your rescue crew is called to the scene of a 35-year-old female complaining of a severe headache and blurred vision. You arrive to find the patient sitting in a darkened room. She states she is 8 months pregnant with her fourth child. She has received no prenatal care. On examination, you note that the patient's face is swollen and her blood pressure is 164/98.

Questions 20–22

20. Which of the following conditions would be consistent with your findings?

(A) Preeclampsia
(B) Placenta previa
(C) Abruptio placenta
(D) Ectopic pregnancy

21. The correct position and mode of transportation for this patient is

(A) patient on her left side, transport rapidly with lights and siren
(B) patient in a knee-chest position, transport rapidly with lights and siren
(C) patient on her left side, transport without lights and siren, and dim the lights in the patient area of the ambulance
(D) patient on her back with her head lower than her feet (Trendelenburg), transport rapidly with lights and siren

22. If this patient's condition worsens, she is at risk of

(A) having a seizure
(B) placenta previa
(C) a diabetic emergency
(D) losing her feet due to inadequate circulation

Your ambulance crew is called to transport a 38-year-old female patient complaining of vaginal bleeding. She is 38 weeks pregnant with her fifth child. Upon examination, you observe that the patient has lost approximately 200–300 milliliters of bright red blood in the last 10 minutes. According to the patient, her bag of waters has not ruptured. She denies any recent trauma or any pain associated with the bloody discharge. Her vital signs are as follows: pulse 116 beats per minute with moderate strength, blood pressure 108/72, respirations 16 breaths per minute.

Questions 23–24

23. Which of the following is consistent with this patient's presentation?

(A) Eclampsia
(B) Placenta previa
(C) Abruptio placenta
(D) First stage of labor

24. Management of this patient should include

(A) instruct the patient to bear down and prepare for home delivery of the infant
(B) insert a tampon to stop the bleeding, administer oxygen by nonrebreather mask, position the patient on her left side, transport promptly
(C) apply sanitary napkins to the outside of the vagina, administer oxygen by nonrebreather mask, position the patient on her left side, transport promptly
(D) place the patient in a knee-chest position, insert a gloved hand into the birth canal to create an airway for the infant, administer oxygen by nonrebreather mask, transport promptly

Your rescue crew is dispatched to a motor vehicle collision on a local highway. Information at the time of dispatch is that there are three cars involved, and the accident "appears serious."

Questions 25–27

25. Your first action when arriving on the scene should be to

(A) perform a scene size-up
(B) begin immediate extrication of all trapped patients
(C) perform an initial assessment on all critical patients
(D) perform a rapid physical examination on all unconscious patients

26. You are assigned to assess and treat a 32-year-old female patient who was the driver of one of the vehicles involved. She tells you she was not wearing her seat belt and was traveling about 40 miles per hour when another car pulled out in front of her. She is alert and answering all questions appropriately. She is in severe distress. Which of the following findings would be consistent with an abruptio placenta?

(A) Elevated blood pressure, pedal edema, and severe headache
(B) Nausea, vomiting, elevated blood pressure, and subsequent seizures
(C) Painless bright red bloody discharge from the vagina and signs of shock
(D) Severe abdominal pain, dark red bloody discharge from the vagina, and signs of shock

27. Appropriate interventions for this patient would be

(A) position the patient sitting upright, high-flow oxygen, and rapid transport
(B) full spinal immobilization with the backboard tilted to the left, high-flow oxygen, and rapid transport
(C) position the patient on her left side, high-flow oxygen, and transport slowly without lights or siren
(D) full spinal immobilization with the head of the backboard elevated, high-flow oxygen, and transport

Your rescue crew is called to the home of a 34-year-old female patient whose bag of waters has broken. You arrive to find the patient supine on the floor of her apartment. The baby's head can be seen at the birth canal. You decide to remain on the scene and deliver the baby.

Questions 28–30

28. After the head has emerged from the birth canal, you should

(A)   instruct the mother to give one last big push
(B)   suction the mouth and nose with a bulb syringe
(C)   apply gentle traction to the head to ease delivery of the shoulder
(D)   apply a pediatric oxygen mask to the baby and flow the oxygen at 5 liters per minute (LPM)

29. As soon as the entire baby has been delivered, you should immediately

(A)   clamp the umbilical cord
(B)   clamp and cut the umbilical cord
(C)   begin warming, drying, and stimulating the baby
(D)   place the infant approximately 2–3 feet below the level of the birth canal

30. Evaluation of this infant's condition after birth is conducted using which of the following acronyms?

(A)   AVPU
(B)   APGAR
(C)   SAMPLE
(D)   A-NU-BABY

ANSWERS AND RATIONALES

1-A. The almond-shaped ovaries are the organs that produce estrogen and progesterone and release eggs. Each month of her reproductive years, a woman typically releases one egg (except while pregnant).

2-D. The fallopian tubes receive and transport the egg to the uterus after ovulation. If fertilization occurs, the developing fetus (unborn infant) implants itself in the uterine wall and develops there.

3-B. At the end of each menstrual period, the uterus again begins to prepare to receive a fertilized egg. Generally, ovulation (release of an egg) occurs 14 days before the beginning of the next menstrual cycle. If the egg does not implant, the lining of the uterus will again shed.

4-C. The area between the anus and the vagina is the perineum. To help prevent tearing of the perineum, you may apply gentle pressure to the top of the infant's head as it emerges from the vagina. Be careful not to touch the fontanelles, the areas of the skull that have not yet formed. The pressure you apply should not halt delivery of the infant, but control it. "Colon" is another term for the large intestine. The cervix is the neck of the uterus. During pregnancy, it contains the mucus plug that protects the uterus from the invasion of bacteria. The passage of the plug may account for a light bloody show in the first stage of labor. The labia majora is the term given to the outermost folds of skin that enclose the vulva.

5-C. The placenta is a specialized structure of pregnancy that begins to develop about 2 weeks after fertilization occurs. It attaches to the mother at the inner wall of the uterus and to the fetus by the umbilical cord. The placenta is responsible for the exchange of oxygen and carbon dioxide between the blood of the mother and fetus, removal of waste products, transport of nutrients from the mother to the fetus, and production of a special hormone of pregnancy that maintains the pregnancy and stimulates changes in the mother's breasts, cervix, and vagina in preparation for delivery. The placenta also provides a barrier against harmful substances and transfers heat from the mother to the fetus.

6-A. The preferred position for a pregnant (more than 20 weeks) female patient is left lateral recumbent. Positioning the patient on the left side prevents the developing fetus from compressing the major blood vessels of the abdomen (abdominal aorta and inferior vena cava).

7-B. Viability may begin as early as 20 weeks' gestation. Statistically, however, long-term viability generally starts at 24 to 28 weeks. Preterm infants often have respiratory difficulty due to immature lung development. One of the most critical interventions when caring for a premature infant is the prevention of hypothermia (lowering of the body temperature). Premature infants rapidly lose body heat and may not have the compensatory mechanism to generate heat. Regardless of gestational age at time of birth, hypothermia is a major contributor to infant distress, but it is easily prevented. Prewarm the ambulance and have ample towels, blankets, and draft protection (aluminum foil, plastic wrap, etc.) readily available. Do not wrap the infant in wet towels or blankets. Leave only the face exposed.

8-D. Until proven otherwise, any female patient in her reproductive years who complains of severe one-sided (left or right) lower abdominal pain should be suspected of and treated for an ectopic pregnancy. Treatment is geared toward slowing the progression of shock. Elevate the legs, provide high-flow oxygen, and transport rapidly to an emergency department.

9-B. While it is possible that delivery is imminent, it is more likely that the patient has plenty of time left. The first stage of labor for a woman pregnant for the first time averages 8–12 hours. For women who have had multiple births, the length of the first stage of labor is less, about 6–8 hours, and it may sometimes be as little as 1 hour. Always be prepared for the immediate delivery of a compromised infant.

10-A. If the placenta delivers before arrival at the receiving facility, you must retain the placenta for inspection. The placenta should be inspected for completeness. Complications may arise from the incomplete delivery of the placenta. Do not pull on the umbilical cord. Always attempt to keep the infant at the same level as the placenta until the cord is clamped. If you hold the infant below the placenta, blood will flow from the placenta to the infant. If you hold the infant above the placenta, blood will flow out of the infant into the placenta.

11-D. The placenta will normally deliver about 10–20 minutes after the infant is born. If it delivers in the field, retain it. If it does not deliver, make sure you pass that information on to medical personnel at the receiving facility. You should not be preoccupied or overly concerned about delivering the placenta. You should be treating and assessing the mother and child.

12-C. If the cord is wrapped around the neck (a nuchal cord), you should first attempt to loop the cord back over the head. If this cannot be accomplished, carefully clamp the cord in 2 places about 3 inches apart. Protect the infant from the scissors by placing your hand between the cord and the infant; then cut the cord. Do not use a scalpel or knife because of the risk of cutting the infant or yourself. The infant should then be free for delivery.

13-A. Meconium is the substance that lines the bowel of the fetus. If the fetus becomes distressed, he or she may pass meconium in the amniotic fluid. If the bag of waters ruptured before your arrival, you should ask about the characteristics of the fluid. Normal amniotic fluid is clear. If meconium is present in the amniotic fluid, it is particularly important to suction the infant's airway after the head emerges (before delivery of the shoulders). If the infant inhales meconium into the lungs, serious complications may arise. Make sure that you inform the receiving facility about the presence of meconium. It is normal for an infant to have a pulse rate of

160 beats per minute, a respiratory rate of 40 to 60 breaths per minute, a vigorous cry, and resistance to straightening.

14-C. This condition is called a prolapsed umbilical cord. Definitive care is achieved at the hospital. Your treatment should be aimed at ensuring adequate blood flow through the cord to the infant and providing oxygen therapy to the mother. To relieve the pressure of the infant on the cord, first place the mother in a knee-chest position (prone with the buttocks up and the head down). In this position, gravity will assist in moving the infant's head away from the birth canal. Using a gloved hand, gently apply pressure to the presenting part of the infant (usually the top of the head) until a pulse can be felt in the umbilical cord. Be mindful of the fontanelles (areas where the skull has not yet developed). The cord should be kept moist with warm (not hot), sterile water or normal saline.

15-C. Definitive care will be provided at the hospital. This is not an indication for field delivery. By positioning the patient with her head lower than her pelvis, the pressure on the infant is decreased. Transport rapidly to the hospital.

16-B. Spinal immobilization is indicated due to the trauma to the head. Here are some guidelines for dealing with alleged sexual assault. It is not your job to determine the truth of the patient's statements. It is also not your job to be judgmental or critical of the patient. You are dealing with a patient who has multiple injuries: an injured head, possible injuries to the pelvic area, and the very real injury to her psyche. Rape is a traumatic event both physically and emotionally. Be professional and supportive. Be thorough in your history-taking but not intrusive. Be supportive, but not chatty. If available, have a crew member of the same gender interact with the patient. Be gentle and brief in conducting a physical examination. Examination of the patient's genitalia should only be done if profuse bleeding is present. If the suspected injury is not so significant that you would need to treat it, visualizing the area only makes the patient more uncomfortable and may result in the damage of important evidence. Ensure your documentation is accurate and complete.

17-A. Since this patient is conscious and alert, questioning her about her medical history and current condition before performing a physical examination is most appropriate. A rapid physical examination would be indicated if the patient were not conscious and alert. Baseline vital signs may be assessed during or after the focused history and physical examination (depending on the size/resources of your crew).

18-C. Pregnancy is divided into trimesters (three trimesters). Each trimester lasts approximately 90 days. The third trimester is from the seventh through the ninth month of pregnancy.

19-B. Do not allow the patient to sit on the toilet to have a bowel movement. When the fetus enters the birth canal, it presses against the rectum. This sensation is often confused with the need to move one's bowels. Frequent urination is generally present throughout pregnancy due to the increasing size of the uterus pressing against the urinary bladder. Do not allow this patient to lie flat on her back. Dizziness and weakness are likely to occur because of the compression of the abdominal blood vessels by the fetus. If left on her back for a sustained period, perfusion to the fetus will be compromised. The contractions associated with imminent delivery generally last 45– 60 seconds and occur every 2–3 minutes.

20-A. Preeclampsia is a hypertensive disorder associated with pregnancy. Signs and symptoms of preeclampsia include abnormal weight gain (due to fluid retention); swelling of the face, hands, and lower back; visual disturbances; headaches; irritability; right upper quadrant abdominal pain; and increased blood pressure (greater than 140/90). The other conditions listed will be discussed in the rationales of other questions.

21-C. The appropriate position for this patient is left lateral recumbent. Although this patient has a serious medical complication, you must transport without lights and siren because stimulation from the flashing lights and loud siren may cause a seizure in this patient.

22-A. Preeclampsia may deteriorate into eclampsia. Eclampsia is the presence of grand mal (full body) seizures in a preeclamptic patient. Eclampsia is a medical emergency. During the active convulsions, treat the mother as you would any other seizure patient and prevent the patient from injuring herself. After the seizure, position the patient on her left side, maintain an open airway (suctioning may be necessary), provide high-flow oxygen (by nonrebreather mask if breathing is adequate or by bag-valve mask if breathing is inadequate), and transport promptly but without excessive stimuli (lights or sirens).

23-B. The painless discharge of blood during the last trimester of pregnancy is most often associated with a placenta previa. Placenta previa develops if the placenta implants too low in the uterine wall. The lower portion of the uterus stretches and contracts in preparation for delivery. If the placenta has implanted in this area, it may tear. The fetus depends on the placenta for nourishment and oxygen.

24-C. While there is commonly a "bloody show" associated with normal delivery (from the passage of the mucus plug), it is not normal for 200 to 300 milliliters (mL) of blood to be discharged before delivery of the infant. This patient should not be told to bear down because this may increase the size of the tear. Never place anything in the vagina (such as a tampon) because it hides the extent of bleeding. Apply sanitary napkins to the exterior of the vaginal opening to absorb the bleeding, provide high-flow oxygen, position the patient on her left side, and transport rapidly. Retain used sanitary napkins for the hospital, as they indicate the extent of bleeding.

25-A. Your initial responsibility is to assess the scene. Your scene assessment should address the number of patients, the mechanism of injury, the need for additional resources, safety (for you, your crew, the patients, and bystanders), and body substance isolation precautions. After the size-up, you can begin gaining access to and evaluating patients.

26-D. Abruptio placenta may occur from trauma, high blood pressure, or multiple pregnancies. An abruptio placenta is the premature separation of the placenta from the uterine wall during the last trimester of pregnancy. Patients with this condition have severe abdominal pain. Bleeding may be present or absent depending on the location of the tear. Patients may also complain of decreased or absent fetal movement. Severe hypoxia slows the activity of the fetus.

27-B. Since your patient has been involved in a motor vehicle collision, spinal immobilization is indicated. You must ensure that the fetus does not compress the blood vessels of the abdomen. To prevent this compression, tilt the entire backboard to the left. Provide high-flow oxygen and transport rapidly to the closest appropriate facility.

28-B. After the head emerges, instruct the mother to "breathe through" the next contraction until you can clear the infant's airway. Clear the airway with a bulb syringe. Make sure you depress (squeeze) the syringe before you put it in the infant's mouth and nose. Once the nose and mouth have been suctioned adequately, you may lower the infant's head slightly to ease delivery of the top shoulder. Then lift up slightly to deliver the bottom shoulder. The shoulders are the widest part of the infant's body. Once the shoulders deliver, the rest of the baby will deliver rapidly. Be gentle but supportive as the infant emerges.

29-C. Leave the infant at the level of the birth canal and immediately begin warming, drying, and stimulating the infant. Regardless of the infant's presentation (whether pink and crying or blue and slow to respond), warming, drying, and stimulating are always the first steps in the resuscitation of a newborn.

30-B. Newborns are evaluated using the Apgar scale: **A**ppearance (color), **P**ulse (heart rate), **G**rimace (irritability), **A**ctivity (muscle tone), and **R**espirations (breathing rate). Each category is rated from 0 to 2 (with 2 being normal/healthy) for a total of 10 possible points. The scale is evaluated at 1 minute and 5 minutes postbirth. If the 5-minute evaluation is less than 7, continue evaluating every 5 minutes. AVPU is an acronym for assessing the level of consciousness for adults or children. SAMPLE is the history-taking acronym. A-NU-BABY is not an accepted acronym.

BIBLIOGRAPHY

Caroline NL: *Emergency Care in the Streets*, 4th ed. Boston, Little, Brown, 1991.

Crosby LA, Lewallen DG (eds): *Emergency Care and Transportation of the Sick and Injured*, 6th ed. Rosemont, IL, American Academy of Orthopaedic Surgeons, 1995.

Grant HD, Murray RH Jr, Bergeron JD: *Emergency Care*, 7th ed. Englewood Cliffs, NJ, Prentice-Hall, 1995.

Hafen BQ, Karren KJ, Mistovich JJ: *Prehospital Emergency Care*, 5th ed. Upper Saddle River, NJ, Prentice-Hall, 1996.

Henry MC, Stapleton ER, Judd RL: *EMT: Prehospital Care*. Philadelphia, WB Saunders, 1992.

McSwain NE, White RD, Paturas JL, et al (eds): *The Basic EMT: Comprehensive Prehospital Patient Care*. St. Louis, Mosby-Year Book, 1996.

Miller RH, Wilson JK: *Manual of Prehospital Emergency Medicine*. St. Louis, Mosby-Year Book, 1992.

Sanders MJ: *Mosby's Paramedic Textbook*. St. Louis, Mosby-Year Book, 1994.

Sheehy SB, Lombardi JE: *Manual of Emergency Care*, 4th ed. St. Louis, Mosby-Year Book, 1995.

Stoy WA: *Mosby's EMT-Basic Textbook*. St. Louis, Mosby-Year Book, 1996.

United States Department of Transportation, National Highway Traffic Safety Administration: *Emergency Medical Technician: Basic. National Standard Curriculum*, 1994.

TRAUMA

FIVE

BLEEDING AND SHOCK

25

25-1 Describe the structure and function of the cardiovascular system.

25-2 Establish the relationship between body substance isolation and bleeding.

25-3 Differentiate among arterial, venous, and capillary bleeding.

25-4 State methods of emergency medical care of external bleeding.

25-5 Establish the relationship between airway management and the trauma patient.

25-6 Establish the relationship between the mechanism of injury and internal bleeding.

25-7 List the signs of internal bleeding.

25-8 List the steps in the emergency medical care of the patient with signs and symptoms of internal bleeding.

25-9 List signs and symptoms of shock (hypoperfusion).

25-10 State the steps in the emergency medical care of the patient with signs and symptoms of shock (hypoperfusion).

CARDIOVASCULAR SYSTEM REVIEW

ANATOMY REVIEW

1. The cardiovascular system consists of the heart, blood vessels, and blood.
2. **Heart**
   a. The right side of the heart receives oxygen-poor blood from the body and pumps it to the lungs to be re-oxygenated.

● MOTIVATION FOR LEARNING ●

Bleeding and shock (hypoperfusion) are conditions that must be identified during the initial assessment. After performing the scene size-up, ensuring personal safety, and evaluating and managing airway and breathing, the EMT-Basic should control arterial or venous bleeding, if present. The EMT-Basic must understand the relationship between mechanisms of injury and the signs and symptoms of bleeding and shock to appropriately manage patients.

b. The left side of the heart receives oxygen-rich blood from the lungs and pumps it to the body.

3. Arteries
    a. Arteries carry blood away from the heart to the body.
    b. All arteries, except the pulmonary arteries, carry oxygen-rich blood.
    c. The walls of arteries have thick muscular and elastic layers that allow the arteries to carry blood under high pressure.
    d. The aorta is the largest artery of the body.

4. Arterioles
    a. The arterioles are the smallest branches of arteries leading to capillaries.
    b. Smooth muscle in the vessel walls allows the vessel to narrow and widen.
        (1) Narrowing of the vessels is called vasoconstriction.
        (2) Widening of the vessels is called vasodilation.
    c. The arterioles are important in controlling the amount of blood flow to specific tissues.

5. Capillaries
    a. Capillaries are microscopic vessels that are one cell thick.
    b. They serve as vessels for exchange of wastes, fluids, and nutrients between the blood and tissues.
    c. They connect arterioles and venules.

6. Venules are the smallest branches of veins leading to capillaries.

7. Veins
    a. Veins carry oxygen-poor blood from the body to the right side of the heart.
    b. All veins, except the pulmonary veins, carry oxygen-poor blood.
    c. The walls of veins are thinner than arteries.
    d. Many veins in the extremities and neck contain valves arranged to allow blood flow in one direction, toward the heart.

8. Blood
    a. Formed elements
        (1) Red blood cells (erythrocytes) are the transport vehicles for oxygen and carbon dioxide in the blood.
            (a) Red blood cells transport oxygen to body cells.
            (b) Each red blood cell contains hemoglobin.
                (i) Hemoglobin is an iron-containing protein.
                (ii) Hemoglobin carries oxygen from the lungs to the tissues.
                (iii) Hemoglobin contains a pigment that gives blood its red color.
            (c) Red blood cells also transport carbon dioxide away from body cells.
        (2) White blood cells (leukocytes) defend the body from microorganisms.
        (3) Platelets (thrombocytes) are essential for the formation of blood clots and function to stop bleeding and repair ruptured blood vessels.
    b. Plasma
        (1) Plasma is the clear, straw-colored liquid component of blood (blood minus its formed elements).
        (2) It carries nutrients to the cells and waste products from the cells.

PHYSIOLOGY

1. Pulse
    a. When the left ventricle contracts, a wave of blood is sent through the arteries, causing them to expand and recoil.
    b. A **pulse** is the regular expansion and recoil of an artery caused by the movement of blood from the heart as it contracts.
    c. A pulse can be felt anywhere an artery simultaneously passes near the skin surface and over a bone.
    d. Central pulses are located close to the heart and include the carotid and femoral pulses *(Figure 25-1)*.
    e. Peripheral pulses are located farther from the heart and include the radial, brachial, posterior tibial, and dorsalis pedis pulses.

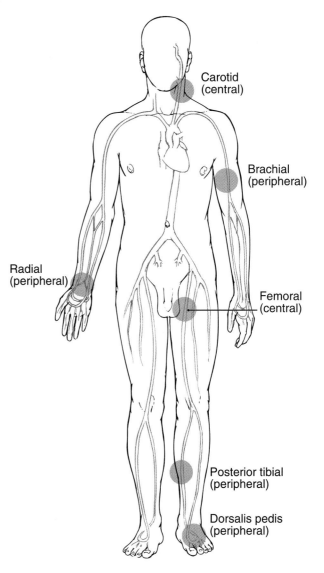

Fig. 25-1. Central and peripheral pulses.

2. **Blood pressure**
   a. **Blood pressure** is the force exerted by the blood on the inner walls of the heart and blood vessels.
   b. **Systolic blood pressure** is the pressure exerted against the walls of the arteries when the left ventricle contracts.
   c. **Diastolic blood pressure** is the pressure exerted against the walls of the arteries when the left ventricle is at rest.
3. **Perfusion**
   a. **Perfusion** is the circulation of blood through an organ or a part of the body.
   b. Perfusion delivers oxygen and other nutrients to the cells of all organ systems and removes waste products.
   c. **Hypoperfusion (shock)** is inadequate circulation of blood through an organ or a part of the body.

EXTERNAL BLEEDING

BODY SUBSTANCE ISOLATION (BSI) PRECAUTIONS

1. BSI precautions must be routinely taken to avoid skin and mucous membrane exposure to body fluids.

2. BSI precautions include eye protection, gloves, gown, and mask.

3. Wash hands after each patient contact.

SEVERITY

1. Normal blood volumes
   a. Adult: 5 liters (L)
   b. Child 8 years of age and younger: 2000 milliliters (mL)
   c. Child 6 years of age and younger: 1600 mL
   d. Infant: 800 mL

2. Blood loss is considered severe when:
   a. An adult loses 1 liter (1000 mL) of blood
   b. A child loses ½ liter (500 mL) of blood
   c. An infant loses 100–200 mL of blood

3. **Example.** A one-year-old has a blood volume of approximately 800 mL. A loss of 150 mL is considered major blood loss.

4. Severity of blood loss should be based on the patient's signs and symptoms.

5. If the patient exhibits signs and symptoms of shock, the bleeding is considered serious.

6. The natural response to bleeding is blood vessel constriction and clotting.
   a. Clotting normally occurs within 6 to 10 minutes.
   b. A serious injury may prevent effective clotting from occurring.
   c. Some medications can also interfere with blood clotting, such as aspirin and Coumadin® (a "blood-thinning," or anticoagulant, drug)
   d. Hemophilia is a disorder in which the blood does not clot normally.

7. Uncontrolled bleeding or significant blood loss may lead to shock and, possibly, death.

TYPES OF BLEEDING (FIGURE 25-2)

1. **Arterial bleeding**
   a. The blood from an artery is bright red, oxygen-rich blood.
   b. Blood spurts from the wound.
   c. Arterial bleeding is life threatening.
   d. It is difficult to control because of the pressure at which arteries bleed.
   e. As the patient's blood pressure drops, the amount of spurting may also drop.

2. **Venous bleeding**
   a. Blood from a vein is dark red or maroon, oxygen-poor blood.
   b. Blood flows as a steady stream.
   c. Bleeding occurs more often from veins than arteries because veins are closer to the skin's surface.
   d. Venous bleeding is usually easier to control than arterial bleeding because it is under less pressure.
   e. Bleeding from deep veins (such as those in the trunk or thigh) can cause profuse bleeding that is hard to control.

3. **Capillary bleeding**
   a. Blood from capillaries is dark red.
   b. Blood oozes from wound.
   c. Bleeding often clots by itself.

ASSESSMENT OF THE PATIENT WITH EXTERNAL BLEEDING

1. Take body substance isolation precautions.

2. During scene size-up, evaluate the mechanism of injury or nature of the illness.

3. Maintain spinal immobilization if needed.

4. Assess the patient's mental status.

5. Assess the patient's airway.

6. Assess breathing.

7. Assess circulation. Severe bleeding must be controlled during the initial assessment.

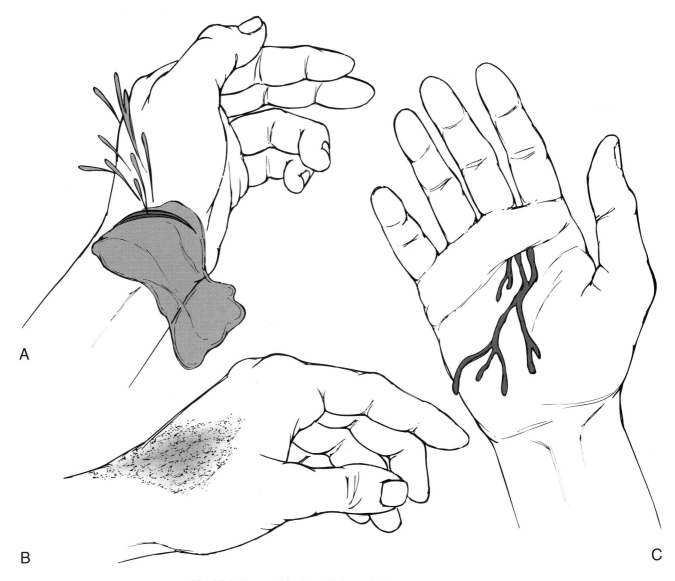

Fig. 25-2. Types of bleeding. *(A)* Arterial, *(B)* capillary, *(C)* venous.

8. Identify any life-threatening conditions and provide care based on these findings.
9. Establish patient priorities.
    a. Priority patients are those who:
        (1) Give a poor general impression
        (2) Have severe pain anywhere
        (3) Have uncontrolled bleeding
        (4) Have signs and symptoms of shock
        (5) Are unresponsive with no gag reflex or cough
    b. Advanced-life-support (ALS) assistance should be requested as soon as possible for priority patients.
    c. If ALS personnel are not available, the patient should be transported promptly to the closest appropriate facility.
10. **Focused history and physical examination**
    a. If the patient is unresponsive:
        (1) Perform a rapid physical examination
        (2) Follow with evaluation of baseline vital signs and gathering of the patient's medical history

b. If the patient is responsive, gather information about the patient's medical history before performing the physical examination.

METHODS OF CONTROLLING EXTERNAL BLEEDING

1. **Direct pressure**
   a. Direct pressure on the bleeding site slows blood flow and allows clotting to occur.
   b. Place a sterile gauze pad or trauma dressing over the injury site.
      (1) If a sterile dressing is not available, apply direct pressure to the site with a gloved hand.
      (2) Continue direct pressure until a dressing can be applied to the bleeding site.
   c. Apply pressure directly on the bleeding point.
   d. Large open wounds may require packing with sterile gauze and direct hand pressure if direct fingertip pressure does not control bleeding.
   e. If bleeding does not stop:
      (1) Remove dressing
      (2) Reassess for bleeding point
      (3) Apply direct pressure
      (4) If diffuse bleeding is discovered, apply additional pressure

2. **Elevation**
   a. Elevation may help control bleeding of an extremity.
   b. Elevate the extremity above the level of the heart if possible.
   c. Do not elevate the extremity if pain, swelling, or deformity is present until after it is splinted.

3. **Pressure points**
   a. Pressure points may be used to slow severe bleeding in an arm or leg.
   b. The brachial artery is pressed against the humerus to slow bleeding in the arm.
   c. The femoral artery is pressed against the pelvis to slow bleeding in the leg.

4. **Splints**
   a. Splinting decreases motion, reducing the amount of tissue damage and bleeding associated with painful, swollen, or deformed bone or joint injuries.
   b. Pressure splints
      (1) The use of air pressure splints can help control severe bleeding associated with lacerations of soft tissue or when bleeding is associated with broken bones.
      (2) Pneumatic counter-pressure devices [pneumatic antishock garment (PASG)] can be used as an effective pressure splint to help control severe bleeding due to massive soft tissue injury to the lower extremities (leg compartments only) or traumatic pelvic hemorrhage (abdominal and lung compartments).
      (3) Follow local protocol.

5. **Tourniquet**
   a. Use ONLY as a last resort to control bleeding of an amputated extremity when all other methods of bleeding control have failed.
   b. Application of a tourniquet can cause permanent damage to nerves, muscles, and blood vessels, resulting in the loss of an extremity.
   c. To apply a tourniquet:
      (1) Use a bandage at least 4 inches wide and 6–8 layers deep
      (2) Wrap the bandage around the extremity twice at a point proximal to the bleeding but as distal on the extremity as possible
      (3) Tie one knot in the bandage and place a stick or rod on top of the knot
      (4) Tie the ends of the bandage over the stick in a square knot
      (5) Twist the stick until the bleeding stops
      (6) After the bleeding has stopped, secure the stick or rod in place
      (7) Notify other emergency personnel who may care for the patient that a tourniquet has been applied

    (8)   Document the use of a tourniquet and the time it was applied in the pre-hospital care report

  d. A continuously inflated blood pressure cuff may be used as a tourniquet. The cuff should be placed above the elbow and inflated above the patient's systolic blood pressure to stop arterial and venous blood flow.

  e. Precautions with the use of a tourniquet

    (1)   Always use a wide bandage. Never use wire, rope, a belt, or any other material that may cut into the skin and underlying tissue.

    (2)   Tourniquet must be applied tightly enough to stop bleeding.

    (3)   Do not remove or loosen the tourniquet once it is applied unless directed to do so by medical direction.

    (4)   Leave the tourniquet in open view so it is readily seen by others.

    (5)   Do not apply a tourniquet directly over any joint, but as close to the injury as possible.

EMERGENCY MEDICAL CARE OF THE PATIENT WITH EXTERNAL BLEEDING

1. Take body substance isolation precautions.

2. Establish and maintain an open airway.

3. Administer oxygen as needed.

  a. If breathing is adequate, apply oxygen by nonrebreather mask at 15 liters per minute (LPM) if not already done.

  b. If breathing is inadequate, provide positive-pressure ventilation with 100% oxygen and assess adequacy of ventilations delivered.

4. Control bleeding by using direct pressure, elevation, pressure points, splints, and, as a last resort, tourniquet.

5. If signs of shock are present, treat for shock.

BLEEDING FROM THE NOSE, EARS, OR MOUTH

1. Possible causes include:

  a. Skull injury

  b. Facial trauma

  c. Digital trauma (nose picking)

  d. Sinusitis and other upper respiratory tract infections

  e. Hypertension (high blood pressure)

  f. Clotting disorders

2. Bleeding from the ears or nose may occur because of a skull fracture.

  a. If the bleeding is the result of trauma, do not attempt to stop the blood flow.

  b. Collect the drainage with a loose dressing, which may also limit exposure to sources of infection.

3. Emergency medical care for nosebleed (epistaxis):

  a. Place the patient in a sitting position

  b. Have the patient lean forward

  c. Apply direct pressure by pinching the fleshy portion of the nostrils together

  d. Keep the patient calm and quiet

  e. Monitor the airway and be prepared for vomiting

INTERNAL BLEEDING

SEVERITY

1. Internal bleeding can result in blood loss severe enough to cause shock and death.

2. Common sources of internal bleeding:

  a. Injured or damaged internal organs

  b. Painful, swollen, deformed extremities

3. Suspicion and severity of internal bleeding should be based on the mechanism of injury and the patient's signs and symptoms.

ASSESSMENT OF THE PATIENT WITH INTERNAL BLEEDING

1. Take body substance isolation precautions.
2. **Scene size-up**
  a. Evaluate the mechanism of injury or nature of the illness.
  b. Mechanisms of injury in which internal bleeding should be suspected (*Table 25-1*):
   (1) Blunt trauma
     (a) Falls
     (b) Motorcycle crashes
     (c) Pedestrian impacts
     (d) Automobile collisions
     (e) Blast injuries
   (2) Penetrating trauma
  c. Ensure the scene is safe before entering.
3. **Initial assessment**
  a. Maintain spinal immobilization if needed.
  b. Assess the patient's mental status
  c. Assess the patient's airway.
  d. Assess breathing.
  e. Assess circulation.
  f. Identify any life-threatening conditions and provide care based on those findings.
  g. Establish patient priorities.
   (1) Priority patients are those who:
     (a) Give a poor general impression
     (b) Have severe pain anywhere
     (c) Have uncontrolled bleeding
     (d) Have signs and symptoms of shock
     (e) Are unresponsive with no gag reflex or cough
   (2) ALS assistance should be requested as soon as possible for priority patients.
   (3) If ALS personnel are not available, the patient should be transported promptly to the closest appropriate facility.
4. **Focused history and physical examination**
  a. If the patient is unresponsive:
   (1) Perform a rapid physical examination and look for evidence of contusions, abrasions, deformity, impact marks, and swelling
   (2) Follow with evaluation of baseline vital signs and gathering of the patient's medical history
  b. If the patient is responsive:

Table 25-1. Mechanisms of Injury in Which Internal Bleeding Should Be Suspected

Blunt trauma
  Falls
  Motorcycle crashes
  Pedestrian impacts
  Automobile collisions
  Blast injuries
Penetrating trauma

(1) Gather information about the patient's medical history before performing the physical examination

(2) Look for evidence of contusions, abrasions, deformity, impact marks, and swelling

SIGNS AND SYMPTOMS OF INTERNAL BLEEDING

Signs and symptoms of internal bleeding include:

1. Pain, tenderness, swelling, or discoloration of the skin (bruising) in the injured area
2. Bleeding from the mouth, rectum, or vagina, or other body opening
3. Vomiting bright red blood or dark, "coffee-ground" blood
4. Dark, tarry stools or stools with bright red blood
5. Tender, rigid, and/or distended abdomen
6. Signs and symptoms of internal bleeding that indicate shock:
   a. Anxiety, restlessness, combativeness, or altered mental status
   b. Weakness, faintness, or dizziness
   c. Thirst
   d. Shallow, rapid breathing
   e. Rapid, weak pulse
   f. Pale, cool, clammy skin
   g. Capillary refill greater than 2 seconds (infants and children younger than 6 years of age only)
   h. Decreasing blood pressure (late sign)
   i. Dilated pupils that are slow to respond to light
   j. Nausea and vomiting

EMERGENCY MEDICAL CARE OF THE PATIENT WITH INTERNAL BLEEDING

1. Take body substance isolation precautions.
2. Establish and maintain an open airway.
3. Administer oxygen.
   a. If breathing is adequate, apply oxygen by nonrebreather mask at 15 LPM if not already done.
   b. If breathing is inadequate, provide positive-pressure ventilation with 100% oxygen and assess adequacy of ventilations delivered.
4. Control external bleeding. If bleeding is suspected in an extremity, control bleeding by direct pressure and application of a splint.
5. Treat for shock.
6. Transport promptly.
   a. Immediate transport is critical for patient with signs and symptoms of shock.
   b. If the patient is stable, perform ongoing assessments every 15 minutes.
   c. If the patient is unstable, perform ongoing assessments every 5 minutes.

SHOCK (HYPOPERFUSION)

SEVERITY

1. Shock is caused by:
   a. Failure of the heart to pump sufficient blood (pump failure)
      (1) The heart muscle fails to pump blood effectively to all parts of the body.
      (2) This failure can occur as a result of a heart attack.
      (3) This type of shock is called **cardiogenic shock.**
   b. Severe blood or fluid loss so that there is insufficient blood for the heart to pump through the system (fluid failure)
      (1) **Hemorrhagic shock** is shock caused by severe bleeding.
      (2) **Hypovolemic shock** is shock caused by either a loss of plasma (e.g., ex-

cessive sweating, dehydration due to vomiting or diarrhea, burns) or blood.

    (3) Trauma patients develop shock from the loss of blood from both internal and external sites.

  c. Enlargement of blood vessels so that there is insufficient blood to fill them (container failure)

    (1) This type of shock is caused by loss of blood vessel control by the nervous system.

    (2) This type of shock is called **neurogenic shock.**

2. Shock results in:

  a. Inadequate perfusion of cells with oxygen and nutrients

  b. Inadequate removal of metabolic waste products

3. Cell and organ malfunction and death can result from shock. Without adequate perfusion:

  a. The heart, brain, and lungs will suffer damage after 4 to 6 minutes

  b. The kidneys and liver will suffer damage after 45 to 90 minutes

  c. The skin and muscles will suffer damage after 4 to 8 hours

4. Prompt recognition and treatment are essential to patient survival.

SIGNS AND SYMPTOMS OF SHOCK (TABLE 25-2)

1. Mental status

  a. Restlessness

  b. Anxiety

  c. Altered mental status

2. Peripheral perfusion

  a. Pale, cool, clammy skin

  b. Weak, thready, or absent peripheral pulses

  c. Delayed capillary refill greater than 2 seconds in normal ambient air temperature (in infants and children younger than 6 years of age only)

3. Vital signs

  a. Increased pulse rate (early sign), weak and thready

  b. Increased breathing rate: shallow, labored, and irregular

  c. Decreased blood pressure (late sign)

4. Other signs and symptoms

  a. Dilated pupils

  b. Marked thirst

  c. Nausea and vomiting

  d. Pallor with cyanosis of the lips

5. Infants and children

  a. Infants and children can maintain their blood pressure until their blood volume is more than half gone.

  b. By the time their blood pressure drops, they are close to death.

EMERGENCY CARE OF THE PATIENT WITH SIGNS AND SYMPTOMS OF SHOCK

1. Take body substance isolation precautions.

2. Establish and maintain an open airway.

Table 25-2. Signs and Symptoms of Shock

Early	Late
Restlessness, anxiety	Altered mental status
Increased heart rate	Marked sweating
Pale, cool, moist skin	Decreased blood pressure
Thirst	Increased respiratory rate
Weakness	Cold, pale skin

3. Administer oxygen.
   a. If breathing is adequate, apply oxygen by nonrebreather mask at 15 LPM if not already done.
   b. If breathing is inadequate, provide positive-pressure ventilation with 100% oxygen and assess adequacy of ventilations delivered.
4. Control external bleeding. If bleeding is suspected in an extremity, control bleeding by direct pressure and application of a splint.
5. Apply and inflate the PASG if:
   a. Approved by medical direction
   b. Signs of shock are present and the lower abdomen is tender and pelvic injury is suspected, with no evidence of chest injury
6. Elevate the lower extremities approximately 8–12 inches. If the patient has serious injuries to the pelvis, lower extremities, head, chest, abdomen, neck, or spine, keep the patient supine.
7. Splint any suspected bone or joint injuries.
8. Prevent heat loss by covering the patient with a blanket when appropriate.
9. Transport promptly.
   a. Immediate transport is critical for the patient with signs and symptoms of shock.
   b. Perform ongoing assessments every 5 minutes.

REVIEW QUESTIONS

Directions: Each of the numbered items or incomplete statements in this section is followed by answers or by completions of the statement. Select the ONE lettered answer or completion that is BEST in each case.

1. Tourniquets should be used only as a last resort to control excessive bleeding when all other measures have failed. When a tourniquet is applied, the rationale is "save the life but lose the limb." Which of the following would be the most appropriate improvised tourniquet device?

   (A) A shoelace
   (B) A power cord
   (C) A bandana
   (D) A clean rope

2. Shock (hypoperfusion) is a condition that develops as a response to injury or insult. Which of the following organs will suffer damage earliest as a result of shock?

   (A) The skin
   (B) The brain
   (C) The kidneys and liver
   (D) The large muscles of the arms and legs

3. Which of the following regarding the response to shock in children and infants is correct?

   (A) Children and infants will compensate much longer than adults
   (B) Children and infants will show the signs of shock much earlier than adults
   (C) Children and infants will show the signs of shock at the same rate as adults
   (D) Children and infants have healthy hearts and blood vessels and never go into shock

4. Shock is generally attributed to failure of one of three components of the cardio-vascular system: the pump (heart), the container (blood vessels), and the fluid (blood). Another name for failure of the pump is

   (A) Neurogenic shock
   (B) Cardiogenic shock
   (C) Hypovolemic shock
   (D) Hemorrhagic shock

5. Your ambulance has been called to the home of an 8-month-old female patient. Her mother informs you the child has had diarrhea for the last 3 days and has re-fused her bottle for the last 36 hours. The child is pale with a capillary refill time of 3 to 4 seconds. This child is most likely

   (A) not in shock
   (B) in shock due to fluid failure
   (C) in shock due to pump failure
   (D) in shock due to container failure

6. Which of the following patients is most likely to be in shock?

   (A) A 6-year old child who was hit by a car
   (B) A 23-year-old man complaining of chest pain
   (C) A 47-year-old diabetic woman who stopped taking her insulin 5 days ago
   (D) All of these patients should be considered to be in shock

Directions: Each of the numbered questions or incomplete statements in this section refers to a scenario that precedes them. The numbered questions or incomplete statements are followed by answers or by completions of the statement. Select the answer or completion of the statement that is BEST in each case.

Your rescue crew has been called to the scene of a "domestic dispute" between family members. You request that local law enforcement respond. After the scene is secured by law enforcement personnel, you arrive to find a 43-year-old male patient complaining of severe abdominal pain. He states he was "hit in the stomach with a bar stool." He denies any other injury. While examining the abdomen, you observe a bruise beginning to de-velop on his left upper abdominal quadrant.

Questions 7–9

7. Which of the following would be consistent with your suspicion that this patient may be bleeding internally?

   (A) The patient is anxious, pale, and cool to touch
   (B) The patient exhibits a slow pulse rate of 64 beats per minute
   (C) The patient has numbness and tingling in the hands and no sensation or movement in the legs
   (D) The patient's blood pressure is 140/92 when supine (flat on back) and is 144/92 when standing erect

8. Which of the following would be considered a late sign that this patient is going into shock?

   (A) Altered mental status
   (B) Rapid, shallow breathing
   (C) Dropping blood pressure
   (D) Persistent rapid, weak pulse

9. As your physical examination continues, the patient becomes more distressed. His vital signs are weak pulse of 132 beats per minute, blood pressure 86/54, respirations 24 breaths per minute. The patient's skin is cool and pale and his pupils are slow to react. Treatment for this patient should include

   (A) oxygen by nasal cannula, loosen or remove clothing, and transport sitting upright
   (B) oxygen by nasal cannula, prevent loss of body heat, elevate legs 24–36 inches, and transport
   (C) oxygen by nonrebreather mask, elevate the legs 8–12 inches, prevent loss of body heat, and transport
   (D) oxygen by nonrebreather mask, begin cooling the body to slow metabolism, elevate legs 8–12 inches, and transport

Your ambulance crew has been called to the home of a 28-year-old male patient complaining of a nosebleed. You arrive to find the patient in the bathroom with his head tilted back. There are about 20 slightly bloodied tissues on the counter and floor. He tells you he gets nosebleeds every year about this time. He denies any recent trauma and has no pertinent medical history.

Questions 10–12

10. The normal clotting time for bleeding is

    (A) 1–2 minutes
    (B) 6–10 minutes
    (C) 10–12 minutes
    (D) 30–60 minutes

11. To assist in controlling the nosebleed, you should

    (A) pinch the bridge of the nose and tilt the head back
    (B) pack the patient's nose with tissue and tilt the head back
    (C) pinch the fleshy portion of the nostrils and have the patient sit up and lean forward
    (D) instruct the patient to blow his nose forcefully every 2–5 minutes and then reapply a tissue

12. Which of the following regarding nosebleeds is correct?

    (A) Nose picking will not cause a nose to bleed
    (B) If the nosebleed is not due to trauma, no true medical emergency exists
    (C) Some medications may influence the amount of time required for a nose to stop bleeding
    (D) Nosebleeds associated with trauma should be treated by packing the nostrils with tissue or gauze

Your rescue crew is called to a construction site for a 28-year-old male patient who cut his hand with a saw. You arrive to find the patient holding a blood-soaked towel over his left hand. He states that blood was "spurting out with every heartbeat."

Questions 13–14

13. This type of bleeding is consistent with

    (A) laceration of a vein
    (B) laceration of a tendon
    (C) laceration of an artery
    (D) laceration of a capillary bed

14. The first step in controlling the bleeding associated with the injury is

(A)   apply a tourniquet
(B)   apply direct pressure at the injury site
(C)   apply pressure to the nearest pressure point
(D)   apply a blood pressure cuff to the upper arm and inflate until the bleeding stops

ANSWERS AND RATIONALES

1-C. An ideal tourniquet is at least 4 inches wide and 6–8 layers deep. Shoelaces, wire, rope, or other such material may fail as the extremity swells.

2-B. The brain, the heart, and the lungs are among the organs most sensitive to oxygen deprivation. Within 4 to 6 minutes, these organs will begin to suffer as a result of hypoperfusion. Because the brain is so sensitive to oxygen deprivation, one of the first signs of hypoperfusion is an altered mental status (anxiety, restlessness, confusion). The skin and muscles will suffer damage after about 4 to 8 hours, and the kidneys and liver will suffer damage after about 45 to 90 minutes.

3-A. Typically, children and infants have a more efficient compensatory mechanism than adults. Children can compensate for massive blood loss, for example, much longer than an adult can. Adults will typically maintain a somewhat normal blood pressure until 10% of the total blood volume is lost. Then, the blood pressure will begin to creep down. Children may not show hemodynamic (blood pressure) compromise until 25% of the total blood volume is lost. By the time a child begins to exhibit the more measurable signs of shock, he or she may be very deep into the progression of shock. Do not let a good blood pressure and healthy appearance fool you into undertreating a child.

4-B. Cardiogenic shock is shock brought on by the inability of the heart (the pump) to keep up with the body's demand. Neurogenic shock is "container failure" shock that occurs when the impulse from the brain to the arteries is cut off (e.g., when the spinal cord is damaged). In the absence of a nervous impulse, the vessels of the body relax and dilate. When the vessels are fully dilated, the average body can hold approximately five times its normal volume of blood. Hypovolemic shock occurs from a loss of fluid, either blood or plasma. Hemorrhagic shock occurs from the loss of blood.

5-B. A patient does not have to bleed to be in shock from "fluid failure." The body may also become depleted of fluid by excessive sweating, urinating, vomiting, diarrhea, or burn injury.

6-D. Not every patient you encounter will be having a heart attack. Not every patient you encounter will have life-threatening wounds. However, it is important to understand that EVERY patient you see may be in shock. Shock is both physical and psychological. Treating for shock begins with establishing rapport with the patient: you should be competent, compassionate, and professional. Treating for shock also means understanding the factors that influence the patient's condition (such as the mechanism of injury, past medical history, history of present illness, and the subtle signs of distress) and treating these patients appropriately.

7-A. Anxiety, pallor, and cool skin temperature are consistent with internal bleeding. Some of the other signs and symptoms associated with internal bleeding are dizziness, thirst, shallow, rapid breathing, rapid, weak pulse, sluggish pupil response, and nausea. A pulse rate of 64 beats per minute is not associated with significant internal bleeding; however, certain medications (e.g., beta-blockers such as Corgard® and Inderal®) may inhibit the body's ability to increase the heart rate to compensate for bleeding. Numbness and tingling or loss of sensation in the extremities in trauma patients is most commonly associated with nerve damage. Comparing blood pressure changes to changes in the patient's body position is referred to as "orthostatics." Patients with significant blood loss (either internal or external) may exhibit a great disparity between blood pressures taken when supine versus taken when standing (with a drop in pressure when standing due to gravity's effect on a lesser circulating blood volume). This patient's blood pressure actually goes up when standing.

8-D. Decreasing blood pressure values are a late sign of shock. Adults may lose about 10% of their total blood volume before the blood pressure starts to fall. Blood pressure may actually go up initially because of the increase in heart rate. Altered mental status (anxiety, dizziness, restlessness) is an early sign since the brain is one of the first organs to be affected by hypoperfusion. Shallow, rapid breathing and a rapid, weak pulse are also early signs as compared to blood pressure.

9-C. When treating for shock, you should provide high-flow oxygen therapy. If breathing is adequate, use a nonrebreather mask connected to oxygen at 15 liters per minute (LPM). If breathing is inadequate, assist ventilations with bag-valve mask connected to oxygen at 15 LPM. If spinal immobilization is not indicated, elevating the legs 8–12 inches decreases the amount of work required of the heart. Spinal immobilization is indicated if the patient sustained head or neck trauma, if the mechanism of injury is uncertain, or if the mechanism of injury suggests spinal injury. The patient's body temperature should be preserved so that heat loss does not further compromise this patient's injury.

10-B. Normal clotting time is 6–10 minutes. However, as evident by the number of tissues used, this patient keeps disturbing the clot before it has time to stop bleeding. Other factors such as disease (hemophilia) and medication reactions (aspirin or Coumadin®) may affect clotting time.

11-C. The correct method for stopping a nosebleed is to pinch the fleshy portion of the nostrils, sit up, and lean forward. Leaning back or tilting the head up causes blood to flow into the stomach. Blood in the stomach usually leads to nausea and vomiting. Vomiting increases the pressure on the clot, and bleeding may resume. If the nose is blown, the clot is disturbed, and the clock is reset (another 6–8 minutes for the formation of a clot).

12-C. As stated earlier, some medications affect the body's ability to form a clot. Patients with a history of coronary vascular disease (heart problems) or cerebral vascular accident (stroke) may be prescribed "blood thinners" to decrease the chances of an embolus (clot) cutting off the circulation to the heart or brain. Nose picking may actually cause a nose to bleed by disrupting the delicate capillary beds of the nasal cavity. While a nosebleed following head trauma may be suggestive of a skull fracture, nontraumatic nosebleeds may also present as a medical emergency. For example, during hypertensive crisis (severe, uncontrolled high blood pressure episode), a patient may rupture a vessel in the nose. Controlling these nosebleeds can be challenging and may require extensive hospital intervention (to stop the bleeding and bring the blood pressure down). If a nosebleed results from head trauma, your efforts should be aimed toward protecting the airway. In certain cases of head trauma, blood may leak from the nose or ears as a result of swelling in the brain. Do not attempt to halt the flow of blood from the nose, as this may result in increasing the amount of pressure on the brain.

13-C. Arteries flow blood under high pressure (as compared to veins). Blood flowing through the arteries of the body is oxygenated and bright red. Therefore, arterial bleeds are characterized by the spurting of bright red blood. Veins carry deoxygenated blood from the cells of the body back to the heart. Deoxygenated blood is darker than oxygenated blood, and veins do not flow blood under as high pressure as arteries. Venous bleeding is characterized by the constant flow of dark red or maroon colored blood. Capillaries are very small vessels. Red blood cells literally line up single file to flow through capillaries. Bleeding associated with capillary injury is an oozing of plasma with a scant amount of blood (like a "carpet burn").

14-B. The steps to control bleeding are: first, apply direct pressure at the bleeding point. If possible, elevate the injury above the level of the heart. If applicable, splint the extremity to decrease movement. If the wound continues to bleed uncontrollably, locate the nearest arterial pressure point. Apply pressure to the pressure point while still maintaining direct pressure on the wound. An arterial pressure point is a point where an artery comes close to the surface of the skin and runs over a bone. By compressing the arterial pressure point, the flow of blood to the injury will decrease. If direct pressure, elevation, splinting, and indirect pressure fail to control bleeding, a tourniquet may be considered. If you have the means to contact medical direction, do so before applying a tourniquet.

BIBLIOGRAPHY

Barber JM, Dillman PA: *Emergency Patient Care for the EMT-A*. Reston, Virginia, Reston Publishing Company, 1981.

Crosby LA, Lewallen DG (eds): *Emergency Care and Transportation of the Sick and Injured*, 6th ed. Rosemont, IL, American Academy of Orthopaedic Surgeons, 1995.

Grant HD, Murray RH Jr, Bergeron JD: *Emergency Care*, 7th ed. Englewood Cliffs, NJ, Prentice-Hall, 1995.

Hafen BQ, Karren KJ, Mistovich JJ: *Prehospital Emergency Care*, 5th ed. Upper Saddle River, NJ, Prentice-Hall, 1996.

Henry MC, Stapleton ER, Judd RL: *EMT: Prehospital Care*. Philadelphia, WB Saunders, 1992.

McSwain NE, White RD, Paturas JL, et al (eds): *The Basic EMT: Comprehensive Prehospital Patient Care*. St. Louis, Mosby-Year Book, 1996.

Sanders MJ: *Mosby's Paramedic Textbook*. St. Louis, Mosby-Year Book, 1994.

Sheehy SB, Lombardi JE: *Manual of Emergency Care*, 4th ed. St. Louis, Mosby-Year Book, 1995.

Sloane E: *Anatomy and Physiology: An Easy Learner*. Boston, Jones and Bartlett, 1994.

Solomon EP and Phillips GA: *Understanding Human Anatomy and Physiology*. Philadelphia, WB Saunders, 1987.

Stoy WA: *Mosby's EMT-Basic Textbook*. St. Louis, Mosby-Year Book, 1996.

Thibodeau GA, Patton KT: *The Human Body in Health and Disease*. St. Louis, Mosby-Year Book, 1992.

Tortora GJ, Grabowski SR: *Principles of Anatomy and Physiology*, seventh ed. New York, HarperCollins, 1993.

United States Department of Transportation, National Highway Traffic Safety Administration: *Emergency Medical Technician: Basic. National Standard Curriculum*, 1994.

26 SOFT TISSUE INJURIES

26

OBJECTIVES

26-1 State the major functions of the skin.

26-2 List the layers of the skin.

26-3 List the types of closed soft tissue injuries.

26-4 Establish the relationship between body substance isolation (BSI) and soft tissue injuries.

26-5 Describe the emergency medical care of the patient with a closed soft tissue injury.

26-6 State the types of open soft tissue injuries.

26-7 Describe the emergency medical care of the patient with an open soft tissue injury.

26-8 Discuss the emergency medical care considerations for a patient with a penetrating chest injury.

26-9 State the emergency medical care considerations for a patient with an open wound to the abdomen.

26-10 Differentiate the care of an open wound to the chest from an open wound to the abdomen.

26-11 Describe the emergency medical care of a patient with an impaled object.

26-12 Describe the emergency medical care of a patient with an amputation.

26-13 List the functions of dressing and bandaging.

26-14 Describe the purpose of a bandage.

MOTIVATION FOR LEARNING

Soft tissue injuries are not often life threatening, although they are common. Injuries range from bruises and abrasions to amputations and full-thickness burns. The EMT-Basic will manage soft tissue injuries after performing the initial patient assessment, unless bleeding is life threatening. The EMT-Basic must be able to differentiate types of soft tissue injuries and provide appropriate management, including control of bleeding, prevention of further injury, and reducing contamination.

26-15 Describe the steps in applying a pressure bandage.

26-16 Describe the effects of improperly applied dressings, splints, and tourniquets.

*26-17 List the structures of the eye and describe the function of each.

26-18 List the classifications of burns.

26-19 Define a superficial burn.

26-20 List the characteristics of a superficial burn.

26-21 Define a partial-thickness burn.

26-22 List the characteristics of a partial-thickness burn.

26-23 Define full-thickness burn.

26-24 List the characteristics of a full-thickness burn.

26-25 Describe the emergency medical care of the patient with a superficial burn.

26-26 Describe the emergency medical care of the patient with a partial-thickness burn.

26-27 Describe the emergency medical care of the patient with a full-thickness burn.

26-28 Describe the emergency care for a chemical burn.

26-29 Describe the emergency care for an electrical burn.

26 30 Establish the relationship between airway management and the patient with chest injury, burns, and blunt and penetrating injuries.

ANATOMY REVIEW

FUNCTIONS OF THE SKIN

1. The skin is the body's first line of defense against bacteria and other organisms, ultraviolet rays from the sun, and harmful chemicals, and cuts and tears.
2. The skin helps regulate body temperature.
3. It senses heat, cold, touch, pressure, and pain; nerves in the skin transmit this information to the brain and spinal cord.
4. The skin is the site where vitamin D is produced.
5. Sweat glands in the skin excrete excess water and some wastes.

LAYERS OF THE SKIN (FIGURE 26-1)

1. **Epidermis**
   a. The **epidermis** is the outermost skin layer.
   b. It consists of four or five layers.
      (1) New cells are continuously formed in the deeper layers of the epidermis.
      (2) Older cells are pushed upward and sloughed off.
   c. The epidermis contains keratin, a waterproofing protein.
2. The **dermis** is the deeper and thicker layer of skin containing sweat and sebaceous glands, hair follicles, blood vessels, and nerve endings.
3. **Subcutaneous (fatty) layer**
   a. The **subcutaneous layer** helps conserve body heat.
   b. Fat can be used as an energy source when adequate food is not available.

ACCESSORY STRUCTURES OF THE SKIN

Accessory structures of the skin include:
1. Hair
2. Nails
3. Sweat glands
4. Sebaceous (oil) glands

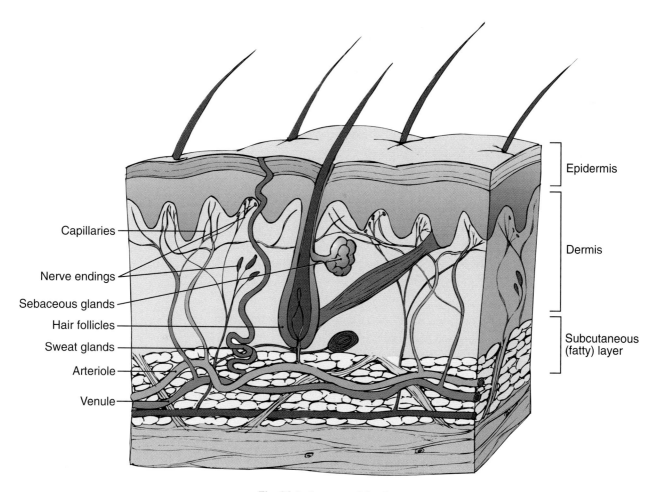

Capillaries

Nerve endings

Sebaceous glands

Hair follicles

Sweat glands

Arteriole

Venule

Epidermis

Dermis

Subcutaneous
(fatty) layer

Fig. 26-1. Anatomy of the skin.

CLOSED SOFT TISSUE INJURIES

OVERVIEW

1. **Closed soft tissue injuries** occur because of blunt trauma.
2. In **blunt trauma,** a forceful impact occurs to the body, but there is no break in the skin.
3. In a closed soft tissue injury, there is no actual break in the skin, but the tissues and vessels may be crushed or ruptured.
4. When assessing a closed soft tissue injury, it is important to evaluate surface damage and consider possible damage to the organs and major vessels beneath the area of impact.

TYPES OF CLOSED SOFT TISSUE INJURIES

1. **Contusion (bruise)**
   a. In a **contusion,** the epidermis remains intact.
   b. Cells are damaged and blood vessels torn in the dermis.
   c. Localized swelling and pain are typically present.
   d. Blood accumulation causes discoloration (**ecchymosis**).
2. **Hematoma**
   a. A **hematoma** is the collection of blood beneath the skin.
   b. A larger amount of tissue is damaged compared to a contusion.
   c. Larger blood vessels are damaged.

d. Hematomas frequently occur with trauma sufficient to break bones.

e. The patient may lose 1 or more liters of blood under the skin.

3. **Crush injuries**

a. Crush injuries are caused by a crushing force applied to the body.

b. These injuries can cause internal organ rupture.

c. Internal bleeding may be severe and lead to shock.

EMERGENCY MEDICAL CARE FOR CLOSED SOFT TISSUE INJURIES

1. Take body substance isolation (BSI) precautions.

a. Wear gloves and other personal protective equipment as needed.

b. Wash hands after each patient contact.

2. Establish and maintain an open airway.

3. Administer oxygen as needed.

a. If breathing is adequate, apply oxygen by nonrebreather mask at 15 liters per minute (LPM) if not already done.

b. If breathing is inadequate, provide positive-pressure ventilation with 100% oxygen and assess adequacy of ventilations delivered.

4. If signs of shock are present or if internal bleeding is suspected, treat for shock.

5. Splint a painful, swollen, deformed extremity.

6. Transport.

OPEN SOFT TISSUE INJURIES

OVERVIEW

1. In **open soft tissue injuries,** a break occurs in the continuity of the skin.

2. Because of the break in the skin, open injuries are susceptible to external hemorrhage and infection.

TYPES OF OPEN SOFT TISSUE INJURIES

1. **Abrasion**

a. In an **abrasion,** the outermost layer of skin (epidermis) is damaged by shearing forces (e.g., rubbing or scraping).

b. Although these injuries are superficial, abrasions can be very painful.

c. Because the pain associated with the injury is similar to that from a second-degree burn, an abrasion is often called "road rash," "rug burn," or "friction burn."

d. Little or no oozing of blood (capillary bleeding) occurs.

2. **Laceration**

a. A **laceration** is a break in skin of varying depth.

b. A laceration may be linear (regular) or stellate (irregular).

c. Lacerations may occur in isolation or with other types of soft tissue injury.

d. They are caused by a forceful impact with a sharp object (e.g., knife, razor blade, glass).

e. Bleeding may be severe.

3. **Puncture**

a. A **puncture** results when the skin is pierced with a pointed object such as a nail, pencil, ice pick, splinter, piece of glass, bullet, or a knife.

b. Little or no external bleeding may occur.

c. Internal bleeding may be severe.

d. Puncture wounds carry an increased risk of infection.

e. Injury to underlying structures must be considered.

    (1) In gunshot and stab wounds, assess for entrance and exit wounds. Exit wounds are usually larger than entrance wounds.

    (2) Evaluate the patient closely for signs and symptoms of shock if the puncture wound occurred to the chest or abdomen.

f. An object that remains embedded in the open wound is called an **impaled object.**

4. **Avulsion**
   a. In an **avulsion,** a flap of skin or tissue is torn loose or pulled completely off.
   b. Tissue is usually pulled away where it separates from a different tissue (e.g., skin from subcutaneous tissue or subcutaneous tissue from muscle).
   c. Bleeding is usually significant.
   d. In a **degloving avulsion** injury, the skin and fatty tissue are stripped away.
5. **Amputations**
   a. In an **amputation,** extremities or other body parts are severed from the body.
   b. Massive bleeding may be present, or bleeding may be limited.
6. **Crush injuries**
   a. In a crush injury, soft tissue and internal organs are damaged.
   b. These injuries may cause painful, swollen, deformed extremities.
   c. External bleeding may be minimal or absent.
   d. Internal bleeding may be severe.

EMERGENCY MEDICAL CARE FOR OPEN SOFT TISSUE INJURIES

1. Take BSI precautions.
   a. Wear gloves, eye protection, and other personal protective equipment as needed.
   b. Wash hands after each patient contact.
2. Establish and maintain an open airway.
3. Administer oxygen as needed.
   a. If breathing is adequate, apply oxygen by nonrebreather mask at 15 liters per minute (LPM) if not already done.
   b. If breathing is inadequate, provide positive-pressure ventilation with 100% oxygen and assess adequacy of ventilations delivered.
4. Expose the wound.
5. Control bleeding.
6. Prevent further contamination.
7. Apply a dry sterile dressing to the wound and bandage securely in place.
8. Keep the patient calm and quiet.
9. Treat for shock if signs and symptoms are present.
10. Splint a painful, swollen, deformed extremity.
11. Transport.

SPECIAL CONSIDERATIONS

1. **Penetrating chest injury**
   a. Apply an occlusive (airtight) dressing to the open wound.
   b. Tape the dressing on three sides (flutter-valve effect) *(Figure 26-2)*.
      (1) The dressing is sucked over the wound as the patient inhales, preventing air from entering.
      (2) The open end of the dressing allows air to escape as the patient exhales.
   c. Administer oxygen if not already done.
   d. Place the patient in a position of comfort if no spinal injury is suspected.
   e. If spinal injury is suspected, immobilize the patient to a long backboard.
2. **Abdominal evisceration** (organs protruding through an abdominal wound) *(Figure 26-3)*
   a. Do not touch or try to replace the exposed organ.
   b. Carefully remove clothing from around the wound.
   c. Cover exposed organs and wound.
      (1) Apply a large sterile dressing, moistened with sterile water or saline, over the organs and wound.

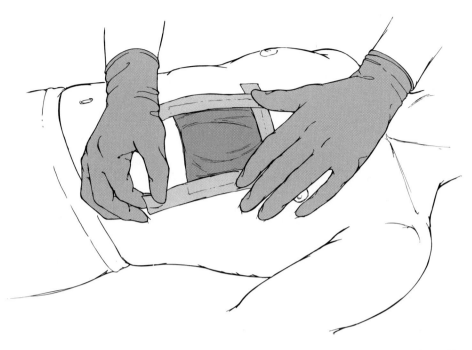

Fig. 26-2. For an open chest wound, apply an occlusive dressing and tape it to the chest on three sides.

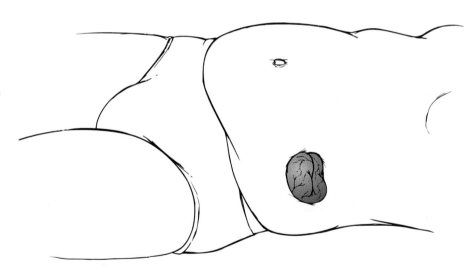

Fig. 26-3. Abdominal evisceration.

    (2)   Secure the dressing in place with a large bandage to retain moisture and prevent heat loss.

   d. Flex the patient's hips and knees, if they are uninjured and spinal injury is not suspected, to decrease tension on the abdominal muscles.

3. Impaled objects *(Figure 26-4)*

   a. Do not remove the impaled object unless the object:

    (1)   Is impaled through the cheek

    (2)   Would interfere with chest compressions

    (3)   Interferes with transport

   b. Manually secure the object to prevent movement.

   c. Expose the wound area.

   d. Control bleeding with direct pressure around the wound edges.

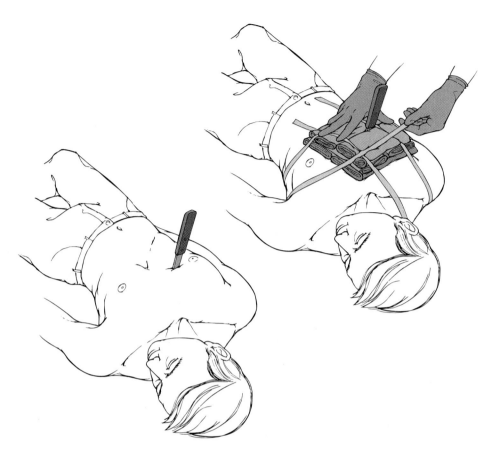

Fig. 26-4. Impaled object. Manually secure the object. Expose the wound area. Control bleeding. Use a bulky dressing to help stabilize the object.

    e. Stabilize the object with bulky dressings.
    f. Secure in place.
4. Care of an amputated body part
    a. Wrap the amputated part in a sterile dressing. Follow local protocol to determine medical direction preference for a dry or moist dressing.
    b. Wrap or bag the amputated part in plastic and keep cool.
        (1) Do not use dry ice.
        (2) Do not allow the part to freeze.
        (3) Do not place the amputated part directly on ice or in water.
    c. Transport the amputated part with the patient.
    d. Do not complete partial amputations.
    e. Immobilize the injured area to prevent further injury.
    f. Treat for shock.
    g. Maintain body temperature.
    h. Transport to an appropriate facility.
5. Large, open neck injury
    a. This type of injury may cause an air embolism.
    b. Place a gloved palm over the wound until an occlusive dressing can be applied.
    c. Cover the wound with an occlusive dressing.
    d. Apply a bulky dressing over the occlusive dressing and apply pressure over the dressing with a gloved hand to control bleeding.
    e. Compress the carotid artery only if absolutely necessary to control bleeding.
    f. Never apply pressure to both sides of the neck at the same time.

DRESSING AND BANDAGING

FUNCTIONS

The functions of dressing and bandaging wounds include:
1. Stop bleeding
2. Protect wounds from further damage
3. Prevent further contamination and infection

DRESSINGS

1. A **dressing** is any material that covers a wound.
2. A sterile dressing should be used when possible.
3. Types of dressings include:
   a. Gauze pads (e.g., 2×2, 4×4, 5×9)
   b. Universal (multitrauma) dressing
   c. Adhesive-type dressing
   d. Occlusive (airtight) dressing

BANDAGES

1. A **bandage** is used to secure a dressing in place.
2. A bandage should be tight enough to control bleeding but not so tight as to interfere with circulation.
3. Types of bandages include:
   a. Self-adherent bandages
   b. Elastic bandage (e.g., Ace® bandage, elastic wrap)
   c. Gauze rolls
   d. Triangular bandages
   e. Adhesive tape
   f. Air splint

PRESSURE BANDAGE

1. A **pressure bandage** is a bandage with which enough pressure is applied over a wound site to control bleeding.
2. **Applying a pressure bandage**
   a. Cover the wound with several sterile gauze dressings or a bulky dressing.
   b. Apply direct pressure to the wound until bleeding is controlled.
   c. Secure the dressing firmly in place with a bandage.
   d. Assess distal circulation.
   e. If possible, do not cover fingers or toes so you can determine if the bandage is too tight.
   f. A bandage may be too tight if:
      (1) Fingers or toes become cold to the touch
      (2) Fingers or toes begin to turn pale or blue
      (3) The patient complains of numbness in the extremity
   g. If blood soaks through the dressing, do not remove it; apply additional dressings and another bandage.

ENRICHMENT—EYE INJURIES

ANATOMY OF THE EYE (FIGURE 26-5)

1. The eyes are globe shaped and approximately 1 inch in diameter.
2. **Orbits** (eye sockets)

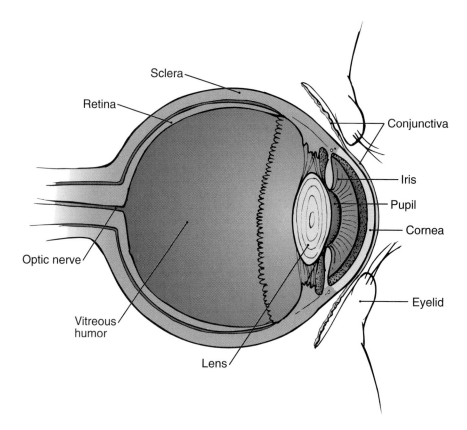

Fig. 26-5. Anatomy of the eye.

a. The **orbits** are the cavities in the front of the skull that contain the eyeballs.

b. They are formed from the bones of the forehead, temple, and upper jaw.

c. Trauma to these bones may result in injury to the eyes.

3. Eyebrows protect the eye from sweat.

4. Eyelids provide protection from trauma, intense light, and foreign particles.

5. **Conjunctiva**

a. The **conjunctiva** is the mucous membrane that covers the front surface of the sclera and the inner eyelid.

a. It serves as protection for the eye.

b. Pinkeye is an inflammation of the conjunctiva, caused by infection of the eyelid.

6. **Lacrimal glands and ducts**

a. **Lacrimal glands** produce tears that act as a lubricant between the eyelid and the cornea and flood foreign material out of the eye.

b. The tears are drained away by lacrimal ducts that are found in the inner corner of the eye.

7. **Sclera**

a. The **sclera** is the outermost layer of the eye.

b. It is sometimes called the "white" of the eye.

c. The cornea is the clear, transparent part of the sclera over the iris.

(1) The cornea is often called the "window of the eye."

(2) It protects the lens.

(3) It is responsible for allowing light to enter the interior of the eye.

8. **Retina**

a. The **retina** is the innermost layer of the eye.

b. It converts light into impulses that are transmitted by the optic nerve to the brain.

9. **Pupil**

  a. The pupil is the rounded opening in the iris through which light enters the interior of the eye.

  b. In dim light, the pupil dilates (widens) to allow more light to enter the eye.

  c. In bright light, the pupil constricts (narrows) to limit the amount of light entering the eye.

10. **Iris**

  a. The **iris** is the visible, colored part of the eye.

  b. It consists of muscles that control the diameter of the pupil, thus controlling the amount of light entering the eye.

11. **Lens**

  a. The **lens** is located directly behind the pupil.

  b. It changes shape to focus images on the retina.

  c. Its ability to change shape decreases with age.

12. **Eye fluids**

  a. The **aqueous humor** is the fluid in the anterior chamber in front of the lens; it nourishes the lens and cornea.

  b. The **vitreous humor** is the fluid in the posterior chamber behind the lens; it maintains the shape of the eye.

13. The optic nerve transmits visual messages to the brain.

EYE INJURIES

1. **Foreign bodies**

  a. Foreign bodies may include dirt, sand, and metal or wood slivers.

  b. Pain is often severe.

  c. Emergency medical care

   (1) Follow local protocol.

   (2) Take BSI precautions.

   (3) Flush the foreign body away from the unaffected eye using normal saline or sterile water.

   (4) Eyelid may be rolled back and a moistened cotton-tipped swab used to remove the object.

   (5) If unable to remove the foreign body, cover both eyes and transport the patient.

2. **Chemical burns**

  a. Chemical burns are the most urgent eye injury.

  b. Damage depends on the type and concentration of the chemical, length of exposure, and elapsed time until treatment.

  c. Emergency medical care

   (1) Follow local protocol.

   (2) Take BSI precautions.

   (3) Immediately flush the eye with water or normal saline. An intravenous bag of saline solution connected to intravenous tubing is an effective means of performing irrigation.

   (4) Continue irrigation for at least 20 minutes.

   (5) Irrigate away from unaffected eye (e.g., from medial to lateral).

   (6) Continue irrigation throughout transport.

   (7) Transport promptly.

3. **Nonchemical burns**

  a. Nonchemical burns can be caused by heat, radiation, lasers, infrared rays, and ultraviolet light.

  b. Patient will complain of severe pain in the eyes.

  c. Emergency medical care

   (1) Cover both eyes.

   (2) Transport the patient for further evaluation and treatment.

4. **Emergency medical care for an impaled object**

  a. Never remove an impaled object in the eye.

    b. Stabilize the object in place with bulky dressings.

    c. Do NOT apply pressure.

    d. Cover the other eye to limit movement.

    e. Transport promptly.

5. **Blunt trauma to the eye.** Blunt trauma can cause hyphema, a black eye, a blow-out fracture, and retinal detachment.

    a. Hyphema is hemorrhage into the anterior chamber of the eye.

    b. A black eye is discoloration, swelling, and tenderness of tissue surrounding the eye; the eye itself may also be damaged.

    c. A **blow-out fracture** is a fracture of the bones that make up the orbit. Signs and symptoms include:

       (1) Double vision

       (2) Loss of sensation above the eyebrow or over the cheek

       (3) Nasal discharge of mucus

       (4) Tenderness on palpation

       (5) Paralysis of upward gaze (e.g., the patient's eyes will not be able to follow your finger upward)

    d. Retinal detachment may be caused by blunt (e.g., boxing) or penetrating trauma.

       (1) It usually occurs months or years after the original injury.

       (2) The patient experiences light flashes, floating black specks in front of the eyes, and complains of something blocking the field of vision.

       (3) During transport, every effort should be made to avoid bumps, bounces, or sudden stops.

    e. Emergency medical care

       (1) Follow local protocol.

       (2) Call for advanced-life-support (ALS) assistance as needed.

       (3) Take BSI precautions.

       (4) Maintain spinal immobilization.

       (5) Cover both eyes.

       (6) Treat any associated injuries.

       (7) Keep the patient quiet.

       (8) Transport the patient for further evaluation and treatment.

6. **Extruded (avulsed) eyeball**

    a. The eye "pops out" of the eye socket.

    b. Avulsion of the eyeball usually occurs because of a high impact injury.

    c. Emergency medical care

       (1) Follow local protocol.

       (2) Take BSI isolation precautions.

       (3) Maintain spinal immobilization as needed.

       (4) Do NOT attempt to replace the eyeball in the eye socket.

       (5) Cover the extruded eyeball with a moist, sterile dressing.

       (6) Place a protective covering (e.g., metal shield or cone shaped from cardboard) over the affected eye.

       (7) Cover the uninjured eye.

       (8) Encourage the patient to remain quiet.

       (9) Treat any associated injuries.

       (10) Transport the patient for further evaluation and treatment.

ENRICHMENT—INJURIES OF THE FACE AND THROAT

MOUTH AND JAW TRAUMA

1. **Fracture of the lower jaw (mandible)**

    a. Because the tongue is attached to the lower jaw, disruption of the lower jaw anatomy (e.g., fracture), may allow the tongue to fall against the back of the throat, occluding the airway. Therefore, fracture of the mandible can cause severe airway compromise.

  b. The mandible is likely to be broken in at least two places.

  c. Assessment findings depend on the area of the mandible affected but often include tenderness, bruising, and swelling.

2. Fracture of the upper jaw (maxilla)

  a. The maxilla is often fractured in high-speed crashes.

  b. The face is thrown forward into the windshield, steering wheel, and dashboard.

  c. Signs and symptoms

    (1) A maxilla fracture is often accompanied by a black eye.

    (2) The face may appear elongated.

    (3) The patient's bite is uneven.

    (4) Swelling is usually present.

  d. Emergency medical care

    (1) Follow local protocol.

    (2) Call for ALS assistance as needed.

    (3) Take BLS precautions.

    (4) Maintain spinal immobilization.

    (5) Establish and maintain an open airway.

    (6) Examine for and remove any teeth, blood, vomitus, etc.

      (a) Suction as necessary.

      (b) Examine the mouth for broken or missing teeth.

        (i) If dentures or missing teeth are found, transport with the patient.

        (ii) Rinse tooth with saline, wrap in moistened sterile gauze, and transport with patient.

    (7) Administer oxygen.

    (8) Assist ventilations as necessary.

    (9) Control bleeding.

    (10) Treat for shock if indicated.

    (11) Transport.

FACIAL FRACTURES

1. Signs and symptoms of facial fractures include:

  a. Bleeding from the nose and mouth

  b. Limited jaw motion

  c. Inability to swallow or talk

  d. Numbness or pain

  e. Increased salivation

  f. Loss of teeth

  g. Distortion of facial features

2. Emergency medical care

  a. Follow local protocol.

  b. Take BSI precautions.

  c. Maintain spinal immobilization.

  d. Establish and maintain an open airway.

  e. Administer oxygen.

  f. Assist ventilations as necessary.

  g. Control bleeding.

  h. Treat for shock if indicated.

  i. Transport.

INJURIES TO THE EAR

1. Blunt trauma

  a. Blunt trauma can result in bruising of the external ear.

      b. Severe blows can result in damage to the eardrum with pain or bleeding or both.

      c. Blood or fluid drainage from the ear should be considered a sign of a possible skull fracture. Place a sterile dressing loosely over the ear to absorb the drainage.

      d. Never pack the ear to control bleeding.

2. Cuts, lacerations, and avulsions

      a. Save the avulsed part and transport with patient.

      b. Treat as for other soft tissue injuries.

3. Injuries of the throat

      a. Causes include:

          (1) Hanging

          (2) Steering wheel impact

          (3) "Clothesline" injuries (e.g., person runs into a stretched wire or cord and strikes the throat)

          (4) Knife or gunshot wounds

      b. Signs and symptoms of neck injury include:

          (1) Stridor

          (2) Shortness of breath

          (3) Hoarseness

      c. Emergency medical care

          (1) Follow local protocol.

          (2) Call for ALS assistance as needed.

          (3) Take BSI precautions.

          (4) Maintain spinal immobilization.

          (5) Establish and maintain an open airway.

          (6) Administer oxygen.

          (7) Assist ventilations as necessary.

          (8) Control bleeding.

          (9) Treat for shock if indicated.

          (10) Transport.

BURNS

CLASSIFICATION OF BURNS BY DEPTH *(FIGURE 26-6)*

1. Superficial burns

      a. Superficial burns are also called **first-degree burns** or superficial partial-thickness burns.

      b. Characteristics of superficial burns include:

          (1) Involvement of only the epidermis

          (2) Reddened skin

          (3) Pain at the site

          (4) Healing in 7 to 10 days (generally)

2. Partial-thickness burns

      a. Partial-thickness burns are also called **second-degree burns** or deep partial-thickness burns.

      b. These burns commonly result from contact with hot liquids or flash burns from gasoline flames.

      c. Characteristics of partial-thickness burns include:

          (1) Involvement of both the epidermis and the dermis, but not underlying tissue

          (2) White to red skin that is moist and mottled

          (3) Blisters

          (4) Intense pain

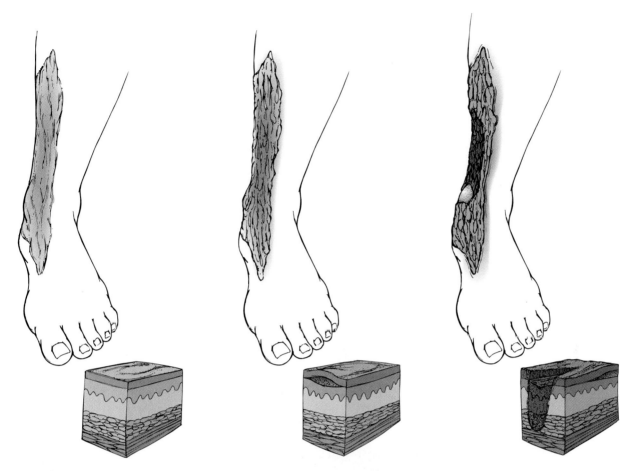

Fig. 26-6. Types of burns. *(A)* Superfical burn. *(B)* Partial-thickness burn. *(C)* Full-thickness burn.

     (5)   Swelling
     (6)   Skin sensitivity to air current
     (7)   Healing in 14 to 21 days (generally)

3. Full-thickness burns
  a. Full-thickness burns are also called **third-degree burns.**
  b. These burns are commonly caused by fire, prolonged exposure to hot liquids, contact with hot objects, or electricity and require skin grafting.
  c. Characteristics of full-thickness burns include:
     (1)   Extension through all the dermal layers; may involve subcutaneous layers, muscle, bone, or organs
     (2)   Dry and leathery skin
     (3)   White, dark brown, or charred skin
     (4)   Loss of sensation, i.e., little or no pain, hard to the touch, pain at periphery

DETERMINING BURN SEVERITY

1. Burn severity depends on:
  a. Depth or degree of the burn (superficial, partial thickness, or full thickness)
  b. Percentage of body surface area (BSA) burned
     (1)   The size of the patient's hand is equal to 1% of the body surface area.
     (2)   **Rule of nines—adult** *(Figure 26-7)*
         (a) Head and neck: 9%
         (b) Each upper extremity: 9%
         (c) Anterior trunk: 18%

          (d) Posterior trunk: 18%
          (e) Each lower extremity: 18%
          (f) Genitalia: 1%
      (3) **Rule of nines—infant**
          (a) Head and neck: 18%
          (b) Each upper extremity: 9%
          (c) Anterior trunk: 18%
          (d) Posterior trunk: 18%
          (e) Each lower extremity: 14%
  c. Location of the burn
      (1) Face and upper airway burns
      (2) Burns of the hands
      (3) Burns of the feet
      (4) Burns of the genitalia
  d. Preexisting medical conditions
  e. Age of the patient. Burns are severe if they occur in patients who are:
      (1) Younger than 5 years of age

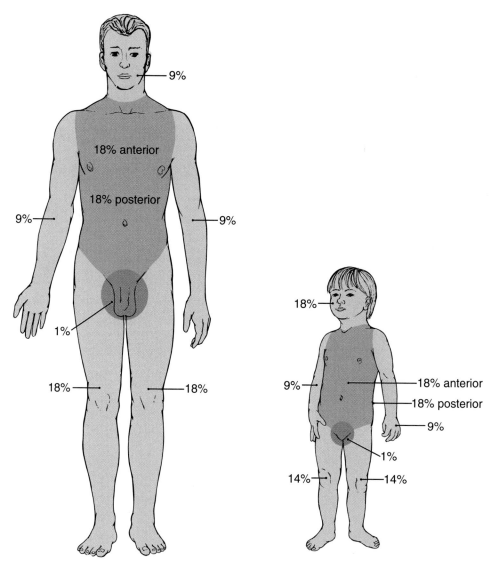

Fig. 26-7. Rule of nines.

(2) Older than 55 years of age
2. **Infant and child considerations**
   a. Relative size of the infant and child compared with adults influences the severity of burns.
      (1) Children have a larger surface area in relationship to the total body size.
      (2) This larger surface area results in greater fluid and heat loss.
   b. Children are at higher risk for shock (hypoperfusion), airway problems, or hypothermia than adults.
   c. Consider possibility of child abuse when treating a burned child.
   d. Any full-thickness burn or partial-thickness burn greater than 20%, or burn involving the hands, feet, face, airway, or genitalia is considered a critical burn in a child.
   e. Any partial-thickness burn of 10 to 20% is considered a moderate burn in a child.
   f. Any partial-thickness burn less than 10% is considered a minor burn in a child.
3. **Categories of burn severity**
   a. Critical burns include:
      (1) Full-thickness burns involving the hands, feet, face, or genitalia
      (2) Burns associated with respiratory injury
      (3) Full-thickness burns covering more than 10% of the body surface
      (4) Partial-thickness burns covering more than 30% of the body surface area
      (5) Burns complicated by a painful, swollen, deformed extremity
      (6) Moderate burns in young children or elderly patients
      (7) Burns encompassing any body part (e.g., arm, leg, or chest)
   b. Moderate burns include:
      (1) Full-thickness burns of 2% to 10% of the body surface area excluding hands, feet, face, genitalia and upper airway
      (2) Partial-thickness burns of 15% to 30% of the body surface area
      (3) Superficial burns of greater than 50% body surface area
   c. Minor burns include:
      (1) Full-thickness burns of less than 2% of the body surface area
      (2) Partial-thickness burns of less than 15% of the body surface area

EMERGENCY MEDICAL CARE FOR BURNS

1. Ensure scene safety.
2. Take BSI precautions.
3. Stop the burning process, initially with room temperature water or saline.
4. Remove smoldering clothing and jewelry, but do not attempt to remove clothing stuck to the patient.
5. Establish and maintain an open airway and continually monitor the airway for evidence of closure.
6. Administer oxygen.
   a. If breathing is adequate, apply oxygen by nonrebreather mask at 15 LPM if not already done.
   b. If breathing is inadequate, provide positive-pressure ventilation with 100% oxygen and assess adequacy of ventilations delivered.
7. Determine the severity of the burn.
   a. If the burn is critical, transport the patient immediately.
   b. Know local protocols for transport to an appropriate local facility.
8. Prevent further contamination.
   a. Follow local protocol.
   b. Cover the burned area with a dry, sterile dressing or sterile burn sheet.
   c. Do not use any type of ointment, lotion, or antiseptic on the burn.
   d. Do not break blisters.
9. Transport promptly to the appropriate facility.

CHEMICAL BURNS

1. Take the necessary scene safety precautions to protect yourself from exposure to hazardous materials.
2. Wear gloves and eye protection.
3. **Emergency medical care**
   a. Dry powders should be brushed off before flushing.
   b. Immediately begin to flush the skin with large amounts of water.
   c. Continue flushing the contaminated area while en route to the receiving facility.
   d. Do not contaminate uninjured areas when flushing.

ELECTRICAL BURNS

1. Ensure scene safety.
2. Do not attempt to remove the patient from the electrical source unless trained to do so.
3. If the patient is still in contact with the electrical source or you are unsure, do not touch the patient.
4. **Emergency medical care**
   a. Administer oxygen if indicated.
   b. Monitor the patient closely for respiratory and cardiac arrest [consider need for automated external defibrillator (AED)].
   c. These burns are often more severe than external indications.
   d. Treat the soft tissue injuries associated with the burn.
   e. Look for both an entrance and exit wound.

REVIEW QUESTIONS

Directions: Each of the numbered items or incomplete statements in this section is followed by answers or by completions of the statement. Select the ONE lettered answer or completion that is BEST in each case.

1. Blunt trauma generally results in

   (A) a puncture
   (B) a laceration
   (C) an abrasion
   (D) a contusion

2. Which of the following regarding a hematoma is correct?

   (A) Hematomas cause profuse external bleeding
   (B) Hematomas result in less tissue damage than contusions
   (C) A patient may lose 1 or more liters of blood under the skin
   (D) Patients will rarely have a broken bone near a hematoma

3. Your ambulance crew is called to a cabinetry shop for a 54-year-old male patient who cut off his index finger and thumb while using a band saw. Appropriate treatment for the amputated parts would include

   (A) pack the parts in ice and transport with the patient
   (B) submerse the parts in distilled water and transport with the patient
   (C) submerse the parts in a salt solution and transport with the patient

(D)   wrap the parts in a sterile dressing, keep them cool and dry, and transport with the patient

4. You have been called to the home of a 3-year-old child who was burned while getting into a bathtub. His mother states the child burned himself because the water was too hot. The child is conscious and crying. Both legs show scald-type burns up to the buttocks. The percent of body surface area burned would be

(A)   18%
(B)   28%
(C)   45%
(D)   54%

5. Which of the following statements regarding facial trauma is true?

(A)   Patients with facial trauma should not be given oxygen
(B)   Never suction the mouth of a patient with facial trauma
(C)   Patients with suspected facial bone fractures should have an oropharyngeal airway (OPA) inserted to protect their airway
(D)   Injuries to the face may complicate airway management due to increased salivation and decreased movement

6. Your rescue crew has been called to the scene of a high-speed vehicle collision. While triaging the patients, you note that one patient has an eyeball dangling out of its socket (an extruded eyeball). Appropriate management of this injury would include

(A)   replace the eyeball in the socket and cover both eyes
(B)   submerge the eyeball in water and cover the affected eye
(C)   replace the eyeball in the socket and cover the affected eye
(D)   cover the eyeball with a moist sterile dressing, protect from further injury, and cover both eyes

7. Patients with a nonchemical burn to an eye (e.g., heat, radiation, infrared burns) should be treated by

(A)   covering both eyes
(B)   covering only the affected eye
(C)   leaving both eyes uncovered
(D)   irrigating both eyes with water

8. Your ambulance has been called to a local elementary school for a 9-year-old female patient who injured her eye. You find the patient in the nurse's office with a pencil imbedded in her eyeball. Appropriate treatment for this injury would include

(A)   breaking off the end of the pencil, covering both eyes, positioning the patient sitting up, and transport
(B)   stabilizing the pencil with medical tape, covering both eyes, positioning the patient sitting up, and transport
(C)   stabilizing the pencil with a bulky dressing, covering both eyes, positioning the patient supine, and transport
(D)   attempting to remove the pencil once but stopping if resistance is met, covering both eyes, and transport

9. When treating an eye injury due to a chemical burn, it is important to

(A)   immediately cover both eyes
(B)   continuously irrigate with normal saline for at least 20 minutes

(C)   immediately attempt to neutralize the chemical by correcting its pH
(D)   continuously irrigate with bicarbonate of soda for at least 20 minutes

---

Directions: Each of the numbered items or incomplete statements in this section is negatively phrased, as indicated by a capitalized word such as NOT, LEAST, or EXCEPT. Select the ONE lettered answer or completion that is BEST.

---

10. Which of the following does NOT necessarily influence the severity of a burn?

(A)   The patient's age
(B)   The location of the burn
(C)   The temperature of the heat source
(D)   The patient's preexisting medical conditions

Directions: Each of the numbered questions or incomplete statements in this section refers to a scenario that precedes them. The numbered questions or incomplete statements are followed by answers or by completions of the statement. Select the answer or completion of the statement that is BEST in each case.

Your ambulance crew is called to the scene of an assault at a local pub. Local law enforcement has already secured the scene. You arrive to find your patient holding a dish towel over his left eye. He tells you he was cut with a broken bottle.

Questions 11–12

11. While assessing the wound, you note it appears to be a straight cut parallel to the eyebrow and about 2–3 inches in length. You may classify this wound as

(A)   a puncture
(B)   a laceration
(C)   an avulsion
(D)   an abrasion

12. To protect this wound from further contamination, you put a(n) _____ over the wound and secure it with _____.

(A)   rag/duct tape
(B)   bandage/a dressing
(C)   dressing/a bandage
(D)   occlusive bandage/a dressing

Your rescue crew is called to the scene of a domestic dispute. Local law enforcement has already secured the scene. Your patient is a 34-year-old male who was cut with a knife. Blood is pouring from his jaw and throat. He is conscious and alert.

Questions 13–14

13. Ideally, this injury should be covered with

(A)   a gloved hand

    (B)   a cervical collar
    (C)   sterile gauze pads
    (D)   an occlusive dressing

14. If direct pressure fails to control the bleeding, you should

    (A)   compress both carotid arteries and transport immediately
    (B)   compress the carotid artery on the injured side and transport immediately
    (C)   compress the carotid artery on the unaffected side and transport immediately
    (D)   wrap a pressure bandage around the neck and transport immediately

Your rescue crew is called to an apartment complex for a fight. Local law enforcement has secured the scene. Your patient is a 16-year-old male adolescent complaining of chest pain and severe difficulty breathing. He states he was stabbed several times in the back. Upon examination, you find five stab wounds to the upper back and a knife protruding from one of the wounds. There is also a 3-inch laceration to the patient's lower left abdominal quadrant.

Questions 15–17

15. The wounds on the patient's upper back should be covered with

    (A)   sterile gauze and wrap
    (B)   occlusive dressing and elastic wrap
    (C)   occlusive dressing taped on one side
    (D)   occlusive dressing taped on three sides

16. According to bystanders, the knife's blade is about 3–4 inches long. About 1 inch of the blade is exposed, the rest is in the patient. You should

    (A)   stabilize the knife with bulky dressings and secure in place
    (B)   seat the knife (push it in the remaining 1 inch), then secure in place
    (C)   remove the knife if it compromises the ability to immobilize the patient's spine
    (D)   attempt to remove the knife once, but stop and secure in place if you meet any resistance

17. While examining the abdominal injury, you note a loop of what appears to be intestine is hanging out about 2 inches. To appropriately manage this injury, you should

    (A)   push the loop back into the abdominal cavity
    (B)   cover the loop with dry, sterile gauze and secure with tape
    (C)   cover with a large, sterile dressing moistened with sterile saline, secure with a large bandage, and prevent heat loss
    (D)   cover the loop with an occlusive dressing, apply ice packs or cool compresses, and secure with a gauze wrap

Your ambulance has been called to the scene of a high-rise fire. You are assigned responsibility of a 66-year-old male patient with burns to his chest and arms. You note that the jacket he is wearing is still smoldering. He is conscious and alert but complains of difficulty breathing and severe arm pain.

Questions 18–19

18. Which of the following should be done first?

    (A)   Remove the patient's burning clothing

    (B)   Attempt to calculate the total burn area
    (C)   Cover the burns with a dry sterile dressing
    (D)   Begin high-flow oxygen therapy with a nonrebreather mask if breathing status is adequate

19. The burns to the patient's upper arms are red and blistered while the burns to the lower arms and hands are dry and leathery. The burns to the upper arms are most likely _____ while the burns to the lower arms are probably _____.

    (A)   full thickness/superficial
    (B)   superficial /full thickness
    (C)   superficial/partial thickness
    (D)   partial thickness/full thickness

20. Calculate the percent of body surface area burned if the patient has burns covering both arms and the anterior trunk.

    (A)   18%
    (B)   27%
    (C)   36%
    (D)   45%

ANSWERS AND RATIONALES

1-D. Blunt trauma generally results in closed skin injury. Punctures, lacerations, and abrasions are open skin injuries. A contusion, commonly known as a bruise, results when damage occurs to the blood vessels and cells of the dermal layer (the middle layer) of skin.

2-C. A hematoma, a closed skin injury, results when large vessels and large amounts of tissues are injured. A hematoma may be described as a severe contusion. Large volumes of blood (up to 1 liter or more) may leak into the damaged tissue. The trauma involved with the formation of a hematoma may be significant enough to cause bones to break (fracture).

3-D. When handling amputated body parts, care should be taken to preserve the part for possible reattachment. The part(s) should be wrapped in sterile gauze (dry or moist according to local protocol), placed in a plastic wrap or bag, and kept cool but not ice-cold. Do not attempt to freeze the amputated parts. Never submerse the amputated part in fluid, as destruction of cells is likely.

4-B. The rule of nines differs for children and infants because their heads are proportionately larger than the heads of adults. The head has twice the adult value, or 18%. The anterior trunk (chest and abdomen), posterior trunk (back), arms, and genitalia have the same values for infants/children and adults. The infant/child legs have a value of 14% each (rather than 18% each for the adult). The percentage of body surface area burned for this patient is 28%. Another aspect of this burn should catch your attention: if the water was too hot, why would the patient put both legs completely under the surface of the water? The "story" from the parent does not make sense. When treating injured dependent patients (e.g., children, elderly, mentally challenged), be aware that abuse is a possibility. While it is not the role of an EMT-Basic to investigate abuse, it is your responsibility to notify the appropriate agency (law enforcement or medical direction) of circumstances that suggest abuse.

5-D. Constant attention to airway status must be maintained in a patient with a suspected facial fracture. Anticipate the need for frequent suctioning. An oropharyngeal airway (OPA) may be inserted if the patient is unconscious and does not have a gag reflex; however, the insertion of an OPA does not preclude the need to constantly reevaluate the patient's airway status.

6-D. Replacing the eyeball may cause further damage and would increase the opportunity for infection. Do not attempt to replace misplaced body parts. Instead, keep the eyeball moist and protected.

7-A. When treating an injured eye, both eyes should be wrapped. Bandaging both eyes prevents movement by the unaffected eye from causing further damage to the affected eye. If irrigation of the eyes is needed, sterile saline solution should be used.

8-C. The eyeball contains two different fluids. The anterior (front) chamber contains aqueous humor, and the posterior chamber contains vitreous humor. Imagine the eye socket is like a cup. Positioning the patient supine maximizes the holding capacity of the cup. Stabilizing the pencil with bulky dressings and covering both eyes are critical to ensuring that further harm does not occur from the movement of the pencil or the eye.

9-B. Chemical injuries to the eyes are considered the most serious eye injury. Immediate and continuous irrigation of the affected eye(s) is critical to the long-term outcome for the patient. Twenty minutes is the minimum amount of time required for irrigation. Preferably, you should continuously irrigate the eye until the patient arrives at the receiving facility. If only one eye is affected, irrigate away from the unaffected eye. You may need to open the eye to facilitate irrigation. Open the eye by gently rolling the lid back. Make sure that you have provided for your safety. The minimum level of personal protective clothing for this type of patient would include medical gloves, arm protection, and face protection (e.g., goggles and mask). Individual chemicals may dictate the need for a higher level of protection.

10-C. Factors that influence the severity of a burn include the degree or depth of the burn, the percent of body surface area burned, the location of the burn, the patient's preexisting medical condition, and the patient's age. The temperature of the heat source does not necessarily influence the severity of the burn. If this were so, a superficial burn from the sun would be the most severe burn.

11-B. A laceration is a break in the skin of varying depth. They may be linear or irregular. The force of impact is generally associated with a sharp object like a knife or glass. A puncture is a wound created when a pointed object pierces the skin. A laceration is a "slashing"-type injury, whereas a puncture is a "stabbing"-type injury. An avulsion is characterized by a flap of skin or tissue at the injury site. An abrasion occurs because of rubbing or scraping. An example of an abrasion is a "skinned knee."

12-C. Dressings cover wounds, and bandages hold dressings in place. Rags may be used in extreme cases when sterile dressings cannot be found; however, avoid the use of duct tape when the tape must contact the patient's skin. Duct tape may cause further trauma during removal. Occlusive dressings are used to form an airtight seal, which is not necessary with a simple laceration.

13-D. Occlusive dressings are designed to create an airtight seal over a wound. Because this injury involves the neck and possibly the major blood vessels of the neck, an airtight dressing is essential to reduce the risk of an air embolism. A gloved hand should be used if there is any delay in applying an occlusive dressing. A cervical collar would be used if spinal immobilization were needed. Sterile gauze pads would allow air to enter the wound and therefore would not prevent an air embolism.

14-C. Compressing the carotid artery should be avoided. However, if life-threatening injury persists despite direct pressure, you may apply pressure to the carotid artery on the affected side. Never compress both carotid arteries or apply a pressure bandage around the neck, as these measures may cut off blood flow to the brain.

15-D. Air will always follow the path of least resistance. If there is a hole in the chest wall, air will enter the hole during inhalation. This air may become trapped in the chest cavity, leading to life-threatening compromise (pneumothorax or tension pneumothorax). An airtight barrier is critical. Sealing the occlusive dressing on three sides creates an airtight seal while allowing a route (the unsecured fourth side) for trapped air to escape.

16-A. The proper technique for securing an impaled object is to wrap the object with a bulky dressing, then secure the bulky dressing. Pushing the knife in further may cause additional harm. Removing the knife to perform spinal immobilization is not appropriate. In this case, spinal immobilization would be indicated since the possibility exists that the spinal cord may have been lacerated. However, you must improvise immobilization to facilitate transporting the patient with the knife in place. You may have to immobilize the patient on his side.

17-C. Never touch or attempt to replace exposed abdominal organs. Protect the organs from further harm by applying a large, sterile dressing over the area moistened with sterile water or saline. Retain moisture and preserve body heat by securing with a large bandage. Replacing the organs in the abdomen increases the risk of infection. Allowing the organs to dry out or freeze may necessitate surgical removal of the affected section of bowel.

18-A. Your immediate concern should be to protect the patient from further harm. You must stop the burning process and move the patient to a safe place. Calculating the burn area, applying sterile dressings, and initiating oxygen therapy should be done only after ensuring the safety of the patient. Note: While oxygen is not flammable, it does support and accelerate combustion. Do not use oxygen around an open or smoldering flame (including cigarettes).

19-D. Partial-thickness burns, also known as second-degree burns, are characterized by painful red or mottled skin that ultimately develops blisters. Both the epidermis and dermis are damaged in a partial-thickness burn, whereas a superficial burn only involves damage to the epidermis. Full-thickness burns, also known as third-degree burns, may appear white, brown, or charred. Since the dermal layer is destroyed in full-thickness burns, pain is not associated with these burns (the nerves that sense pain in the skin are located in the dermal layer).

20-C. The rule of nines for an adult divides the body into regions that equal 9% of the total body surface area (or a multiple of 9%). The head and each arm are given a value of 9%. The anterior trunk (chest and abdomen), the posterior trunk (the back), and each leg are given a value of 18%. The genitalia is considered 1%. This patient's percent of body surface area burned is 36%.

BIBLIOGRAPHY

Barber JM, Dillman PA: *Emergency Patient Care for the EMT-A.* Reston, Virginia, Reston Publishing Company, 1981.

Crosby LA, Lewallen DG (eds): *Emergency Care and Transportation of the Sick and Injured,* 6th ed. Rosemont, IL, American Academy of Orthopaedic Surgeons, 1995.

Grant HD, Murray RH Jr, Bergeron JD: *Emergency Care,* 7th ed. Englewood Cliffs, NJ, Prentice-Hall, 1995.

Hafen BQ, Karren KJ, Mistovich JJ: *Prehospital Emergency Care,* 5th ed. Upper Saddle River, NJ, Prentice-Hall, 1996.

Henry MC, Stapleton ER, Judd RL: *EMT: Prehospital Care.* Philadelphia, WB Saunders, 1992.

McSwain NE, White RD, Paturas JL, et al (eds): *The Basic EMT: Comprehensive Prehospital Patient Care.* St. Louis, Mosby-Year Book, 1996.

Sanders MJ: *Mosby's Paramedic Textbook.* St. Louis, Mosby-Year Book, 1994.

Sheehy SB, Lombardi JE: *Manual of Emergency Care,* 4th ed. St. Louis, Mosby-Year Book, 1995.

Sloane E: *Anatomy and Physiology: An Easy Learner.* Boston, Jones and Bartlett, 1994.

Solomon EP and Phillips GA: *Understanding Human Anatomy and Physiology.* Philadelphia, WB Saunders, 1987.

Stoy WA: *Mosby's EMT-Basic Textbook.* St. Louis, Mosby-Year Book, 1996.

Thibodeau GA, Patton KT: *The Human Body in Health and Disease.* St. Louis, Mosby-Year Book, 1992.

Tortora GJ, Grabowski SR: *Principles of Anatomy and Physiology,* 7th ed. New York, Harper-Collins, 1993.

United States Department of Transportation, National Highway Traffic Safety Administration: *Emergency Medical Technician: Basic. National Standard Curriculum,* 1994.

27-1 Describe the function of the muscular system.

27-2 Describe the function of the skeletal system.

27-3 List the major bones or bone groupings of the:

    a. Spinal column

    b. Thorax

    c. Upper extremities

    d. Lower extremities

27-4 Differentiate between an open and a closed painful, swollen, deformed extremity.

27-5 List the emergency medical care for a patient with a painful, swollen, deformed extremity.

27-6 State the reasons for splinting.

27-7 List the general rules of splinting.

27-8 List the complications of splinting.

ANATOMY REVIEW

MUSCULAR SYSTEM

1. **Function**
    a. The muscular system provides for movement.
        (1) Muscle cells (fibers) shorten (contract) when stimulated by a nerve impulse.
        (2) Muscle cells shorten by converting energy obtained from food (chemical energy) into movement (mechanical energy).

● MOTIVATION FOR LEARNING ●

The EMT-Basic will frequently encounter musculoskeletal injuries. The EMT-Basic must recognize a musculoskeletal injury and provide appropriate management including prevention of further injury, reducing pain, and decreasing the likelihood of permanent damage.

  (a) Skeletal muscles produce motion of the bones to which they are attached.

  (b) Other muscles produce movement within the body's internal organs.

 b. The muscular system gives the body shape.

 c. It protects internal organs.

 d. It contributes to heat production.

2. Types of muscle

 a. Skeletal muscle

  (1) **Skeletal muscle** is also called striated or voluntary muscle.

  (2) These muscles form the major muscle mass of the body.

  (3) The actions of skeletal muscles are under conscious control of the nervous system and brain.

  (4) They can be contracted and relaxed at will.

  (5) They produce rapid, forceful contractions.

  (6) Parts of a skeletal muscle include:

   (a) The origin, the stationary attachment of the muscle to a bone

   (b) The insertion, the movable attachment to a bone

   (c) The body, the main part of the muscle

  (7) **Location** *(Figure 27-1)*

   (a) Skeletal muscles are attached to bones by tendons.

   (b) Tendons create a pull between bones when muscles contract.

   (c) Ligaments connect bone to bone.

  (8) **Function**

   (a) Skeletal muscles move the skeleton.

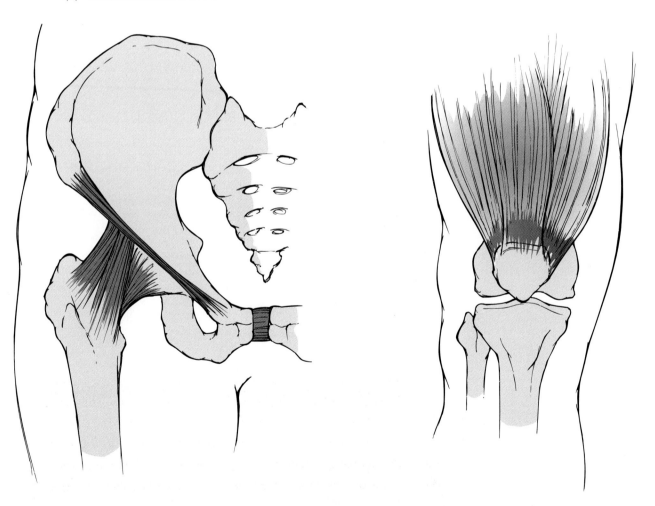

Fig. 27-1. *(A)* Muscles are attached to bones by tendons. *(B)* Ligaments connect bone to bone.

(b) They produce heat (i.e., help maintain constant body temperature).

(c) They maintain posture.

b. Smooth muscle

(1) **Smooth muscle** is also called visceral or involuntary muscle.

(2) Contraction of smooth muscle is not under voluntary control.

(3) Smooth muscles perform the work of all internal organs except the heart.

(4) They are found in blood vessels, the walls of hollow organs, and in the walls of tubular structures.

c. Cardiac muscle

(1) Cardiac muscle is found only in the heart.

(2) Cardiac muscle can tolerate interruption of blood supply for only very short periods.

SKELETAL SYSTEM

1. Function

a. The skeletal system gives the body shape, support, and form.

b. It protects vital internal organs.

(1) The skull protects the brain.

(2) The rib cage protects the heart and lungs.

(3) The lower ribs protect most of the liver and spleen.

(4) The spinal canal protects the spinal cord.

c. It works with muscles to provide for body movement.

d. It stores minerals (calcium, phosphorus).

e. It produces red blood cells.

2. Divisions *(Figure 27-2)*

a. Axial skeleton

(1) **Skull**

(a) Bones of the cranium include:

(i) Frontal (forehead) bones

(ii) Parietal (top sides of cranium) bones

(iii) Temporal (lower sides of cranium) bones

(iv) Occipital (back of skull) bone

(v) Sphenoid (central part of floor of cranium) bone

(vi) Ethmoid (floor of cranium, nasal septum) bone

(b) Bones of the face include:

(i) Orbits (eye sockets)

(ii) Nasal bones (upper bridge of nose)

(iii) Maxilla (upper jaw)

(iv) Mandible (lower jaw)

(v) Zygomatic bones (cheek bones)

(c) Ear bones

(2) **Spine**

(a) The spine consists of 33 separate but connected bones (vertebrae).

(b) The vertebrae are organized as follows:

(i) Seven cervical (neck) vertebrae

(ii) Twelve thoracic (upper back) vertebrae

(iii) Five lumbar (lower back) vertebrae

(iv) Five sacral (back wall of the pelvis) vertebrae (fused into one vertebra in an adult)

(v) Four coccyx (tailbone) vertebrae (fused into one vertebra in an adult)

(3) **Chest**

(a) **Ribs**

(i) All of the ribs are attached posteriorly by ligaments to the thoracic vertebrae.

(ii) Pairs 1–10 are attached anteriorly to the sternum.

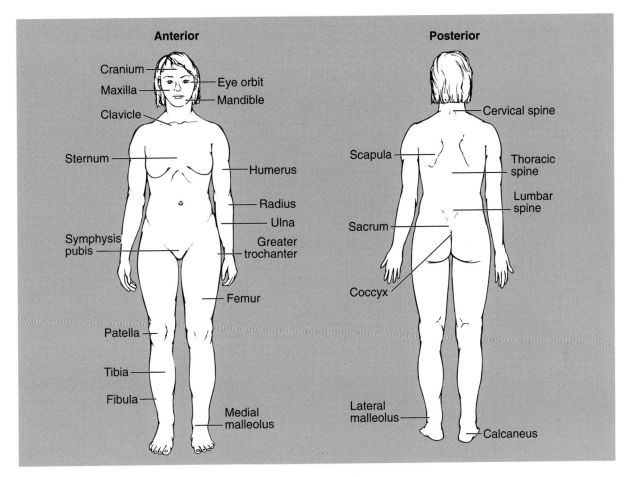

Fig. 27-2. Topographic anatomy.

(iii) Pairs 1–7 are attached anteriorly to the sternum by cartilage (true ribs).
(iv) Pairs 8–10 are attached to the cartilage of the 7th ribs (false ribs).
(v) Pairs 11 and 12 are not attached to the sternum anteriorly (floating ribs).
(b) Sternum
(i) Manubrium (superior portion)
(ii) Body (middle portion)
(iii) Xiphoid process (piece of cartilage that makes up the inferior portion)
(4) Hyoid bone
(a) The hyoid bone is the only bone in the body that does not connect to another bone.
(b) The tongue is anchored to the hyoid bone.
b. Appendicular skeleton
(1) Upper extremities
(a) The shoulder girdle consists of:
(i) Clavicle (collar bone)
(ii) Scapula (shoulder blade)
(b) Humerus (upper arm)
(c) Radius (thumb side of forearm)
(d) Ulna (little finger side of forearm)
(e) Olecranon (elbow)

        (f) Carpals (wrist)

        (g) Metacarpals (hand)

        (h) Phalanges (fingers)

    (2) **Lower extremities**

        (a) The pelvis (hip bone) consists of:

            (i) Iliac crest (wings of pelvis)

            (ii) Pubis (anterior portion of pelvis)

            (iii) Ischium (inferior portion of pelvis)

        (b) Femur (thigh)

        (c) Patella (kneecap)

        (d) Tibia (shinbone)

        (e) Fibula (little toe side of lower leg)

        (f) Tarsals (ankle)

        (g) Metatarsals (foot)

        (h) Phalanges (toes)

3. Joints *(Figure 27-3)*

  a. Ball-and-socket joint

    (1) Ball-and-socket joints allow movement in all directions.

    (2) Examples include the hip (pelvic bone and femur) and shoulder (scapula and humerus).

  b. Hinge joint

    (1) Hinge joints allow movement in only one plane.

    (2) Examples include the elbow (humerus and ulna) and knee (femur and tibia).

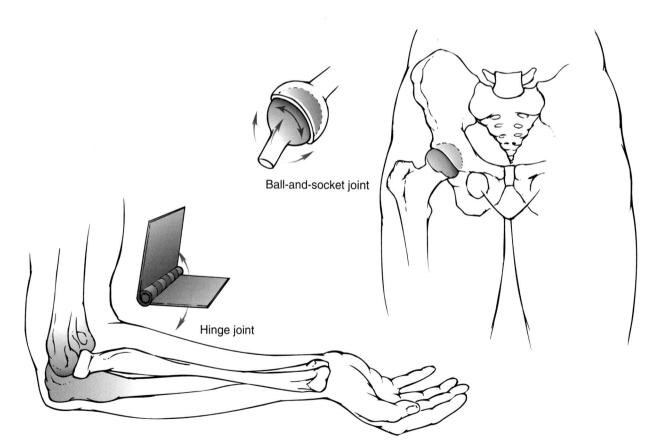

Fig. 27-3. Types of joint: Ball-and-socket joint and hinge.

INJURIES TO BONES AND JOINTS

MECHANISM OF INJURY

1. Direct force causes injury at the point of impact (*Figure 27-4*).
2. Indirect force causes injury at a site other than the point of impact.
3. Twisting force causes one part of the extremity to remain stationary while the rest twists.

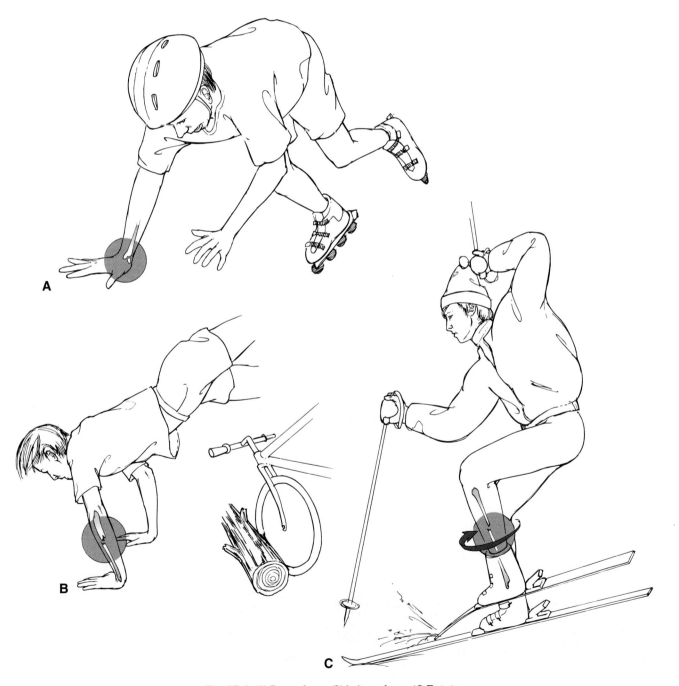

Fig. 27-4. *(A)* Direct force. *(B)* Indirect force. *(C)* Twisting.

BONE AND JOINT INJURIES

1. **Types of Bone and Joint Injuries** (*Figure 27-5*)
   a. Open
      (1) In open bone and joint injuries, the continuity of the skin is broken.
      (2) The bone may or may not protrude through the wound.
      (3) These injuries can result in serious blood loss.
      (4) Risk of infection is increased.
   b. Closed
      (1) In closed bone and joint injuries, the continuity of the skin is not broken.
      (2) However, these injuries can result in serious blood loss due to internal bleeding.
        (a) A broken femur can result in the loss of up to 1 liter of blood.
        (b) Two broken femurs can result in life-threatening hemorrhage.
        (c) A broken pelvis can damage nerves, tear the bladder, or cause internal hemorrhage by tearing large blood vessels (*Figure 27-6*).

2. Signs and symptoms of bone and joint injuries include:
   a. Pain
   b. Swelling
   c. Grating (crepitus)
   d. Loss of sensation
   e. Loss of distal pulse
   f. Exposed bone ends
   g. Bruising (ecchymosis)
   h. Deformity or angulation
   i. Joint locked into position
   j. Inability to move affected area

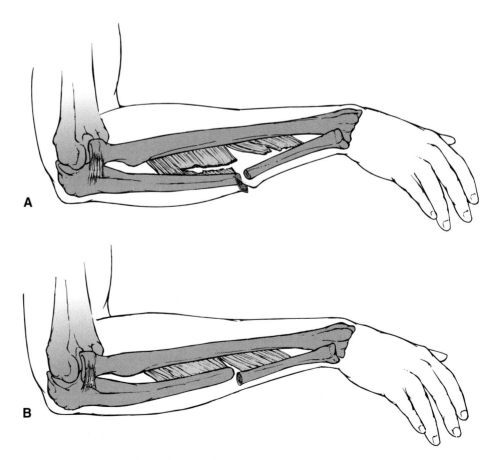

Fig. 27-5. Types of bone injury. *(A)* Open. *(B)* Closed.

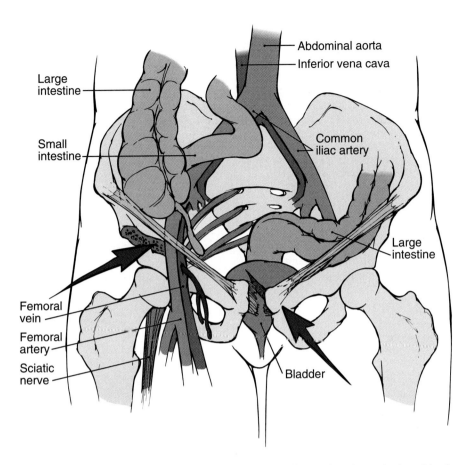

Fig. 27-6. A broken pelvis can tear the bladder or cause internal hemorrhage by tearing large blood vessels.

     k. Point tenderness at site of injury
     l. Numbness or tingling sensation (paresthesia)
  3. Emergency medical care
     a. Take appropriate body substance isolation (BSI) precautions.
     b. Provide specific treatment based on the patient's signs and symptoms.
     c. Maintain spinal immobilization if indicated.
     d. Establish and maintain an open airway.
     e. Administer oxygen if not already done and indicated.
     f. Control bleeding if present.
     g. Treat for shock if indicated.
     h. After life threats have been controlled, splint injuries in preparation for transport.
     i. Apply cold pack to a painful, swollen, deformed extremity to reduce swelling.
     j. If spinal injury is not suspected, elevate the extremity.
     k. Transport.

SPLINTING

REASONS FOR SPLINTING A BONE OR JOINT INJURY (BOX 27-1)

1. Splinting prevents motion of bone fragments, bone ends, or dislocated joints.
2. Splinting minimizes the following complications:
     a. Damage to muscles, nerves, or blood vessels caused by broken bones

---

Box 27-1. **Reasons for Splinting**

- Prevent motion of bone fragments, bone ends, or dislocated joints
- Minimize damage to muscles, nerves, or blood vessels caused by broken bones
- Minimize the chance of converting closed painful, swollen, deformed extremity to an open painful, swollen, deformed extremity
- Minimize restriction of blood flow due to bone ends or dislocations compressing blood vessels
- Minimize bleeding due to tissue damage caused by bone ends
- Minimize pain associated with movement of bone ends of dislocated bones
- Minimize the chance of paralysis of extremities due to a damaged spine

---

b. Conversion of a closed painful, swollen, deformed extremity to an open painful, swollen, deformed extremity
c. Restriction of blood flow due to bone ends or dislocations compressing blood vessels
d. Excessive bleeding due to tissue damage caused by bone ends
e. Increased pain associated with movement of bone ends or dislocated bones
f. Paralysis of extremities due to a damaged spine

GENERAL RULES OF SPLINTING

1. Assess pulse, motor, and sensation distal to the injury before and after splint application.
   a. Marking the pulse site with a pen to identify where it was last felt may be helpful.
   b. Assess every 15 minutes.
   c. Record findings.
2. Immobilize above and below the injury.
   a. If a bone injury, immobilize the joint above and below the injury.
   b. If a joint injury, immobilize the bone above and below the injury.
3. Remove jewelry from the injured area and remove or cut away clothing before splinting.
4. Cover open wounds with a sterile dressing.
5. If there is a severe deformity, or the distal extremity is cyanotic or lacks pulses, align with gentle traction before splinting.
   a. Gently grasp the extremity above and below the break.
   b. Apply traction steadily and smoothly.
   c. Maintain traction while the splint is applied.
   d. Reassess distal pulse and sensation.
   e. If resistance is felt, stop and splint in position found.
   f. Do not intentionally replace protruding bones.
   g. Pad each splint to prevent pressure and discomfort to the patient.
   h. Splint the injury before moving the patient when feasible and no life threats.
   i. When in doubt about whether an injury is present, splint the injury.
   j. If the patient shows signs of shock, align the patient in normal anatomical position on a long backboard, treat for shock, and transport.

EQUIPMENT

Equipment for splinting includes:
1. Rigid splints
2. Traction splints
3. Pneumatic splints (air, vacuum)
4. Improvised splints, pillow
5. Pneumatic anti-shock garment (as a splint)

HAZARDS OF IMPROPER SPLINTING (BOX 27-2)

Hazards of improper splinting include:
1. Compression of nerves, tissues, and blood vessels from the splint
2. Delay in transport of a patient with life-threatening injury
3. Splint applied too tight on the extremity, reducing distal circulation
4. Aggravation of the bone or joint injury
5. Cause or aggravation of tissue, nerve, vessel, or muscle damage from excessive bone or joint movement

SPECIAL CONSIDERATIONS OF SPLINTING

1. **Long bone splinting procedure**
   a. Take BSI precautions.
   b. Manually stabilize bone in position found.
   c. Assess pulse, motor, and sensory function below the injured area.
   d. If there is a severe deformity, or the distal extremity is cyanotic or lacks pulses, align the extremity with gentle traction before splinting.
      (1) Gently grasp the extremity above and below the break.
      (2) Apply traction steadily and smoothly.
      (3) Maintain traction while splint is applied.
      (4) Reassess distal pulse and sensation.
      (5) If resistance is felt, stop and splint in position found.
   e. Measure splint for proper length.
   f. Apply splint, immobilizing the bone and joint above and below the injury.
   g. Pad spaces between the extremity and the splint.
   h. Secure entire injured extremity.
   i. Immobilize a hand or foot in the position of function.
   j. Reassess pulse, motor, and sensation after application of splint.
      (a) Assess every 15 minutes.
      (b) Record findings.
2. **Splinting a joint injury**
   a. Take BSI precautions.
   b. Manually stabilize the joint in the position found.
   c. Assess pulse, motor, and sensory function below the injured area.
   d. Align with gentle traction if distal extremity is cyanotic or lacks pulses and no resistance is met.
   e. Immobilize the site of injury.
   f. Immobilize bone above and below the site of injury.
   g. Reassess pulse, motor, and sensation after application of splint.
      (1) Assess every 15 minutes.
      (2) Record findings.
3. **Traction splinting**
   a. Indication for use is a painful, swollen, deformed midthigh with no joint or lower leg injury.
   b. Do NOT use a traction splint if:
      (1) Injury is close to the knee
      (2) Injury to the knee exists

Box 27-2. Hazards of Improper Splinting

- Delay in transport of a patient with life-threatening injury
- Compression of nerves, tissues, and blood vessels from the splint
- Reduced distal circulation if extremity splint applied too tightly
- Aggravation of the bone or joint injury
- Tissue, nerve, vessel, or muscle damage from excessive bone or joint movement

(3) There is injury to the hip

(4) The pelvis has been injured

(5) There is partial amputation or avulsion with bone separation, and the distal limb is connected only by marginal tissue. Traction would risk separation.

(6) Lower leg or ankle injury

c. Traction splinting procedure

(1) Assess pulse, motor, and sensation distal to the injury and record.

(2) Take BSI precautions.

(3) Manually stabilize the injured leg.

(4) Apply manual traction (required when using a bipolar traction splint).

(5) Prepare/adjust splint to proper length.

(6) Position splint under injured leg.

(7) Apply proximal securing device (ischial strap).

(8) Apply distal securing device (ankle hitch).

(9) Apply mechanical traction.

(10) Position/secure support straps.

(11) Reevaluate proximal/distal securing devices.

(12) Reassess pulse, motor, and sensation after application of splint.

    (a) Assess every 15 minutes.

    (b) Record findings.

(13) Secure torso to long backboard to immobilize hip.

(14) Secure splint to long backboard to prevent movement of splint.

REVIEW QUESTIONS

Directions: Each of the numbered items or incomplete statements in this section is followed by answers or by completions of the statement. Select the ONE lettered answer or completion that is BEST in each case.

1. After splinting a wound, you should reassess motor, sensory, and circulation in the affected limb at least every

(A) 1–2 minutes

(B) 5 minutes

(C) 15 minutes

(D) 1 hour

Directions: Each of the numbered items or incomplete statements in this section is negatively phrased, as indicated by a capitalized word such as NOT, LEAST, or EXCEPT. Select the ONE lettered answer or completion that is BEST in each case.

2. Which of the following is NOT a reason for splinting an injury?

(A) To set the fracture

(B) To minimize the pain of the injury

(C) To minimize damage to surrounding tissues

(D) To prevent movement of bone ends, bone fragments, or dislocated joints

Directions: Each of the numbered questions or incomplete statements in this section refers to a scenario that precedes them. The numbered questions or incomplete statements are followed by answers or by completions of the statement. Select the answer or completion of the statement that is BEST in each case.

Your ambulance crew has been called to the scene of a 47-year-old female patient who has fallen from a ladder. You arrive to find this patient sitting on the ground holding her right wrist.

Questions 3–7

3. Upon examination, you note that her wrist is swollen and deformed. There is a cut at the site of the swelling, but you do not see any bone ends protruding through the cut. What type of injury is this?

    (A) Open
    (B) Closed
    (C) Epiphyseal
    (D) Greenstick

4. When should this injured limb be splinted?

    (A) During the initial assessment
    (B) After arrival at the receiving facility
    (C) After life-threatening injuries have been addressed
    (D) Immediately upon arrival at the scene to prevent further damage

5. If you suspect the bones of the forearm have been damaged, you should immobilize

    (A) the forearm only
    (B) from the wrist to the elbow
    (C) from the fingers to the shoulder
    (D) from the forearm to the shoulder

6. Before splinting, you should

    (A) apply ice directly to the wound
    (B) look inside the cut for the presence of bone ends or foreign fragments
    (C) assess the circulation, sensation, and movement of the affected limb
    (D) assess the circulation, sensation, and movement of the unaffected limb

7. While preparing to splint this extremity, you note that the patient has a large diamond ring on her ring finger. Which of the following would be appropriate?

    (A) Remove the ring in case swelling begins
    (B) Wrap the finger with an elastic bandage to decrease swelling
    (C) Leave the ring in place if the fingers are not swollen
    (D) Apply ice to the finger to ensure that swelling will not be a factor

Your rescue crew is called to the scene of a car-versus-motorcycle collision and assigned responsibility to treat the motorcyclist. Bystanders state that a vehicle T-boned the motorcyclist at about 35 miles per hour. He was wearing a helmet and is found lying on the ground screaming in pain. As you approach, he tells you that his right leg is "all messed up."

8. Which of the following should be done first?

    (A) Begin splinting the right leg
    (B) Remove the patient's helmet
    (C) Perform an initial assessment
    (D) Perform a rapid trauma assessment

9. After the appropriate initial assessment and interventions, you are considering the use of a traction splint for the patient's right leg. Which of the following is an indication for use of the traction splint?

    (A) An isolated pelvic injury with no damage to the leg
    (B) An isolated knee injury with no damage to the pelvis
    (C) An isolated midthigh injury with no joint or lower leg injuries present
    (D) An isolated lower leg injury with no joint or upper leg injuries present

10. When securing the traction splint to the patient, there are three basic points of attachment: the groin, the leg, and the ankle. The proper order for securing the device is

    (A) groin, then ankle, finally leg
    (B) groin, then leg, finally ankle
    (C) ankle, then leg, finally groin
    (D) leg, then ankle, finally groin

ANSWERS AND RATIONALES

1-C. You may opt to reevaluate a splinted extremity more often, but minimally you should reassess motor, sensory, and circulatory statuses every 15 minutes. Do not forget to include these reassessments in your documentation [e.g., "0835 hours: motor, sensory, and circulation intact distal (away from) to injury"].

2-A. EMT-Basics should not attempt to "set" a fracture. Setting fractures is the responsibility of trained, authorized personnel and is generally accomplished after reviewing X-ray results. Proper splinting should prevent further damage; prevent movement; allow for proper blood flow; and minimize bleeding, pain, and the chances of nerve damage.

3-A. If the continuity of the skin is broken at or near the injury site, then the wound is classified as open. Open wounds present an additional hazard to the patient because contaminants can now enter the body. When treating open injuries, you must cover them with a sterile dressing prior to splinting. Epiphyseal and greenstick injuries are specific types of fractures associated with pediatric patients. The epiphyseal plate, also known as the growth plate, is an immature area of the bone where growth takes place. A greenstick fracture is an incomplete fracture of the bone characterized by a splintering effect of the bone (similar to the effect when a branch is bent, hence the name greenstick).

4-C. Splinting should occur after life-threatening conditions have been addressed and managed. Rescuers are often lured into immediately treating musculoskeletal injuries due to the grotesque presentation of some fractures and dislocations. While these injuries are certainly disturbing and painful, splinting should be performed only after truly life-threatening conditions have been stabilized.

5-B. When dealing with a bone injury, you must splint the joint above and below the injury. In this case, you need to splint from the wrist to the elbow. When dealing with a joint injury, you must splint the bone above and below the affected joint. For example, if the elbow were injured, a splint should be applied from the upper arm (humerus bone) to the lower arm (radius and ulna bones).

6-C. Before splinting any injury, it is imperative that you evaluate the motor, sensory, and circulation of the affected area. This monitoring gives you a baseline with which you can compare motor, sensory, and circulation after applying the splint. If motor, sensory, and circulation are intact before application of the splint but are not present after application, you need to immediately reassess your splinting technique. Applying ice to the injury may help reduce swelling and decrease pain; however, ice should never be applied directly to the skin as it may cause further tissue damage.

7-A. Anticipate that the fingers are going to swell in all upper extremity injuries. Preferably, the ring should be removed while you are still at the patient's house so that it may be secured in the house. Do not get in the habit of "holding" personal effects for the patient. Even those rescuers with the best intentions may find themselves in an awkward position.

8-C. Immediately after the scene size-up (which should include body substance isolation precautions), you should begin the initial assessment to evaluate the patient's mental, airway, breathing, and circulation status as well as any life-threatening conditions that may exist. Removing the helmet may be appropriate if it complicates assessment of the airway. A rapid trauma assessment should be performed after the initial assessment for unconscious patients. Since this patient is conscious, a focused history and physical examination should follow the initial assessment.

9-C. Traction splints are indicated for use in the lower extremity if the injury is isolated to the midthigh (midfemur). The device reduces the pain associated with midthigh fractures and also reduces the chance of further tissue damage. The device should not be applied if there is any significant injury to the lower leg, the knee, or the pelvis, since the force of traction necessary to stabilize a thigh injury may increase the extent of trauma to these other body regions.

10-A. First, the traction splint is secured to the anchor-point of the body, the groin. Once it is anchored to the body, the ankle hitch is applied and the traction increased until the amount of mechanical traction equals the amount of manual traction being applied by a second rescuer. Once the splint is sized correctly for the amount of traction necessary, the leg straps should be applied. Avoid applying leg straps directly over the kneecap as they may interrupt the flow of blood to the lower leg.

BIBLIOGRAPHY

Butman AM, Martin SW, Vomacka RW, et al (eds): *Comprehensive Guide to Pre-Hospital Skills: A Skills Manual for EMT-Basic, EMT-Intermediate, EMT-Paramedic.* Akron, Ohio, Emergency Training, 1995.

Campbell JE (ed): *Basic Trauma Life Support for Paramedics and Advanced EMS Providers*, 3rd ed. Englewood Cliffs, NJ, Prentice-Hall, 1995.

Crosby LA, Lewallen DG (eds): *Emergency Care and Transportation of the Sick and Injured*, 6th ed. Rosemont, IL, American Academy of Orthopaedic Surgeons, 1995.

Grant HD, Murray RH Jr, Bergeron JD: *Emergency Care*, 7th ed. Englewood Cliffs, NJ, Prentice-Hall, 1995.

Hafen BQ, Karren KJ, Mistovich JJ: *Prehospital Emergency Care*, 5th ed. Upper Saddle River, NJ, Prentice-Hall, 1996.

Henry MC, Stapleton ER, Judd RL: *EMT: Prehospital Care*. Philadelphia, WB Saunders, 1992.

McSwain NE, White RD, Paturas JL, et al (eds): *The Basic EMT: Comprehensive Prehospital Patient Care*. St. Louis, Mosby-Year Book, 1996.

Sanders MJ: *Mosby's Paramedic Textbook*. St. Louis, Mosby-Year Book, 1994.

Sheehy SB, Lombardi JE: *Manual of Emergency Care*, 4th ed. St. Louis, Mosby-Year Book, 1995.

Sloane E: *Anatomy and Physiology: An Easy Learner*. Boston, Jones and Bartlett, 1994.

Solomon EP and Phillips GA: *Understanding Human Anatomy and Physiology*. Philadelphia, WB Saunders, 1987.

Stoy WA: *Mosby's EMT-Basic Textbook*. St. Louis, Mosby-Year Book, 1996.

Thibodeau GA, Patton KT: *The Human Body in Health and Disease*. St. Louis, Mosby-Year Book, 1992.

Tortora GJ, Grabowski SR: *Principles of Anatomy and Physiology*, 7th ed. New York, Harper-Collins, 1993.

United States Department of Transportation, National Highway Traffic Safety Administration: *Emergency Medical Technician: Basic. National Standard Curriculum*, 1994.

INJURIES TO THE HEAD AND SPINE

OBJECTIVES

28-1 List the functions of the central nervous system.

28-2 State the components of the nervous system.

28-3 Define the structure of the skeletal system as it relates to the nervous system.

28-4 Relate the mechanism of injury to potential injuries of the head and spine.

28-5 Describe the implications of not properly caring for potential spine injuries.

28-6 State the signs and symptoms of a potential spine injury.

28-7 Describe the method of determining if a responsive patient may have a spine injury.

28-8 Relate the airway emergency medical care techniques to the patient with a suspected spine injury.

28-9 Describe how to stabilize the cervical spine.

28-10 Discuss indications for sizing and using a cervical spine immobilization device.

28-11 Establish the relationship between airway management and the patient with head and spine injuries.

28-12 Describe a method for sizing a cervical spine immobilization device.

28-13 Describe how to log roll a patient with a suspected spine injury.

28-14 Describe how to secure a patient to a long spine board.

28-15 List instances when a short spine board should be used.

28-16 Describe how to immobilize a patient using a short spine board.

28-17 Describe the indications for rapid extrication.

28-18 List steps in performing rapid extrication.

28-19 State the circumstances when a helmet should be left on the patient.

28-20 Discuss the circumstances when a helmet should be removed.

MOTIVATION FOR LEARNING

The EMT-Basic must be able to recognize and appropriately manage the patient with potential injury to the head and spine. Knowledge and practice of the techniques and equipment used in spinal immobilization are essential to minimize the risk of permanent disability or death from a spinal injury.

28-21   Identify different types of helmets.

28-22   Describe the unique characteristics of sports helmets.

28-23   Explain the preferred methods to remove a helmet.

28-24   Discuss alternative methods for removal of a helmet.

28-25   Describe how the patient's head is stabilized to remove the helmet.

28-26   Differentiate how the head is stabilized with a helmet compared to without a helmet.

ANATOMY REVIEW

NERVOUS SYSTEM (FIGURE 28-1)

1. The nervous system controls the voluntary and involuntary activities of the body.
2. **Central nervous system (CNS)**
    a. **Brain** (*Figure 28-2*)
        (1)   The brain is the controlling organ of the body.

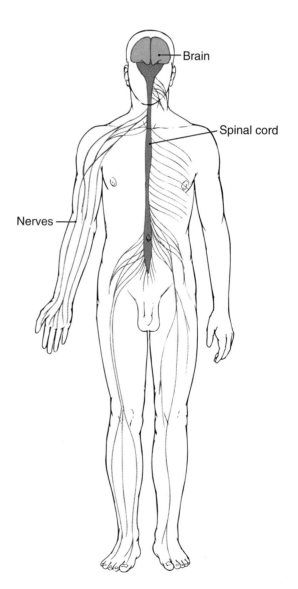

Fig. 28-1. The nervous system.

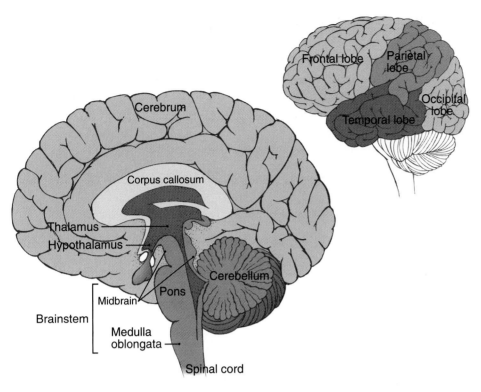

Fig. 28-2. Side view of the brain.

(2)   It is the center of consciousness.
(3)   It occupies the entire space within the cranium.
(4)   Protective coverings of the brain include:
  (a)   Skull
  (b)   Meninges, the three layers of connective tissue coverings that surround the brain and spinal cord. They include:
    (i)   Pia mater, the innermost layer
    (ii)   Arachnoid layer, the middle layer
    (iii)   Dura mater, the tough, outermost layer that adheres to the inner surface of the cranium
(5)   **Cerebrospinal fluid (CSF)**
  (a)   CSF surrounds the brain and spinal cord.
  (b)   It acts as a shock-absorber.
  (c)   It provides a means of exchange of nutrients and wastes among the blood, brain, and spinal cord.
(6)   **Cerebrum**
  (a)   The cerebrum is the largest part of the human brain.
  (b)   It consists of two cerebral hemispheres.
  (c)   Each hemisphere has four lobes:
    (i)   The frontal lobe, which controls motor function
    (ii)   The parietal lobe, which receives and interprets nerve impulses from sensory receptors
    (iii)   The occipital lobe, which controls eyesight
    (iv)   The temporal lobe, which controls hearing and smell
(7)   **Cerebellum**
  (a)   The cerebellum is the second largest part of the human brain.
  (b)   It is responsible for precise control of muscle movements, maintenance of posture, and maintaining balance.
(8)   **Brain stem**
  (a)   The midbrain acts as a relay for auditory and visual impulses.

(b) The pons connects parts of the brain with one another by means of tracts and influences respiration.

(c) The medulla oblongata is involved in the regulation of heart rate, blood vessel diameter, respiration, coughing, swallowing, and vomiting.

b. Spinal cord *(Figure 28-3)*

(1) The spinal cord is made up of long tracts of nerves that join the brain with all body organs and parts.

(2) It is the center for many reflex activities of the body.

(3) It is protected by the spinal column.

3. Peripheral nervous system (PNS)

a. Sensory nerves send information to the brain about the activities of the different parts of the body relative to their surroundings.

b. Motor nerves leave the brain and cause stimulation of a muscle or organ.

THE SKELETAL SYSTEM

1. Function

a. The skeletal system gives the body shape, support, and form.

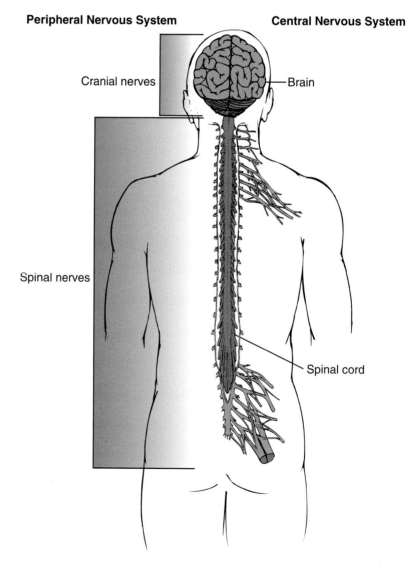

Fig. 28-3. The spinal cord is made up of long tracts of nerves that join the brain with all body organs and parts.

    b. It protects vital internal organs.
- **(1)** The skull protects the brain.
- **(2)** The rib cage protects the heart and lungs.
- **(3)** The lower ribs protect most of the liver and spleen.
- **(4)** The spinal canal protects the spinal cord.

    c. It works with muscles to provide for body movement.
    d. It stores minerals (calcium, phosphorus).
    e. It produces red blood cells.

2. Selected components of the skeletal system include:
    a. The skull
    b. The spinal column, which consists of 33 bones and surrounds and protects the spinal cord

INJURIES TO THE SPINE

MECHANISM OF INJURY

1. Compression
    a. Compression can drive the weight of the head or pelvis into the stationary neck or torso.
    b. Compression results from:
- **(1)** Contact sports
- **(2)** Motor vehicle crashes
- **(3)** Diving into shallow water
- **(4)** Falls from moving vehicles or falls from a height of more than 10 to 20 feet onto head or legs

2. Excessive extension (hyperextension)
    a. Hyperextension is a severe backward movement of the head or neck.
    b. Hyperextension results from:
- **(1)** Diving into shallow water
- **(2)** Impact of the face into windshield in motor vehicle crashes
- **(3)** Falling and striking face or chin (usually seen in an elderly person)

3. Excessive flexion (hyperflexion)
    a. Hyperflexion is a severe forward movement of the head onto the chest.
    b. Hyperflexion results from:
- **(1)** Diving into shallow water
- **(2)** Sudden deceleration of a motor vehicle
- **(3)** Being thrown from a horse or motorcycle

4. Rotation
    a. Severe rotation of the torso or head and neck can move one side of the spinal column against the other.
    b. Rotation results from:
- **(1)** Motorcycle crash
- **(2)** Rollover motor vehicle crash

5. Lateral bending
    a. Lateral bending is a sudden side impact that moves the torso sideways. The head remains in place until moved along by its attachments to the cervical spine.
    b. Lateral bending results from:
- **(1)** Contact sports
- **(2)** "T-bone" or angular motor vehicle crashes

6. Distraction
    a. Distraction is a pulling apart of the spine.
    b. Distraction results from:
- **(1)** Hangings

    (2)   Schoolyard or playground accidents

    (3)   Snowmobile or motorcycle under rope or wire

7. Penetrating trauma

    a. Penetrating trauma can occur to the head, neck, or torso

    b. Penetrating trauma results from:

        (1)   Stab wounds

        (2)   Gunshot wounds

SCENE SIZE-UP

1. Determine the mechanism of injury from the patient, family members, or bystanders and inspection of the scene.

2. Determine if it is safe to approach the patient.

3. Maintain a high index of suspicion of spinal injury if the mechanism of injury suggests any of the following (*Box 28-1*):

    a. Fall

    b. Hanging

    c. Blunt trauma

    d. Diving accident

    e. Electrical injury

    f. Motorcycle crash

    g. Motor vehicle crash

    h. Unconscious trauma victim

    i. Pedestrian–vehicle collision

    j. Penetrating trauma to head, neck, or torso

4. In infants and children, maintain a high index of suspicion of spinal injury if the mechanism of injury suggests any of the following (see *Box 28-1*):

    a. Falls over 10 feet (or three times body height)

    b. Bicycle collision

    c. Vehicle collision at a medium speed

    d. Any vehicle collision where the infant or child was unrestrained

5. Do NOT rule out the possibility of spinal column or cord damage in a patient walking about at the scene.

INITIAL ASSESSMENT

1. If the mechanism of injury suggests the possibility of spinal injury, maintain in-line spinal immobilization until the patient is secured to a long backboard.

2. Assess the patient's mental status.

Box 28-1. Significant Mechanisms of Injury

- Ejection from a vehicle
- Death in the same passenger compartment
- Falls from more than 20 feet (or three times body height)
- Rollover of a vehicle
- High-speed vehicle collision
- Pedestrian–vehicle collision
- Motorcycle crash
- Unresponsive or altered mental status
- Penetrations of the head, chest, or abdomen
- Hidden injuries from seat belts or airbags

Infants and children:
- Falls from more than 10 feet in infants and children (or three times body height)
- Bicycle collision
- Vehicle collision at a medium speed
- Any vehicle collision where the infant or child was unrestrained

3. Assess the patient's airway (jaw-thrust maneuver).
4. Assess breathing.
5. Assess circulation.
6. Identify any life-threatening conditions and provide care based on these findings.
7. Establish patient priorities. Priority patients are those:
   a. Who give a poor general impression
   b. With severe pain anywhere
   c. With uncontrolled bleeding
   d. Experiencing difficulty breathing
   e. With signs and symptoms of shock
   f. Are unresponsive with no gag reflex or cough
   g. Are responsive and are unable to follow commands
8. ALS assistance should be requested as soon as possible.
9. If ALS personnel are not available, the patient should be transported promptly to the closest appropriate facility.

FOCUSED HISTORY AND PHYSICAL EXAMINATION

1. If no significant mechanism of injury exists (e.g., cut finger):
   a. Perform a focused physical examination based on:
      (1) Patient's chief complaint
      (2) Mechanism of injury
      (3) Initial (rapid) assessment findings
   b. Assess baseline vital signs
   c. Obtain SAMPLE history
2. If a significant mechanism of injury exists:
   a. Continue in-line spinal stabilization
   b. Consider ALS request
   c. Reconsider transport decision
   d. Reassess mental status
   e. Perform rapid trauma assessment to determine life-threatening injuries
   f. In the responsive patient, symptoms should be sought before and during the trauma assessment
   g. Assess baseline vital signs
   h. Obtain SAMPLE history
3. **Assessment of the patient with a possible spine injury**
   a. If awake, instruct the patient not to move during the examination.
   b. Inspect and palpate the head, neck, chest, abdomen, pelvis, extremities, and posterior body for:
      (1) Deformities
      (2) Contusions (bruises)
      (3) Abrasions (scrapes)
      (4) Penetrations
      (5) Burns
      (6) Tenderness
      (7) Lacerations (cuts)
      (8) Swelling
      (9) Instability
      (10) Crepitation (grating)
      (11) Distal pulses, motor function, and sensation of each extremity
         (a) Assess motor function of each extremity. If the patient is awake, assess equality of strength of extremities.
            (i) Use the hand grip (have the patient squeeze your fingers).
            (ii) Have the patient gently push feet against your hands.
         (b) Assess sensation of each extremity.
            (i) If the patient is awake, ask if he or she can feel you touch his or her fingers and toes. Ask, "Can you feel me touching your

finger/toe? Which hand/foot and finger/toe am I touching?"

(ii) If the patient is unresponsive, note if the patient responds when you pinch the fingers and toes.

c. Assess baseline vital signs.

d. Obtain a SAMPLE history.

> **Note:** The ability to walk, move the extremities, or feel sensation or a lack of pain to the spinal column does NOT rule out the possibility of spinal column or spinal cord damage.

---

(1) **Signs and symptoms.** Signs and symptoms of possible spine injury include (*Box 28-2*):

    (a) Tenderness in the area of injury

    (b) Pain associated with moving

      (i) Do not ask the patient to move to try to elicit a pain response.

      (ii) Do not move the patient to test for a pain response.

    (c) Pain independent of movement or palpation along the spinal column or lower legs (may be intermittent)

    (d) Obvious deformity of the spine on palpation

    (e) Soft tissue injuries associated with trauma

      (i) Injuries to the head and neck suggest injury to the cervical spine.

      (ii) Shoulder, back, or abdominal injury may indicate trauma to the thoracic or lumbar spine.

      (iii) Injury to the lower extremities may indicate trauma to the lumbar or sacral spine.

    (f) Numbness, weakness, or tingling in the extremities

    (g) Loss of sensation or paralysis below the suspected level of injury

    (h) Loss of sensation or paralysis in the upper or lower extremities

    (i) Incontinence

(2) **Allergies.** Determine if the patient has any allergies to medications or other substances and materials.

(3) **Medications.** Determine if the patient is taking any medications (prescription and over-the-counter).

    (a) Determine if the patient takes his or her medications regularly and his or her response to them.

    (b) Determine if there has been any recent change in medications (additions, deletions, or change in dosages).

    (c) Provide all information obtained to the receiving facility.

Box 28-2. **Signs and Symptoms of Possible Spinal Injury**

- Tenderness in the area of injury
- Pain independent of movement or palpation along the spinal column or lower legs (may be intermittent)
- Obvious deformity of the spine on palpation
- Soft tissue injuries associated with trauma
- Numbness, weakness, or tingling in the extremities
- Loss of sensation or paralysis below the suspected level of injury
- Loss of sensation or paralysis in the upper or lower extremities
- Incontinence

(4) **Pertinent past medical history.** Ascertain whether the patient has any of the following conditions:
   (a) Diabetes
   (b) Seizures
   (c) Stroke
(5) **Last oral intake.** Determine the patient's last oral intake.
(6) **Events.** Determine the events leading to the present situation by asking:
   (a) What happened?
   (b) When did the injury occur?
   (c) Where does it hurt?
   (d) Does your neck or back hurt?
   (e) Were you wearing a seat belt?
   (f) Did you pass out before the accident?
   (g) Did you move or did someone move you before we arrived?
   (h) Have your symptoms changed from the time of the injury until the time we arrived?

COMPLICATIONS OF SPINE INJURY

Complications of spinal injury include:
1. Paralysis
2. Inadequate breathing effort
   a. Injuries to the cervical and thoracic spine may affect the patient's ability to breathe.
   b. An injury involving the lower cervical or upper thoracic portion of the spinal cord may result in paralysis of the intercostal muscles.
      (1) An injury around the 4th cervical vertebra usually results in paralysis of the diaphragm.
      (2) If the diaphragm is paralyzed, you will observe abdominal breathing that is usually shallow.
      (3) These patients require assisted ventilation with 100% oxygen.
3. Inadequate circulation
   a. Disruption of the nervous system can cause widespread dilation of the blood vessels.
   b. Normally, the body responds to widespread dilation of the blood vessels by increasing the heart rate, constricting the blood vessels, and increasing the strength of the heart's contractions.
   c. In the patient with a spinal injury:
      (1) Blood pools in the dilated blood vessels resulting in normal skin color and temperature
      (2) Heart rate is within normal range or slow despite a low blood pressure

EMERGENCY MEDICAL CARE FOR SUSPECTED SPINAL INJURY

1. Take body substance isolation (BSI) precautions.
2. Establish and maintain in-line immobilization.
   a. Place the head in a neutral in-line position unless the patient complains of pain or the head is not easily moved into position.
   b. Place the head in alignment with the spine.
   c. Maintain constant manual in-line immobilization until the patient is properly secured to a backboard with the head immobilized.
3. Establish and maintain an open airway.
   a. Whenever possible, airway control must be done with in-line immobilization.
   b. Insert an oropharyngeal airway (OPA) or nasopharyngeal airway (NPA) as needed.
   c. Suction as necessary.
4. Administer oxygen.

    a. If the patient's breathing is adequate, apply oxygen by nonrebreather mask at 15 liters per minute (LPM) if not already done.

    b. If the patient's breathing is inadequate, provide positive-pressure ventilation with 100% oxygen.

        (1) Whenever possible, artificial ventilation must be done with in-line immobilization.

        (2) Assess the adequacy of the ventilations delivered.

5. Assess pulse, motor, and sensation in all extremities.

6. Assess the cervical region and neck before applying a rigid, cervical immobilization device.

    a. Properly size the cervical immobilization device (an improperly fitted immobilization device will do more harm than good).

    b. If it does not fit, use a rolled towel or blanket.

        (1) Tape the towel/blanket roll to the board.

        (2) Maintain manual in-line stabilization.

7. Immobilize the patient to a long backboard.

8. Reassess pulses, motor function, and sensation in all extremities and record.

9. Transport promptly.

    a. If the patient is stable, perform ongoing assessments every 15 minutes.

    b. If the patient is unstable, perform ongoing assessments every 5 minutes.

FOUR-PERSON LOG ROLL

1. Take appropriate BSI precautions.

2. Rescuer # 1 kneels at the patient's head, maintaining manual in-line immobilization of the head and spine and directing the movement of the patient.

3. A rigid cervical immobilization device is applied (if not already done).

4. The patient is positioned with legs extended and arms (palms inward) extended at his or her sides (if the arms are uninjured).

5. Rescuer # 2 positions a long backboard at one side of the patient.

6. Rescuers # 2, # 3, and # 4 control the movement of the rest of the patient's body.

    a. Rescuer # 2 supports the shoulders, rescuer # 3 supports the hips, and rescuer # 4 supports the lower extremities.

    b. If only two additional rescuers are available, rescuer # 2 is positioned at the midchest and rescuer # 3 is positioned at the hips to support the hips and lower extremities.

7. When everyone is ready, rescuer # 1 gives the order to roll the patient.

    a. Rescuer # 1 maintains the head and neck in a neutral position.

    b. Rescuers # 2, # 3, and # 4 roll the patient on his or her side toward them.

    c. The patient's head, shoulders, and pelvis are kept in-line during the roll.

8. The patient's posterior body is quickly assessed, if not already done.

9. The long backboard is positioned under the patient.

10. When everyone is ready, rescuer # 1 gives the order to roll the patient onto the backboard.

    a. If the backboard was angled, the patient and backboard are lowered to the ground together.

    b. Do not rotate the patient's head, shoulders, or pelvis when moving the patient onto the backboard.

11. If necessary, the patient's position is adjusted so that he or she is centered on the board.

    a. Do not move the patient from side to side to adjust his or her position.

    b. Slide the patient lengthwise to maintain alignment of the spine.

IMMOBILIZING A SUPINE PATIENT ON A LONG BACKBOARD

1. Take appropriate BSI precautions.

2. Position the long backboard at the patient's side.

3. Move the patient onto the backboard by log rolling.
   a. One EMT-Basic must maintain manual in-line immobilization of the head and spine.
   b. The EMT-Basic at the head directs the movement of the patient.
   c. One to three other EMT-Basics control the movement of the rest of the body.
   d. Quickly assess the patient's posterior body, if not already done.
4. Position the long backboard under the patient during the log roll.
   a. Place the patient onto the backboard at the command of the EMT-Basic at the head.
   b. Use a slide, proper lift, log roll, or scoop stretcher to keep movement to a minimum.
   c. Which method to use must be decided based upon the situation, scene, and available resources.
5. Pad voids (spaces) between the patient and the board as necessary.
   a. For an adult, pad under the head and torso, being careful to avoid extra movement.
   b. For an infant or child, pad under the shoulders to the toes to maintain a neutral position.
6. Immobilize the patient's torso to the board.
   a. Immobilize the upper torso to the board with one strap over the chest or, preferably, two straps in an "X" fashion.
   b. Immobilize the lower torso (pelvis) to the board with one strap centered over the iliac crests or a pair of groin loops.
7. Evaluate and pad under the patient's head as necessary.
8. Immobilize the patient's head to the board with a head immobilizer or blanket rolls.
   a. Place a strap or tape snugly across the lower forehead.
   b. Place another strap or tape snugly across the anterior portion of the cervical collar.
9. Secure the patient's legs to the board.
   a. Secure the upper legs with a strap across the legs above the knees.
   b. Secure the lower legs with a strap across the legs below the knees.
10. Secure the patient's arms to the board (arms extended, palms in toward the patient's side).
12. Reassess security of the straps.
13. Reassess pulses, motor function, and sensation in all extremities and record.

IMMOBILIZING A SEATED PATIENT WITH A VEST-TYPE EXTRICATION DEVICE

1. If the patient is found in a sitting position, immobilize with a vest-type immobilization device, transfer the patient to and then immobilize the patient on a long backboard.
2. Take BSI precautions.
3. Maintain manual in-line immobilization of the head and spine.
4. Apply a cervical collar.
5. Assess pulses, motor function, and sensation in all extremities.
6. Position the patient.
   a. While supporting the spine, move the patient forward on the seat until there is adequate space between the patient's back and the seat to allow the device to be inserted.
   b. If the patient is slumped forward:
      (1) Rescuer # 1 maintains in-line stabilization of the head and spine.
      (2) Rescuer # 2 supports the patient's midchest.
      (3) At the direction of the rescuer at the head, together both rescuers move the patient's upper body until he or she is sitting upright.
7. Position the device behind the patient.
   a. Slide the flat side of the device behind the patient's back and the seat back.

b. Center the device on the patient's back and raise it until the side flaps are snugly up in each armpit.

8. Secure the device to the patient's torso.
   a. Fasten all straps (top, middle, and lower) across the patient's torso.
   b. Tighten the middle and lower torso straps until they are snug.
   c. Do not tighten the top strap at this time.
   d. Fasten and tighten both leg straps.
   (1) Loop each leg strap around the leg on the same side and back to the buckle on the same side.
   (2) Fasten snugly.
9. Check all torso straps to be sure they are secure and adjust as necessary without excessive movement of the patient.
10. Evaluate and pad behind the patient's head as necessary to maintain neutral in-line immobilization.
11. Secure the patient's head to the device.
    a. Bring the head flaps around to the side of the head.
    b. Secure the forehead strap.
    c. Secure the lower head strap over the cervical collar.
    d. Fasten the ends of the straps to the Velcro on the head flaps snugly, but not too tightly.
    e. Ensure that the position of the straps does not prevent the mouth from being opened.
12. Tighten the top torso strap.
13. Insert a long backboard under the patient's buttocks and rotate and lower him or her onto it.
14. Secure the vest-type device to the long backboard and loosen the top torso strap to allow adequate chest rise.
15. Secure the upper legs to the board with a strap placed above the knees.
16. Secure the lower legs to the board with a strap placed below the knees.
17. Secure the arms to the board (arms extended, palms in toward the patient's side).
18. Reassess pulses, motor function, and sensation in all extremities and record.

IMMOBILIZING A STANDING PATIENT

1. Take appropriate BSI precautions.
2. Provide manual in-line immobilization.
3. Apply a cervical collar.
4. Position the long backboard behind patient.
5. One rescuer is positioned on each side of the patient with one additional rescuer at the foot facing the patient.
6. The rescuers on either side of the patient reach with the hand closest to the patient under the arm to grasp the board, and use the hand farthest from the patient to secure the head.
7. Once the position is assured, place the leg closest to the board behind the board and begin slowly tipping the board backward.
8. The rescuer at the foot of the board secures the board and the patient to prevent them from sliding.
9. The board is then lowered to the ground.
10. Once the board is on the ground, one rescuer maintains manual in-line stabilization while the patient is assessed by the other rescuers.

INJURIES TO THE BRAIN AND SKULL

INJURIES TO THE SCALP

1. Scalp wounds may occur because of blunt or penetrating trauma.

2. They may or may not be associated with brain injury.
3. The scalp has a rich supply of blood vessels.
   a. When injured, the scalp may bleed heavily.
   b. The amount of blood loss from a scalp wound may be enough to produce shock in children.
   c. In adults, shock is usually not due to a scalp wound but rather to an injury elsewhere.
4. Assess the scalp carefully for lacerations (cuts) because some are not easy to detect.
5. Control bleeding with direct pressure; however, do not apply pressure to an open or depressed skull injury.

SKULL INJURIES

1. Skull injuries may occur from blunt or penetrating trauma.
2. Open injury: scalp is not intact and risk of infection is increased.
3. Closed injury: scalp is unbroken (intact).
4. Types of skull injuries include:
   a. Linear: line crack in the skull
   b. Depressed: pieces of bone are pushed inward pressing on and sometimes causing tearing of brain tissue
   c. Basilar: fractures of the base of the skull
   d. Comminuted: multiple cracks radiate from the center of impact
   e. Penetrating: foreign object penetrates the skull or brain
5. Signs and symptoms of skull injury include (*Figure 28-4*):

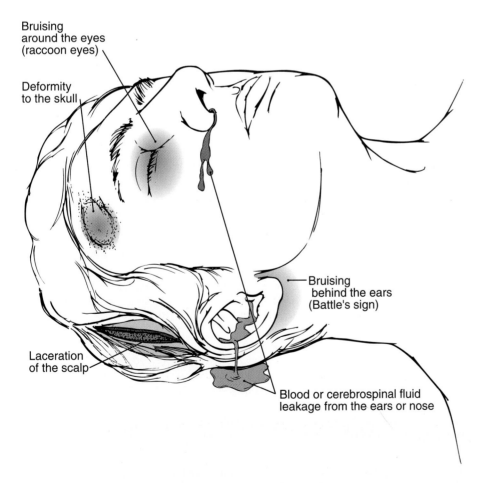

Bruising around the eyes (raccoon eyes)

Deformity to the skull

Bruising behind the ears (Battle's sign)

Laceration of the scalp

Blood or cerebrospinal fluid leakage from the ears or nose

Fig. 28-4. Signs and symptoms of skull injury.

    a. Mechanism of injury (trauma)
    b. Contusions, lacerations, hematomas to the scalp
    c. Deformity to the skull
    d. Blood or fluid (cerebrospinal fluid) leakage from the ears or nose
    e. Bruising around the eyes (raccoon eyes)
    f. Bruising behind the ears (mastoid process) [Battle's sign]

BRAIN INJURIES

1. A brain injury or bleeding into the skull will cause an increase in the pressure within the skull.
2. **Nontraumatic injuries**
   a. Nontraumatic injuries may occur due to clots or hemorrhaging.
   b. They can be a cause of altered mental status.
   c. Their signs and symptoms are similar to those of traumatic injuries.
3. **Traumatic injuries**
   a. Types of traumatic brain injuries include:
       (1) Concussion: temporary loss of function in some or all of the brain
       (2) Contusion: bruising of the brain; bleeding and swelling of brain tissue
       (3) Cerebral hematoma: bleeding within the brain
   b. Consider mechanism of injury, such as:
       (1) Deformity of windshield
       (2) Deformity of helmet

OPEN HEAD INJURY

1. Consider mechanism of injury, such as:
   a. Deformity of windshield
   b. Deformity of helmet
2. Signs and symptoms of open head injury include:
   a. Contusions, lacerations, hematomas to the scalp
   b. Deformity to the skull
   c. Penetrating injury (do not remove impaled objects in the skull)
   d. Soft area or depression upon palpation
   e. Exposed brain tissue
   f. Bleeding from the open bone injury
   g. Blood or fluid (cerebrospinal fluid) leakage from the ears and nose
   h. Bruising around the eyes
   i. Bruising behind the ears (mastoid process) [Battle's sign]
   j. Nausea and/or vomiting
   k. Possible signs and symptoms of a closed head injury, if brain injury has occurred

SCENE SIZE-UP

1. Determine the mechanism of injury from the patient, family member, or bystanders and inspection of the scene.
2. Determine if it is safe to approach the patient.

INITIAL ASSESSMENT

1. If the mechanism of injury suggests the possibility of spinal injury, maintain in-line spinal immobilization until the patient is secured to a long backboard.
2. Assess the patient's mental status.
3. Assess the patient's airway (jaw-thrust maneuver).
4. Assess breathing.
5. Assess circulation.
6. Identify any life-threatening conditions and provide care based on these findings.
7. Establish patient priorities. Priority patients are those:

    a. Who give a poor general impression

    b. With severe pain anywhere

    c. With uncontrolled bleeding

    d. Experiencing difficulty breathing

    e. With signs and symptoms of shock

    f. Are unresponsive with no gag reflex or cough

    g. Are responsive and are unable to follow commands

8. ALS assistance should be requested as soon as possible.

9. If ALS personnel are not available, the patient should be transported promptly to the closest appropriate facility.

FOCUSED HISTORY AND PHYSICAL EXAMINATION

1. If no significant mechanism of injury exists (e.g., cut finger):

    a. Perform a focused physical examination based on:

        (1) Patient's chief complaint

        (2) Mechanism of injury

        (3) Initial (rapid) assessment findings

    b. Assess baseline vital signs

    c. Obtain SAMPLE history

2. If a significant mechanism of injury exists:

    a. Continue in-line spinal stabilization

    b. Consider ALS request

    c. Reconsider transport decision

    d. Reassess mental status

    e. Perform rapid trauma assessment to determine life-threatening injuries

    f. In the responsive patient, symptoms should be sought before and during the trauma assessment

    g. Assess baseline vital signs

    h. Obtain SAMPLE history

3. **Assessment of the patient with a possible head injury**

    a. If awake, instruct the patient not to move during the examination.

    b. Inspect and palpate the head, neck, chest, abdomen, pelvis, extremities, and posterior body for:

        (1) Deformities

        (2) Contusions (bruises)

        (3) Abrasions (scrapes)

        (4) Penetrations

        (5) Burns

        (6) Tenderness

        (7) Lacerations (cuts)

        (8) Swelling

        (9) Instability

        (10) Crepitation (grating)

        (11) Distal pulses, motor function, and sensation

    c. Assess baseline vital signs.

    d. Obtain a SAMPLE history.

        (1) **Signs and symptoms.** Signs and symptoms of traumatic head injury include *(Figure 28-5):*

            (a) Altered or decreasing mental status

                (i) Confusion, disorientation, or repetitive questioning

                (ii) Conscious to deteriorating mental status

                (iii) Unresponsive

            (b) Irregular breathing pattern

            (c) Contusions, lacerations, hematomas to the scalp

            (d) Deformity to the skull

            (e) Blood or fluid (CSF) leakage from the ears and nose

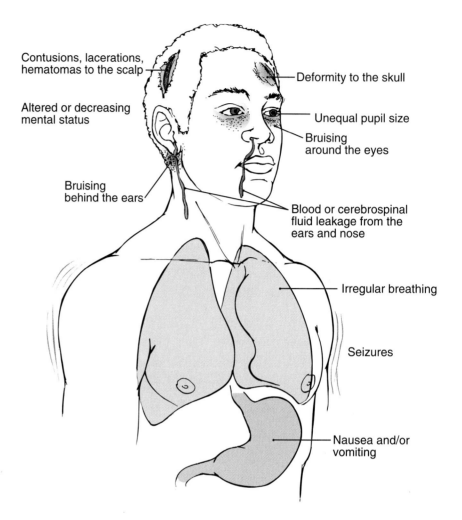

Contusions, lacerations, hematomas to the scalp

Deformity to the skull

Altered or decreasing mental status

Unequal pupil size

Bruising around the eyes

Bruising behind the ears

Blood or cerebrospinal fluid leakage from the ears and nose

Irregular breathing

Seizures

Nausea and/or vomiting

Fig. 28-5. Signs and symptoms of traumatic head injury.

    (f)   Bruising around the eyes
    (g)   Bruising behind the ears
    (h)   Nausea and/or vomiting
    (i)   Unequal pupil size with altered mental status
    (j)   Possible seizure activity

(2) **<u>A</u>llergies.** Determine if the patient has any allergies to medications or other substances and materials.

(3) **<u>M</u>edications.** Determine if the patient is taking any medications (prescription and over-the-counter).
    (a)   Determine if the patient takes his or her medications regularly and his or her response to them.
    (b)   Determine if there has been any recent change in medications (additions, deletions, or change in dosages).
    (c)   Provide all information obtained to the receiving facility.

(4) **<u>P</u>ertinent <u>p</u>ast medical history.** Ascertain whether the patient has any of the following conditions:
    (a)   Diabetes
    (b)   Seizures
    (c)   Stroke

(5) **<u>L</u>ast oral intake.** Determine the patient's last oral intake.

(6) **<u>E</u>vents.** Determine the events leading to the present situation by asking:
    (a)   What happened?

(b) When did the injury occur?
(c) Where does it hurt?
(d) Does your neck or back hurt?
(e) Were you wearing a seat belt?
(f) Did you pass out before the accident?
(g) Did you move or did someone move you before we arrived?
(h) Have your symptoms changed from the time of the injury until the time we arrived?

EMERGENCY MEDICAL CARE FOR A HEAD INJURY

1. Take BSI precautions.
2. Establish and maintain in-line immobilization.
   a. Place the head in a neutral in-line position unless the patient complains of pain or the head is not easily moved into position.
   b. Maintain constant manual in-line immobilization until the patient is properly secured to a backboard with the head immobilized.
3. Establish and maintain an open airway.
   a. Whenever possible, airway control must be done with in-line immobilization.
   b. Insert an OPA or NPA as needed.
   c. Suction as necessary.
4. Administer oxygen.
   a. If the patient's breathing is adequate, apply oxygen by nonrebreather mask at 15 LPM if not already done.
   b. If the patient's breathing is inadequate, provide positive-pressure ventilation with 100% oxygen.
      (1) Whenever possible, artificial ventilation must be done with in-line immobilization.
      (2) Assess the adequacy of the ventilations delivered.
5. Closely monitor the airway, breathing, pulse, and mental status for deterioration.
6. Control bleeding.
   a. Do not apply pressure to an open or depressed skull injury.
   b. Dress and bandage an open wound as indicated in the treatment of soft tissue injuries.
   c. Do not attempt to stop the flow of blood or CSF from the ears or nose. Cover the area with a loose sterile dressing to absorb drainage.
   d. Do not remove penetrating objects; rather, stabilize in place with bulky dressings.
7. Assess pulse, motor function, and sensation in all extremities.
8. With any head injury, the EMT-Basic must suspect spinal injury.
   a. Immobilize the spine.
   b. Assess the cervical region and neck before applying a rigid, cervical immobilization device.
9. If a medical condition or nontraumatic injury exists, place the patient on the left side.
10. Be prepared for changes in patient condition (e.g., seizures).
11. Transport promptly.
    a. If the patient is stable, perform ongoing assessments every 15 minutes.
    b. If the patient is unstable, perform ongoing assessments every 5 minutes.

IMMOBILIZATION

CERVICAL SPINE IMMOBILIZATION DEVICES (CERVICAL COLLARS)

1. Indications include:
   a. Any suspected injury to the spine based on mechanism of injury, history or signs and symptoms

b. Use with short and long backboards

2. **Sizing**
    a. Various types of rigid cervical immobilization devices exist; therefore, sizing is based on the specific design of the device.
    b. An improperly sized immobilization device has a potential for further injury.
    c. Do not obstruct the airway with the placement of a cervical immobilization device.
    d. If it does not fit, use a rolled towel, tape to the board, and manually support the head.
    e. An improperly fitted device will do more harm than good.

3. **Precautions**
    a. Cervical immobilization devices alone do not provide adequate in-line immobilization.
    b. Manual immobilization must always be used with a cervical immobilization device until the head is secured to a board.

SHORT BACKBOARDS

1. Several different types of short board immobilization devices exist, including:
    a. Vest-type devices
    b. Rigid short board
2. Short backboards provide stabilization and immobilization to the head, neck, and torso.
3. They are used to immobilize noncritical sitting patients with suspected spinal injuries.
4. **General application**
    a. Provide manual in-line immobilization.
    b. Assess pulses, motor function, and sensation in all extremities.
    c. Assess the cervical area.
    d. Apply a cervical immobilization device.
    e. Position the short board immobilization device behind the patient.
    f. Secure the device to the patient's torso.
    g. Evaluate torso and groin fixation and adjust as necessary without excessive movement of the patient.
    h. Evaluate and pad behind the patient's head as necessary to maintain neutral in-line immobilization.
    i. Secure the patient's head to the device.
    j. Release manual immobilization of head.
    k. Rotate or lift the patient to the long backboard.
    l. Immobilize the patient to the long backboard.
    m. Reassess pulses, motor function, and sensation in all extremities.

LONG BACKBOARDS (FULL-BODY SPINAL IMMOBILIZATION DEVICES)

1. Several different types of long board immobilization devices exist.
2. Long backboards provides stabilization and immobilization to the head, neck and torso, pelvis, and extremities.
3. They are used to immobilize patients found in a lying, standing, or sitting position.
4. They are sometimes used with short backboards.
5. **General application**
    a. Provide manual in-line immobilization.
    b. Assess pulses, motor function, and sensation in all extremities.
    c. Assess the cervical area.
    d. Apply a cervical immobilization device.
    e. Position the device.
    f. Move the patient onto the device by log roll, suitable lift or slide, or scoop stretcher.

g. Pad voids between the patient and the board.
   (1) For adults, pad under the head and under the torso as needed.
   (2) For infants and children, pad under the shoulders to the toes to establish a neutral position.
h. Immobilize the torso to the board by applying straps across the chest and pelvis and adjust as needed.
i. Immobilize the patient's head to the board.
j. Secure the legs with straps above and below the knees.
k. Reassess pulses, motor function, and sensation and record.

SPECIAL CONSIDERATIONS

INDICATIONS FOR RAPID EXTRICATION

1. The scene is unsafe.
2. Unstable patient condition warrants immediate movement and transport.
3. Patient blocks the EMT-Basic's access to another, more seriously injured, patient.
4. Rapid extrication is based on time and the patient, not the EMT-Basic's preference.

HELMET REMOVAL

1. Special assessment needs for patients wearing helmets include:
   a. Airway and breathing
   b. Fit of the helmet and patient's movement within the helmet
   c. Ability to gain access to airway and breathing
2. Indications for leaving the helmet in place include:
   a. Good fit with little or no movement of the patient's head within the helmet
   b. No impending airway or breathing problems
   c. Removal would cause further injury to the patient
   d. Proper spinal immobilization could be performed with the helmet in place
   e. No interference with the EMT-Basic's ability to assess and reassess airway and breathing
3. Indications for removing the helmet include:
   a. Inability to assess and/or reassess airway and breathing
   b. Restriction of adequate management of the airway or breathing
   c. Improperly fitted helmet allowing for excessive patient head movement within the helmet
   d. Proper spinal immobilization cannot be performed due to the helmet
   e. Cardiac arrest
4. Types of helmets
   a. Sports helmets are typically open anteriorly and provide easier access to the airway.
   b. Motorcycle helmets include full-face and shield helmets.
5. General rules for removal of a helmet
   a. The technique for removal of a helmet depends on the type of helmet worn by the patient.
   b. Take BSI precautions.
   c. Remove the patient's eyeglasses, if present, before removal of the helmet.
   d. EMT-Basic **# 1** stabilizes the helmet by placing his or her hands on each side of the helmet with the fingers on the mandible to prevent movement.
   e. EMT-Basic **# 2** loosens the helmet strap.
   f. EMT-Basic **# 2** places one hand on the lower jaw at the angle of the jaw and the other hand behind the head at the occipital region.
   g. EMT-Basic **# 1** pulls the sides of the helmet apart and gently slips the helmet halfway off the patient's head and then stops.

h. EMT-Basic **#** 2 slides the hand supporting the occipital region toward the top of the patient's head to prevent the head from falling back after complete helmet removal.

i. EMT-Basic **#** 1 removes the helmet completely and proceeds with spinal immobilization.

INFANTS AND CHILDREN

1. Immobilize the infant or child on a rigid board appropriate for size (short, long, or padded splint).

2. Pad from the shoulders to the heels of the infant or child, if necessary, to maintain neutral immobilization.

3. Properly size the cervical immobilization device.

a. If it does not fit, use a rolled towel, tape to the board, and manually support head.

b. An improperly fitted immobilization device will do more harm than good.

REVIEW QUESTIONS

Directions: Each of the numbered items or incomplete statements in this section is followed by answers or by completions of the statement. Select the ONE lettered answer or completion that is BEST in each case.

1. Your rescue crew has been called to a motor vehicle collision. Upon arrival at the scene, you observe that a passenger van has rear-ended a four-door sedan. Your patient is a 47-year-old woman complaining of neck pain. Based on this mechanism of injury, when can you rule out the possibility of spinal column or cord damage?

(A) During the initial assessment
(B) If the patient is able to walk without difficulty
(C) During the focused history and physical examination
(D) Only after examination by the receiving medical facility

2. For adults, a fall from 20 feet or more is considered significant, while for a child, a fall from 10 feet or more is considered significant. Regardless of age, another indicator of a significant fall is

(A) a fall from twice the body's height
(B) a fall from three times the body's height
(C) a fall from four times the body's height.
(D) a fall from five times the body's height

3. The correct technique for opening the airway of an unconscious patient with a suspected spinal injury is

(A) the head-tilt, chin-lift maneuver
(B) the modified neck lift
(C) the neck-thrust, jaw-lift maneuver
(D) jaw-thrust maneuver

4. Which of the following is a life-threatening complication associated with spinal cord injuries around the 4th cervical vertebra?

   (A) Sudden cardiac arrest
   (B) Paralysis of the diaphragm
   (C) Inability to move the lower extremities (legs)
   (D) Inability to move the upper extremities (arms)

5. There are several types of short backboards used to assist in maintaining spinal immobilization. The most common types are the rigid short backboard and vest-type devices such as the Kendrick Extrication Device (KED). Which of the following patients would be a candidate for the application of such a device?

   (A) A motor vehicle collision patient who is found in the back seat of a passenger van and who is not breathing
   (B) A motorcycle rider who has been "T-boned" at an intersection and found unconscious in the street lying on his back
   (C) A motor vehicle collision patient complaining of neck pain who is found sitting in her vehicle in a low level of distress
   (D) A victim of assault who is found standing in the doorway of her apartment complaining of neck pain after being hit in the head with a lamp

6. Your rescue crew is called to the scene of an assault. Your patient is a 34-year-old man found unconscious in a parking lot. Bystanders state that the patient was hit with a bat several times. While performing a rapid trauma assessment, you note that blood is leaking out of both ears. Appropriate management of this finding would be

   (A) pack the ears with a gauze dressing
   (B) pack the ears with sterile cotton balls
   (C) cover the ears with an occlusive dressing
   (D) loosely cover the external ear canal with an absorbent dressing

7. Which of the following is true regarding the sizing of cervical collars?

   (A) It is better to have a collar too big than one too small
   (B) It is better to have a collar too small than one too big
   (C) An improperly sized cervical collar may do more harm than good
   (D) If you do not have the correct size, do not attempt to immobilize the cervical spine

8. Your ambulance crew is called to the scene of a motor vehicle collision near a railroad track. You arrive to find one vehicle positioned on the tracks, and a train is approaching and less than 2 minutes from the scene. Your patient is unconscious and may have severe spinal compromise. This is an indication for

   (A) positioning the ambulance between the train and the victim's car
   (B) rapid extrication possibly without the use of any immobilization device
   (C) use of a cervical collar and long backboard for extrication and immobilization
   (D) use of a cervical collar and short backboard for extrication and immobilization

Directions: Each of the numbered items or incomplete statements in this section is negatively phrased, as indicated by a capitalized word such as NOT, LEAST, or EXCEPT. Select the ONE lettered answer or completion that is BEST in each case.

9. Your ambulance is called to the scene of a vehicle-versus-bicycle collision. Your patient is a 23-year-old man complaining of upper back pain. Which of the following is NOT consistent with spinal cord compromise?

(A) Loss of bowel or bladder control
(B) Deformity at the spinal column in the area of pain
(C) Numbness, weakness, and tingling in the extremities
(D) Loss of movement and sensation above the level of the injury

Directions: Each of the numbered questions or incomplete statements in this section refers to a scenario that precedes them. The numbered questions or incomplete statements are followed by answers or by completions of the statement. Select the answer or completion of the statement that is BEST in each case.

Your rescue crew is called to the scene of a motor vehicle collision. Your patient is a 17-year-old girl complaining of neck pain and tingling in the feet and hands. She was not wearing her seat belt when her vehicle was rear-ended by another vehicle traveling about 35 miles per hour. There was no loss of consciousness, and the patient answers all questions completely and appropriately. She is out of the vehicle lying on the grass by the side of the road as you arrive on the scene. There is only one other patient, and he is being treated by another crew.

Questions 10–13

10. Which of the following should you do first?

(A) Immobilize the patient to a long backboard
(B) Manually immobilize the patient's head and neck
(C) Take appropriate body substance isolation (BSI) precautions
(D) Inspect the airway to ensure that it is patent (clear and open)

11. When log rolling this patient to put her on a long backboard, who is in charge of calling the commands for moving the patient?

(A) The patient
(B) The EMT-Basic maintaining in-line stabilization of the head and neck
(C) The EMT-Basic positioned at the patient's lower extremities
(D) The EMT-Basic positioned at the patient's chest and abdomen

12. In what order should the patient be secured to the backboard?

(A) From head to toe
(B) From toe to head
(C) Trunk (chest and abdomen), head, then extremities
(D) Trunk (chest and abdomen), extremities, then head

13. Which is the LAST step in securing this patient to a long backboard?

(A) Apply a cervical collar
(B) Secure the patient's arms to the backboard
(C) Secure the patient's head to the backboard
(D) Reassess pulses, motor function, and sensation in all extremities

Your ambulance crew is called to the scene of a motor vehicle collision in the parking lot of a local mall. You arrive to find your patient, a 57-year-old man, sitting behind the steering wheel with his seat belt still in place. He tells you that another vehicle hit his car head on at less than 10 miles per hour. The other vehicle has fled the scene. The patient is complaining of severe lower back pain. After evaluation, you decide to use a vest-type extrication device.

Questions 14–15

14. Which of the following should you do first?

    (A) Apply a cervical collar
    (B) Position the device behind the patient
    (C) Maintain manual in-line immobilization of the head and spine
    (D) Assess pulses, motor function, and sensation in the upper and lower extremities

15. There are three different body regions that this device attaches to: the head, the chest, and the legs/groin. In which order should the straps be secured?

    (A) Head, chest, legs/groin
    (B) Head, legs/groin, chest
    (C) Chest, legs/groin, head
    (D) Legs/groin, chest, head

Your ambulance is called to a local park for an unconscious patient with an unknown medical problem. You arrive to find an unconscious male patient lying on his side. It appears that he has been involved in a fight, and a small amount of blood is leaking from his ears.

Questions 16–18

16. Which of the following signs would be consistent with a skull injury?

    (A) The patient has two black eyes
    (B) The patient's breath has a fruity odor
    (C) The patient's abdomen is firm on palpation
    (D) The patient's trachea is deviated to the right

17. Your entire crew has taken appropriate body substance isolation (BSI) precautions. Which of the following should be performed first?

    (A) Immobilize the patient's head and neck with a cervical collar
    (B) Open the patient's airway with the head-tilt, chin-lift maneuver
    (C) Open the patient's airway with a jaw thrust
    (D) Immobilize the patient's head and spine by applying a long backboard

18. While transporting this patient to the hospital, his breathing status changes. While reassessing this patient, you observe that his respiratory effort is erratic and gasping with a rate of 6 breaths per minute. You have already begun oxygen therapy with a nonrebreather mask at 12 liters per minute (LPM) of supplemental oxygen. Appropriate management would include

    (A) begin cardiopulmonary resuscitation (CPR)
    (B) assist ventilations with a bag-valve mask without supplemental oxygen
    (C) increase the liter flow on the nonrebreather mask to 15 to 20 LPM
    (D) assist ventilations with bag-valve mask connected to supplemental oxygen

Your rescue crew is called to the scene of a "motorcycle down." You arrive to find one patient in the middle of the street lying on his back. Bystanders inform you that a vehicle bumped the patient's motorcycle, then fled the scene. The speed limit in the area is 45 mph.

Questions 19–20

19. After taking the appropriate body substance isolation (BSI) measures, you assess your patient's mental status and find him to be unconscious. Which of the following would be an indication that his helmet must be removed?

(A) Helmets are always removed
(B) The helmet must be removed if it does not have a face shield
(C) The helmet must always be removed if you are going to immobilize the spine
(D) The helmet must be removed if it interferes with your ability to assess the airway

20. It takes a minimum of two EMT-Basics to remove a helmet properly. Which of the following statements regarding helmet removal is correct?

(A) The helmet should be cut away with trauma scissors
(B) The patient's head should be turned to the side to facilitate removal of the helmet
(C) The helmet should be removed in one swift motion as soon as the chin strap is released
(D) The patient's head should be supported so that it does not drop to the backboard when the helmet is removed

ANSWERS AND RATIONALES

1-D. EMT-Basics should not "clear" the spine of any patient complaining of neck or back pain. This is true regardless of the position the patient is found in (standing, sitting, walking, etc.). If the patient is complaining of traumatic neck pain, you should immediately begin manual in-line immobilization until full spinal immobilization is in place.

2-B. Regardless of the patient's size, a fall from three times his or her body height is considered significant. However, falls from less than three times the patient's body height can also be significant. Many factors come into play: the surface the patient fell on, the position at impact, the medical history of the patient, the patient's age, and the cause of the fall all must be evaluated and weighed.

3-D. The jaw thrust is the correct technique for opening the airway of a patient with a suspected spinal injury. Ideally, the jaw thrust is achieved by kneeling or lying at the patient's head. Your elbows should be firmly on the ground. Both of your thumbs should be placed on the patient's cheeks and your index and middle fingers positioned at the angle of the patient's jaw. You would then lift the jaw perpendicular to the patient's axis, being careful not to manipulate the spine. The head-tilt, chin-lift maneuver is the preferred technique for opening the airway of patients without possible spinal compromise.

4-B. The diaphragm is the primary muscle of breathing. The nerves that send impulses to the diaphragm exit the spine at about the 4th cervical vertebra. Damage to the spinal cord in or above this area may result in paralysis of the diaphragm and subsequent apnea (no breathing). A helpful jingle to remember when dealing with these patients is: "C-3-4-5 keep the diaphragm alive." C-3-4-5 refers to the 3rd, 4th, and 5th cervical vertebrae. Certainly an injury at the level of the 4th cervical vertebra may impact both the upper and lower extremities; however, paralysis of the arms and legs is not as life-threatening as is paralysis of the breathing muscles. Sudden cardiac arrest is not typically associated with isolated neck trauma, although if you do not monitor the patient's breathing status closely, respiratory and cardiac arrest may follow.

5-C. Short backboards are used to immobilize noncritical sitting patients with suspected spinal injuries. Since it may take up to 5 additional minutes to immobilize a patient if you are using a short backboard, these devices are not indicated for use on critically injured patients.

6-D. One of the signs of a skull injury is the leakage of blood or cerebrospinal fluid from the ears. If the leakage is halted (as with packing the ears), the pressure in the skull may increase. Think of the ears and the nose as "emergency bypass valves" that help release pressure from inside the skull.

7-C. If you are not able to properly size a patient with a cervical collar, it is better to use an improvised device rather than a cervical collar of the wrong size. Cervical collars that are too small do not provide the necessary support, and collars that are too big may manipulate the spine or complicate airway control. Improvisation may be accomplished by using towel rolls, blanket rolls, or rolled-up clothing.

8-B. This scene is immediately unsafe for the patient and the crew. You should attempt to perform rapid extrication of the patient. Remember that the safety of yourself and your crew comes before the safety of the patient. If adequate time does not exist to rapidly extricate the patient, do not stay in the hazard area! Other situations that dictate the need for rapid extrication are if the patient is acutely unstable or if a patient is in the way of accessing another more seriously injured patient.

9-D. Information travels from the brain down the spinal cord and to the body. It is not typical for patients with true spinal injuries to have neurological compromise above the level of the injury. This does not, however, rule out spinal compromise. Other signs and symptoms associated with spinal compromise/damage include: loss of bowel or bladder control; deformity at the spinal column in the area of pain; numbness, weakness, and tingling in the extremities; loss of movement and sensation below the level of the injury; and priapism (in males).

10-C. No member of your crew should come in contact with the patient without first addressing body substance isolation (BSI) precautions. Ideally, you should have addressed BSI prior to approaching the patient so that the initiation of treatment and stabilization is not delayed.

11-B. The rescuer positioned at the patient's head is in charge of directing the movement of the patient. This is true regardless of rank (provided the rescuer at the head understands his or her responsibility). Therefore, it is not ideal to put an inexperienced or untrained person at the patient's head. Moves should be coordinated and carefully choreographed efforts.

12-C. The trunk is secured first because it carries the bulk of the patient's weight. The head is next, followed by the extremities (legs first, then arms). If there are sufficient rescue personnel, all three regions are often secured simultaneously.

13-D. It is imperative that the patient's circulatory, sensory, and muscular/movement status be evaluated before and immediately after any splinting technique. By initially assessing, you may gather valuable information about the patient's condition due to the motor vehicle collision. Reassessing circulation, sensation, and movement after immobilization is complete allows you the opportunity to ensure that your treatment has not caused further harm to the patient. These assessments should be included in your documentation (e.g., "Motor and sensory functions and circulation in arms and legs intact before and after full spinal immobilization").

14-C. After taking body substance isolation (BSI) precautions, begin manual immobilization of the patient's head and spine. This is best achieved by positioning a rescuer behind the patient to hold the patient's head and neck with both hands. Then, motor function, sensation, and circulation should be evaluated in all four extremities. The neck should then be visualized and palpated for injury and a cervical collar put on. The patient is positioned and the device is then placed behind the patient for application.

15-C. The correct order for securing this device to the patient is the chest (generally there are three chest/abdomen straps), the legs/groin (one strap for each leg), then the head (one strap for the forehead and one for the chin). Make sure that any voids (spaces) are padded. The device should not be so tight that breathing or opening the mouth is impaired.

16-A. Bilateral black eyes, also known as raccoon's eyes, may be indicative of a skull fracture. Other findings associated with skull injuries include: contusions (bruises), lacerations (cuts), hematomas to the scalp, deformity to the skull, blood or fluid (cerebrospinal fluid) leaking from the ears or nose, and bruising behind the ears (also known as Battle's sign). A fruity odor on the patient's breath may be attributed to a diabetic emergency (hypoglycemia); a firm abdomen is generally indicative of trauma to the abdomen; and tracheal deviation is a late sign that a lung has collapsed.

17-C. Since this patient is unconscious and may have spinal cord damage, the patient's airway should be opened using a jaw thrust before application of a cervical collar or long backboard. Unlike the head-tilt, chin-lift maneuver, the jaw thrust allows the airway to be opened without manipulating the spinal cord.

18-D. It is not uncommon for patients with serious head or neck trauma to have respiratory compromise. This patient's respiratory rate and effort are terribly deficient. Ventilations should be assisted with a bag-valve mask connected to supplemental oxygen. Merely increasing the flow of oxygen through a nonrebreather mask is not likely to change this patient's condition. Cardiopulmonary resuscitation (CPR) should be initiated only if the patient is apneic and pulseless.

19-D. Indications for removal of a helmet include: inability to assess and/or reassess airway and breathing, restriction of adequate management of the airway or breathing, improperly fitted helmet allowing for excessive patient head movement within the helmet, proper spinal immobilization cannot be performed due to the helmet, and cardiac arrest. If the helmet does not interfere with airway, breathing, or immobilization and is well-fitted, it should be left in place and secured to the backboard.

20-D. Removing a helmet is a carefully coordinated effort between two knowledgeable rescuers. Strict attention must be paid to ensure that the spine is not manipulated. The head and spine should be maintained in a neutral in-line position throughout the procedure. The use of a cutting device should be avoided as it increases the length of time necessary to remove the helmet and the possibility of manipulating the spine.

BIBLIOGRAPHY

Butman AM, Martin SW, Vomacka RW, et al (eds): *Comprehensive Guide to Pre-Hospital Skills: A Skills Manual for EMT-Basic, EMT-Intermediate, EMT-Paramedic.* Akron, Ohio, Emergency Training, 1995.

Campbell JE (ed): *Basic Trauma Life Support for Paramedics and Advanced EMS Providers*, 3rd ed. Englewood Cliffs, NJ, Prentice-Hall, 1995.

Crosby LA, Lewallen DG (eds): *Emergency Care and Transportation of the Sick and Injured*, 6th ed. Rosemont, IL, American Academy of Orthopaedic Surgeons, 1995.

Grant HD, Murray RH Jr, Bergeron JD: *Emergency Care*, 7th ed. Englewood Cliffs, NJ, Prentice-Hall, 1995.

Hafen BQ, Karren KJ, Mistovich JJ: *Prehospital Emergency Care*, 5th ed. Upper Saddle River, NJ, Prentice-Hall, 1996.

Henry MC, Stapleton ER, Judd RL: *EMT: Prehospital Care*. Philadelphia, WB Saunders, 1992.

McSwain NE, White RD, Paturas JL, et al (eds): *The Basic EMT: Comprehensive Prehospital Patient Care*. St. Louis, Mosby-Year Book, 1996.

Sanders MJ: *Mosby's Paramedic Textbook*. St. Louis, Mosby-Year Book, 1994.

Sheehy SB, Lombardi, JE: *Manual of Emergency Care*, 4th ed. St. Louis, Mosby-Year Book, 1995.

Sloane E: *Anatomy and Physiology: An Easy Learner*. Boston, Jones and Bartlett, 1994.

Solomon EP and Phillips GA: *Understanding Human Anatomy and Physiology*. Philadelphia, WB Saunders, 1987.

Stoy WA: *Mosby's EMT-Basic Textbook*. St. Louis, Mosby-Year Book, 1996.

Thibodeau GA, Patton KT: *The Human Body in Health and Disease*. St. Louis, Mosby-Year Book, 1992.

Tortora GJ, Grabowski SR: *Principles of Anatomy and Physiology*, 7th ed. New York, Harper-Collins, 1993.

United States Department of Transportation, National Highway Traffic Safety Administration: *Emergency Medical Technician: Basic. National Standard Curriculum*, 1994.

OBJECTIVES

*29-1 List the contents of the chest cavity.

*29-2 List two classifications of chest injuries.

*29-3 State the signs and symptoms and describe the emergency medical care for:

    a. Rib fractures

    b. Flail chest

    c. Simple pneumothorax

    d. Tension pneumothorax

    e. Hemothorax

    f. Cardiac tamponade

    g. Traumatic asphyxia

    h. Pulmonary contusion

    i. Myocardial contusion

    j. Open pneumothorax

*29-4 List the contents of the abdominal cavity.

*29-5 State the signs and symptoms of a possible abdominal injury.

*29-6 Describe the emergency medical care for a patient with:

    a. Abdominal evisceration

    b. Impaled object in the abdomen

    c. Blunt abdominal injury

*29-7 List the components of the male external genitalia.

*29-8 List the components of the female external genitalia.

*29-9 Describe the emergency medical care for injuries to the external male genitalia.

*29-10 Describe the emergency medical care for injuries to the external female genitalia.

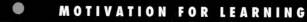

MOTIVATION FOR LEARNING

The information in this chapter is enrichment material provided to assist the EMT-Basic in learning the types of injuries that may result from trauma to the chest, abdomen, and genitalia.

ENRICHMENT—CHEST INJURIES

ANATOMY OF THE CHEST (THORACIC) CAVITY

1. The chest is the upper part of the trunk between the diaphragm and the neck.
2. It contains the **mediastinum** and pleural cavities.
   a. The mediastinum is the area between the lungs that extends from the sternum to the vertebral column.
   b. The mediastinum includes all of the contents of the chest cavity (except the lungs), including the esophagus, trachea, heart, and large blood vessels.
   c. The right lung is in the right pleural cavity; the left lung is in the left pleura cavity.
3. The chest is protected by the rib cage and the upper portion of the spine (*Figure 29-1*).
   a. The rib cage includes the ribs, thoracic vertebrae, and the sternum.
   b. The ribs are connected to the vertebrae in back.
   c. All but two of the ribs are connected by cartilage to the sternum in the front.
   d. The rib cage encloses the lungs and heart.
   e. Damage to the ribs can result in damage to these organs.

CATEGORIES OF CHEST INJURIES

1. **Closed chest injuries**
   a. In closed chest injuries, no break occurs in the skin over the chest wall.
   b. These injuries are usually the result of blunt trauma.
   c. Underlying structures (e.g., heart, lungs, great vessels) may sustain significant injury.
2. **Open chest injuries**
   a. In open chest injuries, a break occurs in the skin over the chest wall.
   b. These injuries result from penetrating trauma, such as:
      (1) Gunshot wounds
      (2) Stabbings
      (3) Impaled object

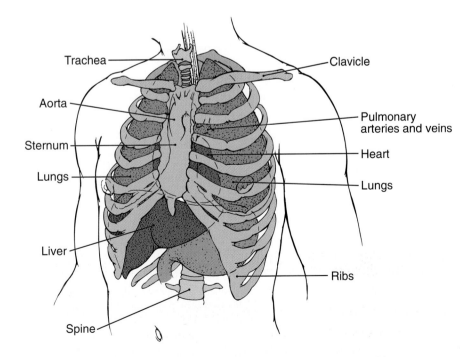

Fig. 29-1. Damage to the ribs can result in damage to the heart and lungs.

CLOSED CHEST INJURIES

1. Rib fractures
   a. A fracture is a break in the continuity of a bone.
   b. Rib fractures are the most frequent injury to the chest.
   c. The presence of rib fractures suggests significant force caused the injury.
   d. Pathophysiology
      (1) Rib fractures are most frequently caused by blunt trauma.
      (2) They may be associated with injury to the underlying lung or the heart.
      (3) Seriousness of the injury increases with age, the number of fractures, and the location of the fractures.
         (a) Children are less likely to sustain rib fractures than adults because a child's chest wall is more flexible than that of an adult.
         (b) Rib fractures most commonly occur in the elderly because the ribs of the elderly patient are more brittle and rigid.
         (c) Ribs 4–9 are the most commonly fractured because these ribs are long, thin, and poorly protected.
         (d) Ribs 1–3 are protected by the shoulder girdle.
            (i) Fractures of ribs 1 and 2 are associated with significant trauma.
            (ii) These fractures are often associated with injury to the head, neck, spinal cord, lungs, and the major blood vessels.
         (e) Consider the possibility of injury to underlying structures with lower rib fractures.
            (i) Fractures of ribs 9–11 on the left are associated with rupture of the spleen.
            (ii) Fractures of ribs 5–9 on the right are associated with injury to the liver.
         (f) Multiple rib fractures may result in inadequate ventilation and pneumonia.
         (g) Posterior rib fractures are usually the result of deceleration accidents.
   e. Signs and symptoms of rib fracture include:
      (1) Localized pain at the fracture site that worsens with deep breathing, coughing, or moving
      (2) Pain that often causes the patient to "splint" the injury by holding his or her arm close to the chest
      (3) Pain on inspiration
      (4) Shallow breathing (to decrease the pain associated with breathing)
      (5) Tenderness on palpation
      (6) Deformity of chest wall
      (7) Crepitus (grating sound produced by bone fragments rubbing together)
      (8) Swelling and/or bruising at the fracture site
      (9) Possible subcutaneous emphysema
         (a) Subcutaneous emphysema is a crackling sensation under the fingers felt while palpating the chest.
         (b) It suggests laceration of a lung and the leakage of air into the pleural space.
   f. Emergency medical care
      (1) Take body substance isolation (BSI) precautions.
      (2) If spinal injury is suspected, maintain manual in-line stabilization until the patient is secured to a long backboard.
      (3) Establish and maintain an open airway.
      (4) Administer oxygen.
         (a) If the patient's breathing is adequate, apply oxygen by nonrebreather mask at 15 liters per minute (LPM) if not already done.
         (b) If the patient's breathing is inadequate, provide positive-pressure ventilation with 100% oxygen and assess the adequacy of the ventilations delivered.

(5) Encourage the patient to breathe deeply.

(6) Reassess frequently for development of a pneumothorax or hemothorax.

(7) Do not apply tape or straps to the ribs or chest wall; applying tape or straps limits chest wall motion and reduces the effectiveness of ventilation.

(8) Transport.

2. Flail chest

a. A flail chest is a life-threatening injury.

b. Flail chest most commonly occurs in vehicle crashes but may also occur because of:

(1) Falls from a height

(2) Assault

(3) Industrial accidents

(4) Birth trauma

c. Pathophysiology

(1) Flail chest occurs when three or more adjacent ribs are fractured in two or more places or when the sternum is detached *(Figure 29-2)*.

(2) The section of the chest wall between the fractured ribs becomes free-floating because it is no longer in continuity with the thorax.

(3) This free-floating section of the chest wall is called the "flail segment."

(4) The injured portion of the chest wall (flail segment) does not move with the rest of the rib cage when the patient attempts to breathe (paradoxical movement).

    (a) When the patient inhales, the flail segment is drawn inward instead of moving outward.

    (b) When the patient exhales, the flail segment moves outward instead of moving inward.

(5) The forces necessary to produce a flail chest cause bruising of the underlying lung (pulmonary contusion).

(6) Although instability of the chest wall results in paradoxical movement of the chest wall during breathing, it is the bruising of the underlying lung and pain associated with breathing that contribute to hypoxia.

(7) Respiratory failure may occur due to:

    (a) Bruising of the underlying lung and associated hemorrhage of the alveoli, reducing the amount of lung tissue available for gas exchange

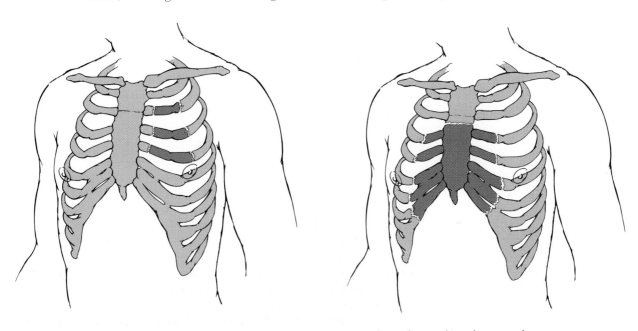

Fig. 29-2. A flail chest occurs when three or more adjacent ribs are fractured in at least two places.

   (b) Instability of the chest wall and pain associated with breathing, lead-
         ing to decreased ventilation and hypoxia
   (c) Interference with the normal "bellows" action of the chest, resulting
         in inadequate gas exchange
   (8) A flail chest may be associated with other injuries including:
      (a) Bruising of the underlying lung (pulmonary contusion)
      (b) Bruising of the heart muscle (myocardial contusion)
      (c) Hemothorax
      (d) Pneumothorax
d. Signs and symptoms of flail chest include:
   (1) Crepitus
   (2) Breathing difficulty
   (3) Bruising of the chest wall
   (4) Increased heart rate (tachycardia)
   (5) Pain and splinting of the affected side
   (6) Increased respiratory rate (tachypnea)
   (7) Pain in the chest associated with breathing
   (8) Paradoxical chest wall movement
      (a) Paradoxical movement is probably most readily observed in the un-
            conscious patient.
      (b) In patients with thick or muscular chest walls, it may be difficult to
            observe paradoxical movement.
      (c) In some conscious patients, spasm and splinting of the chest muscles
            may cause paradoxical motion to go unnoticed.
e. Emergency medical care of flail chest
   (1) Take BSI precautions.
   (2) Maintain manual in-line stabilization until the patient is secured to a long
         backboard.
   (3) Establish and maintain an open airway.
   (4) Administer oxygen.
      (a) If the patient's breathing is adequate, apply oxygen by nonrebreather
            mask at 15 LPM if not already done.
      (b) If the patient's breathing is inadequate, provide positive-pressure
            ventilation with 100% oxygen and assess the adequacy of the ventila-
            tions delivered.
   (5) Stabilize the flail segment (follow local protocol).
      (a) Provide initial stabilization with manual pressure.
      (b) After the patient has been placed on a backboard, apply bulky dress-
            ings over the affected area and tape to the chest wall.
      (c) Extend the tape to both sides of the chest.
   (6) Continually monitor and reassess respiratory rate, rhythm, depth, and ef-
         fort; vital signs; degree of paradoxical chest movement; and skin tempera-
         ture, color, and condition (moisture).
   (7) Transport promptly to the closest appropriate facility, reassessing vital
         signs at least every 5 minutes en route.
3. Simple pneumothorax
   a. A simple pneumothorax may occur because of blunt or penetrating chest
        trauma.
   b. Pathophysiology
      (1) Air enters the chest cavity causing a loss of negative pressure and a partial
            or total collapse of the lung.
      (2) Air may enter the chest cavity through a hole in the chest wall (sucking
            chest wound) or a hole in the lung tissue, bronchus, or the trachea (*Figure
            29-3*).
      (3) As air enters and fills the pleural space, lung tissue is compressed, reduc-
            ing the amount of lung tissue available for gas exchange.

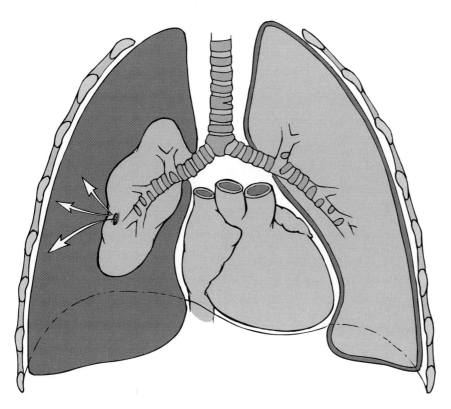

Fig. 29-3. Simple pneumothorax.

    (4) Signs and symptoms depend on the size of the pneumothorax.
        (a) Small tears may self-seal, resolving by themselves; the patient may not experience dyspnea or other signs of respiratory distress.
        (b) Larger tears may progress, resulting in signs and symptoms of respiratory distress.
  c. Signs and symptoms of a simple pneumothorax include:
    (1) Sudden onset of sharp pain in the chest associated with breathing
    (2) Shortness of breath
    (3) Difficulty breathing
    (4) Decreased or absent breath sounds on the affected side
    (5) Increased respiratory rate (tachypnea)
    (6) Increased heart rate (tachycardia)
    (7) Subcutaneous emphysema (but may not be present)
  d. Emergency medical care
    (1) Take BSI precautions.
    (2) If spinal injury is suspected, maintain manual in-line stabilization until the patient is secured to a long backboard.
    (3) Establish and maintain an open airway.
    (4) Administer oxygen.
        (a) If the patient's breathing is adequate, apply oxygen by nonrebreather mask at 15 LPM if not already done.
        (b) If the patient's breathing is inadequate, provide positive-pressure ventilation with 100% oxygen and assess the adequacy of the ventilations delivered.
    (5) Reassess frequently for signs of tension pneumothorax.
    (6) Transport promptly to the closest appropriate facility.
4. Tension pneumothorax
  a. Tension pneumothorax is a life-threatening injury.

b. It can occur because of blunt or penetrating trauma or as a complication of treatment of an open pneumothorax.

c. Pathophysiology

    (1) Air enters the pleura during inspiration and progressively accumulates under pressure.

    (2) The flap of injured lung acts as a one-way valve, allowing air to enter the pleural space during inspiration, but trapping it during expiration.

    (3) The injured lung collapses completely.

    (4) Pressure rises, forcing the trachea, heart, and major blood vessels to be pushed toward the opposite side *(Figure 29-4)*.

        (a) Shifting of the trachea to the side opposite the injury is called tracheal deviation.

        (b) Shifting of the heart and major blood vessels to the side opposite the injury is called mediastinal shift.

    (5) Shifting of the major blood vessels causes them to kink, resulting in a backup of blood into the venous system.

    (6) The backup of blood into the venous system results in:

        (a) Jugular venous distention (JVD)

        (b) Decreased blood return to the heart

        (c) Signs of shock

d. Signs and symptoms of tension pneumothorax include:

    (1) Cool, clammy skin

    (1) Increased pulse rate

    (1) Cyanosis (late sign)

    (2) JVD

    (3) Decreased blood pressure

    (4) Severe respiratory distress

    (5) Agitation, restlessness, anxiety

    (6) Bulging of intercostal muscles on the affected side

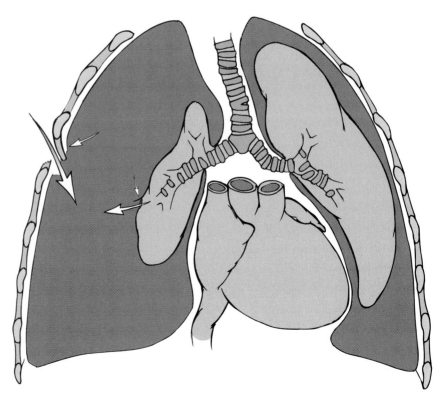

Fig. 29-4. In a tension pneumothorax, pressure rises, forcing the trachea, heart, and major blood vessels toward the opposite side.

(7) Decreased or absent breath sounds on the affected side
(8) Tracheal deviation toward the unaffected side (late sign)
(9) Possible subcutaneous emphysema in the face, neck, or chest wall
e. Emergency medical care
(1) Take BSI precautions.
(2) If spinal injury is suspected, maintain manual in-line stabilization until the patient is secured to a long backboard.
(3) Establish and maintain an open airway.
(4) Administer oxygen.
(a) If the patient's breathing is adequate, apply oxygen by nonrebreather mask at 15 LPM if not already done.
(b) If the patient's breathing is inadequate, provide positive-pressure ventilation with 100% oxygen and assess the adequacy of the ventilations delivered.
(5) If an open chest wound was bandaged with an occlusive dressing, release the dressing.
(a) If air is present under tension, air will rush out of the wound.
(b) Once the air is released, reseal the wound again with a dressing taped on three sides.
(6) Transport promptly to the closest appropriate facility, reassessing vital signs at least every 5 minutes en route.
5. Hemothorax
a. A hemothorax most commonly occurs because of penetrating chest trauma, but it may also occur because of blunt trauma.
(1) Rib fractures are a frequent cause of a hemothorax.
(2) A hemothorax is often seen with a simple or tension pneumothorax.
b. Pathophysiology
(1) A hemothorax is a collection of blood in the pleural space that may result from injury to the chest wall, the major blood vessels, or the lung due to penetrating or blunt trauma *(Figure 29-5)*.

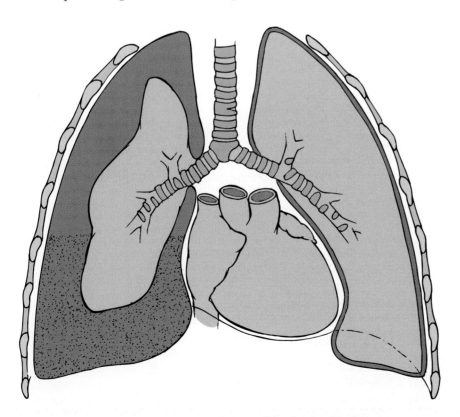

Fig. 29-5. A hemothorax is a collection of blood in the pleural space.

    (2)   The term massive hemothorax is used to describe blood loss of more than 1500 milliliters (mL) in the chest cavity.

        (a) The chest cavity can hold 2000–3000 mL of blood.

        (b) A massive hemothorax is a life-threatening injury.

  c. Signs and symptoms of hemothorax include:

    (1)   Cool, clammy skin

    (2)   Weak, thready pulse

    (3)   Restlessness, agitation, anxiety

    (4)   Hemoptysis (coughing up blood)

    (5)   Rapid, shallow breathing (tachypnea)

    (6)   Flat neck veins (due to hypovolemia)

    (7)   Decreasing blood pressure (hypotension)

    (8)   Decreased or absent breath sounds on the affected side

  d. Emergency medical care

    (1)   Take BSI precautions.

    (2)   If spinal injury is suspected, maintain manual in-line stabilization until the patient is secured to a long backboard.

    (3)   Establish and maintain an open airway.

    (4)   Administer oxygen.

        (a) If the patient's breathing is adequate, apply oxygen by nonrebreather mask at 15 LPM if not already done.

        (b) If the patient's breathing is inadequate, provide positive-pressure ventilation with 100% oxygen and assess the adequacy of the ventilations delivered.

    (5)   Treat for shock.

    (6)   Reassess frequently for development of a tension pneumothorax.

    (7)   Transport promptly to the closest appropriate facility, reassessing vital signs at least every 5 minutes en route.

6. Cardiac (pericardial) tamponade

  a. Pericardial tamponade is a life-threatening injury.

  b. It most frequently occurs because of penetrating chest trauma, but it can occur because of blunt trauma to the chest.

  c. Pathophysiology

    (1)   Pericardial tamponade occurs when blood enters the pericardial sac because of:

        (a) Laceration of a coronary blood vessel

        (b) Ruptured coronary artery

        (c) Laceration of a chamber of the heart

        (d) Significant cardiac contusion

    (2)   The blood in the pericardial sac compresses the heart, decreasing the amount of blood the heart can pump out with each contraction.

    (3)   The patient's signs and symptoms depend on how quickly blood collects in the pericardial sac.

  d. Signs and symptoms of pericardial tamponade include:

    (1)   Cool, clammy skin

    (2)   Normal breath sounds

    (3)   Narrowing pulse pressure

    (4)   Trachea in midline position

    (5)   Increased heart rate (tachycardia)

    (6)   Cyanosis of head, neck, upper extremities

    (7)   Muffled heart sounds (often difficult to assess in the field)

    (8)   Distended neck veins (may not be present in hypovolemia)

  e. Emergency medical care

    (1)   Take BSI precautions.

    (2)   If spinal injury is suspected, maintain manual in-line stabilization until the patient is secured to a long backboard.

(3) Establish and maintain an open airway.
(4) Administer oxygen.
    (a) If the patient's breathing is adequate, apply oxygen by nonrebreather mask at 15 LPM if not already done.
    (b) If the patient's breathing is inadequate, provide positive-pressure ventilation with 100% oxygen and assess the adequacy of the ventilations delivered.
(5) Transport promptly to the closest appropriate facility, reassessing vital signs at least every 5 minutes en route.

7. Traumatic asphyxia
  a. Pathophysiology
    (1) Traumatic asphyxia occurs because of a severe compression injury to the chest, such as:
      (a) Steering wheel injury
      (b) Compression of the chest under a heavy object
    (2) Blood backs up into the vessels of the head and neck.
      (1) Jugular veins fill with blood.
      (2) Capillaries rupture.
  b. Signs and symptoms of traumatic asphyxia include:
    (1) JVD
    (2) Swelling of the tongue and lips
    (3) Eyes may appear bloodshot and bulging
    (4) Blue/purple discoloration of the face and neck
    (5) Low blood pressure once the compression is released
    (6) Skin below the level of the crush injury remains pink (unless other injuries are present)
  c. Emergency medical care
    (1) Take BSI precautions.
    (2) If spinal injury is suspected, maintain manual in-line stabilization until the patient is secured to a long backboard.
    (3) Establish and maintain an open airway.
    (4) Administer oxygen.
      (a) If the patient's breathing is adequate, apply oxygen by nonrebreather mask at 15 LPM if not already done.
      (b) If the patient's breathing is inadequate, provide positive-pressure ventilation with 100% oxygen and assess the adequacy of the ventilations delivered.
    (5) Control any bleeding, if present.
    (6) Treat for shock.
    (7) Transport promptly to the closest appropriate facility, reassessing vital signs at least every 5 minutes en route.

8. Pulmonary contusion
  a. Pulmonary contusion is a potentially life-threatening injury.
  b. A pulmonary contusion (bruising of the lung) is the most common chest injury resulting from blunt trauma.
  c. It is frequently missed due to presence of other associated injuries.
  d. Pathophysiology
    (1) The alveoli fill with blood and fluid because of bruising of the lung tissue.
    (2) The area of the lung available for gas exchange is decreased.
    (3) Severity of signs and symptoms depends on the amount of lung tissue injured.
    (4) Bleeding from a pulmonary contusion may result in a blood loss of 1000–1500 mL.
  e. Signs and symptoms of pulmonary contusion include:
    (1) Evidence of blunt chest trauma
    (2) Apprehension, anxiety

      (3)   Increased respiratory rate
      (4)   Increased heart rate
      (5)   Cough
      (6)   Hemoptysis (coughing up blood)
      (7)   Difficulty breathing
      (8)   Cyanosis

   f. Emergency medical care
      (1)   Take BSI precautions.
      (2)   Maintain manual in-line stabilization until the patient is secured to a long backboard.
      (3)   Establish and maintain an open airway.
      (4)   Administer oxygen.
         (a) If the patient's breathing is adequate, apply oxygen by nonrebreather mask at 15 LPM if not already done.
         (b) If the patient's breathing is inadequate, provide positive-pressure ventilation with 100% oxygen and assess the adequacy of the ventilations delivered.
      (5)   Transport promptly to the closest appropriate facility, reassessing vital signs at least every 5 minutes en route.

9. Myocardial (cardiac) contusion
   a. Myocardial contusion is a potentially life-threatening injury.
   b. Myocardial contusion (bruising of the heart) occurs because of blunt chest trauma, such as:
      (1)   Chest compressions during cardiopulmonary resuscitation (CPR)
      (2)   Acceleration/deceleration injuries
      (3)   Associated injuries
      (4)   Fractures of the sternum
      (5)   Fractures of ribs 1–3
   c. Signs and symptoms of myocardial contusion include:
      (1)   Chest pain
      (2)   Increased heart rate
      (3)   Irregular heart rhythm
   d. Emergency medical care
      (1)   Take BSI precautions.
      (2)   Maintain manual in-line stabilization until the patient is secured to a long backboard.
      (3)   Establish and maintain an open airway.
      (4)   Administer oxygen.
         (a) If the patient's breathing is adequate, apply oxygen by nonrebreather mask at 15 LPM if not already done.
         (b) If the patient's breathing is inadequate, provide positive-pressure ventilation with 100% oxygen and assess the adequacy of the ventilations delivered.
      (5)   Transport promptly to the closest appropriate facility.
      (6)   Reassess frequently.

OPEN CHEST INJURIES—OPEN PNEUMOTHORAX

1. An open pneumothorax is a life-threatening injury.
2. An open pneumothorax ("sucking chest wound") is caused by penetrating trauma, such as:
   a. Blast injuries
   b. Knife wounds
   c. Impaled objects
   d. Gunshot wounds
   e. Motor vehicle collisions
3. Pathophysiology

    a. Air enters the chest cavity through an open wound in the chest wall into the pleural space.

    b. The severity of an open pneumothorax depends on the size of the wound.

    c. If the diameter of the chest wound is more than two-thirds the diameter of the patient's trachea, air will enter the chest wound rather than through the trachea with each breath.

    d. A sucking or gurgling sound is heard as air moves in and out of the pleural space through the open chest wound.

    e. If the flap of chest wall closes during expiration, air will become trapped inside the pleural space. As air collects in the pleural space, pressure will build with each inspiration, eventually resulting in a tension pneumothorax.

4. Signs and symptoms of an open pneumothorax include:

    a. Shortness of breath

    b. Increased heart rate

    c. Pain at the site of injury

    d. Increased respiratory rate

    e. Subcutaneous emphysema

    f. Sucking sound on inhalation

    g. Open wound in the chest wall

    h. Decreased breath sounds on the affected side

5. Emergency medical care

    a. Take BSI precautions.

    b. Maintain manual in-line stabilization until the patient is secured to a long backboard.

    c. Establish and maintain an open airway.

    d. Promptly close the chest wall defect with an occlusive (airtight) dressing.

        (1) Plastic wrap, petroleum gauze, or a defibrillation pad are examples of dressings that may be used.

        (2) Tape the dressing on three sides (flutter-valve effect).

            (a) The dressing is sucked over the wound as the patient inhales, preventing air from entering.

            (b) The open end of the dressing allows air to escape as the patient exhales.

    e. Administer oxygen.

        (1) If the patient's breathing is adequate, apply oxygen by nonrebreather mask at 15 LPM if not already done.

        (2) If the patient's breathing is inadequate, provide positive-pressure ventilation with 100% oxygen and assess the adequacy of the ventilations delivered.

    f. Transport promptly to the closest appropriate facility.

    g. Reassess frequently, monitoring for development of a tension pneumothorax.

ENRICHMENT—ABDOMINAL INJURIES

ANATOMY OF THE ABDOMEN

1. The abdomen contains the stomach, small intestine, much of the large intestine, liver, gallbladder, pancreas, spleen, kidneys, and ureters.

2. The pelvis contains the urinary bladder, part of the large intestine, and in females, the reproductive organs.

3. Digestive system (*Figure 29-6*)

    a. Function

        (1) Ingestion: brings nutrients, water, and electrolytes into the body

        (2) Digestion: chemically breaks down food into small parts so absorption can occur

(3) Absorption: facilitates the movement of nutrients, water, and electrolytes into the circulatory system so they can be used by body cells

(4) Defecation: eliminates undigested waste

b. Organs of digestion

(1) The primary organs include the mouth, pharynx, esophagus, stomach, small intestine, large intestine, rectum, and anal canal.

(2) Accessory organs include the teeth and tongue, salivary glands, liver, gallbladder, and pancreas.

c. Peristalsis is an involuntary wavelike contraction of smooth muscle that moves material through the digestive tract.

4. **Urinary system** (*Figure 29-7*)

a. The urinary system produces and excretes urine from the body.

b. The urinary system consists of the kidneys, ureters, urinary bladder, and urethra.

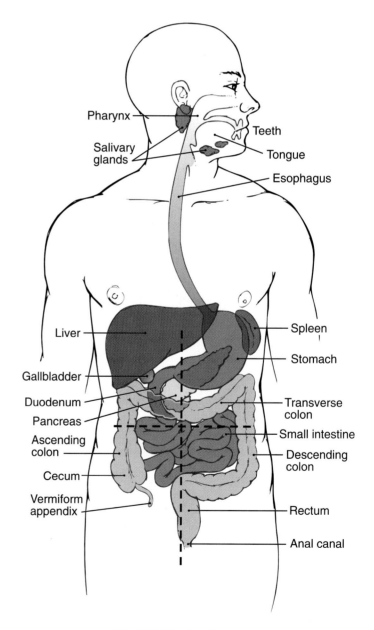

Fig. 29-6. The digestive system.

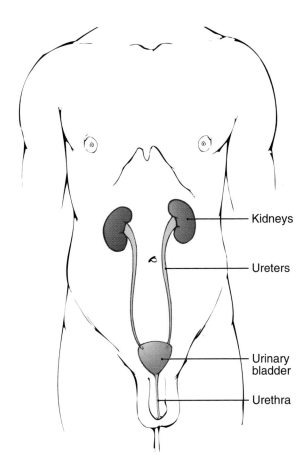

Fig. 29-7. The urinary system.

5. **Reproductive system** (*Figure 29-8*)
   a. **Male**
      (1)   The gonads (testes) produce sperm and the hormone testosterone.
      (2)   Reproductive ducts allow passage of sperm and include the:
         (a) Epididymis
         (b) Ductus (vas) deferens
         (c) Ejaculatory duct
         (d) Urethra
      (3)   Accessory glands include:
         (a) Seminal vesicles, which secrete fluid that nourishes and protects sperm
         (b) The prostate gland, which secretes fluid that enhances sperm motility and neutralizes the acidity of the vagina during intercourse
         (c) Bulbourethral (Cowper's) glands, which secrete mucuslike fluid
      (4)   External genitalia include:
         (a) The penis, which serves as the outlet for sperm and urine
         (b) The scrotum, the loose sac of skin that houses the testes
   b. **Female**
      (1)   The gonads (ovaries) produce the hormones estrogen and progesterone.
      (2)   Fallopian tubes (oviducts) receive and transport the egg to the uterus after ovulation.
      (3)   The uterus is a hollow, muscular organ in which a fertilized egg (ovum) implants and receives nourishment until birth.
      (4)   The vagina (birth canal) receives the penis during intercourse and serves as the passageway for menstrual flow and delivery of an infant.

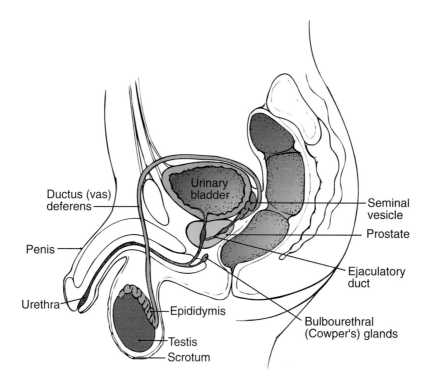

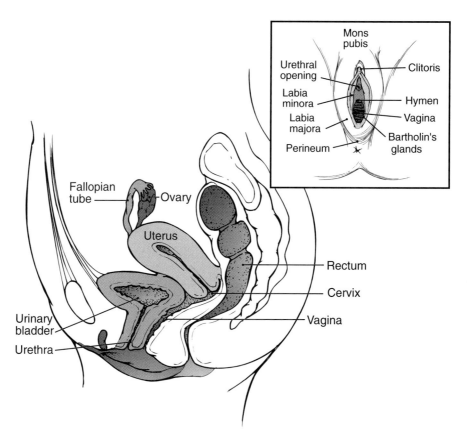

Fig. 29-8. *(A)* Male reproductive organs. *(B)* Female reproductive organs.

(5) Mammary glands (breasts) are accessory organs that function in milk production after delivery of an infant.

(6) External genitalia include:

  (a) The mons pubis, clitoris, urethral opening, vagina, labia minora, labia majora, and hymen

  (b) The perineum, the area between the vaginal opening and anus

INJURIES TO THE ABDOMEN

1. Types of abdominal injuries include:
   a. Open injuries, in which the skin is broken
   b. Closed injuries, in which the skin is not broken
2. **Hollow and solid organs** (*Figure 29-9*)
   a. The abdomen contains both hollow and solid organs.
   b. If hollow organs are cut or rupture, their contents spill into the abdominal cavity, causing inflammation.
   c. Severe bleeding may result if a solid organ is cut or ruptures.
   d. Closed or open wounds to the abdomen may involve major blood vessels and quickly result in death.

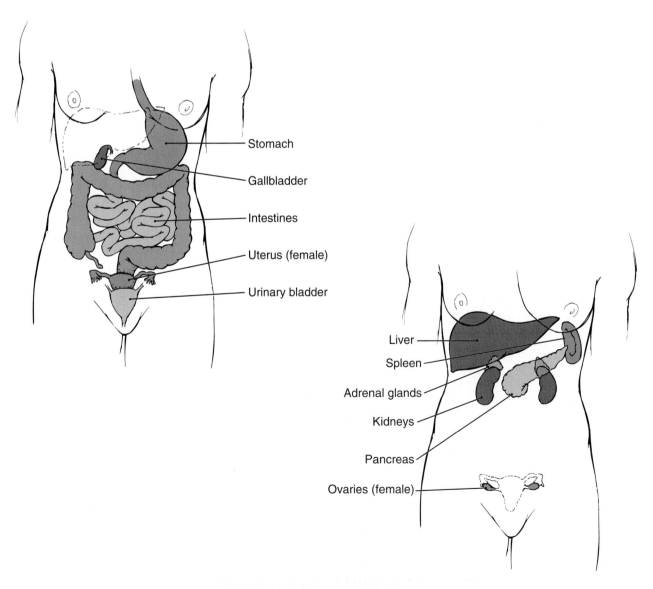

Fig. 29-9. *(A)* Hollow organs. *(B)* Solid organs.

    e. Hollow organs include:
        (1) Stomach
        (2) Intestines
        (3) Gallbladder
        (4) Urinary bladder
        (5) Uterus (female)
    f. Solid organs include:
        (1) Liver
        (2) Spleen
        (3) Pancreas
        (4) Kidneys
        (5) Adrenal glands
        (6) Ovaries (female)

3. Signs and symptoms of abdominal injury include:
    a. Patient lies still, usually with the legs drawn up to the chest (fetal position)
    b. Nausea
    c. Vomiting blood (hematemesis)
    d. Possible blood in the urine (hematuria)
    e. Possible skin wounds and penetrations
    f. Abdominal pain
    g. Rigid abdominal muscles
    h. Distended abdomen
    i. Rapid, shallow breathing
    j. Signs of shock
    k. Protruding organs (evisceration)

4. Emergency medical care
    a. Take BSI precautions.
    b. Establish and maintain an open airway.
    c. Administer oxygen.
        (1) If the patient's breathing is adequate, apply oxygen by nonrebreather mask at 15 LPM if not already done.
        (2) If the patient's breathing is inadequate, provide positive-pressure ventilation with 100% oxygen and assess the adequacy of the ventilations delivered.
    d. Control any external bleeding.
    e. If signs of shock are present or if internal bleeding is suspected, treat for shock.
    f. Do not remove penetrating objects; rather, stabilize in place with bulky dressings.
    g. Do not touch protruding organs.
        (1) Carefully remove clothing from around the wound.
        (2) Apply a large sterile dressing, moistened with sterile water or saline, over the organs and wound.
        (3) Secure the dressing in place with a large bandage to retain moisture and prevent heat loss.
    h. Flex the patient's hips and knees, if they are uninjured and spinal injury is not suspected, to decrease tension on the abdominal muscles.
    i. Transport promptly.

ENRICHMENT—INJURIES TO THE GENITALIA

MALE

1. Injuries to the external male genitalia include bruises, lacerations, penetrating objects, and avulsions.

2. Emergency medical care
    a. Take BSI precautions.
    b. Administer oxygen by nonrebreather mask at 15 LPM.

c. Control bleeding by direct pressure.

d. A cold pack may be used to decrease swelling and pain.

e. Do not remove penetrating objects.

f. Manage avulsed or amputated parts as other soft tissue injuries.

g. Protect the patient's modesty.

h. Transport.

FEMALES

1. **Internal genitalia**
   a. The internal female genitalia are rarely injured except in the pregnant female.
   b. Blunt injuries may rupture the uterus, cause loss of life of the fetus, and severe hemorrhage.
2. **External genitalia.** Injuries to the external female genitalia are usually due to straddle injuries or sexual assault.
3. **Emergency medical care**
   a. Take BSI precautions.
   b. Administer oxygen by nonrebreather mask at 15 LPM.
   c. Control bleeding by direct pressure.
   d. A cold pack may be used to decrease swelling and pain.
   e. Do not remove penetrating objects.
   f. Manage avulsed or amputated parts as other soft tissue injuries.
   g. Nothing should be placed in the vagina.
   h. Protect the patient's modesty.
   i. Transport.

REVIEW QUESTIONS

Directions: Each of the numbered items or incomplete statements in this section is followed by answers or by completions of the statement. Select the ONE lettered answer or completion that is BEST in each case.

1. Your rescue crew is called to the scene of a motor vehicle accident. Your patient is a 43-year-old woman complaining of pain in the area of her lower ribs on the left anterior chest wall. Which of the following abdominal organs is most likely to have been injured?

   (A)   The liver
   (B)   The heart
   (C)   The spleen
   (D)   The gallbladder

2. Crepitus is a sign associated with rib fractures. Which of the following best defines this finding?

   (A)   The absence of breath sounds on the affected side
   (B)   The presence of blood in the patient's sputum (cough)
   (C)   The grating sound created when bone ends rub together
   (D)   The crackling sensation felt on palpation due to leakage of air into surrounding tissues

3. The abdomen contains both solid and hollow organs. The liver, for example is considered solid, while the stomach is considered hollow. Perforation of a solid abdominal organ is most commonly associated with

    (A) paralysis
    (B) severe hemorrhage
    (C) tension pneumothorax
    (D) inflammation and infection

4. Perforation of a hollow abdominal organ is most commonly associated with

    (A) paralysis
    (B) severe hemorrhage
    (C) tension pneumothorax
    (D) inflammation and infection

5. Your rescue crew has been called to the scene of a sexual assault. Local law enforcement personnel have secured the scene. The police inform you that while trying to commit a rape, a 34-year-old man had his penis severed from his body. The amputated body part is on the ground. The patient is bleeding lightly from the groin. Appropriate management would include

    (A) control bleeding with a tourniquet, leave the amputated part at the crime scene, and transport the patient to the emergency department
    (B) control bleeding with a tourniquet, pack the amputated part in a bag filled with ice, and transport the patient and the bag to the emergency department
    (C) control bleeding with direct pressure, submerge the amputated part in a cup of water, and transport the patient and the cup to the emergency department
    (D) control bleeding with direct pressure, wrap the amputated part in sterile gauze, place in a plastic bag and keep cool, and transport the patient and the bag to the emergency department

6. Which of the following regarding a hemothorax is true?

    (A) Jugular venous distention (JVD) accompanies a hemothorax due to the accumulation of blood around the heart
    (B) Hemothorax is always caused by penetrating trauma (stabbing, gunshot wound) and never by blunt trauma (assault, motor vehicle collision)
    (C) Signs and symptoms of a hemothorax may include coughing up blood, shallow breathing, and decreased breath sounds on the affected side
    (D) By assisting ventilations with a bag-valve mask, the blood accumulating in the pleural space will be driven back into the vessels of the circulatory system

7. Your rescue crew is called to a local recreation area for a 23-year-old female patient who injured herself while mountain biking. The patient states that she slipped off the seat while going over a bump and landed on the bar. There is a slow stream of blood accumulating in her groin. She tells you that there is a 1-inch laceration between her vagina and anus. Appropriate management of this injury would include

    (A) apply ice directly to the wound
    (B) pack the vaginal opening with sterile gauze
    (C) control bleeding with external pressure and sterile gauze
    (D) protect the patient's modesty by not evaluating or treating the injury

Directions: Each of the numbered questions or incomplete statements in this section refers to a scenario that precedes them. The numbered questions or incomplete statements are followed by answers or by completions of the statement. Select the answer or completion of the statement that is BEST in each case.

Your ambulance crew is called to the scene for a 15-year-old male patient injured in a gang fight. Local law enforcement personnel have secured the scene. Your patient is found sitting against a wall clutching his chest. Bystanders state that he was hit several times with a metal bar.

Questions 8–10

8. During the focused history and physical examination, you observe that the patient's right chest wall is tender to palpation and that multiple bruises are forming. Which of the following findings may be directly attributed to a fractured rib(s)?

   (A) There is blood in the vomit
   (B) Jugular venous distention (JVD) is present
   (C) The patient has shallow breathing with pain on inspiration
   (D) The patient has unequal pupils that are slow to respond to light

9. While watching the patient's respiratory effort, you note that one section of his chest wall appears to move independently and in the opposite direction than the rest of the chest. This finding is indicative of

   (A) a flail chest
   (B) a simple pneumothorax
   (C) a tension pneumothorax
   (D) pericardial tamponade

10. After providing high-flow supplemental oxygen by nonrebreather mask, appropriate management of this injury would include

   (A) apply tape around the entire chest wall after the patient has inhaled
   (B) apply tape around the entire chest wall after the patient has exhaled
   (C) apply bulky dressings over the affected area and tape to the chest wall
   (D) apply an occlusive dressing to the chest wall and secure on three sides

Your ambulance crew is called to the scene of a construction accident. A 28-year-old man was injured when an air compressor ruptured, sending metal shrapnel flying. He was struck in the right upper chest wall where there is a laceration (cut) about 1 inch wide. The shrapnel is not visible at the wound's surface. The patient is conscious and alert.

Questions 11–15

11. The moment air began to leak into the patient's chest cavity, which of the following immediately developed?

   (A) Flail chest
   (B) Hemothorax
   (C) Simple pneumothorax
   (D) Pericardial tamponade

12. While examining the wound, you note that air is drawn through the wound into the chest cavity during inhalation. The term given this finding is

   (A) dyspnea
   (B) tachypnea
   (C) sucking chest wound
   (D) subcutaneous emphysema

13. Appropriate management of this injury would include

   (A) tape around the entire chest wall after the patient has inhaled
   (B) cover the wound with a bulky dressing and tape to the chest wall

(C) cover the wound with an occlusive dressing secured on three sides
(D) probe the wound for the presence of shrapnel and remove it if found

14. While en route to the emergency department, this patient's difficulty breathing increases. It is difficult for you to assess lung sounds due to the noise of the ambulance. His trachea is deviated to the left, and jugular venous distention (JVD) is present. The patient's mental status is altered. You should immediately

(A) stop the ambulance and reassess the patient
(B) apply more dressing and tape over the wound
(C) insert an oropharyngeal airway (OPA) and increase the liter flow of oxygen
(D) temporarily remove the dressing from the wound to allow air to escape

15. While en route to the emergency department, this patient's respiratory rate increases to 40 breaths per minute with extremely low tidal volume (the amount of air moved in and out of the lungs). Appropriate management would include

(A) provide supplemental oxygen by nasal cannula
(B) provide supplemental oxygen by nonrebreather mask
(C) assist ventilations with a bag-valve mask at a rate of 40 breaths per minute
(D) assist ventilations with a bag-valve mask at a rate of 1 breath every 5 seconds

Your rescue crew is called to a construction site for a 34-year-old female patient injured in a trench collapse. The patient has been extricated by the fire department's technical rescue team and brought to a treatment area. She is unconscious.

Questions 16–18

16. After the scene size-up, you should immediately turn your attention to

(A) performing a focused history
(B) performing an initial assessment
(C) performing a rapid trauma assessment
(D) providing high-flow oxygen therapy by nonrebreather mask

17. Upon examination, you note that the patient's eyes and tongue appear engorged with blood and her face and neck are swollen. You suspect

(A) hemothorax
(B) traumatic asphyxia
(C) pericardial tamponade
(D) tension pneumothorax

18. This patient is apneic (not breathing) and pulseless. Based on the mechanism of injury, you should

(A) ventilate only (do not do chest compressions)
(B) perform cardiopulmonary resuscitation (CPR) with the head-tilt, chin-lift technique
(C) perform CPR with the jaw-thrust technique
(D) perform CPR with the jaw-thrust technique but only compress the chest 0.5 inch rather than the full 1.5 to 2 inches.

ANSWERS AND RATIONALES

1-C. The spleen is located in the left upper quadrant of the abdominal cavity. Situated just below the diaphragm and largely protected by the ribs, the spleen is vulnerable to injury when the ribs are broken. The majority of the liver is located in the right upper quadrant of the abdomen, as is the gallbladder. The heart is located on the left side of the body and may be damaged if ribs are broken; however, the heart is not an abdominal organ.

2-C. Crepitus, noted on palpation or auscultation, is the sensation or sound created when bone ends rub together. Conscious patients generally experience intense pain associated with crepitus. The presence of blood in the sputum is called hemoptysis. The crackling sensation felt on palpation due to the leakage of air into the surrounding tissues is called subcutaneous emphysema.

3-B. The solid organs of the abdominal cavity (the spleen, liver, pancreas, and kidneys) are extremely vascular structures. Damage to these organs commonly results in significant blood loss. The abdominal organs may be injured by either penetrating or blunt trauma. For example, unrestrained patients in motor vehicle accidents are highly susceptible to spleen damage from striking the steering wheel during impact. Paralysis is most commonly associated with nerve damage, while a tension pneumothorax is a thoracic (chest) injury.

4-D. The hollow organs of the abdominal cavity (the large and small intestine, gallbladder, gall ducts, urinary bladder, and ureters) all contain matter which, if leaked, can cause inflammation and infection. Damage to these structure is most commonly associated with penetrating trauma.

5-D. Amputated genital organs are treated like any other amputation injury, with a more concerned emphasis placed on patient modesty and privacy. Bleeding should be controlled with direct pressure. Cold packs (not direct ice application) may relieve pain and swelling. The amputated body part should be wrapped in sterile gauze, placed in a bag, kept cool, and transported with the patient. As with all crime scenes, you must communicate closely with local law enforcement.

6-C. A hemothorax results when blood accumulates in the chest cavity (outside the lung space) either due to penetrating or blunt trauma. The signs and symptoms associated with a hemothorax include coughing up blood (hemoptysis); hypoperfusion (shock); rapid, shallow breathing; flat neck veins from blood loss; decreased breath sounds; and decreasing blood pressure. Assisting ventilatory effort with a bag-valve mask may improve tidal volume and oxygenation but will not drive the fluids back into the damaged vessels.

7-C. This injury is treated like any other soft tissue injury: apply direct pressure with a sterile dressing. Protecting the patient's modesty is important; however, not treating the patient due to the location of the injury is inappropriate. If possible, have a female rescuer examine and treat this injury. Be professional. Ice should never be applied directly to any wound due to the possibility of tissue damage. Vaginal bleeding should never be treated with the internal application of gauze or any other product.

8-C. Patients with rib fractures generally have associated pain with deep inspiration or movement; therefore, breathing will be shallow. To compensate for the shallow breathing, the respiratory rate is increased. Blood in the vomitus is generally associated with bleeding in the gastrointestinal tract. Blood in the sputum is consistent with a rib fracture. In the presence of chest trauma, jugular venous distention (JVD) is most commonly associated with damage or compromise to the heart (as with a tension pneumothorax or cardiac tamponade). In a trauma patient, unequal pupils is considered a sign of head trauma.

9-A. This sign is commonly referred to as "paradoxical movement," since the chest wall simultaneously moves in opposite directions. Paradoxical movement may occur when three or more adjacent ribs are broken in two or more places, thus creating an "island" of bone, muscle, and tissue. A simple pneumothorax, tension pneumothorax, or pericardial tamponade may ultimately develop from this injury.

10-C. Your treatment should be directed at minimizing the amount of paradoxical movement, thus decreasing pain and the chance of further damage to the surrounding structures (lungs, blood vessels, muscle, nerves). You must, however, be cautious not to impede the patient's ability to breathe. The best method to use is to apply bulky dressings (e.g., a folded towel, several abdominal gauze pads) over the flail segment, and tape the dressing to the chest without wrapping the circumference of the chest. An occlusive dressing would be indicated if the wound were open (skin not intact).

11-C. The presence of air in the chest cavity outside the lung space (also known as the pleural space) is a simple pneumothorax. The presence of blood in the pleural space is termed a hemothorax. A flail chest occurs when three or more ribs are fractured in two or more places, and a pericardial tamponade is the presence of blood in the sac that surrounds the heart (the pericardium).

12-C. A sucking chest wound is evident if air is drawn through an open injury in the chest wall. A sucking chest wound is also called an open pneumothorax. Air always takes the path of least resistance. If there is less resistance keeping the air from entering the wound than there is from air entering via the mouth and nose, air will be drawn in the wound on inhalation. However, on exhalation, less air typically escapes through the wound than was drawn in. Therefore, the air begins to accumulate in the pleural space.

13-C. Your treatment should be directed at keeping air from entering the chest cavity through the wound. An occlusive (air tight) dressing will facilitate this aim. An example of an occlusive dressing is petroleum jelly-impregnated gauze. The occlusive dressing should be secured on three sides. This technique will hold the dressing over the wound yet will allow air to escape the injury, thus decreasing the amount of air build up in the pleural space.

14-D. Air may continue to accumulate in the chest cavity outside the lung space. This patient exhibits the classic signs and symptoms of a tension pneumothorax: tracheal deviation and jugular venous distention (JVD). You may be able to effectively reduce the air build up by "burping" the occlusive dressing. Ideally, the dressing should cover the wound during inhalation and be lifted during exhalation. It would also be a good idea to reassess the chest to make sure you did not overlook a second open pneumothorax. Since definitive care will be done in the emergency department, you should not delay transport, and the application of more dressings over the wound will not relieve the air buildup. If the patient is semiconscious, an oropharyngeal airway (OPA) would probably induce vomiting.

15-D. This patient is in severe respiratory distress and on the verge of cardiopulmonary arrest. You need to quickly and aggressively manage his airway and breathing. At 40 respirations per minute with shallow tidal volume, this patient is not getting sufficient oxygenation. You need to assist his ventilatory effort at a rate of 12 breaths per minute (1 every 5 seconds) with slow, deep ventilations via a bag-valve mask and supplemental oxygen. By assisting ventilations, you may also effectively slow the progression (worsening) of this patient's pneumothorax.

16-B. The first step after the scene size-up is the initial assessment of the patient's mental status, airway, breathing, and circulation status and life-threatening conditions. A rapid trauma assessment would be the next step for this unconscious patient. If the patient were conscious, a focused history and physical examination would follow the initial assessment. Oxygen therapy should be considered after evaluating the patient's breathing.

17-B. Due to the mechanism of injury and the patient's presentation, traumatic asphyxia is the most likely cause. Traumatic asphyxia results when the chest is severely compressed and blood is suddenly and violently forced into the upper torso and head. This causes jugular venous distention (JVD), capillary rupture of the upper torso and head, swelling of the tongue and lips, bulging eyes, and low blood pressure once the compressive force is released.

18-C. Since this is a trauma patient, the airway should be opened using the jaw thrust and cardiopulmonary resuscitation (CPR) should be performed as normal. The adult depth of compression is 1.5 to 2 inches at a rate of 80 to 100 compressions per minute. Ventilations should be delivered slowly and deeply once every 5 seconds.

BIBLIOGRAPHY

Campbell JE (ed): *Basic Trauma Life Support for Paramedics and Advanced EMS Providers*, 3rd ed. Englewood Cliffs, NJ, Prentice-Hall, 1995.

Crosby LA, Lewallen DG (eds): *Emergency Care and Transportation of the Sick and Injured*, 6th ed. Rosemont, IL, American Academy of Orthopaedic Surgeons, 1995.

Grant HD, Murray RH Jr, Bergeron JD: *Emergency Care*, 7th ed. Englewood Cliffs, NJ, Prentice-Hall, 1995.

Hafen BQ, Karren KJ, Mistovich JJ: *Prehospital Emergency Care*, 5th ed. Upper Saddle River, NJ, Prentice-Hall, 1996.

Henry MC, Stapleton ER, Judd RL: *EMT: Prehospital Care*. Philadelphia, WB Saunders, 1992.

McSwain NE, White RD, Paturas JL, et al (eds): *The Basic EMT: Comprehensive Prehospital Patient Care*. St. Louis, Mosby-Year Book, 1996.

Miller RH, Wilson JK: *Manual of Prehospital Emergency Medicine*. St. Louis, Mosby-Year Book, 1992.

Stoy WA: *Mosby's EMT-Basic Textbook*. St. Louis, Mosby-Year Book, 1996.

United States Department of Transportation, National Highway Traffic Safety Administration: *Emergency Medical Technician: Basic. National Standard Curriculum*, 1994.

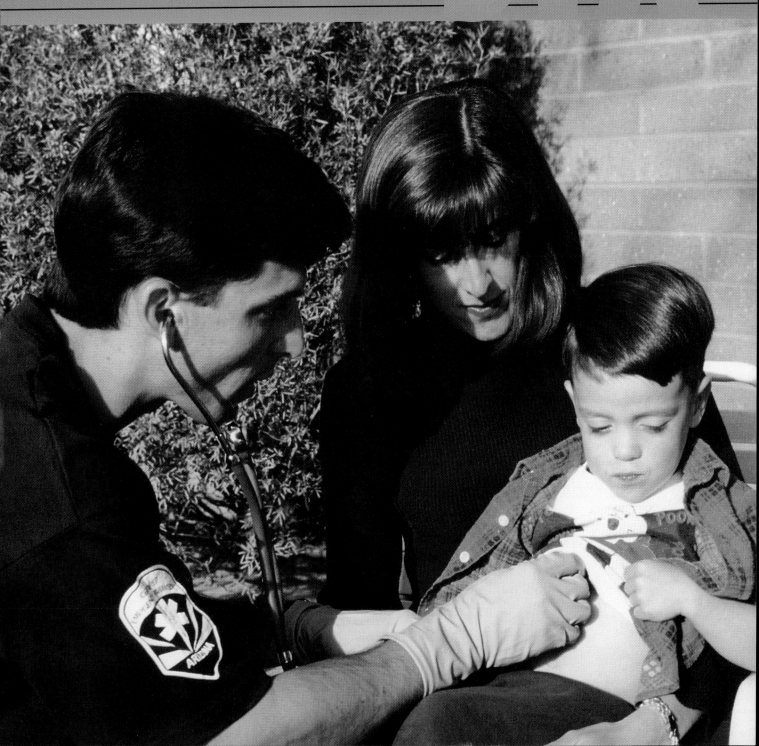

SIX

INFANTS AND CHILDREN

OBJECTIVES

30-1 Identify the developmental considerations for the following age groups:
   a. infants
   b. toddlers
   c. preschool children
   d. school-age children
   e. adolescents

30-2 Differentiate the response of the ill or injured infant or child (age specific) from that of an adult.

30-3 Describe differences in anatomy and physiology of the infant, child, and adult patient.

30-4 List the steps in the management of foreign-body airway obstruction.

30-5 Indicate various causes of respiratory emergencies.

30-6 State the usual cause of cardiac arrest in infants and children versus adults.

30-7 Differentiate between respiratory distress and respiratory failure.

30-8 Summarize emergency medical care strategies for respiratory distress and respiratory failure.

30-9 List the common causes of seizures in the infant and child patient.

30-10 Describe the management of seizures in the infant and child patient.

*30-11 List possible causes of altered mental status in the infant and child patient.

*30-12 Describe management of the infant or child with an altered mental status.

*30-13 List the common poisonous substances ingested by children.

MOTIVATION FOR LEARNING

The EMT-Basic may experience anxiety when treating children because of a lack of experience in treating children, a fear of failure, and/or identifying the patient with his or her own children. It is important to learn the physical and developmental attributes of infants and children of different ages and the methods to use to approach these patients for evaluation.

*30-14 List the questions that should be asked when obtaining a SAMPLE history in a situation in which a child has been exposed to a poisonous substance.

*30-15 Describe the management of poisoning in an infant and child patient.

*30-16 List common causes of fever in an infant or child.

*30-17 Describe the management of fever in an infant or child.

*30-18 List the common causes of shock in infants and children.

*30-19 Identify the signs and symptoms of shock (hypoperfusion) in the infant and child patient.

30-20 Describe the methods of determining end organ perfusion in the infant and child patient.

*30-21 Describe the management of shock in the infant and child patient.

*30-22 Define the terms drowning and near-drowning.

*30-23 Identify the signs and symptoms of near-drowning.

*30-24 Describe the management of the infant or child victim of a submersion incident.

*30-25 Define Sudden Infant Death Syndrome (SIDS) and apparent life-threatening events (ALTEs).

*30-26 Discuss factors associated with SIDS.

*30-27 Identify the signs and symptoms of SIDS.

*30-28 Describe the management of SIDS.

30-29 Differentiate among injury patterns in adults, infants, and children.

*30-30 Identify the signs and symptoms of head injury in an infant or child.

30-31 Discuss the field management of the infant and child trauma patient.

*30-32 Discuss the use of the pneumatic anti-shock garment (PASG) in infants and children.

30-33 Summarize the indicators of possible child abuse and neglect.

30-34 Describe the medical–legal responsibilities in suspected child abuse.

*30-35 Discuss the emergency care of infants and children with special needs including the care of an infant or child with a:

a. tracheostomy tube

b. home artificial ventilator

c. central line

d. gastrostomy tube

e. shunt

30-36 Recognize the need for EMT-Basic debriefing following a difficult infant or child transport.

DEVELOPMENTAL STAGES

DEFINITIONS

1. **Neonate:** first 4 weeks of life
2. **Infant:** birth to 1 year of age
3. **Toddler:** 1–3 years of age
4. **Preschooler:** 3–6 years of age
5. **School age:** 6–12 years of age
6. **Adolescent:** 12–18 years of age

INFANTS (BIRTH TO 1 YEAR OF AGE)

1. **Young infant** (0 to 6 months of age)
   a. Young infants are unafraid of strangers.
   b. They have no modesty.
2. **Older infant** (6 months to 1 year of age)
   a. Older infants begin to experience stranger anxiety.
   b. They do not like to be separated from parents (separation anxiety).
   c. They show little modesty.
   d. They may be threatened by direct eye contact with strangers.
3. **Suggested strategies for the EMT-Basic**
   a. Keep the infant warm; make sure hands and stethoscope are warmed before touching the infant.
   b. Smile while using a calm, soothing voice.
   c. Provide comfort measures as needed (e.g., use of a pacifier).
   d. If possible, involve the caregiver in the care of the infant.
   e. If possible, assess the infant in the arms of the caregiver.
   f. Begin with examination of the trunk (e.g., heart and lungs) and examine the head last.
      (1) Obtain heart and lung sounds before the infant becomes agitated.
      (2) Assess breathing from a distance (observe rate, chest rise, skin color, level of activity).
   g. Be careful not to leave small objects within the infant's reach.

TODDLERS (1–3 YEARS OF AGE)

1. Favorite words are "no" and "mine."
2. Toddlers fear pain and separation from caregiver and special objects (e.g., blanket, toy).
3. They are distrustful of strangers.
   a. They are likely to resist examination and treatment.
   b. They may scream, cry, or kick when touched.
4. Toddlers do not like having clothing removed.
5. They view illness/injury as punishment.
6. They are afraid of needles.
7. **Suggested strategies for the EMT-Basic**
   a. A child of this age may experience emotional problems as a result of the illness or injury.
   b. Approach the child slowly and talk to him or her at eye level.
      (1) Use simple words and phrases and a reassuring tone of voice. The child will understand your tone, even if he or she does not understand your words.
      (2) Assure the child that he or she was not bad and is not being punished.
      (3) Reassure the child that it is all right to cry but not to kick, hit, or bite.
   c. When possible, talk with the caregiver first. The child may be more at ease if he or she sees that the adult is not threatened.
   d. Provide the child with a security object (e.g., teddy bear, blanket).
   e. Use equipment or toys as distractions.
      (1) Ask the child to "blow out the light" on a pen light.
      (2) Use a blown-up exam glove as a balloon.
   f. When possible, allow the child to remain on the caregiver's lap. If not possible, try to keep the caregiver within the child's line of vision.
   g. Examine the child from trunk to head.
      (1) Examine the child before he or she becomes agitated.
      (2) Remove clothing, examine the child, then replace clothing.
      (3) Limit the examination to the essentials.
      (4) Restrain the child as little as possible. If restraints are necessary, use hands rather than mechanical devices.

(5)   Reward the child for cooperative behavior (e.g., praise, stickers).

(6)   Transport with a special toy, blanket.

PRESCHOOLERS (3–6 YEARS OF AGE)

1. Preschoolers often view illness or injury as their fault.

2. Preschoolers:

    a. Are modest

    b. Do not like to be touched

    c. Do not like being separated from parents

    d. Do not like having clothing removed

    e. Fear being suffocated by an oxygen mask

    f. Fear pain and permanent injury

    g. Are afraid of blood and needles

        (1)   Afraid their skin will burst open like a balloon

        (2)   Believe the entire needle and syringe go inside their skin

        (3)   Believe the needle leaves a large hole

3. Suggested strategies for the EMT-Basic

    a. Approach the child slowly and talk to him or her at eye level.

        (1)   Use simple words and phrases and a reassuring tone of voice.

        (2)   Assure the child that he or she was not bad and is not being punished.

        (3)   Do NOT say, "Big kids don't cry."

    b. Tell the child how things will feel and what is to be done immediately before doing it.

    c. Examine the child from trunk to head.

        (1)   The child often feels more in control if examined in a sitting or standing position.

        (2)   The child usually prefers presence of caregiver during examination.

        (3)   Respect the child's modesty.

            (a) Remove clothing, examine child, then replace clothing.

            (b) Consider that children have been told not to let strangers touch them.

            (c) Use of a doll or a stuffed animal may be helpful when explaining procedures.

            (d) Encourage the child's participation.

            (e) The child may want to hold or examine equipment.

            (f) It may be helpful to "pretend" about a procedure (e.g., when assessing blood pressure, "I'm seeing how strong your muscles are.")

            (g) Reward the child for cooperative behavior (e.g., praise, stickers).

SCHOOL-AGE CHILDREN (6–12 YEARS OF AGE)

1. School-age children are usually cooperative.

2. School-age children:

    a. Are afraid of blood and prolonged separation from caregiver

    b. Fear pain, permanent injury, and disfigurement

    c. Are very modest

        (1)   They do not like their bodies exposed to strangers.

        (2)   Consider that children have been told not to let strangers touch them.

    d. May still view illness or injury as punishment (e.g., ran across the street without looking, tore clothing, damaged bicycle)

3. Suggested strategies for the EMT-Basic

    a. Talk to the child at eye level.

        (1)   Talk directly to the child about what happened, even if you also obtain a history from the caregiver.

        (2)   Prepare the child for procedures with simple explanations of what will take place, but do it just before the procedure so he or she does not have long to think about it.

b. Do not threaten the child if he or she is uncooperative.

c. Do not belittle the child's pain or fears.

d. Respect the child's modesty.

   (1) Remove clothing, examine the child, then replace clothing.

   (2) Younger child may prefer the presence of caregiver; older child may prefer privacy.

e. Enlist the child's cooperation and involve him or her in care as much as possible.

f. Reward the child for his or her cooperation (e.g., praise, stickers).

ADOLESCENT (12–18 YEARS OF AGE)

1. Adolescents:

   a. Fear pain, permanent injury, disfigurement, and death

   b. Can be very modest

   c. May react hysterically

   d. Expect to be treated as adults

2. Suggested strategies for the EMT-Basic

   a. Talk directly to the child about what happened, even if you also obtain a history from the caregiver.

   b. When possible, an EMT-Basic of the same gender should provide direct patient care.

   c. Recognize the tendency for overreaction and do not become angry with the emotional patient.

   d. Do not tease or embarrass the patient.

   e. Give full explanations and allow time for questions.

   f. The adolescent may desire to be assessed privately, away from caregiver.

   g. The adolescent may prefer to have a peer close by for reassurance.

ANATOMICAL DIFFERENCES (FIGURE 30-1)

HEAD

1. The child's head is proportionately larger and heavier than an adult's until approximately 4 years of age. Trauma may result in flexion and extension injuries.

2. Bones of the skull

   a. The bones of the skull allow for growth as the brain grows.

   b. There are two main fontanels ("soft spots") in the skull (*Figure 30-2*).

   (1) The posterior fontanel closes between 2 and 6 months of age.

   (2) The anterior fontanel closes between 12 and 18 months of age.

   c. Soft spots are normally nearly level with the skull.

   (1) Coughing, crying, or lying down may cause the soft spots to bulge temporarily.

   (2) A bulging soft spot suggests increased pressure within the skull.

   (3) A markedly sunken (depressed) soft spot suggests dehydration.

3. Neck muscles are less developed in infants.

AIRWAY

1. Nose

   a. Nasal passages are small and easily obstructed.

   b. Newborns and young infants (less than 6 months of age) are obligate nose breathers (e.g., they do not automatically open their mouths to breathe when their noses become obstructed).

   c. Suctioning the nose can improve breathing problems in an infant.

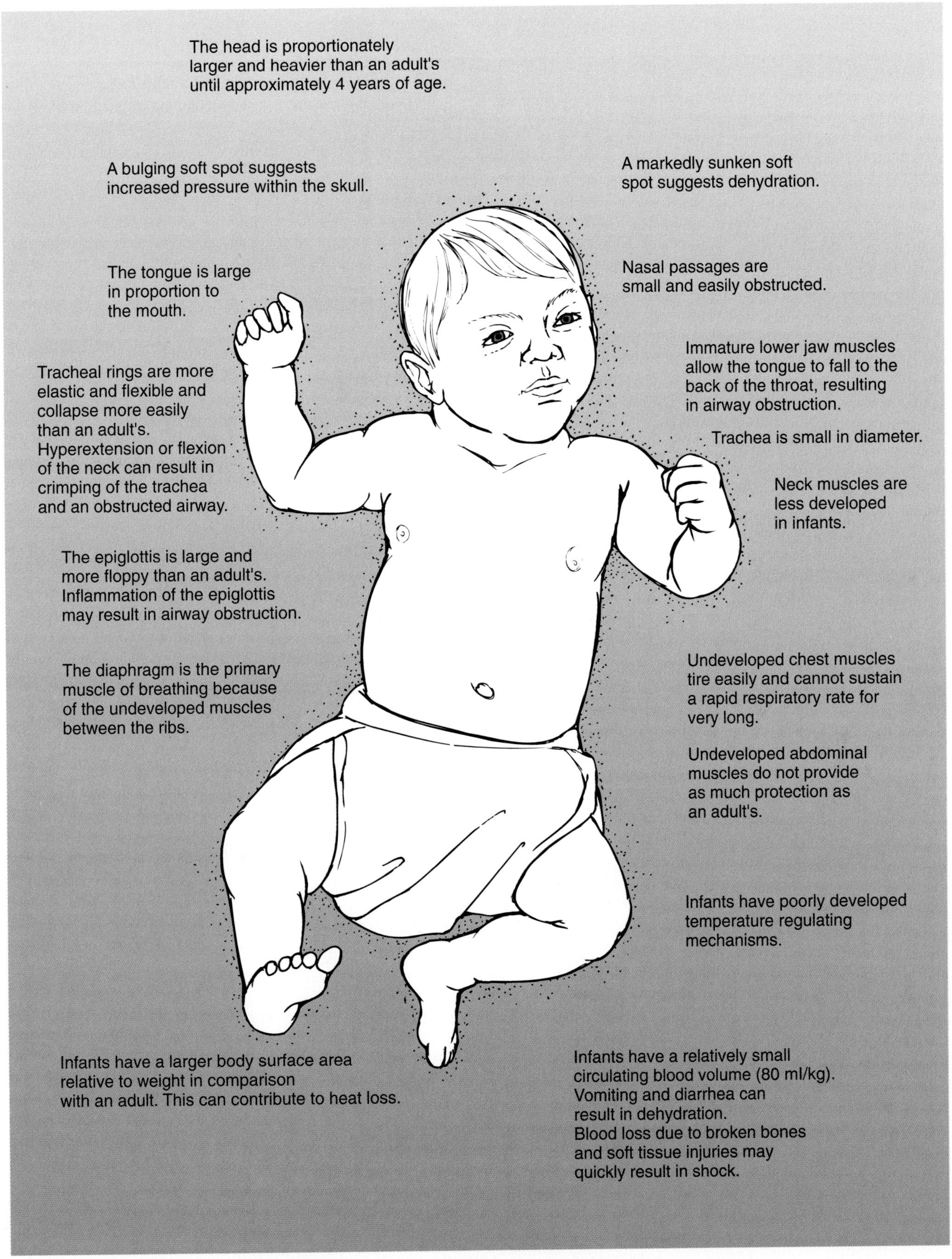

The head is proportionately larger and heavier than an adult's until approximately 4 years of age.

A bulging soft spot suggests increased pressure within the skull.

A markedly sunken soft spot suggests dehydration.

The tongue is large in proportion to the mouth.

Nasal passages are small and easily obstructed.

Immature lower jaw muscles allow the tongue to fall to the back of the throat, resulting in airway obstruction.

Tracheal rings are more elastic and flexible and collapse more easily than an adult's. Hyperextension or flexion of the neck can result in crimping of the trachea and an obstructed airway.

Trachea is small in diameter.

Neck muscles are less developed in infants.

The epiglottis is large and more floppy than an adult's. Inflammation of the epiglottis may result in airway obstruction.

The diaphragm is the primary muscle of breathing because of the undeveloped muscles between the ribs.

Undeveloped chest muscles tire easily and cannot sustain a rapid respiratory rate for very long.

Undeveloped abdominal muscles do not provide as much protection as an adult's.

Infants have poorly developed temperature regulating mechanisms.

Infants have a larger body surface area relative to weight in comparison with an adult. This can contribute to heat loss.

Infants have a relatively small circulating blood volume (80 ml/kg). Vomiting and diarrhea can result in dehydration. Blood loss due to broken bones and soft tissue injuries may quickly result in shock.

Fig. 30-1. Anatomical differences between children and adults.

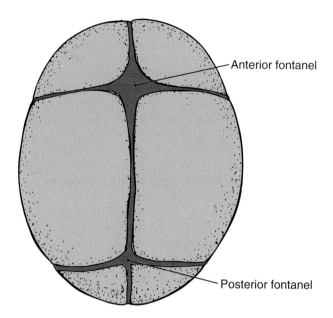

Fig. 30-2. There are two main fontanels ("soft spots") in the skull. The posterior fontanel closes between 2 and 6 months of age. The anterior fontanel closes between 12 and 18 months of age.

2. **Mouth**
   a. The tongue is large in proportion to the mouth.
   b. Immature lower jaw (mandible) muscles allow the tongue to fall to the back of the throat, resulting in airway obstruction.
   c. The tongue is the most common cause of upper airway obstruction in the unconscious child.

3. **Trachea**
   a. The trachea is small in diameter when compared with an adult's.
      (1) The diameter of the trachea of an infant is approximately 4 millimeters (mm) compared with the 20-mm tracheal diameter of an adult trachea.
      (2) The smallest diameter is at the cricoid cartilage in children up to about 8 years of age (the narrowest portion of an adult's airway is at the vocal cords).
      (3) Because of its small diameter, the trachea can be easily obstructed by swelling.
   b. Tracheal rings are more elastic and flexible and collapse more easily than an adult's.
      (1) Hyperextension or flexion of the neck can result in crimping of the trachea and an obstructed airway.
      (2) The head of the infant or young child should be placed in a neutral or "sniffing" position.

4. **Larynx and epiglottis**
   a. The larynx is anterior in comparison with an adult's and is positioned higher in the neck.
   b. The epiglottis (which protects the trachea during swallowing) is large and more floppy than in an adult. Inflammation of the epiglottis may result in airway obstruction.

5. **Chest**
   a. In children, the diaphragm is the primary muscle of breathing because the muscles between the ribs (intercostal muscles) are undeveloped.
      (1) Use of the diaphragm results in abdominal breathing.
      (2) Undeveloped chest muscles tire easily and cannot sustain a rapid respiratory rate for very long.
   b. The ribs are more flexible than in an adult.
      (1) Accidental rib fracture is rare.

      (2)   Retractions are often present with respiratory distress.

6. Abdomen

    a. Undeveloped abdominal muscles do not provide as much protection as an adult's. Abdominal organs (e.g., liver) are more prone to injury.

    b. Young children are abdominal breathers; observe the rise and fall of the abdomen, rather than the chest, to count respirations.

    c. The abdomen distends with air with crying and bag-valve-mask ventilation.

        (1)   Abdominal distention puts pressure on the diaphragm and limits movement.

        (2)   Because infants and young children depend on the diaphragm for breathing, respiratory distress will result if movement of the diaphragm is limited.

7. Skin

    a. Infants and young children are susceptible to heat- and cold-related emergencies.

    b. A child has a larger body surface area relative to weight in comparison with an adult. The larger body surface area contributes to heat loss.

    c. Infants have thin skin with little subcutaneous fat.

    d. Infants have poorly developed temperature-regulating mechanisms.

        (1)   They are unable to shiver in cold temperatures.

        (2)   Their sweating mechanism is immature in warm temperatures.

8. Circulatory system

    a. Blood volume

        (1)   Infants and young children have a relatively small circulating blood volume [80 milliliters per kilogram (mL/kg)].

        (2)   Most of an infant's body weight is water, so vomiting and diarrhea can result in dehydration.

        (3)   Blood loss due to broken bones and soft tissue injuries may quickly result in shock.

            (a)   Sudden loss of 1/2 liter (500 mL) of blood in a child and 100–200 mL of the blood volume in an infant is considered serious.

            (b)   A 1-year-old has a blood volume of approximately 800 mL; thus, a loss of 150 mL is considered major blood loss.

    b. An increased heart rate (tachycardia) may be present in an infant or child in response to a lack of oxygen, decreased volume (hypovolemia), fever, pain, or anxiety, among many other causes.

    c. A decreased heart rate (bradycardia) may occur as a result of a lack of oxygen.

9. Compensatory mechanisms

    a. Children can compensate well for short periods.

    b. Infants and children compensate for a lack of oxygen (hypoxia) by increasing their breathing rate and effort of breathing. Compensation is followed rapidly by decompensation due to rapid respiratory muscle fatigue and general fatigue of the infant or child.

    c. Infants and children compensate for a loss of blood or fluid by first increasing heart rate and constricting the blood vessels of the skin. A low blood pressure will not be observed until the infant or child is no longer able to compensate.

AIRWAY

OPENING THE AIRWAY

1. Head-tilt, chin-lift maneuver

    a. Do NOT use if trauma is suspected.

    b. Place the hand closest to the child's head on the forehead.

    c. Tilt the head gently back into a neutral or slightly extended position.

    d. Place the fingers (not the thumb) of the other hand under the bony part of the lower jaw at the chin.

    e. Lift upward and outward.

    f. Do not push on the soft tissues under the chin; doing so may obstruct the airway.

2. **Jaw-thrust maneuver with spinal stabilization**

    a. The jaw thrust is the procedure of choice for opening the airway when trauma is suspected.

    b. Ideally, the airway should be managed with two rescuers.

        (1) One rescuer opens the airway with the jaw-thrust maneuver.

        (2) The second rescuer maintains manual in-line stabilization of the cervical spine.

    c. While maintaining manual cervical spine stabilization, grasp the angles of the patient's lower jaw with both hands, one on each side.

    d. Using upward pressure, thrust the patient's lower jaw forward.

SUCTIONING

1. **Bulb syringe**

    a. The bulb syringe is used to remove secretions from the mouth or nose.

    b. Administer oxygen before, between, and after suctioning.

    c. Technique

        (1) Take body substance isolation (BSI) precautions.

        (2) Depress (squeeze) the bulb before inserting.

        (3) With the bulb depressed, insert the syringe into the nose or mouth and release.

        (4) Remove the syringe and empty the contents.

        (5) Apply suction for no more than 5 seconds at a time.

    d. Precautions. Do not stimulate the back of the throat; it may cause gagging, vomiting, or result in severe slowing of heart rate.

2. **Soft, flexible catheter**

    a. The soft, flexible catheter is used to clear the mouth and nose and to remove secretions from an endotracheal tube in intubated patients.

    b. It is available in many sizes.

    c. Its inside diameter is smaller than that of a rigid catheter.

    d. Administer oxygen before, between, and after suctioning.

    e. Technique

        (1) Take BSI precautions.

        (2) Preoxygenate the patient if possible; if suctioning an intubated patient, preoxygenation is essential.

        (3) Measure the catheter from the tip of the nose to the tip of the ear and do not insert past the base of the tongue (in patients without an endotracheal tube in place).

        (4) Turn on the suction unit.

        (5) Attach the catheter to the suction unit.

        (6) Insert the catheter WITHOUT applying suction.

        (7) Apply intermittent suction by closing the side opening while withdrawing the catheter in a side-to-side motion.

        (8) Avoid touching the back of the throat.

        (9) Apply suction for no more than 5 seconds at a time.

        (10) Periodically rinse the catheter and tubing with water.

        (11) Administer oxygen after suctioning.

3. **Rigid catheter**

    a. The rigid catheter is used to clear the mouth and oropharynx of an unresponsive patient.

    b. Use in conscious or semiconscious patients may cause vomiting.

    c. The rigid catheter can suction large amounts of fluid rapidly.

d. Administer oxygen before, between, and after suctioning.

e. Technique
   (1) Take BSI precautions.
   (2) Preoxygenate the patient if possible.
   (3) Turn on the suction unit.
   (4) Attach the catheter to the suction unit.
   (5) Insert the suction device into the mouth WITHOUT applying suction.
      (a) It should be inserted only as far as you can see.
      (b) Do not insert past the base of the tongue.
   (6) Once the suction tip is in contact with secretions, apply suction for no more than 5 seconds at a time.
   (7) Avoid touching the back of the throat.
   (8) Periodically rinse the catheter and tubing with water.
   (9) Administer oxygen after suctioning.

AIRWAY OBSTRUCTION

1. **Partial airway obstruction**
   a. Infant or child may still be alert, pink, with good peripheral perfusion.
   b. Stridor, crowing, or otherwise noisy breathing may be present.
   c. Retractions on inspiration may be seen.
2. **Complete airway obstruction**
   a. The child will be unable to cry or talk.
   b. Cough is ineffective or absent.
   c. The child may have an altered mental status or may be unresponsive.
   d. Cyanosis may be present.

CLEARING A COMPLETE FOREIGN-BODY AIRWAY OBSTRUCTION

1. **Infants (younger than 1 year of age)**
   a. A combination of back blows and chest thrusts is recommended.
   b. Technique
      (1) Place the infant face down with the head lower than the trunk over the rescuer's forearm.
      (2) Using the heel of one hand, deliver up to 5 back blows forcefully between the shoulder blades.
      (3) Position the infant face up with the head lower than the trunk and deliver up to 5 chest thrusts. Use the tips of two fingers positioned one finger-width below the nipple line.
      (4) Open the infant's mouth and look for the foreign body.
         (a) If it is visible, remove it.
         (b) If it is not visible, do not perform a blind finger sweep.
      (5) Open the airway and attempt to ventilate.
         (a) If the chest does not rise, reposition the head and reattempt to ventilate.
         (b) If the airway remains obstructed (no chest rise):
            (i) Repeat back blows, chest thrusts, and attempts to ventilate twice and then transport immediately
            (ii) Continue resuscitation efforts until the object is removed and rescue breathing is effective or until arrival at the receiving facility
2. **Children (1 to 8 years of age)**
   a. Conscious child
      (1) Ask, "Are you choking?"
      (2) Deliver abdominal thrusts.
         (a) Make a fist by grasping your thumb with the right hand.
         (b) Stand behind the child and place the thumbside of the fist against the

child's abdomen in the midline slightly above the umbilicus.

   (c) Grasp your fist with your other hand and deliver inward and upward abdominal thrusts.

   (d) Continue until the foreign body is expelled or the child becomes unconscious.

b. Unconscious child

  (1) Establish unresponsiveness.

  (2) Open the airway and assess breathing.

  (3) Attempt to ventilate.

  (4) If there is no chest rise, reposition the head and reattempt to ventilate.

  (5) If the airway remains obstructed, kneel beside the child or straddle the child's hips.

    (a) Place the heel of one hand on the child's abdomen in the midline slightly above the umbilicus.

    (b) Place the other hand on top of the first.

  (6) Deliver up to 5 abdominal thrusts, pressing both hands into the abdomen with quick, upward thrusts directed toward the midline of the child's body.

  (7) Move to the child's head and open the airway.

  (8) If the foreign body is seen, remove it. Do not perform a blind finger sweep.

  (9) If the airway remains obstructed (no chest rise), repeat the abdominal thrusts and attempts to ventilate until the object is removed and rescue breathing is effective.

  (10) When the obstruction is removed, assess for breathing.

    (a) If breathing is present:

      (i) Place the child on his or her side (if trauma is not suspected)

      (ii) Continue to assess breathing and pulse while maintaining an open airway

      (iii) If breathing is adequate, administer oxygen by nonrebreather mask at 15 liters per minute (LPM)

      (iv) If breathing is inadequate, perform positive-pressure ventilation with 100% oxygen

    (b) If breathing is absent but a pulse is present, deliver 1 breath every 3 seconds (20 breaths per minute) and monitor the pulse frequently.

    (c) If breathing is absent and there is no pulse, begin cardiopulmonary resuscitation (CPR).

AIRWAY ADJUNCTS

1. Oropharyngeal airway

  a. The oropharyngeal airway is also called an oral airway or OPA.

  b. Use

    (1) It should only be used in an unconscious infant or child who does not have a gag reflex.

    (2) Should be used if procedures to open the airway (head-tilt, chin-lift or jaw-thrust maneuvers) in the unconscious infant or child fail to provide and maintain an open airway.

    (3) Use in conscious or semiconscious patients may stimulate the back of the throat when the back of the tongue or throat is touched, resulting in gagging or vomiting.

  c. Proper size is determined by aligning the airway on the side of the face and selecting an airway that extends from the corner of the mouth to the angle of the jaw.

  d. Technique of insertion

    (1) Take BSI precautions.

    (2) The OPA should be inserted using a tongue depressor (blade).

(3) Insert the tongue depressor to the base of tongue.
(4) Push down against the tongue while lifting upward.
(5) Insert the OPA directly without rotation.
(6) Maintain proper head position.
2. **Nasopharyngeal airway (NPA)**
   a. The NPA may be used in the conscious or semiconscious patient.
   b. Proper size is determined by aligning the airway on the side of the patient's face and selecting an airway that extends from the tip of the nose to the earlobe.
   c. Technique of insertion
   (1) Take BSI precautions.
   (2) Generously lubricate the outside of the airway with a water-soluble lubricant.
   (3) Using gentle pressure, slide the airway along the floor of the nostril into the back of the throat behind the tongue.
   (4) If resistance is felt, do NOT force.
   d. The NPA should not be used in head trauma.

OXYGEN THERAPY

OXYGEN DELIVERY

1. **Nonrebreather mask**
   a. In the nonrebreather mask, a one-way valve between the reservoir bag and the mask allows exhaled air to escape but prevents room air from being inhaled.
   b. The nonrebreather mask is the preferred method of oxygen delivery in the prehospital setting.
   (1) It allows delivery of high-concentration oxygen to a spontaneously breathing patient.
   (2) At 15 LPM, the oxygen concentration delivered is approximately 90%.
2. **Blow-by (free-flow) oxygen**
   a. Blow-by oxygen refers to blowing oxygen over the face of an infant or child so that the patient breathes oxygen-enriched air.
   b. Method # 1
   (1) Connect oxygen tubing to oxygen set to at least 5 LPM.
   (2) Cup your hand around the tubing over the face of the infant or child.
   (3) Hold the tubing 2 inches from the patient's face.
   c. Method # 2
   (1) Insert the oxygen tubing into a paper cup and direct the tubing at the patient's face.
   (2) Styrofoam cups should not be used because they may crumble and result in an airway obstruction if the particles enter the patient's airway.
   d. Method # 3. Have the caregiver hold an oxygen mask 2 inches from the patient's face.

ARTIFICIAL VENTILATION

1. **Ventilation face masks**
   a. Ventilation face masks should be clear to allow:
   (1) Visualization of the color of the patient's lips
   (2) Visualization of blood, vomitus, or other secretions
   b. They should extend from the bridge of the nose to the cleft of the chin and cover the nose and mouth without putting pressure on the eyes.
   c. A mask that is too large or too small will prevent effective ventilation.
2. **Mask seal**
   a. Two rescuers
   (1) One rescuer uses both hands to open the airway and make an airtight mask-to-face seal.

    (2) A second rescuer squeezes the ventilation bag.

  b. Single rescuer

    (1) Form a "C" with your thumb and index finger to maintain a seal with the mask.

    (2) Hold the lower part of the mask securely against the patient's face with your index finger.

    (3) Hold the upper part of the mask against the patient's face with your thumb.

  c. Do not push the mask into the patient's face; the patient's face should be gently pulled up to the mask while maintaining the head in a neutral position.

3. Mouth-to-mask artificial ventilation

  a. Mouth-to-mask ventilation is the preferred method of ventilation in the prehospital setting because:

    (1) Use of the pocket mask provides a physical barrier between the rescuer and the patient's nose, mouth, and secretions

      (a) The pocket mask reduces the risk of infectious disease exposure.

      (b) Use of a one-way valve at the ventilation port eliminates exposure to the patient's exhaled air.

    (2) If the patient resumes spontaneous breathing, the mask can be used as a simple face mask to deliver 40%–60% oxygen by administering supplemental oxygen through the oxygen inlet on the mask

    (3) A greater tidal volume can be delivered with a pocket mask than with a bag-valve mask

      (a) Both of the rescuer's hands can be used to hold the mask in place while maintaining proper head position.

      (b) This results in greater lung ventilation and less gastric distention.

    (4) With mouth-to-mask ventilation, the rescuer can feel the resistance of the patient's lungs

  b. Technique

    (1) Take BSI precautions.

    (2) Connect a one-way valve to the ventilation port on the mask.

    (3) Connect oxygen tubing to the oxygen inlet on the mask.

    (4) Set the oxygen flow rate for 15 LPM.

    (5) Open the airway with a head-tilt, chin-lift maneuver or, if trauma is suspected, perform the jaw-thrust maneuver.

    (6) Insert an OPA or NPA if needed to maintain an open airway.

    (7) Position yourself at the top of the supine patient's head.

    (8) Place the mask on the patient's face.

      (a) Apply the apex (narrow portion) of the mask over the bridge of the patient's nose and stabilize in place with your thumbs.

      (b) Lower the mask over the patient's face and mouth.

      (c) Use the remaining fingers of both hands to maintain proper head position and stabilize the broad portion of the mask in place over the cleft of the chin (indentation beneath the lower lip).

    (9) Place your mouth around the one-way valve and deliver slow, steady breaths.

      (a) Each breath should be delivered over 1 to 1.5 seconds for an infant or child.

      (b) For infants and children less than 8 years of age, breaths should be delivered once every 3 seconds (20 per minute).

      (c) Use only enough pressure to make the patient's chest rise.

4. Use of a bag-valve mask

  a. The bag-valve mask used should not have a pop-off (pressure-release) valve.

    (1) A pop-off valve may prevent effective ventilation during the resuscitation of an infant or child.

    (2) If a pop-off valve is present, it may be disabled by taping it down.

b. Size

   (1) Bag-valve-mask devices used for ventilating full-term neonates and infants should have a minimum volume of 450 mL.

   (2) In older children and adults, use a bag with a minimum volume of 1000 mL (1 liter).

c. Technique

   (1) Take BSI precautions.

   (2) Open the airway using a head-tilt, chin-lift maneuver or a jaw-thrust maneuver if trauma is suspected.

   (3) Size and insert an OPA or NPA.

   (4) Select the correct mask size.

   (5) Create a face-to-mask seal.

   (6) Connect the bag to the mask if not already done.

   (7) Connect the bag to oxygen at 15 LPM and attach a reservoir.

   (8) Squeeze the bag slowly and evenly, using only enough pressure to make the patient's chest rise.

      (a) Observe the rise and fall of the patient's chest with each ventilation.

      (b) Stop ventilation when adequate chest rise is observed.

      (c) Allow the patient to exhale between breaths.

   (9) Ventilate the patient at a rate of once every three seconds (20 breaths per minute).

ASSESSMENT OF THE INFANT AND CHILD

SCENE SIZE-UP

1. Determine if the emergency is due to trauma or a medical condition.
   a. If due to trauma, determine the mechanism of injury from the patient, family members, or bystanders and inspection of the scene.
   b. If due to a medical condition, determine the nature of the illness from the patient, family members, or bystanders.
2. Observe the patient's environment for clues to the cause of the emergency (e.g., pill bottles, household cleaners, mechanism of injury).

INITIAL ASSESSMENT

1. Maintain spinal immobilization if trauma is suspected.
2. Form a general impression of the patient.
   a. A general impression of a "well" versus a "sick" child can be obtained from the overall appearance and level of activity.
   b. Begin your assessment from a distance.
3. Assess the child's mental status.
   a. Does the child display appropriate behavior for his or her age?
   b. Is the child playing or moving around or does he or she appear drowsy or unaware of his or her surroundings?
   c. Does the child recognize his or her parents/caregiver?
   d. Does the child respond to the parent or caregiver calling his or her name?
   e. Does the child show interest in what is happening?
   f. Is the child agitated or irritable?
   g. Does the child appear confused or combative?
4. Assess the airway. A child who is crying or talking has an open airway.
5. Assess breathing.
   a. Note chest expansion/symmetry.
   b. Listen for:
      (1) Stridor (upper airway obstruction)
      (2) Wheezing (lower airway obstruction)

        (3) Grunting

   c. Look for signs of increased breathing effort, such as:

       (1) Nasal flaring (widening of the nostrils)

       (2) Retractions

       (3) Head bobbing (the child's head drops down with each inspiration and comes up with expansion of the chest)

       (4) Seesaw respirations

       (5) Use of accessory muscles

   d. Assess respiratory rate.

       (1) Observe the abdomen to count the respiratory rate.

       (2) **Normal ranges**

          (a) Infant: 25–50 breaths per minute

          (b) Child: 15–30 breaths per minute

6. Observe the child's skin color.

   a. Red (flushed) skin suggests the presence of a fever or exposure to heat.

   b. Pale, mottled, or grayish skin suggests poor tissue perfusion.

   c. Yellowing of the sclerae of the eyes and skin (jaundice) suggests a liver problem.

   d. Cyanosis may be due to a heart defect or severe respiratory distress.

7. Observe the child's position.

   a. In cases of serious upper airway obstruction, the child may instinctively assume the "sniffing" position (e.g., child seated and jaw thrust forward).

   b. In cases of severe respiratory distress, the child may assume the "tripod" position (e.g., child seated and leaning forward on outstretched arms) to maximize the use of the accessory muscles of respiration.

8. Listen for a change in voice or cry. Hoarseness may be caused by a foreign body or inflammation of the upper airway.

HANDS-ON ASSESSMENT OF THE INFANT OR CHILD PATIENT

1. In the conscious infant or child, begin with a toes-to-head or trunk-to-head approach.

   a. The order of assessment depends on the situation and age of the child.

   b. A toes-to-head or trunk-to-head approach should help reduce the infant or child's anxiety.

2. **Baseline vital signs**

   a. Assess breath sounds.

      (1) Listen below the clavicles in the midclavicular line and under the armpits along the midaxillary line.

      (2) Determine if breath sounds are present or absent.

         (a) Wheezing may be present due to swelling, spasm, secretions, or the presence of a foreign body.

         (b) If air movement is inadequate, wheezing may not be heard.

   b. Assess circulation.

      (1) Assess pulse.

         (a) Assess central and peripheral pulses.

           (i) Use the brachial or femoral pulses in an infant.

           (ii) Use the carotid and radial pulses in a child.

         (b) Note the rate, regularity (rhythm), and quality of the pulse. Pulse regularity normally changes with respirations (increases with inspiration, decreases with expiration).

         (c) Compare the strength of the peripheral pulse with that of the central pulse. A difference in strength between peripheral and central pulses may occur because of hypothermia or shock, among other causes.

      (2) Assess capillary refill in children 6 years of age or younger.

         (a) Normal capillary refill is less than 2 seconds.

         (b) Delayed capillary refill may occur because of shock or hypothermia, among other causes.

(3) Assess blood pressure in children older than 3 years of age.
  (a) Blood pressure is one of the LEAST sensitive indicators of adequate circulation in children.
  (b) A child may have compromised circulation despite a normal blood pressure.
  (c) A properly sized cuff must be used to obtain accurate readings.
    (i) A cuff that is too wide will cause a falsely low reading.
    (ii) A cuff that is too narrow will cause a falsely high reading.
  (d) The width of the cuff should be approximately two-thirds the length of the long bone used (e.g., upper arm, thigh).
  (e) In children older than 1 year of age, the following formula may be used to determine the lower limit of a normal systolic blood pressure: 70 + (2 × child's age in years) = systolic blood pressure.
  (f) The diastolic blood pressure should be approximately two-thirds the systolic pressure.
(4) Assess skin color, temperature, and moisture.
  (a) Hot skin suggests fever or heat exposure.
  (b) Cool skin suggests inadequate circulation or exposure to cold.
  (c) Cold skin suggests extreme exposure to cold.
  (d) Clammy (cool and moist) skin suggests shock, among many other conditions.
  (e) Wet or moist skin may indicate shock (hypoperfusion), a heat-related illness, or diabetic emergency.
  (f) Excessively dry skin may indicate dehydration.

AIRWAY AND BREATHING PROBLEMS IN INFANTS AND CHILDREN

RESPIRATORY DISTRESS AND RESPIRATORY FAILURE

1. The most common cause of cardiac arrent in adults is cardiac in origin. In children, cardiopulmonary arrest is usually the result of progressive deterioration in respiratory and circulatory function.
2. Respiratory distress is increased work of breathing (respiratory effort).
3. Respiratory failure is a condition in which there is inadequate oxygenation of the blood or inadequate elimination of carbon dioxide, or both.
   a. Respiratory failure is often preceded by respiratory distress.
   b. The child's work of breathing increases in an attempt to compensate for a lack of oxygen.
   (1) Respiratory rate increases.
   (2) Depth of breathing increases.
4. Causes of respiratory failure include:
   a. Infection (e.g., croup, epiglottitis, pneumonia)
   b. Foreign-body airway obstruction
   c. Asthma
   d. Smoke inhalation
   e. Trauma
5. Signs and symptoms of early respiratory distress include (*Table 30-1*):
   a. Restlessness
   b. Nasal flaring
   c. Increased heart rate
   d. Increased respiratory rate (tachypnea)
   e. Increased depth of breathing (hyperpnea)
   f. Head bobbing
   g. Seesaw respirations
   h. Grunting

Table 30-1. Signs of Respiratory Distress, Respiratory Failure, and Respiratory Arrest

Respiratory Distress	Respiratory Failure	Respiratory Arrest
Restlessness	Altered mental status	Unresponsiveness
Increased respiratory rate	Respiratory rate > 60/minute	Breathing rate
Increased heart rate	Increased heart rate	<10/minute
Increased depth of breathing	Poor peripheral perfusion	Slow or absent heart
Seesaw respirations	Decreased muscle tone	rate
Stridor	Severe use of accessory muscles	Weak or absent distal
Crowing	Cyanosis	pulses
Nasal flaring	Grunting	Limp muscle tone
Grunting	Head bobbing	
Head bobbing		
Retractions on inspiration		
Audible wheezing		

    i. Stridor
    j. Crowing
    k. Retractions on inspiration
    l. Audible wheezing
6. Emergency medical care for respiratory distress
    a. Keep the child with the caregiver.
    b. Allow the child to assume a position of comfort.
       (1) The child may sit on the caregiver's lap.
       (2) Do not force a conscious child to lie down.
    c. Administer high-flow oxygen.
       (1) Do not agitate the child to administer oxygen by nasal cannula or nonrebreather mask.
       (2) Allow the caregiver to administer blow-by oxygen.
       (3) Limit the physical examination to the essentials.
    d. Maintain normal body temperature.
    e. Transport promptly to the closest appropriate facility.
7. Signs and symptoms of respiratory failure include the signs of respiratory distress and any of the following (see *Table 30-1*):
    a. Respiratory rate greater than 60 breaths per minute
    b. Cyanosis
    c. Decreased muscle tone
    d. Severe use of accessory muscles
    e. Poor peripheral perfusion
    f. Altered mental status
8. Emergency medical care for respiratory failure
    a. Maintain an open airway.
    b. Administer 100% oxygen.
    c. Provide positive-pressure ventilation with 100% oxygen, if necessary.
    d. Maintain normal body temperature.
    e. Transport promptly to the closest appropriate facility.
9. Signs and symptoms of respiratory arrest include (see *Table 30-1*):
    a. Breathing rate less than 10 breaths per minute
    b. Limp muscle tone
    c. Unresponsiveness
    d. Slow or absent heart rate
    e. Weak or absent distal pulses
10. Emergency medical care for respiratory arrest
    a. Establish and maintain an open airway.

b. Provide positive-pressure ventilation with 100% oxygen.

c. Transport rapidly to the closest appropriate facility.

RESPIRATORY EMERGENCIES

1. The EMT-Basic must be able to recognize the difference between upper airway obstruction and lower airway disease.

2. **Upper airway obstruction**
   a. Stridor is heard on inspiration.
   b. Suspect a foreign-body airway obstruction in infants and children with a SUDDEN onset of respiratory distress associated with coughing, gagging, stridor, or wheezing.

3. **Lower airway disease**
   a. Wheezing and increased breathing effort occur on exhalation.
   b. Breathing is rapid (tachypnea) without stridor.
   c. There is no evidence of foreign-body obstruction.

MEDICAL PROBLEMS IN INFANTS AND CHILDREN

SEIZURES

1. Seizures in infants and children may be caused by epilepsy, head injury, infection, fever, poisoning, hypoglycemia, trauma, decreased levels of oxygen, failure to take antiseizure medication. Sometimes, the cause is unknown.

2. Seizures:
   a. May be brief or prolonged
   b. Are rarely life threatening in children who have them frequently
   c. Should be considered life threatening by the EMT-Basic

3. Febrile seizures:
   a. Are caused by a rapid rise in temperature
   b. May occur in healthy children from 6 months to 6 years of age
   c. Usually last less than 15 minutes
   d. Are the most common cause of seizures encountered by prehospital personnel in children younger than 5 years old

4. Assess for the presence of injuries that may have occurred during the seizure.

5. While taking the SAMPLE history, determine the following:
   a. Does the child have a history of seizures?
   b. If yes, is this the child's normal seizure pattern?
   c. Has the child taken his or her antiseizure medication?
   d. How long did the seizure last?
   e. Has the child been sick?
   f. Has the child had any recent immunizations?
   g. If the child has a fever, how long was it present before the seizure?

6. **Emergency medical care**
   a. Ensure an open airway.
   b. Position the child on his or her side if there is no possibility of cervical spine trauma.
   c. Be prepared to suction if necessary.
   d. Administer oxygen.
      (1) If breathing is adequate, administer oxygen at 15 LPM by nonrebreather mask.
      (2) If breathing is inadequate, provide positive-pressure ventilation with 100% oxygen and assess the adequacy of the ventilations delivered.
   e. Protect the child from physical injury.
      (1) Remove or loosen tight clothing.
      (2) Do not try to restrain body movements during the seizure.

    f. Transport promptly to the closest appropriate facility. Although brief seizures are not harmful, they may indicate a more dangerous underlying condition.

ALTERED MENTAL STATUS

1. Altered mental status can be caused by a variety of conditions, including:
   a. Alcohol ingestion (accidental in young child, possible abuse in older child/adolescent)
   b. Epilepsy/environmental conditions
   c. Infection
   d. Overdose (accidental in young child, possible suicide attempt in older child/adolescent)
   e. Uremia (kidney failure)
   f. Trauma/temperature
   g. Insulin (too much or too little)
   h. Psychological causes
   i. Stroke/shock
2. **Emergency medical care**
   a. Maintain spinal immobilization if trauma is suspected.
   b. Secure and maintain an open airway.
   c. Insert an OPA or NPA as needed.
   d. Be prepared to suction if necessary.
   e. Administer oxygen.
      (1) If breathing is adequate, administer oxygen at 15 LPM by nonrebreather mask.
      (2) If breathing is inadequate, provide positive-pressure ventilation with 100% oxygen and assess the adequacy of the ventilations delivered.
   f. Position the patient.
      (1) If the child is sitting or standing, help him or her to the floor.
      (2) If there is no possibility of cervical spine trauma, place the patient in a lateral recumbent (recovery) position.
      (3) If the child is immobilized due to suspected trauma and vomits, the child and backboard should be turned as a unit and the child's airway cleared with suctioning.
   g. Remove or loosen tight clothing.
   h. Maintain body temperature.
   i. Transport.

POISONINGS

1. Poisoning is a common reason for infant and child ambulance calls.
2. Commonly ingested substances include:
   a. Prescription and over-the-counter medications
   b. Cosmetics
   c. Plants
   d. Cleaning products
3. While taking the SAMPLE history, determine the following:
   a. Type of exposure (e.g., ingestion, inhalation, injection, absorption)
   b. Are there other victims?
   c. What substance was involved?
      (1) Look for clues (e.g., bottles, containers, plastic bags, injection equipment).
      (2) Bring container to the receiving facility if possible.
   d. How much of the substance was ingested?
   e. When did the exposure occur?
   f. Has any treatment been given since the exposure? Has any vomiting occurred?
   g. What is the child's weight?

    h. For older children and adolescents, prior suicide or psychiatric history?
4. Emergency medical care
    a. After ensuring the safety of the scene, remove the patient from the source of the poison.
    b. Assess the patient for airway secretions, unusual breath odor and sores on the mouth, tongue, or throat.
    c. Maintain spinal immobilization if trauma is suspected.
    d. If the patient is responsive:
        (1) Contact medical direction or poison center regarding the need to administer activated charcoal if the poison was ingested
        (2) Administer oxygen
            (a) If breathing is adequate, administer oxygen at 15 LPM by nonrebreather mask.
            (b) If breathing is inadequate, provide positive-pressure ventilation with 100% oxygen and assess the adequacy of the ventilations delivered.
        (3) Transport promptly, monitoring the patient closely en route to the receiving facility
    e. If the patient is unresponsive:
        (1) Establish and maintain an open airway
        (2) Be prepared to suction if necessary
        (3) Administer oxygen
            (a) If breathing is adequate, administer oxygen at 15 LPM by nonrebreather mask.
            (b) If breathing is inadequate, provide positive-pressure ventilation with 100% oxygen and assess the adequacy of the ventilations delivered.
        (4) Contact medical direction.
        (5) Perform a rapid trauma assessment to rule out trauma as a cause of the child's altered mental status.
        (6) Transport promptly to the closest appropriate facility.

FEVER

1. Fever is a common reason for infant or child ambulance calls.
2. Elevated body temperature may be caused by:
    a. Infection or inflammation (e.g., meningitis)
    b. Heat exposure
    c. Certain poisonings (e.g., aspirin)
    d. Severe dehydration
    e. Uncontrolled seizures
3. A fever with a rash is a potentially serious condition.
4. Emergency medical care
    a. Follow local protocol.
    b. Remove excess clothing.
    c. Be alert for seizures in infants and young children.
    d. If instructed to begin cooling measures by medical direction, sponge the child with lukewarm water.
    e. Do not use cold or ice water or alcohol to cool the child.
    f. Transport.

SHOCK (HYPOPERFUSION)

1. Shock rarely results from a primary cardiac problem in infants and children.
2. Common causes of shock in infants and children include:
    a. Diarrhea and dehydration
    b. Trauma
    c. Vomiting
    d. Blood loss

  e. Infection

  f. Abdominal injuries

 3. Less common causes of shock include:

  a. Allergic reactions

  b. Poisoning

  c. Cardiac disorders

 4. Signs and symptoms of shock include:

  a. Rapid respiratory rate

  b. Pale, cool, clammy skin

  c. Weak or absent peripheral pulses

  d. Delayed capillary refill

  e. Decreased urine output; measured by asking caregiver about diaper wetting and looking at diaper

  f. Mental status changes

  g. Absence of tears, even when crying

 5. Emergency medical care

  a. Ensure and maintain an open airway.

  b. Administer oxygen.

   (1) If breathing is adequate, administer oxygen at 15 LPM by nonrebreather mask.

   (2) If breathing is inadequate, provide positive-pressure ventilation with 100% oxygen and assess the adequacy of the ventilations delivered.

  c. Control any bleeding if present.

  d. If there is no history of trauma, elevate the patient's legs.

  e. Maintain normal body temperature.

  f. Transport rapidly to the closest appropriate facility.

NEAR-DROWNING

1. Drowning is a submersion injury that leads to death within the first 24 hours.

2. Near-drowning is a submersion injury in which there is survival for at least 24 hours after submersion.

3. Drowning is the second major cause of unintentional death in children.

4. Absence of adult supervision is a factor in most submersion incidents involving infants and children.

5. The near-drowning victim submersed in very cold water [less than 40° Fahrenheit (F) or 5° Celsius (C)] may have an improved survival rate because hypothermia reduces the brain's need for oxygen.

6. Predisposing conditions include:

 a. Seizures

 b. Alcohol ingestion (preadolescents and adolescents)

 c. Trauma, accidental and nonaccidental (e.g., suicide, child abuse, homicide)

7. The major injury from submersion is a lack of oxygen, which affects every organ system.

8. Scene size-up

 a. Study the scene and determine if approaching the patient is safe.

 b. Evaluate the mechanism of injury and determine, if possible:

  (1) Length of submersion

  (2) Cleanliness of the water

  (3) Temperature of the water

 c. Obtain additional help BEFORE contact with the patient, if needed.

 d. Protect the patient from environmental temperature extremes.

9. Initial assessment

 a. Maintain spinal immobilization as needed.

 b. Assess the patient's mental status.

      (1) Mental status may range from awake and alert to combative, difficult to arouse, or unresponsive.

      (2) These variations in mental status may be due to an associated injury or a lack of oxygen from submersion.

  c. Assess the patient's airway.

  d. Assess breathing.

  e. Assess circulation.

  f. Identify any life-threatening conditions and provide care based on those findings.

  g. Establish patient priorities.

10. Signs and symptoms of near-drowning will vary depending on the type and length of submersion and include:

  a. Coughing, vomiting, choking, airway obstruction

  b. Absent or inadequate breathing

  c. Difficulty breathing

  d. Absent, slow or increased heart rate

  e. Seizures

  f. Cool, clammy, pale, or cyanotic skin

  g. Possible gastric distention

11. Determine the events leading to the present situation.

  a. How long was the child submerged?

  b. What was the water temperature?

  c. Where did the incident occur (e.g., lake, pool, bathtub, toilet, bucket)?

  d. Was the child breathing when removed from the water?

  e. Was there a pulse?

  f. Did the child experience any loss of consciousness?

  g. Was the incident witnessed? (This information is useful in determining possible head or spinal injury.)

  h. Does the child have any significant medical problems?

  i. Look for signs of abuse or neglect.

12. Assess baseline vital signs.

13. Perform a focused physical examination, carefully assessing the patient for other injuries.

14. Emergency medical care

  a. Ensure the safety of all rescue personnel.

  b. Remove the patient from the water as quickly and safely as possible.

  c. Any pulseless, nonbreathing patient who has been submerged in cold water should be resuscitated.

  d. Suction as needed.

  e. Administer oxygen.

      (1) If breathing is adequate, administer oxygen at 15 LPM by nonrebreather mask.

      (2) If breathing is inadequate, provide positive-pressure ventilation with 100% oxygen and assess the adequacy of the ventilations delivered.

  f. If gastric distention interferes with artificial ventilation:

      (1) Place the patient on the left side

      (2) With suction immediately available, the EMT-Basic should place his or her hand over the epigastric area of the patient's abdomen and apply firm pressure to relieve the distention. This procedure should only be done if the gastric distention interferes with the ability to ventilate the patient effectively.

  g. Remove wet clothing and dry the patient to prevent heat loss.

  h. Transport promptly.

      (1) All near-drowning victims should be transported to the hospital.

      (2) If the patient is stable, perform ongoing assessments every 15 minutes.

(3) If the patient is unstable, perform ongoing assessments every 5 minutes.

SUDDEN INFANT DEATH SYNDROME

1. **Sudden Infant Death Syndrome** (SIDS) is the sudden and unexpected death of an infant or young child in which a careful autopsy cannot find an adequate cause of death.
   a. SIDS is also called "crib death" or "cot death."
   b. The cause or causes of SIDS are not known.
   c. Approximately 90% of all SIDS deaths occur between 2 and 6 months of age.
   d. By agreement among researchers, deaths in children younger than 1 month or older than 1 year of age are not classified as SIDS.
2. **Apparent life-threatening events**
   a. **Apparent life-threatening events** (ALTEs) were formerly known as "near-miss SIDS."
   b. An ALTE is described as:
      (1) An episode that is frightening to the observer, who feels the child died or would have died without vigorous intervention
      (2) The child has some combination of:
         (a) Apnea (absence of breathing)
         (b) Color change (cyanosis or pallor)
         (c) Marked change in muscle tone, usually extreme limpness
         (d) Choking or gagging
3. **Factors associated with SIDS**
   a. Peak age is between 2 and 4 months of age.
   b. Higher percentage of males are affected than females.
   c. Death occurs during or after periods of presumed sleep (naptime or night).
   d. Incidence increases in winter; peaks in January.
   e. Incidence is higher in Native Americans and African Americans, followed by Caucasians.
   f. Risk of SIDS is increased in low-birth-weight and premature infants and in twins.
   g. Incidence of SIDS is higher in infants born to women younger than 20 years of age.
   h. SIDS occurs in all socioeconomic levels.
   i. SIDS victims appear to be healthy before death.
4. Studies from countries other than the United States link sleeping in a prone position (on the stomach) with an increased risk of SIDS.
   a. It is not known whether sleeping in a prone position is in itself a risk factor or whether it depends on some other condition, such as sleeping on soft bedding.
   b. It has been found that infants sleeping on their stomachs on polystyrene-filled pillows may not be able to move their heads to get fresh air, resulting in suffocation.
   c. In 1992, the American Academy of Pediatrics recommended that babies be placed on their backs to sleep except in a few special situations (e.g., premature babies, babies with upper airway abnormalities).
5. SIDS is not caused by external suffocation, vomiting, or choking.
6. SIDS is not contagious and cannot be predicted or prevented, even by a physician.
7. Only an autopsy can conclusively determine if an infant's death is due to SIDS.
   a. The EMT-Basic should make no assumptions about the cause of death.
   b. The EMT-Basic should know some of the identifying features characteristic of the SIDS victim as opposed to the abused child.
8. **Signs and symptoms of SIDS**
   a. Infant appears well-nourished and well-developed.
   b. Skin may be mottled.
   c. Frothy, sometimes blood-tinged fluid in and around the mouth and nostrils (and bedclothes) is often present.

    d. Vomitus may be present.

    e. Diaper is usually wet and full of stool.

    f. No external signs of injury are present.

9. **Scene size-up**

    a. Observe the environment for signs of:

       (1) Illness (e.g., thermometer, humidifier, medications)

       (2) Possible accidental or intentional injury:

          (a) Recent surface injuries

          (b) Old injuries in various stages of healing

       (3) Suffocation (e.g., large pillow, plastic bed coverings)

       (4) Poisoning:

          (a) Heater (carbon monoxide)

          (b) Household cleaners

          (c) Plants

    b. Note:

       (1) Position of the infant (on back or stomach, covered or uncovered)

       (2) Physical appearance of the infant

       (3) Presence of objects in the crib

       (4) Appearance of the room/house

10. **SAMPLE history**

    a. When obtaining the history:

       (1) Be calm, direct, and nonjudgmental

       (2) Refer to the baby by name

    b. What happened?

    c. Where was the infant found?

    d. What time was the infant put to bed or fell asleep?

    e. When was the infant last fed? Appetite?

    f. Any changes in appetite, sleeping habits, usual routine in last 24–48 hours?

    g. Was CPR started?

    h. Was the infant moved?

    i. Past illnesses, hospitalizations, medications, immunizations?

11. **Emergency medical care**

    a. Begin resuscitation efforts unless there are obvious signs of death, such as:

       (1) Rigor mortis

          (a) Body stiffens after death.

          (b) It takes place quickly in infants (about 3 hours).

       (2) Dependent lividity (discoloration due to the pooling of blood in the lowest body areas after death)

    b. Reactions of caregivers vary.

       (1) Reactions may include anger, hysteria, physical shaking, crying, screaming, denial, or no expression of emotion.

       (2) Caregivers may express that the situation is due to something they did or did not do.

    c. Allow the family to verbalize their emotions.

    d. Avoid any comments that might suggest blame to the parents.

TRAUMA

INJURY PREVENTION

1. Injuries are the leading cause of childhood death and disability in the United States.

2. Common childhood injuries include:

    a. Motor vehicle passenger injuries

    b. Pedestrian injuries

    c. Bicycle injuries
    d. Submersion
    e. Burns
    f. Firearm injuries

MECHANISMS AND PATTERNS OF INJURY

1. **Motor vehicle passenger injuries**
   a. Nearly half of all pediatric injuries and deaths are associated with motor-vehicle–related trauma.
   b. Contributing factors include:
      (1) Failure to use (or improper use of) passenger restraints
      (2) Inexperienced adolescent drivers
      (3) Alcohol abuse
   c. Unrestrained passengers have head and neck injuries.
   d. Restrained passengers have abdominal and lower spine injuries.
2. **Pedestrian injuries**
   a. Pedestrian injuries are the leading cause of death among children 5–9 years of age.
   b. Child is unable to judge the speed of the traffic and typically bolts out into the street.
   c. They are often injured while chasing a toy, friend, or pet into the path of an oncoming vehicle.
   d. A child struck by a car is likely to sustain injury to the head, chest or abdomen, and an extremity (Waddell's triad).
      (1) Vehicle first strikes the left side of the child.
      (2) The bumper contacts the left femur, and the fender strikes left side of the abdomen.
      (3) The child is thrown against the vehicle's hood or windshield.
      (4) The child is thrown to the ground, striking the head on the pavement as the vehicle comes to a stop.
      (5) The child is then often run over by the vehicle.
3. **Bicycle injuries**
   a. Head trauma is the cause of most bicycle-related injuries and death.
   b. Other injuries associated with bicycle crashes include abdominal injuries (from striking the handle bars) and trauma to the face and extremities.
4. **Submersion**
   a. Submersion is a significant cause of death and disability in children younger than 4 years of age.
   b. Alcohol appears to be a significant risk factor in adolescent drowning.
5. **Burns and smoke inhalation**
   a. Approximately 80% of fire and burn-related deaths result from house fires.
   b. Most fire-related deaths occur in private residences, usually in homes without working smoke detectors.
   b. Smoke inhalation, scalds, and contact and electrical burns are especially likely to affect children younger than 4 years of age.
6. **Firearm injuries**
   a. Firearm homicide is the leading cause of death among African-American adolescents and young adults.
   b. Most guns used in unintentional shootings are found in the home and often found loaded in readily accessible places.
   c. The presence of a gun in the home has been linked to an increased likelihood of adolescent suicide.
   d. Injuries caused by a firearm include an entrance wound, exit wound, and an internal wound.
7. **Falls**
   a. Falls are the most common cause of injury in infants and children.

b. Infants and young children have large heads in comparison to their body size, making them more prone to falls

c. Note:

    (1) The distance of the fall; any fall more than three times the child's height should be considered serious

    (2) The surface on which the child landed

        (a) Concrete and asphalt are associated with more severe injuries than other surfaces.

        (b) Children who land on hard ground or concrete sustain more severe injury than those who hit grass, even when the heights of the falls are similar.

    (3) The body area(s) struck

d. If the child fell from a height or was diving into shallow water, suspect injuries to the head and neck.

8. Sports injuries. Sports injuries often involve injuries to the head and neck.

HEAD INJURY

1. Head injury is the most frequent cause of death in the pediatric trauma patient.

2. Most children who experience multiple injuries also have a head injury because:

    a. The child's cranium is thin and provides little protection for the brain

    b. The head makes up a greater percentage of body area and weight, making it susceptible to injury

    c. The cervical spine muscles are poorly developed and provide little support for the head

3. The scalp of an infant and young child is proportionately larger and more vascular than an adult's.

    a. A minor scalp laceration (cut) can cause significant blood loss, resulting in shock.

    b. Direct pressure is usually adequate to control bleeding.

4. Signs and symptoms of head injury (vary according to location and severity of injury) include:

    a. Altered mental status (usually the first sign of head injury)

    b. Headache

    c. Nausea and vomiting

    d. Abnormal behavior

    e. Seizures

    f. Dilation of one pupil

    g. Dilation of both pupils, unresponsive to light (late sign, suggests severe brain injury)

5. The most common cause of hypoxia in the unresponsive head injury patient is the tongue obstructing the airway.

6. If signs and symptoms of shock are present with a closed head injury, look for signs of other injuries (e.g., internal bleeding) that may be the cause of the hypoperfusion.

7. Respiratory arrest is common secondary to severe head injuries and may occur during transport.

CHEST TRAUMA

1. Chest trauma in children most often occurs as a result of blunt trauma (e.g., motor vehicle crashes, falls).

2. Children have an elastic chest wall and soft, pliable ribs. Because the ribs tend to bend, rather than break, rib fractures are less common in infants and young children than in adults.

3. Because of the flexibility of the chest wall and ribs, significant injury may occur to underlying organs and vessels without any external signs of injury.

ABDOMINAL TRAUMA

1. The abdomen is a more common site of injury in children than in adults.
2. The abdominal muscles of an infant and young child are thin and not as well developed as an adult's, providing poor protection for the abdominal organs.
3. The abdomen is often a source of hidden injury.
   a. In children, the spleen is the most commonly injured abdominal organ, followed by the liver.
   b. Injury to the liver is the most common abdominal injury that leads to death.
4. Always consider abdominal injury in the multiple trauma patient who is deteriorating without external signs of injury.
5. The major muscle of respiration in children is the diaphragm.
   a. Excessive air can collect in the stomach (gastric distention) because of positive-pressure ventilation or swallowing air when crying.
   b. Gastric distention interferes with movement of the diaphragm, thus interfering with breathing, and can contribute to vomiting.

EXTREMITY TRAUMA

1. Extremity injuries are common in children and are managed in the same manner as in adults.
2. Three common injuries require close monitoring and immediate care:
   a. Pelvic fractures, which most often occur due to motor vehicle crashes, including pedestrian–motor vehicle crashes
   b. Femur fractures, which can result in significant blood loss; for example, a closed femur fracture may be responsible for 300 to 400 mL of blood loss and can contribute to hypovolemic shock
   c. Open fractures, which carry an increased risk of infection due to contamination

BURNS

1. In children younger than 3 years old, scald burns from hot liquids are the most common cause of burns.
2. When obtaining a history, it is important to determine:
   a. The nature of the burned material
   b. The duration of the exposure
   c. If the exposure occurred in an enclosed space
   d. If the child was found unresponsive, or if the child had a period of unresponsiveness
3. Determine the severity of the burn by considering:
   a. The depth of the burn
   b. Total body surface area burned (rule of nines)
   c. Age of the child
   d. Presence of any preexisting medical conditions
   e. Presence of any associated injuries
4. Transport to an appropriate facility based on the severity of the burn and local protocol.

EMERGENCY MEDICAL CARE FOR TRAUMATIC INJURIES

1. Maintain spinal immobilization.
   a. Any patient with an injury above the clavicles should be assumed to have a spinal cord injury and be immobilized accordingly.
   b. An unresponsive infant or child should always be immobilized, even when the cause is unknown.
   c. Do not use sandbags to stabilize a child's head. If the board needs to be turned because of patient vomiting, the weight of the sandbags on the child's head may cause injury.

2. Establish and maintain an open airway.
   a. Open the airway using a jaw thrust.
   b. Be prepared to suction if necessary with a large-bore suction catheter.
3. Administer oxygen.
   a. If the patient's breathing is adequate, apply oxygen by nonrebreather mask at 15 LPM if not already done.
   b. If the patient's breathing is inadequate, provide positive-pressure ventilation with 100% oxygen and assess the adequacy of the ventilations delivered.
4. Transport to the closest appropriate facility.
   a. Children with the following conditions should be transported as quickly as possible to a pediatric center:
      (1) Unstable airway
      (2) Obvious respiratory insufficiency
      (3) Shock
      (4) Altered mental status
   b. Follow local protocol.

PNEUMATIC ANTI-SHOCK GARMENT (PASG)

1. Use of the PASG is controversial; follow local protocol.
2. Indications include trauma with signs of severe hypoperfusion and pelvic instability.
3. Use the PASG only if the garment fits the child (do not place an infant in one leg of the PASG).
4. Do not inflate the abdominal compartment.
   a. Inflation of the abdominal compartment may limit breathing by interfering with movement of the diaphragm.
   b. It may compress the stomach, resulting in vomiting.
5. The PASG should not be used in children with penetrating wounds to the chest or abdomen.

CHILD ABUSE AND NEGLECT

DEFINITIONS

1. **Child maltreatment** includes intentional physical abuse or neglect, emotional abuse or neglect, and sexual abuse of children, usually by adults.
2. **Neglect** is defined as giving insufficient attention or respect to someone who has a claim to that attention.
   a. Child neglect is the failure of a parent or other person legally responsible for the child's welfare to provide for the child's basic needs and an adequate level of care.
   b. Child neglect is the most common form of maltreatment.
      (1) **Physical neglect** is defined as the lack of necessities such as food, clothing, shelter, medical care, education, and supervision.
      (2) **Emotional neglect** is defined as failure to meet the child's needs for attention, affection, and emotional growth.
3. **Abuse** is improper or excessive action so as to injure or cause harm.
   a. **Physical abuse** is the deliberate act of causing physical injury to a child.
   b. **Emotional abuse** is the deliberate attempt to destroy or impair a child's self-esteem or competence.
   c. **Sexual abuse** is the "use, persuasion, or coercion of any child to engage in sexually explicit conduct (or any simulation of such conduct) for producing any visual depiction of such conduct, or rape, molestation, prostitution, or incest with children" (The Child Abuse and Prevention Act, Public Law 100-294).

SIGNS AND SYMPTOMS OF ABUSE

1. **Bruises and welts**
   a. The pattern of bruises and welts is suggestive of object used (e.g., hand, wire hanger, rope, belt buckle, human bite marks, pinch marks).
   b. Multiple bruises in various stages of healing may be seen.
   c. Bruises on the cheeks, abdomen, back, buttocks, and inner thigh should raise suspicion of abuse.
2. **Burns.** Types of burns seen in abuse include:
   a. Circular burns from a cigarette or cigar
   b. Rope burns on wrists from being bound
   c. Burns in the shape of a household utensil or appliance (e.g., heated fork, spoon, iron)
   d. "Glovelike" or "stockinglike" burns with no associated splash marks
      (1) These burns are caused by immersion in scalding water.
      (2) They are usually present on the buttocks, perineum, genitalia, or extremities.
3. Injury is inconsistent with the mechanism described.
4. Repeated law-enforcement and emergency calls are made to the same address.
5. Parents seem inappropriately unconcerned.
6. Parents or child give conflicting stories about the incident.
7. The child is afraid to discuss how the injury occurred.

SIGNS AND SYMPTOMS OF NEGLECT

Signs and symptoms of neglect include:
1. Lack of adult supervision
2. Unsafe living environment
3. Poor skin hygiene
4. Lack of medical attention for infections or injuries
5. Malnourished-appearing child
6. Untreated medical problems
   a. Lack of necessary immunizations
   b. Failure to provide required medication (e.g., asthmatic child with no medication)

HEAD INJURY DUE TO CHILD ABUSE

1. Head injury is the leading cause of death from child abuse.
2. Most victims are younger than 2 years of age.
3. Head injury occurs as a result of:
   a. Vigorous shaking of an infant (Shaken Baby Syndrome)
   b. Pressure on the carotid arteries of the neck during shaking, resulting in decreased oxygenation of the brain and swelling
   c. A direct blow to the head; the infant is both shaken and struck on the head (Shaken Impact Syndrome)
4. Rib fractures and grip marks on the extremities may be present from violent shaking.
5. Child may experience apnea, seizures, and/or may be slow to respond.

ABDOMINAL TRAUMA DUE TO CHILD ABUSE

1. Abdominal injuries are the second leading cause of death from child abuse.
2. Blunt trauma is the most common type of abdominal trauma in children, usually the result of a punch or kick to the abdomen.
3. Because the child's abdominal wall is elastic and absorbs much of the force, only mild bruising may be seen or there may be no external sign of injury.
4. Child may experience abdominal tenderness, vomiting, and/or signs of shock.

HISTORY AND PHYSICAL EXAMINATION

1. When gathering the history:
   a. Obtain the history in a nonaccusatory manner
   b. Do not accuse the caregiver(s) in the field
      (1) Accusation and confrontation delay transportation and patient care.
      (2) Bring objective information to the receiving facility.
2. When performing the physical examination, consider the following:
   a. Where is the injury?
   b. Is the injury/condition compatible with the history given?
   c. Is this type of injury consistent with what you would expect for the child's age group?
   d. How did the injury occur?
   e. Are there any other unexplained injuries on the child's body?
   f. What are the size and shape of the injury (if applicable)?
   g. Does the child appear clean and well-cared for?
   h. Does there appear to have been a delay in calling for medical attention?

REPORTING REQUIREMENTS

1. Every state has reporting requirements regarding cases of suspected child abuse and neglect.
2. The EMT-Basic must be familiar with the specific procedure for reporting in his or her area.
3. Document objectively.
   a. Describe what you see and hear, NOT what you think.
   b. Describe the environment in which the child was found.
   c. Document the behaviors and interactions between the child and caregiver(s).
   d. Describe each injury.
4. Privately provide a thorough verbal report to appropriate personnel at the receiving facility.

INFANTS AND CHILDREN WITH SPECIAL NEEDS

OVERVIEW

1. Children with special needs may also be referred to as "technology-assisted children."
2. Children experiencing a chronic or terminal illness are being cared for at home with high-technology equipment.
3. Types of children with special needs include:
   a. Premature babies with lung disease
   b. Babies and children with heart disease
   c. Infants and children with neurologic disease
   d. Children with chronic disease or altered function from birth
4. Often, these children will be at home, technologically dependent.

TRACHEOSTOMY TUBES

1. A **tracheostomy** is the creation of a surgical opening into the trachea through the neck, with insertion of a tube to aid passage of air or removal of secretions. The surgical opening created is called a **stoma.**
2. A tracheostomy may be temporary or permanent.
   a. A temporary tracheostomy is sewn closed when no longer needed.
   b. In a permanent tracheostomy, a tube is inserted to keep the stoma open.
3. Tracheostomy tubes come in a variety of types and sizes.
   a. Tubes may be metal or plastic.

b. They may be cuffed or uncuffed.

c. Tube selection depends on the patient's condition and physician preference.

4. Complications that may be encountered by the EMT-Basic include:

    a. Obstruction of the tube by dried secretions, excessive secretions, or airway swelling

    b. Dislodgment from coughing, patient movement, accidental removal, or inability to reinsert after a routine change

    c. Bleeding

    d. Air leak

    e. Infection

5. **Emergency medical care**

    a. Maintain an open airway.

        (1) If the tracheostomy tube has become dislodged and the caregiver is unable to replace it, ventilate the patient as needed with a bag-valve mask.

        (2) Seal the bag-valve mask over the child's mouth and nose and cover the stoma with a gloved hand.

        (3) If unsuccessful, cover the stoma with a small mask and attempt to ventilate through the stoma. At the same time, cover the child's mouth and nose with a gloved hand.

    b. If needed, suction the tracheostomy tube to clear secretions. Limit suctioning to no more than 5 seconds at a time.

    c. If external bleeding is present, apply gentle direct pressure to the bleeding site, being careful not to block the airway or apply pressure to the carotid arteries.

    d. Allow the patient to maintain a position of comfort.

    e. Transport.

HOME MECHANICAL VENTILATORS

1. Mechanical ventilators are used to assist breathing in patients who are unable to breathe adequately on their own.

2. Ventilator equipment is usually managed by a supplier that provides 24-hour emergency service. The home ventilator has an internal backup battery in case of power failure.

3. Ventilator malfunction is usually due to mechanical failure, power outage, or low oxygen supply.

4. **Emergency medical care**

    a. If the ventilator is malfunctioning and the caregiver cannot quickly determine the cause of the problem, disconnect the child from the ventilator.

    b. Establish and maintain an open airway.

    c. Provide positive-pressure ventilation with a bag-valve mask. If the child has a tracheostomy tube in place, the bag-valve device can be connected directly to the tracheostomy tube.

    d. Transport.

CENTRAL LINES

1. A **central line** is an intravenous (IV) line placed near the heart for long-term use.

    a. Central lines may be used to administer medications and nutritional solutions directly into the venous circulation.

    b. Central lines may also be referred to by the manufacturers' name (e.g., Broviac, Hickman, Groshong, Corcath).

    c. Central lines may be placed in the subclavian vein or, often, the femoral vein in children.

2. Peripherally inserted central catheters:

    a. Are also called PICC lines

    b. Are smaller in size than those routinely used for central lines

    c. Are often used for neonates, young children, or those requiring only short-term therapy because of their small size

3. Complications include:
   a. Cracked line
   b. Infection
   c. Clotting off
   d. Bleeding
4. **Emergency medical care**
   a. Establish and maintain an open airway.
   b. Administer oxygen if needed.
   c. If bleeding, apply direct pressure to the site with a sterile dressing.
   d. Transport.

GASTROSTOMY TUBES AND GASTRIC FEEDING

1. A **gastrostomy tube** is a special catheter placed directly into the stomach for feeding. It is most often used for children in whom passage of a tube through the mouth, pharynx, or esophagus is contraindicated or impossible.
2. The usual gastrostomy tube protrudes approximately 12–15 inches from the skin and is sewn in place.
3. A skin-level **"feeding button"** may be used in children who require long-term gastrostomy feedings.
   a. The "button" is small, made of silicone, and protrudes slightly from the abdomen.
   b. The button has a one-way valve that accepts a feeding tube.
   c. It allows the child greater mobility and comfort, and is easier to care for, than customary gastrostomy tubes.
4. **Emergency medical care**
   a. Establish and maintain an open airway.
   b. Be prepared to suction if necessary.
   c. Be alert for changes in mental status. If the child is a diabetic, he or she will become hypoglycemic quickly if he or she cannot be fed.
   d. Administer oxygen as needed.
   e. Transport the patient in a sitting (Fowler's) position or lying on the right side, with the head elevated.

SHUNTS

1. **Hydrocephalus** is a condition in which there is an excess of cerebrospinal fluid (CSF) within the brain.
2. A **ventricular shunt** is a drainage system used to remove the excess CSF (*Figure 30-3*).
   a. A catheter is surgically implanted in the lateral ventricle in the brain.
   b. The catheter is connected to a reservoir that collects the fluid.
      (1) The reservoir can usually be felt through the skin behind the ear.
      (2) A one-way valve prevents fluid from flowing back into the ventricle.
   c. The reservoir is connected to a drainage catheter that empties into the peritoneal cavity.
3. The major complications associated with shunts include infection and malfunction due to obstruction, kinking, plugging, displacement, or separation of the tubing.
   a. If the shunt becomes obstructed, excess CSF will collect in the brain.
   b. Because the skull is a rigid vault, pressure within the skull will increase, producing signs and symptoms similar to those of a patient with a head injury. These include:
      (1) Change in mental status
      (2) Headache
      (3) Irritability
      (4) Vomiting
      (5) Seizures

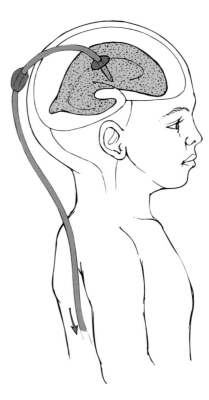

Fig. 30-3. A ventricular shunt is a drainage system used to remove excess cerebrospinal fluid (CSF). A catheter is surgically implanted in the lateral ventricle in the brain. The catheter is connected to a reservoir that collects the fluid. A one-way valve prevents fluid from flowing back into the ventricle. The reservoir is connected to a drainage catheter that empties into the peritoneal cavity.

      (6) Respiratory depression
  4. Emergency medical care
    a. Establish and maintain an open airway.
    b. Be prepared to suction if necessary.
    c. Administer oxygen.
      (1) If the patient's breathing is adequate, apply oxygen by nonrebreather mask at 15 LPM if not already done.
      (2) If the patient's breathing is inadequate, provide positive-pressure ventilation with 100% oxygen.
    d. Transport.

RESPONSES TO ILL AND INJURED INFANTS AND CHILDREN

FAMILY RESPONSE

1. A child cannot be cared for in isolation from the family; therefore, you have multiple patients.
2. Your calm and supportive interaction with the family will result in an improved ability to deal with the child.
    a. Calm parents = calm child
    b. Agitated parents = agitated child
3. Family members experience anxiety because of their concern for their child's pain and fear for the child's well-being. Their anxiety is worsened by a sense of helplessness.
4. Although many parents may not have medical training, they are experts on what is normal or abnormal for their child and what will calm him or her.

a. Allow the parents to remain part of the child's care unless the child's medical condition requires separation.

b. Ask the parents to calm the child.

c. The parents can help the child maintain a position of comfort and administer blow-by oxygen.

THE EMT-BASIC'S RESPONSE

1. You may experience anxiety when treating children because of:
   a. A lack of experience in treating children
   b. A fear of failure
   c. Identifying the patient with your own children
2. To help reduce your anxiety:
   a. Remember that much of what you have learned regarding the care of adults can be applied to children, but you need to keep in mind the differences between adults and children
   b. Prepare in advance
      (1) Practice frequently with equipment.
      (2) Practice examining children.

REVIEW QUESTIONS

Directions: Each of the numbered items or incomplete statements in this section is followed by answers or by completions of the statement. Select the ONE lettered answer or completion that is BEST in each case.

1. The fontanels (soft spots) are areas of the skull that have not fused together. These areas provide a window to the brain when assessing young children for dehydration or closed head trauma. The anterior fontanel, the last to close, closes at approximately what age?

    (A) 1–2 months of age
    (B) 12–18 months of age
    (C) 2–3 years of age
    (D) 13–18 years of age

2. To clear a complete airway obstruction due to foreign body (choking) for an unconscious infant (younger than 1 year of age), the correct technique would be

    (A) continuous abdominal thrusts until the airway is cleared
    (B) repeat series of back blows and chest thrusts until the obstruction is cleared
    (C) repeat series of back blows, chest thrusts, and airway evaluation until the obstruction is cleared
    (D) repeat series of back blows, chest thrusts, and blind finger sweeps until the obstruction is cleared

3. Which of the following regarding the use of bag-valve masks in children is correct?

    (A) A "pop-off" (pressure-release) valve should be used to prevent over-inflation
    (B) To deliver adequate ventilations, the bag-valve mask should be squeezed quickly and evenly

(C) For children younger than 8 years of age, the correct rate of ventilatory assistance is 1 breath every 3 seconds

(D) When ventilating unconscious infants, the patient's chin should be on the chest to maintain a patent (open) airway

4. Which of the following regarding circulation in infants is correct?

(A) Assessment of blood pressure is vital to monitoring the progress of these patients

(B) When assessing peripheral pulses, the correct location is the carotid artery of the neck

(C) Capillary refill assessment provides valuable information about the patient's circulatory status

(D) An early sign of circulatory compromise in these patients is a slow heart rate (less than 100)

5. Your rescue crew has been called to a local flood-control basin for a 12-year-old boy who was swept away by flood waters following a sudden storm. Upon your arrival, the patient is being moved from the water to a treatment area by a team trained in swift-water rescue techniques. The patient is apneic, pulseless, cold, and blue. A swift-water rescue technician informs you that the patient has been in the water for 20 minutes. Appropriate treatment would include

(A) call for the coroner

(B) warm the patient and begin cardiopulmonary resuscitation (CPR) when the patient's rectal temperature reaches 95° Fahrenheit (F)

(C) perform CPR and continue to warm the patient until arrival at the emergency department

(D) perform CPR and keep the patient cool until arrival at the emergency department to slow the child's metabolism

6. Sudden Infant Death Syndrome (SIDS) is caused by

(A) malnutrition
(B) physical abuse
(C) airway obstruction
(D) a yet unknown cause

7. Which of the following regarding children and trauma is correct?

(A) Abdominal injuries are rare in children
(B) Children's skulls are thin and provide little protection for the brain
(C) Children will commonly have fractured ribs following chest trauma
(D) Children in seat belts will seldom be injured as a result of a motor vehicle collision

8. In children, the first sign of a major head injury is

(A) seizures
(B) vomiting
(C) altered mental status
(D) unequal pupil reaction

9. The use of the pneumatic anti-shock garment (PASG) is controversial. If local protocol dictates the application of the PASG, which of the following statements would be correct?

(A) The PASG is effective in stabilizing pelvic fractures
(B) The PASG may be used to stabilize patients with penetrating chest injuries

(C) The abdominal compartment should be fully inflated before inflating the leg compartments

(D) If the patient is too small for the PASG, put both of the patient's legs in one leg of the PASG

Directions: Each of the numbered questions or incomplete statements in this section refers to a scenario that precedes them. The numbered questions or incomplete statements are followed by answers or by completions of the statement. Select the answer or completion of the statement that is BEST in each case.

---

10. Your ambulance crew is called to the home of an 8-year-old girl who fell from her bicycle. This is the fourth time this month you have been to the same house for an injured child. The patient initially tells you she fell off her bike, but then changes her story. Her body is covered with bruises in different stages of healing. You suspect the child has been physically abused. You should

   (A) question the child about the possible abuse
   (B) question the parents about their discipline habits and document your findings
   (C) treat and transport the patient, document all your findings, and express your concerns to the emergency department physician
   (D) treat the child and transport only if medically necessary. If the child is not transported, start keeping a detailed log with regard to your suspicions

11. Your rescue crew is called to the home of a 2-year-old boy with difficulty breathing. Upon arrival, the patient's mother tells you the patient's tracheostomy tube sounds clogged and that he is having difficulty getting his breath. You assess the patient's airway and breathing and conclude that suctioning is necessary. You should

   (A) provide oxygen before and after suctioning and suction for no more than 5 seconds per attempt
   (B) remove the tracheostomy tube, clean it in sterile water or normal saline, then put it back in place
   (C) attempt to dislodge the obstruction with subdiaphragmatic abdominal thrusts (Heimlich maneuver)
   (D) provide oxygen by nonrebreather mask and transport with lights and siren to the closest appropriate facility

Your rescue crew is called to the home of a 2-year-old male child with shortness of breath. You arrive to find this patient conscious and alert in his mother's arms. She informs you that her son has had a three-day history of a productive cough and runny nose. He is not presently taking any medications.

Questions 12–13

12. To make the child more at ease with your presence, you should

   (A) introduce yourself and try to hold him
   (B) develop a rapport with the patient's mother
   (C) inspect the patient's airway with a pen light
   (D) separate the mother and child and perform an initial assessment

13. When performing a focused physical examination, you should

(A) attempt to hold the patient for better control
(B) examine the trunk before examining the head
(C) speak in a harsh tone that demands respect and submission
(D) explain the entire procedure to the child before beginning the examination

Your ambulance crew is called to the home of a 4-month-old female infant with difficulty breathing and a history of an upper respiratory infection. You arrive on scene to find this patient pale and sleepy in her father's arms. There is a considerable amount of viscous (thick), yellow discharge coming from the patient's nose.

Questions 14–16

14. To open the airway of this patient, you should

(A) perform a jaw thrust
(B) hyperextend the head and neck
(C) place the patient's chin on her chest
(D) place the head in the neutral or sniffing position

15. Which of the following is true regarding this patient's airway and breathing?

(A) The tongue is proportionally smaller in children than adults
(B) An early sign of infant respiratory distress is bradypnea (slow respiratory rate)
(C) It is a common and nonsignificant finding for children this age to grunt during exhalation
(D) Children this age are obligate nose breathers and she may not open her mouth to breathe if the nose is obstructed

16. After assessing the airway, you determine a need for suctioning. Which of the following is a correct guideline for suctioning this patient's nasal passages?

(A) Use a rigid catheter and suction for no more than 15 seconds
(B) Use a bulb syringe and suction on insertion for no more than 10 seconds
(C) Use a bulb syringe and suction on withdrawal for no more than 5 seconds
(D) Use a rigid catheter and suction on insertion for no more than 15 seconds

Your rescue crew is called to the home of an 11-month-old male infant experiencing a seizure. The family does not speak English and you have no translator immediately available. When you arrive at the scene, the patient is lying on a couch with his eyes open. He does not respond to you.

Questions 17–19

17. After the scene size-up, your first priority is to

(A) assess vital signs
(B) perform an initial assessment
(C) find someone to translate for you
(D) perform a rapid trauma assessment

18. Which of the following findings would be consistent with a febrile seizure?

(A) The patient's fontanels are bulging
(B) The patient's skin is red and flushed
(C) The patient's mouth is blistered and red
(D) The patient's body is stiff and the extremities turned outward

19. The patient's rectal temperature is 103.5° Fahrenheit (F). He is still unresponsive but is not actively seizing. Appropriate treatment would include

(A) put the patient in an ice-water bath
(B) apply ice to the groin, neck, and armpits
(C) administer acetaminophen (Children's Tylenol®)
(D) remove the patient's clothing and cool with moist towels

Your ambulance crew is called to the home of an 8-month-old female infant. Information at time of dispatch is that "the parents are unable to wake the child."

Questions 20–22

20. Upon arrival, you are met by very distraught parents who ask you to begin cardiopulmonary resuscitation (CPR) to save their baby. You first action should be to

(A) open the baby's airway
(B) perform a scene size-up
(C) assess the baby's mental status
(D) perform a focused history and physical examination

21. Which of the following signs would be consistent with Sudden Infant Death Syndrome (SIDS)?

(A) Bulging fontanels
(B) Blood leaking from the ears
(C) Blood-tinged fluid in the mouth
(D) Multiple bruises about the chest and abdomen

22. Under which circumstances would you consider NOT beginning cardiopulmonary resuscitation (CPR) on this patient?

(A) The infant is cyanotic
(B) The infant has a large amount of vomitus in the airway
(C) The infant has cold extremities and a warm trunk
(D) The infant has pooling of blood where she was in contact with the bed

ANSWERS AND RATIONALES

1-B. While they are present, the fontanels provide quick and valuable information about the patient's brain. Generally, the posterior fontanels close between 2 and 6 months of age. The anterior fontanels close between 12 and 18 months of age. A normal fontanel should be soft and level with or just slightly below the exterior surface of the skull. Bulging fontanels are indicative of increased pressure in the brain cavity. Sunken fontanels are indicative of dehydration (which may occur rapidly in sick infants).

2-C. The correct sequence to follow once you conclude that the airway is obstructed is as follows: five back blows; five chest thrusts; look in the airway; attempt to ventilate; if unsuccessful, reattempt to ventilate; if unsuccessful, begin again with five back blows. If the child were conscious, you would repeat a series of back blows and chest thrusts until the airway is clear or the child becomes unconscious. Never perform blind finger sweeps in infants or children.

3-C. The correct rate at which to assist ventilations for children is 1 ventilation every 3 seconds (20 respirations per minute). A bag-valve mask used for pediatric resuscitation should not have a pop-off valve. If it does have one, the valve should be secured shut. A pop-off valve may not allow effective ventilation. When delivering ventilations (either by bag-valve mask, pocket mask, by mouth-to-mouth/mouth-to-mouth-and-nose ventilation) to any patient regardless of age, the ventilations should be slow and even. This prevents gastric distention (air in the stomach) which decreases expansion of the diaphragm and increases the chances of vomiting and aspiration. The head should be maintained in the neutral or sniffing position.

4-C. While capillary refill in adults is generally considered less than reliable, it is a valuable tool in assessing the perfusion status of children 6 years of age or younger. Normal capillary refill is less than 2 seconds. To assess capillary refill, blanch (pinch) the nail beds, then observe the amount of time necessary for the return of normal color to the nail bed. Blood pressure in children 3 years of age or younger is one of the least sensitive indicators of perfusion status. The brachial artery is the correct area to assess peripheral pulses in infants, and a pulse rate of less than 100 is an ominous sign of imminent circulatory collapse.

5-C. Unless there are obvious indications that this patient is unsalvageable (e.g., exposed brain tissue), begin cardiopulmonary resuscitation (CPR) and attempt to warm the patient en route to the hospital. It is not uncommon for children to recover completely after prolonged submersion in cold water. Provide the best treatment possible and transport rapidly.

6-D. While there are many theories about what may contribute to Sudden Infant Death Syndrome (SIDS) [second-hand smoke, sleeping position, mattress construction, etc.], the exact cause is yet unknown. SIDS is pronounced the cause of death only after all other factors are ruled out.

7-B. Children's heads are proportionally larger, their necks are proportionally weaker, and their skulls are thinner than adults'. Head trauma is a serious and frequent complication associated with motor vehicle accidents, bicycle accidents, and falls. Because the abdominal muscles are less developed and the abdominal organs less protected, abdominal injuries among children are not rare. Blunt or penetrating trauma may severely compromise the pediatric abdomen. Rib fractures among children are rare because of the elasticity of the bones; however, severe damage to underlying structures (e.g., heart, lungs) may result from blunt trauma that leaves little or no external sign of damage. You must carefully consider the mechanism of injury for all pediatric patients.

8-C. While it is sometimes difficult to evaluate, a change in the child's mental status is the first sign of head trauma. One of the most effective techniques for evaluating a child's mental status is to ask a parent or guardian, "Does he or she appear to be acting normally to you?" Subtle changes that may elude health care providers are generally evident to the patient's family and friends. Seizures, vomiting, and unequal pupil reaction may be indicative of a major head injury, but do not occur as early as does an altered mental status.

9-A. Because the pneumatic anti-shock garment (PASG) exerts equal pressure around the entire pelvis, it may be used to stabilize a pelvic fracture. It is, however, contraindicated in patients with penetrating chest or abdominal injuries. Because children rely heavily on the diaphragm for breathing, the abdominal compartment should not be inflated as it may impair lung expansion. The PASG is available in different sizes. If you do not have a size suitable for correct application, do not alter the device or its application—do not apply it at all.

10-C. If you suspect abuse, all efforts should be made to transport the child to an appropriate facility. Attempt to gather as much information as possible without appearing to be too intrusive. It is difficult not to get emotionally involved when a child has been injured, but your professionalism may be the key to getting the matter handled appropriately. If you suspect abuse and the parents/guardian refused transport, discretely contact medical direction and law enforcement as per local protocol. Make sure that your documentation of the incident is complete, accurate, and without drawn conclusions or personal bias.

11-A. As with all pediatric patients, you should suction for a maximum of 5 seconds, and oxygen therapy should be provided between suctioning attempts. A flexible catheter is generally used to clear obstructed tracheostomy tubes. Remember to suction only on withdrawal, not on insertion. If you have problems or questions, consult medical direction. If the patient is in severe respiratory distress and you are unable to correct the obstruction, request advanced-life-support assistance or immediately begin rapid transport.

12-B. At this age, children are very attached to their parents and guardians. You are a perceived threat. If you show that the parent trusts you, the child may open up to you. Attempting to hold him, sticking a light in his eyes, or separating him from his mother may be disastrous (not necessarily for the child's health, but for your ability to evaluate him).

13-B. A child may watch and interact if you assess the abdomen and chest first. If you go straight to the patient's head, again you will be perceived as a threat to his safety. Whenever possible, have the parent hold the patient during the examination. Children understand tone at a very young age. Use a gentle tone and simple explanations. Overexplaining your intentions may only confuse and upset the child. Be gentle, nonthreatening, and kind. Use praise or rewards (e.g., stickers, a "glove balloon").

14-D. A "sleepy" or lethargic presentation in a distressed child is an ominous sign. Infants and children do not generally become sleepy until their compensatory mechanisms are about to fail. The correct manner in which to position an infant's airway is to place the head in a neutral position or with the head slightly elevated ("sniffing" position). Hyperextending the neck may result in trauma to the patient's delicate trachea. Placing the chin on the chest may cause the tongue to obstruct the airway. Since there is no indication or history of trauma, the jaw thrust would not be necessary.

15-D. Until about 6 months of age, infants are obligate nose breathers. They depend on a patent (open) nasal passage for breathing. If the nasal passage is obstructed, these infants may not "think" to breathe through their mouths. The tongue is proportionally larger in children and infants than adults. A slow respiratory rate is a late and ominous sign of distress. Infants and children compensate for distress much longer than adults, but when they crash, they crash fast. Do not wait for measurable signs of injury or illness before initiating treatment. Grunting with each exhalation is a significant sign of possible respiratory collapse. If grunting is present and breathing is adequate, provide high-flow oxygen by nonrebreather mask and continuous reassessment. If breathing is inadequate, assist ventilations with a bag-valve mask and supplemental oxygen.

16-C. Bulb syringes are excellent for suctioning nasal and oral secretions in infants. You should provide oxygen before and immediately after suctioning. To correctly use the bulb syringe, you must first depress the bulb, then insert the tip gently in the patient's mouth or nose, and finally release the bulb. Remove the syringe from the airway, depress the bulb, and repeat as necessary. Do not suction for more than 5 seconds per attempt and provide supplemental oxygen between suctioning attempts if possible.

17-B. The immediate assessment of the patient's mental status, airway, breathing and circulation status, and any life-threatening conditions can be done regardless of the patient's (or the patient's family) ability to converse with you—as long as you are able to obtain consent to treat. Do not forget that body substance isolation (BSI) precautions are considered part of the scene size-up. Finding a translator will ultimately be important for a complete history of the present illness and the patient's past medical history; however, assessment and treatment need not be delayed. A rapid trauma assessment would follow the initial assessment if the patient were unresponsive and the history difficult to obtain.

18-B. Red, flushed skin in infants can be attributed to fever or exposure to heat/humidity. Bulging fontanels would be indicative of increased intracranial pressure (which may also cause seizures). Trauma or burns to the mouth may be indicative of a poisoning or electrical emergency. If this is the cause, reevaluate your scene size-up in an attempt to get more information about the patient's condition. If poisons are found in the area, safely package them and transport to the emergency department with the patient. If the patient's body is stiff and the extremities are turned outward (called decerebrate posturing), you should consider brain damage as a possible cause.

19-D. Attempt to cool this patient by removing the patient's clothing and keeping the skin moist with tepid water. If shivering begins, the patient is being cooled too aggressively. While acetaminophen is commonly given for fever, nothing should be put in the mouth of a semiconscious patient and, more importantly, you are not authorized (as an EMT-Basic) to administer this medication.

20-B. Without being accusatory, you need to rapidly assess the scene. Call for advanced-life-support (ALS) care if it is available in your system. Examine the surroundings. Take full body substance isolation (BSI) precautions. Then begin the initial assessment by first assessing the child's mental status, then airway, breathing, circulation, and life-threatening conditions. A brief history will need to be obtained from the parents, but do not allow this to interfere with your efforts to save this patient.

21-C. It is not uncommon for a Sudden Infant Death Syndrome (SIDS) baby to have a small amount of blood-tinged fluid in or around the mouth. Do not immediately jump to the conclusion that this patient was physically abused. Document (without drawing conclusions) and discuss (privately) your findings with the emergency department physician. Bulging fontanels, blood leaking from the ears, and multiple bruises are all consistent with trauma. These findings should be documented and communicated to the emergency department physician. Never imply or accuse the parents of mistreating the child.

22-D. Pooling in dependent areas (also referred to as lividity) is indicative of a "prolonged down time" (dead for a significant period of time). While the prognosis for the infant is bleak, you may decide to attempt resuscitation even if lividity is present for this reason: the parents will always remember that everything possible was done to save their baby. As with all policies, follow local protocol and instructions from medical direction.

BIBLIOGRAPHY

Campbell JE (ed): *Basic Trauma Life Support for Paramedics and Advanced EMS Providers*, 3rd ed. Englewood Cliffs, NJ, Prentice-Hall, 1995.

Crosby LA, Lewallen DG (eds): *Emergency Care and Transportation of the Sick and Injured*, 6th ed. Rosemont, IL, American Academy of Orthopaedic Surgeons, 1995.

Dietrich AM, Shaner, S: *Pediatric Basic Trauma Life Support*. Oakbrook Terrace, Illinois, Basic Trauma Life Support International, 1995.

Grant HD, Murray RH Jr, Bergeron JD: *Emergency Care*, 7th ed. Englewood Cliffs, NJ, Prentice-Hall, 1995.

Hafen BQ, Karren KJ, Mistovich JJ: *Prehospital Emergency Care*, 5th ed. Upper Saddle River, NJ, Prentice-Hall, 1996.

Henry MC, Stapleton ER, Judd RL: *EMT: Prehospital Care*. Philadelphia, WB Saunders, 1992.

McSwain NE, White RD, Paturas JL, et al (eds): *The Basic EMT: Comprehensive Prehospital Patient Care*. St. Louis, Mosby-Year Book, 1996.

Miller RH, Wilson JK: *Manual of Prehospital Emergency Medicine*. St. Louis, Mosby-Year Book, 1992.

Seidel JS, Henderson DP: *Prehospital Care of Pediatric Emergencies*, 2nd ed. Sudbury, Massachusetts, Jones and Bartlett, 1997.

Stoy WA: *Mosby's EMT-Basic Textbook*. St. Louis: Mosby-Year Book, 1996.

United States Department of Transportation, National Highway Traffic Safety Administration: *Emergency Medical Technician: Basic. National Standard Curriculum*, 1994.

Wong DL: *Essentials of Pediatric Nursing*, 4th ed. St. Louis, Mosby-Year Book, 1993.

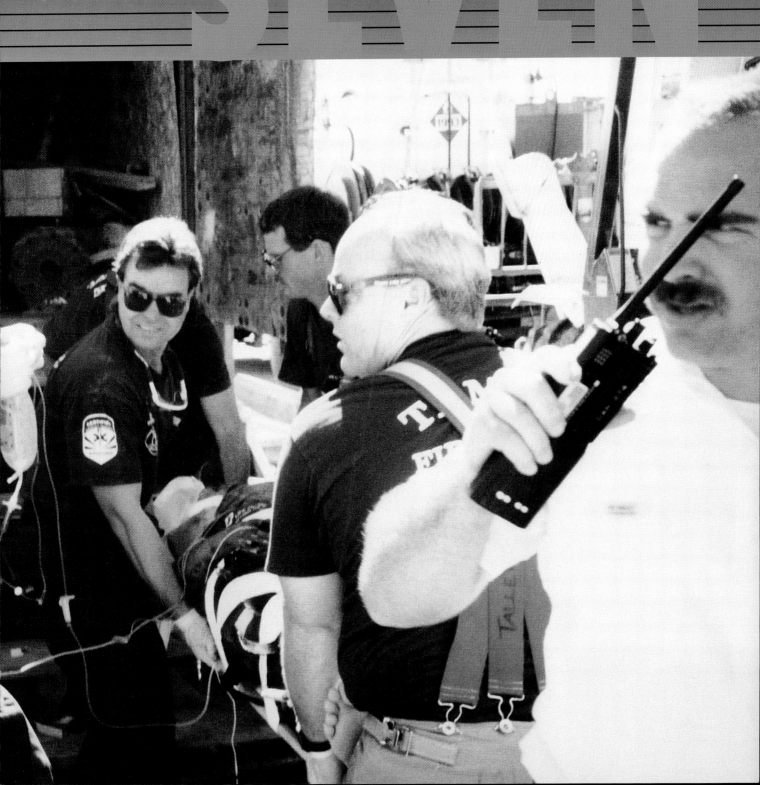

OPERATIONS SEVEN

OBJECTIVES

31-1 Describe the general provisions of state laws relating to the operation of the ambulance and privileges in any or all of the following categories:

    a. Speed   d. Right-of-way

    b. Warning lights   e. Parking

    c. Sirens   f. Turning

31-2 Describe the considerations that should be given to:

    a. Request for escorts   c. Intersections

    b. Following an escort vehicle

31-3 Discuss the medical and nonmedical equipment needed to respond to a call.

31-4 List the phases of an ambulance call.

31-5 State what information is essential to respond to a call.

31-6 Discuss various situations that may affect response to a call.

31-7 Discuss the concept of "due regard for safety of others" while operating an emergency vehicle.

31-8 List contributing factors to unsafe driving conditions.

31-9 Differentiate between the various methods of moving a patient to the unit based upon injury or illness.

31-10 Apply the components of the essential patient information in a written report.

31-11 Explain the importance of preparing the unit for the next response.

31-12 Identify what information is essential for completion of a call.

31-13 Distinguish among the terms cleaning, disinfection, high-level disinfection, and sterilization.

MOTIVATION FOR LEARNING

The **EMT-Basic** must be familiar with emergency vehicle operations, the medical and nonmedical equipment used in patient care, the phases of an emergency call, and appropriate use of air transport services. To minimize the risk of exposure to and transmission of infectious diseases, the **EMT-Basic** must understand the primary methods of decontamination.

31-14 Describe how to clean or disinfect items following patient care.

*31-15 **List situations that may require helicopter transport.**

*31-16 **Describe the factors that must be considered before transporting a patient by helicopter.**

*31-17 **Describe how to properly prepare a helicopter landing zone.**

*31-18 **Describe the basic principles of helicopter safety.**

LAWS, REGULATIONS, AND ORDINANCES

MOTOR-VEHICLE LAWS

1. Review state and local laws, regulations, or ordinances concerning the operations of an emergency vehicle, including:
   a. Vehicle parking or standing regulations
   b. Procedures at red lights, stop signs, and other intersections
   c. Regulations regarding speed limits
   d. Exemptions from following direction of traffic flow or specified turns
   e. Standard emergency or disaster routes
   f. Use of audible warning devices (e.g., sirens)
   g. Use of visual warning devices (e.g., lights)
   h. School buses
2. **Emergency driving privileges**
   a. Laws vary from state to state.
   b. Most states exempt emergency vehicles from normal traffic laws in specific circumstances.
   c. When driving in emergency mode, the operator of an emergency vehicle must follow specific rules:
      (1) Operate all visual and audible warning devices.
      (2) Drive with due regard for the safety of others on the roadway. Due regard means that, in similar circumstances, a reasonable and responsible person would act in a way that is safe and considerate of others.
      (3) Under these conditions, in most states, the emergency vehicle may:
         (a) Exceed the speed limit posted for the area
         (b) Cautiously proceed through a steady red signal, flashing red signal, or stop sign
         (c) Disregard regulations governing the direction of movement or turning in specific directions

ESCORTS AND MULTIPLE-VEHICLE RESPONSES

1. Escorts and multiple-vehicle responses are extremely dangerous.
2. They should be used only if the emergency responders are unfamiliar with the location of patient or receiving facility.
3. Provide a safe following distance (generally a minimum of 500 feet).
4. Use a different siren time and/or tone to help other motorists distinguish multiple emergency vehicles.
5. Recognize hazards of a multiple-vehicle response.
   a. A motorist may see the first emergency vehicle pass and begin to proceed, assuming it was the only emergency vehicle.
   b. An accident may occur with the motorist and the second emergency vehicle.

INTERSECTION CRASHES

1. Intersection crashes are the most common collision involving emergency vehicles.
2. Intersection crashes can occur in the following ways:

a. The motorist arrives at an intersection as the light changes and does not stop.

b. Multiple emergency vehicles are following closely, and a waiting motorist does not expect more than one vehicle.

c. Vision is obstructed by vehicles waiting at an intersection, blocking view of pedestrian.

PHASES OF AN AMBULANCE CALL

PREPARATION FOR THE CALL

1. **Necessary equipment for an emergency call**
   a. Medical equipment includes (*Table 31-1*):
      (1) Basic supplies
      (2) Patient transfer equipment
      (3) Airways
      (4) Suction equipment
      (5) Artificial ventilation devices
      (6) Oxygen inhalation equipment
      (7) Cardiac compression equipment
      (8) Basic wound care supplies
      (9) Splinting supplies
      (10) Childbirth supplies
      (11) Medications
      (12) Automated external defibrillator (AED)
   b. Nonmedical equipment includes (see Table 31-1):
      (1) Personal safety equipment per local, state, and federal standards
      (2) Preplanned routes or comprehensive street maps
   c. Personnel requirements include:
      (1) Available for response
      (2) A minimum of at least one EMT-Basic in the patient compartment (two is preferred)
3. **Daily inspections**
   a. Daily inspection of vehicle systems should include:
      (1) Fuel
      (2) Oil
      (3) Engine cooling system
      (4) Battery
      (5) Brakes
      (6) Wheels and tires

Table 31-1. Emergency Vehicle Equipment

Medical Supplies	Nonmedical Supplies
Basic supplies	Personal safety equipment
Patient transfer equipment	Preplanned routes or comprehensive stree
Airways	maps
Suction equipment	
Artificial ventilation devices	
Oxygen inhalation equipment	
Cardiac compression equipment	
Basic wound care supplies	
Splinting supplies	
Childbirth supplies	
Medications	
Automated external defibrillator (AED)	

      (7) Headlights
      (8) Stop lights
      (9) Turn signals
      (10) Emergency warning lights
      (11) Wipers
      (12) Horn
      (13) Siren
      (14) Doors closing and latching
      (15) Communication system
      (16) Air conditioning/heating system
      (17) Ventilation system
    b. Daily inspection and inventory of emergency care equipment and supplies should ensure that they are:
      (1) Checked and maintained
      (2) Restocked and repaired
      (3) Batteries charged for defibrillator, suction, oxygen, etc.
    c. Cleanliness of interior and exterior of the vehicle should be maintained daily.
4. Before proceeding to a call, safety precautions and seat belts should be put in place.

DISPATCH

1. The Emergency Medical Dispatcher (EMD) is responsible for:
    a. Asking questions of the caller
    b. Radio dispatching
    c. Logistics coordination. The EMD is knowledgeable about the geography of the area, the emergency medical system's (EMS) capabilities, and the activities of other public service agencies.
    d. Providing prearrival instructions to the caller (in some EMS systems)
2. The dispatcher should provide the following information:
    a. Location of the call
    b. Nature of the call
    c. Name, location, and callback number of the caller
    d. Location of the patient
    e. Number of patients and severity of the problem
    f. Other special problems (e.g., hazardous materials)
3. Ask the dispatcher to repeat any information that is unclear.

EN ROUTE

1. Wear seatbelts.
2. Notify dispatch that you are responding to the call *(Figure 31-1)*.
3. Write down the essential information from the dispatcher, including:
    a. Nature of the call
    b. Location of the call
4. Determine what the responsibilities of crew members will be before arriving on the scene.
5. Assign anticipated equipment needs to each crew member.
6. Call for advanced-life-support (ALS) personnel if necessary.
7. Driving the ambulance
    a. It is recommended, and in some states mandated, that the driver of an emergency vehicle attend an approved driving course. Emergency driving programs have been developed by groups including:
      (1) Department of Transportation
      (2) National Safety Council
      (3) Insurance companies
      (4) State or local agencies

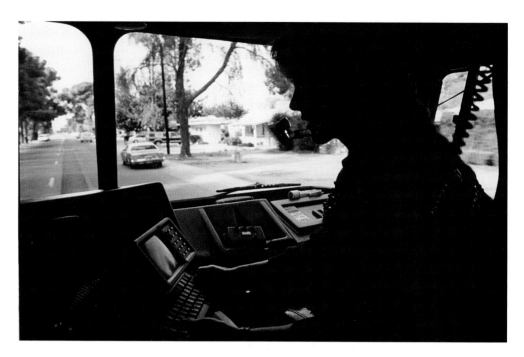

Fig. 31-1. En route to a call. Notify dispatch that you are responding. Write down essential information from the dispatcher, such as the nature and location of the call. Determine what the responsibilities of crew members will be before arriving on the scene. Assign anticipated equipment needs to each crew member.

b. Characteristics of good emergency vehicle operators include:
- **(1)** Physically fit
- **(2)** Mentally fit
- **(3)** Able to perform under stress
- **(4)** Positive attitude about abilities
- **(5)** Tolerant of other drivers

c. Safe driving
- **(1)** Safe driving is an important phase in the emergency medical care of the ill or injured patient.
- **(2)** Seatbelts should be worn by all occupants.
- **(3)** Become familiar with the characteristics of your vehicle before being dispatched to an emergency.
- **(4)** Be alert to changes in weather and road conditions and adjust speed to allow for decreased visibility.
- **(5)** Exercise caution in use of red lights and sirens.
- **(6)** Select an appropriate response route.
  - **(a)** Use preplanned routes and street maps.
  - **(b)** Select the best route based on weather, traffic patterns, and road conditions.
    - **(i)** Note detours, road closings, bridges, railroad crossings, tunnels, schools, heavy traffic areas.
    - **(ii)** Consider time of day, day of week.
  - **(c)** Plan an alternate route if unforeseen conditions are encountered.
- **(7)** Maintain a safe following distance (4-second rule).
  - **(a)** Follow the vehicle ahead at a distance so that an object passed by the first vehicle is passed by the emergency vehicle 4 seconds later.
  - **(b)** Count 4 seconds between the emergency vehicle and the vehicle ahead when passing the same object.
- **(8)** Drive with due regard for the safety of others.
- **(9)** Know state laws regarding the use of lights and sirens.

      (a) Headlights are the most visible warning devices on an emergency vehicle because they are mounted at eye-level of other drivers.

      (b) Most state laws require the use of lights and sirens when exercising emergency driving privileges.

      (c) Use of lights and sirens does not automatically grant right-of-way *(Figure 31-2)*.

          (i) Other drivers may not see or hear the warning devices (e.g., use of air conditioning, stereo equipment).

          (ii) Ensure the driver sees the emergency vehicle before taking the right-of-way.

  d. Contributing factors to unsafe driving conditions include:

    (1) Escorts

    (2) Road surface

    (3) Excessive speed

    (4) Reckless driving

    (5) Weather conditions

    (6) Multiple-vehicle response

    (7) Inadequate dispatch information

    (8) Failing to heed traffic warning signals

    (9) Disregarding traffic rules and regulations

    (10) Failing to anticipate the actions of other motorists

    (11) Failing to obey traffic signals or posted speed limits

8. Positioning the unit

  a. Park with convenient access to the patient. Consider the effects of traffic flow, the roadway, known hazards, the public, and other agencies.

  b. Park in front of or behind a collision *(Figure 31-3)*. Do not park beside the collision site, which may block the movement of other emergency vehicles.

  c. Park a safe distance from wreckage or hazardous scenes.

    (1) Park uphill and upwind from leaking hazards.

    (2) Park a minimum of 100 feet from wreckage or a burning vehicle.

    (3) Park at least 2000 feet from a hazardous substance.

  d. When possible, park in a way that allows for the smooth flow of traffic.

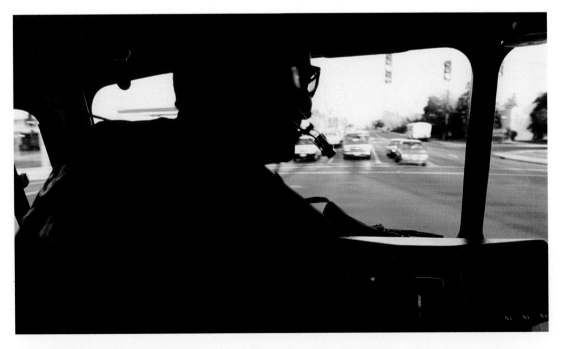

Fig. 31-2. Use of lights and sirens does not automatically grant the right-of-way. Other drivers may not see or hear the warning devices. Ensure that the driver sees the emergency vehicle before proceeding.

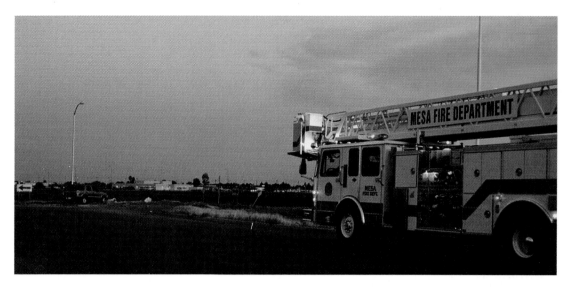

Fig. 31-3. Park in front of or behind a collision. Park a minimum of 100 feet from wreckage or a burning vehicle.

    e. Set parking brake.

    f. Use warning lights.

    g. Shut off headlights unless there is a need to illuminate the scene.

    h. Avoid parking in a location that will hamper your exit from the scene.

ARRIVAL AT THE SCENE

1. Actions at the scene should be rapid and organized, keeping in mind the goal of safe and efficient transport.

2. Notify dispatch.

3. Scene size-up

    a. Take body substance isolation (BSI) precautions.

        (1) BSI precautions should be taken before patient contact.

        (2) Use gloves, gowns, and eyewear when appropriate.

    b. Ensure scene safety.

        (1) Assess the scene for hazards.

            (a) Is the emergency vehicle parked in a safe location?

            (b) Is it safe to approach the patient?

            (c) Does the victim require immediate movement because of hazards?

        (2) Do not enter the scene until it is safe.

    c. Determine mechanism of injury or nature of illness.

        (1) Determine the total number of patients.

            (a) Request additional resources BEFORE patient contact.

            (b) Initiate multiple-casualty-incident (MCI) response if necessary.

            (c) Begin triage.

        (2) If you and your crew can manage the situation, consider spinal precautions (if appropriate) and continue care.

4. Gain access to the patient.

5. Perform an initial assessment and determine priorities of care.

6. Provide essential emergency care.

7. Prepare the patient for transport.

TRANSFERRING THE PATIENT TO THE AMBULANCE

1. Ensure that dressings and splints, if used, are secure.

2. Transfer the patient to the transport vehicle. The lifting and moving method and the device used will depend on the patient's illness or injury and the safety of the scene (e.g., emergency move at an unsafe scene versus stable medical patient).

3. Secure the patient to the stretcher and lock the stretcher in place.

4. Before leaving the scene, the driver should ensure outside compartment doors are closed and secure.

EN ROUTE TO THE RECEIVING FACILITY

1. Wear seatbelts.

2. Notify dispatch when leaving the scene.
   a. Identify the facility destination.
   b. Follow local protocol regarding the communication of additional patient information.

3. The driver should use only the necessary speed, keeping in mind the patient's condition and comfort, and the safety of passengers and crew.

4. Reassure the patient throughout the transport.

5. Perform detailed and ongoing assessments.
   a. Reassess mental status, airway, breathing, perfusion, and vital signs.
      (1) Repeat every 5 minutes if the patient is unstable.
      (2) Repeat every 15 minutes if the patient is stable.
   b. Reassess emergency interventions (e.g., oxygen, dressings, splints) and adjust as needed.

6. Contact the receiving facility, if possible, and use a standardized medical reporting format:
   a. Identify unit's name and level of service [basic life support (BLS), ALS]
   b. Estimated time of arrival
   c. Patient's age and gender
   d. Patient's chief complaint
   e. Brief, pertinent history of the present illness
   f. Major past illnesses
   g. Patient's mental status
   h. Patient's baseline vital signs
   i. Pertinent physical examination findings
   j. Emergency medical care given
   k. Patient's response to emergency medical care

7. Complete the prehospital care report.

AT THE RECEIVING FACILITY

1. Notify dispatch.

2. Give a complete verbal report to appropriate receiving facility personnel at the patient's bedside.
   a. Introduce the patient by name (if known).
   b. Summarize the information already provided by radio or telephone to the receiving facility:
      (1) Patient's chief complaint
      (2) Pertinent patient history that was not previously given
      (3) Emergency medical care given en route and the patient's response to the treatment given
      (4) Vital signs taken en route
   c. Provide any additional information collected en route but not transmitted to the receiving facility.

3. Complete the written prehospital care report and leave a copy at the receiving facility before returning to service.
   a. Essential administrative information includes:
      (1) Time incident reported
      (2) Time unit notified

(3) Time of arrival at patient
(4) Time unit left scene
(5) Time of arrival at destination
(6) Time of transfer of care
b. Essential patient information (minimum data set) includes:
(1) Chief complaint
(2) Mental status (AVPU)
(3) Systolic blood pressure for patients older than 3 years old
(4) Skin perfusion (capillary refill) for patients younger than 6 years old
(5) Skin color and temperature
(6) Pulse rate
(7) Respiratory rate and effort
4. If requested to do so, assist in the transfer of the patient from the ambulance stretcher to the receiving facility bed or stretcher using proper lifting and moving techniques.
5. Exchange any backboards or other items as needed and per local protocol.
6. Wash hands thoroughly with soap and water.

EN ROUTE TO THE STATION

1. Notify dispatch.
2. Prepare for the next call.
   a. Clean and disinfect the ambulance as needed.
   b. Clean and disinfect ambulance equipment.
   c. Restock disposable supplies.
3. Follow biohazard disposal procedures.
4. Return equipment to its storage area.

POSTRUN

1. Refuel the vehicle according to local protocol.
2. Complete and file all reports.
3. Inspect the vehicle, checking tires, lights, and anything unusual noticed during the run.
4. Complete cleaning and disinfecting the vehicle and/or equipment.
5. Replace empty oxygen cylinders.
6. Replace discharged batteries or reconnect to vehicle chargers.
7. Replace supplies used during the run.
8. Change soiled uniforms.
9. Notify dispatch of availability.

DECONTAMINATION

METHODS OF DECONTAMINATION

1. Occupational Safety and Health Administration (OSHA) defines **decontamination** as "the use of physical or chemical means to remove, inactivate, or destroy bloodborne pathogens on a surface or item to the point where they are no longer capable of transmitting infectious particles and the surface or item is considered safe for handling, use, or disposal."
2. Primary methods of decontamination
   a. Disinfection
      (1) Low-level disinfection
         (a) Low-level disinfection destroys most bacteria, some viruses and fungi, but not tuberculosis bacteria or bacterial spores.

   (b) It is used for routine cleaning of surfaces, such as floors, countertops, and ambulance seats, when no body fluids are visible.

   (c) Use a 1:100 solution of household bleach and water or a hospital disinfectant registered with the Environmental Protection Agency (EPA).

   (2) Intermediate-level disinfection

   (a) Intermediate-level disinfection destroys tuberculosis bacteria, vegetative bacteria, and most viruses and fungi, but not bacterial spores.

   (b) It is used for surfaces that contact intact skin and have been visibly contaminated with body fluids, such as blood pressure cuffs, stethoscopes, backboards, and splints.

   (c) Use a 1:10 solution of household bleach and water or an EPA-registered hospital disinfectant that claims it is tuberculocidal.

   (3) High-level disinfection

   (a) High-level disinfection destroys all microorganisms except large numbers of bacterial spores.

   (b) It is used for reusable equipment that has been in contact with mucous membranes, such as laryngoscope blades.

   (c) Use either hot-water pasteurization by placing articles in water 80° to 100° Celsius (C) for 30 minutes or immerse in an EPA-registered chemical sterilizing agent for 10 to 45 minutes according to manufacturer's instructions.

   (d) Items requiring high-level disinfection should first be cleaned with soap and water to remove debris.

b. Sterilization

   (1) Sterilization destroys all microorganisms including highly resistant bacterial spores.

   (2) It is used for instruments that penetrate the skin or contact normally sterile areas of the body during invasive procedures.

   (3) Methods include:

   (a) Autoclave (steam under pressure)

   (b) Immersion in an EPA-registered chemical sterilizing agent for 6 to 10 hours

   (4) Sterilization is usually performed at the hospital.

   (5) Items requiring sterilization should first be cleaned with soap and water to remove debris.

3. Medical equipment should never be disinfected in areas such as the kitchen, bathrooms, or living areas of the station or receiving facility.

INFECTION CONTROL PROCEDURES

1. Personal

   a. Remove contaminated clothing.

   (1) If blood or other potentially infectious material contaminates your clothing, remove it as soon as possible.

   (2) Bag the clothing for decontamination and place in an appropriately designated area or container.

   b. Thoroughly wash your hands, contaminated skin areas, and areas of skin that were not covered by clothing or personal protective equipment.

   (1) Hands should be washed after every patient encounter.

   (2) Remember to wash hands after cleaning and disinfecting procedures are completed.

   c. Put on appropriate personal protective equipment.

   (1) Wear protective gloves (e.g., cleaning gloves) when cleaning up potentially infectious materials.

   (2) If splashing is likely, wear face and eye protection.

2. **Vehicle**
   a. Contaminated sharps must be discarded immediately in an acceptable sharps container.
      (1) If leakage is possible, or if the outside of the container has become contaminated, the sharps container must be placed in a secondary container that is closable, labeled or color-coded, and leak resistant.
      (2) If the sharps container is half to three-fourths full:
         (a) Close and lock the lid
         (b) Follow agency procedures for disposal of the container
   b. Decontaminate the vehicle and large equipment.
      (1) Clean up blood and body fluid spills.
         (a) Use disposable towels.
         (b) Dispose of the towels in a biohazard-labeled bag.
      (2) Decontaminate surfaces with soap and water.
      (3) Wipe or spray with a disinfectant solution as needed and allow disinfected areas to air dry.
   c. Place disposable personal protective equipment worn during decontamination procedures in a properly labeled sealed waste container.
   d. Restock the vehicle.
   e. Make note of any items needing repair or replacement.
3. **Laundry**
   a. Protective gloves and other appropriate personal protective equipment must be worn when handling contaminated laundry.
   b. Laundry contaminated with blood or other potentially infectious materials:
      (1) Should be handled as little as possible
      (2) Must be placed in appropriately marked bags at the location where it was used
      (3) Should be washed according to the uniform or linen manufacturer's recommendations
   c. Contaminated items should always be laundered separately from other laundry to prevent cross-contamination.

AIR MEDICAL TRANSPORT

SITUATIONS FOR POSSIBLE HELICOPTER TRANSPORT

1. Mechanisms of injury that may require helicopter transport include:
   a. Vehicle rollover with unrestrained passengers
   b. Vehicle striking pedestrian at a speed of greater than 10 miles per hour
   c. Falls from more than 15 feet
   d. Motorcyclist thrown from the motorcycle at a speed of more than 20 miles per hour
   e. Multiple victims
2. Time and distance must be considered before transporting by helicopter.
   a. Transport time to a trauma center is more than 15 minutes by ground ambulance.
   b. Transport time to a local hospital by ground ambulance is more than the transport time to a trauma center by helicopter.
   c. Patient is entrapped and extrication will take longer than 15 minutes.
   d. Use of local ground ambulance leaves the local community without ground ambulance coverage.

HELICOPTER (ROTOR-WING) LANDING ZONES

1. The landing zone should measure:
   a. A minimum of 60 feet × 60 feet during daylight hours
   b. A minimum of 100 feet × 100 feet at night

2. The area should be free of overhead obstacles (e.g., wires, trees, light poles).
3. The area should be free of debris and relatively level.
4. The ground should be clear of rocks and grooves and must be firm enough to support the aircraft.
5. Mark the corners of the landing area with secured flares (if there is no danger of fire), light sticks, or cones or use emergency vehicles with headlights directed toward the landing area (not at the approaching aircraft). Contact your local service for landing zone requirements.
6. If the landing area is dirt, lightly moisten the area with water if possible.

SAFETY

1. Never move toward the helicopter until signaled by the flight crew.
2. Always approach from the front where the pilot can see you.
3. Wear ear and eye protection when approaching the helicopter.
4. Never raise your arms or equipment above your head.
5. If the aircraft is parked on a slope, always approach and exit from the downhill side.
6. When moving from one side of the helicopter to the other, always cross in front of the helicopter.
7. Do not open or pull on any part of the aircraft.
8. Do not smoke within 50 feet of the aircraft.
9. Do not allow vehicles or nonaircraft personnel within 60 feet of the aircraft.

REVIEW QUESTIONS

Directions: Each of the numbered items or incomplete statements in this section is followed by answers or by completions of the statement. Select the ONE lettered answer or completion that is BEST in each case.

1. Emergency response units responding together should keep a minimum distance between units of

   (A) 50–100 feet
   (B) 200 feet
   (C) 500 feet
   (D) 1 mile

2. Most collisions involving emergency response units occur

   (A) in intersections
   (B) in school zones
   (C) in residential tracts
   (D) in rural communities

3. Your ambulance has been dispatched to a motor vehicle collision at a major intersection (three lanes of traffic in all directions). Upon arrival, you find that two vehicles have collided and come to rest in the middle of the intersection. Which of the following ambulance positions would be most appropriate?

   (A) Behind the accident
   (B) In a nearby parking lot
   (C) To the side of the accident
   (D) On the opposite side of the street

4. Your rescue crew is responding to a report of an overturned vehicle. Information at the time of dispatch indicates that a truck carrying chlorine has been involved. Which of the following vehicle positions would be most appropriate?

    (A) Park at least 1 mile from the scene
    (B) Park directly behind the chlorine truck
    (C) Park approximately 2000 feet away from the scene
    (D) Drive through the accident scene and park on the far side

Directions: Each of the numbered items or incomplete statements in this section is negatively phrased, as indicated by a capitalized word such as NOT, LEAST, or EXCEPT. Select the ONE lettered answer or completion that is BEST in each case.

5. While en route to an emergency call, responders should do all of the following EXCEPT

    (A) anticipate equipment needs
    (B) decontaminate essential equipment
    (C) determine crew responsibilities/assignments
    (D) call for advanced-life-support (ALS) personnel as necessary

6. Your ambulance crew is transporting a 56-year-old male patient to the emergency department. He is complaining of chest pain. When you arrive at the receiving facility, you should give a complete verbal report. Which of the following should NOT be a component of this report?

    (A) The patient's chief complaint
    (B) Emergency care given en route
    (C) The most recent set of vital signs
    (D) Your diagnosis of the patient's illness

Directions: Each of the numbered questions or incomplete statements in this section refers to a scenario that precedes them. The numbered questions or incomplete statements are followed by answers or by completions of the statement. Select the answer or completion of the statement that is BEST in each case.

Your rescue crew has transported a 43-year-old female patient to the emergency department. After transferring patient care to the receiving facility, you return to your vehicle to make sure that it is ready to go back in service.

Questions 7–9

7. Assuming there is no sign of body fluids present, which of the following solutions would be most appropriate for cleaning the floors, seats, and countertops of the vehicle?

    (A) Clean water
    (B) Window cleaner
    (C) Undiluted bleach
    (D) A 1:100 solution of bleach and water

8. While cleaning equipment, you note that there is a small amount of blood on the blood pressure cuff. Which of the following solutions would be most appropriate for disinfecting this equipment?

(A) Gasoline
(B) Undiluted ammonia
(C) A 1:10 solution of bleach and water
(D) Nothing. This equipment must be thrown away in an approved biohazard waste container

9. While inspecting the backboard used to transport this patient, you notice there is a small amount of blood on one side. You should

(A) gently clean with mild soap and water
(B) wear protective gloves and face and eye protection while cleaning
(C) turn the board over and continue to use it until you have time to disinfect it properly
(D) Nothing. This equipment must be thrown away in an approved biohazard waste container

Your rescue crew is called to a shooting in a remote area. A hunter, cleaning his rifle, accidentally shot himself in the abdomen. By the time you arrive, he is in severe shock. His pulse is 132 beats per minute and weak. The blood pressure is 72/42. Respirations are 24 per minute and very shallow. His skin is pale and moist.

Questions 10–12

10. You should evaluate the possibility of transporting this patient by helicopter if

(A) there is no exit wound present
(B) the patient goes into full cardiopulmonary arrest
(C) it will take you more than 15 minutes to get to a trauma center by ground ambulance
(D) it will take you more than 1 hour to get to a trauma center by ground ambulance

11. When establishing a landing zone for a medical helicopter (during daylight hours), the minimum area secured should be

(A) 20 feet × 40 feet
(B) 60 feet × 60 feet
(C) 200 feet × 200 feet
(D) One mile square

12. Once the helicopter has set down, you should, if necessary, approach

(A) from uphill
(B) from the rear
(C) from the side
(D) from the front

ANSWERS AND RATIONALES

1-C. Units responding to the same scene should maintain a distance of at least 500 feet. If the units fail to keep this distance, other drivers on the road may only recognize or anticipate one unit, even if both units have their lights and sirens activated. Another helpful technique, when responding with multiple units, is to use different or alternating siren tones. This may alert other drivers that other vehicles are present.

2-A. Intersections are by far the most dangerous area for emergency response vehicles. Before proceeding through an intersection, emergency response vehicle operators (drivers) should account for the safety of drivers in all lanes of traffic. When traveling through school zones, be particularly alert for children. Children are often drawn to the lights and excitement associated with emergency response vehicles. Slow down and proceed with caution. Do the same in residential areas. Do not let your guard down when responding in rural areas. Always be prepared to bring your vehicle to a rapid and controlled stop.

3-A. By parking behind the accident, you can warn oncoming drivers that an emergency exists. Your vehicle also acts as a barrier between oncoming traffic and the accident scene. Position the vehicle approximately 100 feet from the accident scene.

4-C. Based on the additional information, you should do several things. First, call for additional help (hazardous materials team and local law enforcement for traffic control and possible evacuation). Second, position your vehicle so that you may gather additional information without becoming a victim. As a rule of thumb, you should position a vehicle 2000 feet from any hazardous scene.

5-B. All equipment should be decontaminated or replaced before going in service. For your safety and the safety of your next patient, do not respond to an emergency scene with contaminated equipment. While en route to an incident, start preparing yourself and your crew. Preparation includes evaluating the dispatch information and making a tentative action plan based on that information. The action plan may involve calling for additional help or assigning on-scene tasks to specific personnel. If possible, have body substance isolation (BSI) precautions in place before or as you are arriving at the scene.

6-D. Given at the patient's bedside, your verbal report should include a summary of your encounter with the patient. You should identify the patient's chief complaint, his past medical history, emergency care given and his response, and vital signs taken en route to the hospital. EMT-Basics are not diagnosticians. The determination of the exact cause of the patient's distress is not as important as the appropriate management of the patient's distress. Avoid saying things such as, "He's having a heart attack" or "She fractured her ribs." Instead, say, "He's having severe chest pain" or "She got hit in the chest with a stick and has severe pain with palpation or deep inspiration."

7-D. This would be considered a "low level" disinfection since no body fluids are visible. The appropriate solution would be a 1:100 solution of bleach and water. This solution will adequately kill most bacteria and some viruses and fungi. Undiluted bleach would kill the same microorganisms, but may also shorten the life span of your equipment.

8-C. A stronger solution of bleach is necessary to disinfect when body fluids are visible. Never use gasoline or other flammables for cleaning.

9-B. Just because the patient is not around does not mean that you cannot be exposed. Until all equipment is disinfected or replaced, the hazard of contamination exists. When cleaning large objects (such as a backboard), the possibility of a splash-type exposure is high. Protect yourself while decontaminating and do not forget to wash your hands after decontaminating. Never use a contaminated piece of equipment.

10-C. Generally, if it will take longer than 15 minutes to transport a critically injured patient to an appropriate facility, you should evaluate the option of calling for an air ambulance.

11-B. The minimum acceptable size for a landing zone is 60 feet × 60 feet during the day and 100 feet × 100 feet at night. All unnecessary personnel should be kept out of the landing zone at all times. There should be no smoking in the landing zone. If you are landing a helicopter in an unpaved area, you may want to consider lightly moistening the ground to prevent a dust cloud "brown out." The landing zone surface should be as level as possible, free of overhead obstructions, and clear of rocks or grooves. Ideally, the landing zone areas should be clearly marked and secured.

12-D. Communication with the helicopter crew is extremely important. Make verbal or eye contact with the pilot before approaching the aircraft. Approach from the front in plain view of the pilot, and exit from the front so the pilot knows your whereabouts. As you approach the aircraft, make sure that you do not have any loose papers, clothing, or hat that may be dislodged due to air turbulence. Do not hold anything above the level of your head. If the helicopter is parked on a slope, approach from the downhill side to ensure clearance from the rotors. Remember, most helicopters have a tail rotor that, when spinning, may appear invisible from some angles. When in doubt about a procedure, ask the flight crew for direction.

BIBLIOGRAPHY

Crosby LA, Lewallen DG (eds): *Emergency Care and Transportation of the Sick and Injured*, 6th ed. Rosemont, IL, American Academy of Orthopaedic Surgeons, 1995.

Grant HD, Murray RH Jr, Bergeron JD: *Emergency Care*, 7th ed. Englewood Cliffs, NJ, Prentice-Hall, 1995.

Hafen BQ, Karren KJ, Mistovich JJ: *Prehospital Emergency Care*, 5th ed. Upper Saddle River, NJ, Prentice-Hall, 1996.

Henry MC, Stapleton ER, Judd RL: *EMT: Prehospital Care*. Philadelphia, WB Saunders, 1992.

McSwain NE, White RD, Paturas JL, et al (eds): *The Basic EMT: Comprehensive Prehospital Patient Care*. St. Louis, Mosby-Year Book, 1996.

Roush WR (ed): *Principles of EMS Systems*, 2nd ed. Dallas, American College of Emergency Physicians, 1994.

Stoy WA: *Mosby's EMT-Basic Textbook*. St. Louis, Mosby-Year Book, 1996.

United States Department of Transportation, National Highway Traffic Safety Administration: *Emergency Medical Technician: Basic. National Standard Curriculum*, 1994.

OBJECTIVES

32-1 Describe the purpose of extrication.

32-2 Discuss the role of the EMT-Basic in extrication.

32-3 Define the fundamental components of extrication.

32-4 Identify the required personal safety equipment for the EMT-Basic.

32-5 Distinguish between simple and complex access.

32-6 Evaluate various methods of gaining access to the patient.

32-7 State the steps that should be taken to protect the patient during extrication.

ROLE OF THE EMT-BASIC IN EXTRICATION

NONRESCUE EMS

1. The role of nonrescue emergency medical services (EMS) providers is to administer necessary care to the patient before extrication and ensure that the patient is removed in a way that minimizes further injury (**extrication** = freeing from entrapment).
2. Patient care precedes extrication unless delayed movement would endanger the life of the patient or rescuer.
   a. Patient care should include attention to life-threatening emergencies.
   b. All patients should be packaged and moved carefully to minimize the danger of further injury or aggravation of existing injuries.
3. The nonrescue EMS provider will need to work with the providers of rescue. The nonrescue EMT-Basic should cooperate with the activities of the rescuers and not allow their activities to interfere with patient care.

MOTIVATION FOR LEARNING

The EMT-Basic must be familiar with the actions necessary to extricate a patient. Knowledge of personal safety equipment and measures that should be taken to protect the patient during extrication is essential.

RESCUE EMS

1. In some instances, the EMS providers are also the rescue providers.
2. A chain of command should be established to assure patient care priorities.
   a. Administer necessary care to the patient before extrication and ensure that the patient is removed in a way that minimizes further injury.
   b. Patient care precedes extrication unless delayed movement would endanger life of the patient or rescuer.

STAGES OF EXTRICATION

SCENE SIZE-UP

1. **Safety**
   a. **Personal safety**
      (1) Personal safety is the number one priority for all EMS personnel.
      (2) Protective clothing that is appropriate for the situation should be used.
   b. **Patient safety.** Following the safety of the EMS responders, the next priority is the safety of the patient.
   c. **Bystander safety.** Following the safety of the patient, the next priority is the safety of bystanders.
2. **Scene size-up**
   a. Determine the number and type of vehicles and extent of damage.
   b. Determine the number of persons injured and types of injury.
   c. Determine the presence of hazards.
3. **Hazard control and safety considerations.** Be alert for any of the following:
   a. Traffic at the scene of an accident
   b. Gasoline spills
   c. Hazardous materials
   d. Exposed or downed electrical wires
   e. Fire or possibility of fire
   f. Explosive materials
   g. Unstable vehicle or structure
   h. Environmental conditions
      (1) Heavy rain
      (2) Heavy snow fall
      (3) Flash floods

STABILIZATION OF VEHICLES AND STRUCTURES

1. **Purpose.** The purpose of stabilization is to:
   a. Eliminate potential movement of vehicle/structure that may cause further harm to entrapped patients or rescuers
   b. Ensure structural integrity
2. Equipment for stabilization includes:
   a. Wood cribbing and wedges
   b. Airbags
   c. Step chocks
   d. Come-along (hand winch)
   e. Hydraulic rams
   f. Jacks
   g. Chains

GAINING ACCESS TO THE PATIENT (*FIGURE 32-1*)

1. **Types of access**
   a. **Simple access** does not require equipment (*Figure 32-2*).

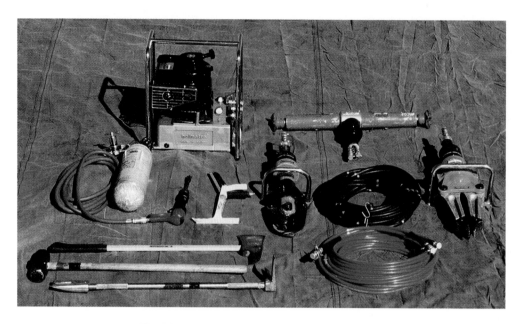

Fig. 32-1. Equipment commonly used for extrication.

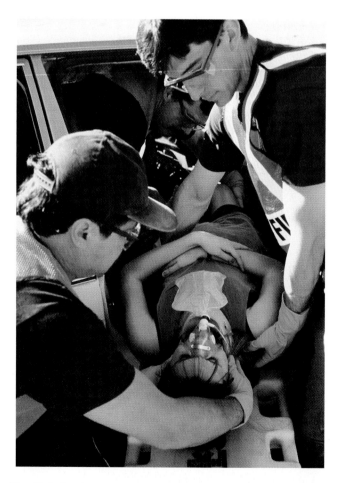

Fig. 32-2. Simple access does not require the use of rescue equipment.

    b. Complex access requires the use of tools, special equipment, and special education and includes (*Figure 32-3*):

       (1)   High-angle rescue

       (2)   Basic vehicle rescue

       (3)   Water and ice rescue

       (4)   Confined space rescue

       (5)   Building collapse rescue

2. The route used to reach the patient is not necessarily the route through which the patient will be removed.

3. Use the path of least resistance.

    a. Try opening each door.

    b. Roll down windows.

    c. Have patient unlock doors.

    d. If these methods are unsuccessful, it may be necessary to break a window to gain access.

       (1)   Windshields of modern vehicles are made of laminated safety glass, which consists of two sheets of plate glass bonded to a sheet of tough plastic.

       (2)   Most modern passenger car side and rear windows are made of tempered glass, which breaks into small rounded pieces instead of sharp shards of glass.

       (3)   Cover/shield the patient with a rescue blanket.

       (4)   Use a side or rear window as far from the patient as possible.

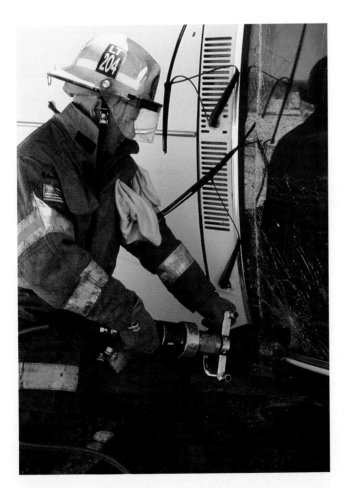

Fig. 32-3. Complex extrication requires special education, skills, and equipment.

PERFORMING CRITICAL INTERVENTIONS

1. Once access has been gained, perform an initial assessment.
2. Perform in-line cervical spine stabilization.
3. Correct life-threatening problems.
4. **Patient safety**
   (1) Protect the patient from broken glass, sharp metal, and other hazards, including the environment, during disentanglement.
   (2) Cover, shield, and pad the patient.

DISENTANGLEMENT

1. **Disentanglement** is the moving or removing of material that is trapping a victim.
2. Remove wreckage from the patient, not patient from the wreckage.
3. As disentanglement progresses, the patient can be prepared for removal.
   a. Maintain cervical spine stabilization.
   b. Dress and bandage open wounds.
   c. Splint or stabilize fractures.
   d. Immobilize spine securely using:
      (1) Short spine board
      (2) Rapid extrication considerations

REMOVAL

1. Move the patient, not the immobilization device.
2. Make sure to use sufficient personnel.
3. Choose the path of least resistance.
4. Continue to protect the patient from hazards.

REVIEW QUESTIONS

Directions: Each of the numbered items or incomplete statements in this section is followed by answers or by completions of the statement. Select the ONE lettered answer or completion that is BEST in each case.

1. Your ambulance crew is dispatched to the scene of a motor vehicle collision. A 26-year-old female patient is trapped in her vehicle. Which of the following is correct regarding the care and handling of this patient?

   (A) Assessment and treatment should always begin before extricating the patient from the vehicle
   (B) Nonrescue EMT-Basics should not begin assessment or treatment until rescue EMT-Basics have extricated the patient
   (C) The patient should always be extricated from the vehicle before the initiation of assessment and treatment
   (D) Unless delayed movement would endanger the life of the patient, assessment and treatment should be initiated before extrication

2. Extrication refers to

   (A) freeing patients from entrapment
   (B) sorting patients according to the severity of their injuries

    (C)   protecting bystanders from injury at motor vehicle collision scenes

    (D)   securing vehicles to prevent movement that may cause further harm to trapped patients or rescue workers

3. Your ambulance crew is called to the scene of a motor vehicle collision. One vehicle was T-boned on the driver's side door. The door cannot be opened manually. Which of the following would be the preferred method for removing this patient?

    (A)   Open the door with a hydraulic tool (e.g., Jaws of Life)

    (B)   Open the passenger side door and remove the patient out the passenger side

    (C)   Cover the patient, cut the roof off the vehicle, and remove the patient vertically

    (D)   Cover the patient, break the driver's side window, and remove the patient out this window

4. Which of the following may assist in assuring that patient care priorities are addressed throughout extrication?

    (A)   Establishing a chain of command

    (B)   Requesting a medical helicopter for transportation

    (C)   Removing all nonrescue EMT-Basics from the immediate area

    (D)   Extricating patients from the most severely damaged vehicle first

---

Directions: Each of the numbered questions or incomplete statements in this section refers to a scenario that precedes them. The numbered questions or incomplete statements are followed by answers or by completions of the statement. Select the answer or completion of the statement that is BEST in each case.

Your rescue crew is called to the scene of a motor vehicle collision on a local four-lane highway. Information at time of dispatch indicates that there are at least five vehicles involved. The posted speed limit is 55 miles per hour. The accident has occurred 45 miles from the nearest hospital.

Questions 5–10

5. Which of the following duties should be performed first?

    (A)   Gain access to the most critically injured patients

    (B)   Triage patients according to the severity of their injuries

    (C)   Determine the number of patients, the types of injuries, and additional resource needs

    (D)   Assess the mental, airway, breathing, and circulation status of all patients, and begin treating life-threatening conditions

6. One of the vehicles has come to rest on its side. There is one occupant in the vehicle. Before gaining access and assessing the occupants, you should consider

    (A)   removing the vehicle's battery

    (B)   siphoning the fuel from the tank

    (C)   cribbing the vehicle with wedges and boards

    (D)   checking to see if the patient can get out of the vehicle without assistance

7. After access has been made to this patient, you determine that he is critically injured and showing late signs of shock. Which of the following should you consider?

   (A) Requesting a medical helicopter
   (B) Application of an automated external defibrillator (AED)
   (C) Rapid removal of the patient without full spinal immobilization
   (D) Rocking the vehicle back over on to its wheels to facilitate rapid extrication

8. To gain full access to this patient, you must go through one of the windows. Which of the following techniques would be indicated?

   (A) Break either the front or rear window
   (B) Cover the patient with a blanket and break the front windshield
   (C) Cover the patient with a blanket and break a window far from the patient
   (D) Cover the patient with a blanket and break the window closest to the patient

9. Once you gain access to this patient, which of the following should be done first?

   (A) Check for a pulse
   (B) Perform an initial assessment
   (C) Perform a rapid trauma assessment
   (D) Apply a nonrebreather mask connected to supplemental oxygen

10. Your crew has successfully applied a short backboard to this patient while he was still in the vehicle. Which of the following is correct regarding the removal of this patient from the vehicle?

   (A) Your crew should grasp the short backboard and pull firmly to remove the patient
   (B) Your crew should move the patient, not the immobilization device, to remove the patient
   (C) Once the short backboard is applied, you should instruct the patient to climb free of the wreckage
   (D) Your crew should grasp the tape and straps used to secure the patient to the backboard and pull firmly to remove the patient

ANSWERS AND RATIONALES

1-D. In most cases, assessment and treatment may (and should) begin prior to and during extrication. Every attempt should be made to complete the initial assessment, treat life-threatening conditions, and stabilize the patient's spine before physically removing the patient from entrapment or entanglement. While nonrescue EMT-Basics (EMT-Basics not trained in extrication practices) should not perform complex extrication techniques, they should be involved in assessing, treating, and stabilizing patients under the supervision of rescue EMT-Basics.

2-A. Extrication is the removal of patients from entrapment. Sorting patients according to the severity of their injuries is the process of triage. Protecting bystanders from injury at motor vehicle scenes is an important aspect of the scene size-up. Finally, securing vehicles to prevent movement that may cause further harm to trapped patients or rescue workers is referred to as stabilization.

3-B. When extricating patients from damaged vehicles, a number of options are usually available: remove the door, cut off the roof, break out the window, etc. The most desirable option is always the simplest method that does not compromise the patient. The old adage of "try before you pry" is true. Before rescue personnel form their plan for extrication, they should analyze the vehicle from all sides.

4-A. Having one person in charge of coordinating the rescue effort is important when multiple tasks or crews are required for patient extrication and care. This person, the Incident Commander, is able to look at the "big picture" to ensure the safety of rescue crews, the appropriate treatment of patients, and the adequacy of the on-scene resources.

5-C. The scene size-up is your first responsibility at the scene. Some of the components of the scene size-up include determining the number of patients, the types of injuries, the need for additional resources, the number of vehicles, and the extent of damage to the vehicles. An important aspect of the size-up is the concern for the safety of yourself, your crew, the patient(s), and bystanders. Do not forget that body substance isolation (BSI) is part of the scene size-up. Gaining access to, triaging, and assessing patients all occur after the scene size-up.

6-C. This vehicle is not secure in its present position (on its side). Before accessing the patient, rescue personnel should immediately begin stabilizing the vehicle with wedges, chocks, jacks, etc. Removing the battery may actually slow your extrication efforts if an electric seat in the vehicle needs to be moved to access the patient more fully. Siphoning fuel from the tank may actually increase the possibility of explosion or exposure. Patients involved in motor vehicle collisions should not be asked to crawl free of the wreckage unless imminent danger exists (e.g., the vehicle is on fire).

7-A. With the closest hospital 45 miles from the accident scene, it is safe to say that ground transport will exceed 15 minutes. This patient is in critical condition, and rapid transportation to an appropriate facility is just as vital as is rapid stabilization and extrication. The automated external defibrillator (AED) may be applied if the patient is apneic and pulseless; currently, this is not the case. Since there is no evidence of imminent danger, this patient should be extricated only after immobilization of the spinal cord has been addressed. Rocking the vehicle back onto its wheels would compromise the patient's spinal immobilization and any other injury that exists.

8-C. Ideally, you should break a window remote from the patient. Modern passenger car side and rear windows are made of tempered glass. When broken, tempered glass fractures into hundreds of small rounded pieces rather than large shards of glass. The front windshield, however, is made of laminated safety glass. This glass is much more difficult to remove because the plates of glass are bonded to a clear laminate. Perhaps the best way to remove the front windshield is to remove the frame and rubber seal, then pop the window out. In any case, patients should be covered during extrication. Putting a rescuer in with the patient is ideal; extrication can be very noisy and frightening for patients of any age. Close communication with the patient is essential.

9-B. Once access is made, an initial assessment should be performed. If the patient is unconscious, a rapid trauma assessment would follow the initial assessment. If the patient is conscious, a focused history and physical examination would follow the initial assessment.

10-B. Immobilization devices are meant to do just that: immobilize the patient. Unless specifically designed to be used as an extrication device, you should use the immobilization device to secure the patient, then move the patient (not the device).

BIBLIOGRAPHY

Crosby LA, Lewallen DG (eds): *Emergency Care and Transportation of the Sick and Injured,* 6th ed. Rosemont, IL, American Academy of Orthopaedic Surgeons, 1995.

Grant HD, Murray RH Jr, Bergeron JD: *Emergency Care,* 7th ed. Englewood Cliffs, NJ, Prentice-Hall, 1995.

Hafen BQ, Karren KJ, Mistovich JJ: *Prehospital Emergency Care*, 5th ed. Upper Saddle River, NJ, Prentice-Hall, 1996.

Henry MC, Stapleton ER, Judd RL: *EMT: Prehospital Care*. Philadelphia, WB Saunders, 1992.

McSwain NE, White RD, Paturas JL, et al (eds): *The Basic EMT: Comprehensive Prehospital Patient Care*. St. Louis, Mosby-Year Book, 1996.

Miller RH, Wilson JK: *Manual of Prehospital Emergency Medicine*. St. Louis, Mosby-Year Book, 1992.

Stoy WA: *Mosby's EMT-Basic Textbook*. St. Louis, Mosby-Year Book, 1996.

United States Department of Transportation, National Highway Traffic Safety Administration: *Emergency Medical Technician: Basic. National Standard Curriculum*, 1994.

● MOTIVATION FOR LEARNING ●

The EMT-Basic may respond to situations involving hazardous materials or multiple patients. The EMT-Basic must be able to recognize that a hazardous materials situation exists to prevent further illness or injury. The EMT-Basic must also understand the basic concepts of incident management and be able to effectively triage patients in multiple-casualty situations.

HAZARDOUS MATERIALS

DEFINITIONS

1. The U.S. Department of Transportation (DOT) defines a **hazardous material** as "any substance or material in a quantity or form which poses an unreasonable risk to health, safety, and property when transported in commerce."

2. The Environmental Protection Agency (EPA) defines a hazardous substance as "any substance designated under the Clean Water Act and Comprehensive Environmental Response Compensation and Liability Act as posing a threat to waterways and the environment when released."

3. The EPA defines hazardous waste as "any waste or combination of wastes which pose a substantial present or potential hazard to human health or living organisms because such wastes are nondegradable or persistent in nature, or because they can biologically magnify, or because they may otherwise cause or tend to cause detrimental cumulative effects."

4. The National Fire Protection Association (NFPA) defines a hazardous material as "any substance that causes or may cause adverse effects on the health or safety of employees, the general public, or the environment: any biological agent and other disease-causing agent, or a waste or combination of wastes."

REGULATIONS AND STANDARDS

1. **Superfund Amendments and Reauthorization Act (SARA), Title III**
   a. This federal legislation was passed in 1986.
   b. It established hazardous chemical requirements for local, state, and federal governments.
   c. Emergency planning section of this legislation was designed to develop state and local preparedness and response capabilities.

2. **Occupational Safety and Health Administration (OSHA) regulation 1910.120**
   a. This regulation was put in place in 1989.
   b. It requires specific training for all emergency medical services (EMS) personnel who might respond to hazardous material incidents.
   c. It specifies the training requirements for five levels of hazardous material incident responders:
      (1) First responder awareness
      (2) First responder operations
      (3) Hazardous materials technicians
      (4) Hazardous materials specialist
      (5) On-scene incident commander

3. **NFPA standards**
   a. NFPA 472—Professional Competence of Responders to Hazardous Materials Incidents
   b. NFPA 473—Competencies for EMS Personnel Responding to Hazardous Materials Incidents
   c. NFPA 704—Hazard Classification System

SAFETY CONCERNS

1. Safety is the primary concern and should be assured for:
   a. EMT-Basic and crew
   b. Patient
   c. Public

2. Do not enter the scene unless you are trained to handle hazardous materials and know how to use the necessary equipment.

3. The EPA has defined four levels of chemical-protective equipment.

a. Level "A" protection
  (1) Level A is the highest level of chemical-protective clothing.
  (2) This level requires an encapsulated, impermeable suit that covers everything including the self-contained breathing apparatus (SCBA).
  (3) This suit is typically used by hazardous material teams for entry into hot zone.

b. Level "B" protection
  (1) Level B protection is typically worn by the decontamination team.
  (2) This level provides the highest level of respiratory protection but a lesser level of skin protection than Level A.
  (3) It is available in encapsulated and nonencapsulated types.
  (4) It does not provide full-body protection against gases.

c. Level "C" protection
  (1) Level C protection is used when the type of airborne substance is known.
  (2) It includes chemically resistant clothing, full-face mask, and a canister-equipped respirator that filters chemicals from the air.
  (3) It does not include a SCBA.

d. Level "D" protection
  (1) Level D protection is firefighter turnout clothing or regular work clothing.
  (2) It provides no respiratory protection and little body protection from chemicals.

SCENE SIZE-UP

1. Incidents that may involve hazardous materials include:
  a. Vehicle crashes
    (1) Commercial vehicles
    (2) Pest control vehicles
    (3) Tankers
    (4) Cars with alternative fuels
    (5) Tractor-trailers
  b. Transportation (e.g., railroads, pipelines)
  c. Storage
    (1) Tanks, storage vessels
    (2) Warehouses
    (3) Hardware or agricultural stores
    (4) Agriculture
  d. Manufacturing operations (e.g., chemical plants)
  e. Acts of terrorism
2. The following may be used to identify the substance:
  a. DOT *Emergency Response Guidebook*
  b. United Nations (UN) classification numbers
  c. Placards and labels
    (1) NFPA 704 placard system
      (a) This system uses a diamond-shaped diagram divided into quadrants.
      (b) The system uses different background colors and numbers ranging from 0 to 4 to indicate the dangers presented by the hazardous material.
        (i) Blue quadrant indicates a health hazard.
        (ii) Red quadrant indicates a flammability hazard.
        (iii) Yellow quadrant indicates a reactivity hazard.
        (iv) White quadrant indicates a specific hazard (e.g., radioactivity, need for protective equipment).
    (2) UN/DOT placards
      (a) The U.S. DOT requires that a placard be displayed on the shipping container and transport vehicle of dangerous materials.
      (b) The color of the placard tells the class of the hazardous material (*Table 33-1*).

Table 33-1. Classes of Hazardous Materials

Class	Color Code
Class 1—explosives/blasting agents	Orange
Class 2—gases compressed, liquified, or dissolved under pressure	Green
Class 3—flammable and combustible liquids	Red
Class 4—flammable solids	White and red stripes
Class 5—oxidizers/organic peroxides	Yellow
Class 6—poisons, irritants, and etiologic agents	White
Class 7—radioactive materials	Yellow over white
Class 8—corrosives	White over black
Class 9—other regulated materials	White

      (c) Presence of a four-digit number allows more specific identification; the four-digit number is keyed to the DOT *Emergency Response Guidebook*.
  d. Shipping papers
  e. Material safety data sheets (MSDS), which provide detailed information about the material, including:
      (1) Name of the substance
      (2) Physical properties of the substance
      (3) Fire and explosion hazard information
      (4) Emergency first-aid treatment
  f. Size and shape of the container. The DOT regulates the design and type of container used and the manner by which the hazardous material may be transported.
  g. Location
3. Establish safety zones
  a. The hot zone is the contamination zone (site of incident).
      (1) It is a dangerous area.
      (2) Only personnel with high-level personal protective equipment enter this area.
  b. The warm zone is the control zone.
      (1) It serves as the entry and decontamination point.
      (2) All personnel must wear appropriate protective gear.
  c. The cold zone is the safe zone and serves as the staging area for personnel and equipment.

GENERAL PROCEDURES

1. Park upwind/uphill from the incident at a safe distance.
2. Keep unnecessary people away from the area.
3. Isolate the area.
  a. Keep people out.
  b. Do not enter unless fully protected with proper equipment and self-contained breathing apparatus.
4. Avoid contact with material.
5. Remove patients to a safe zone, if no risk to EMT-Basic.
6. Do not enter a hazardous material area unless you are trained as a hazardous material technician and have proper training in SCBA.

RESOURCES

Resources that provide information about hazardous materials include:
1. Local hazardous material response team

2. Chemical Transportation Emergency Center (CHEMTREC)
   a. 24-hour hotline: (1-800-424-9300)
   b. The hotline can provide product and emergency action information.
3. *Emergency Response Guidebook*, published by the U.S. DOT
4. Regional poison control center, which can provide detailed information including decontamination methods and treatment
5. Material Safety Data Sheets (MSDS)

MULTIPLE-CASUALTY SITUATIONS (MCS)

TERMINOLOGY

1. A **multiple-casualty situation** (MCS) may also be called a mass-casualty incident (MCI) or multiple-casualty incident.
2. An MCS is any event that places a great demand on resources, be it equipment or personnel.

INCIDENT MANAGEMENT SYSTEM (IMS)

1. **Overview**
   a. An incident management system (IMS) has been developed to assist with the control, direction, and coordination of emergency response resources.
   (1) It provides an orderly means of communication and information for decision making.
   (2) Interactions with other agencies are easier because of the single coordination.
2. **Structure**
   a. After an incident commander (IC) is determined, EMS sectors are established as needed. EMS sectors include:
   (1) Incident command, which performs the following:
     (a) Oversees incident needs
     (b) Establishes objectives/priorities
     (c) Develops an action plan
     (d) Coordinates with other agencies/officials
     (e) Approves, orders, and releases resources
   (2) Extrication sector, which performs the following:
     (a) Determines the type of equipment and resources needed
     (b) Ensures that special safety equipment is available to all personnel (e.g., SCBA, protective clothing)
     (c) Ensures that support materials (e.g., gasoline, electricity, compressed air, etc.) for extrication equipment and materials are readily available
     (d) Works with treatment personnel with extended extrication or special rescue situations
     (e) Coordinates with safety officer, staging, and triage
   (3) Treatment sector, which performs the following:
     (a) Provides additional care as patients are received from the extrication and triage sectors, generally away from the immediate action area
     (b) Provides for secondary triage of patients as they arrive in the treatment sector
     (c) Communicates/coordinates with command, triage, and transportation sectors
     (d) Moves patients to transportation sector
   (4) Transportation sector, which performs the following:
     (a) Establishes ambulance staging and landing zones if necessary
     (b) Determines hospital receiving /treatment capabilities

(c) Coordinates transportation and distribution of patients to hospitals

(d) Tracks patients leaving the site and maintains tracking log with:

    (i) Patient identification

    (ii) Unit transporting

    (iii) Destination facility

(5) Staging sector, which performs the following:

(a) Coordinates with transportation sector for the movement of equipment/personnel to the scene

(b) Confers with command about additional resources needed

(6) Supply (support) sector, which performs the following:

(a) Obtains additional resources including personnel, equipment, and disposable supplies for other sectors

(b) Coordinates with the transportation sector to obtain additional supplies from local facilities

(7) Triage sector, which performs the following:

(a) Works at the incident or action site

(b) Assures initial primary triage is performed to minimize re-triage

(c) Determines site treatment needs and assures initial triage/treatment

(d) Organizes resources to deliver patients to the treatment area

(e) Responsible for supervising safety and treatment of entrapped patients

b. Various individuals/organizations carry out specific duties at the scene.

(1) Individuals at the scene will be assigned to particular roles in one of the sectors.

(2) Upon arrival, the EMT-Basic should report to the sector officer for specific duties.

(3) Once assigned a specific task, the EMT-Basic should complete the task and report back to the sector officer.

BASIC TRIAGE

1. **Triage** is the sorting of multiple casualties into priorities for emergency care or transportation to definitive care.

2. Priorities are given in three levels (*Table 33-2*).

    a. Highest priority patients are those with:

    (1) Airway and breathing difficulties

    (2) Uncontrolled or severe bleeding

    (3) Decreased mental status

    (4) Severe medical problems (e.g., diabetic and cardiac emergencies)

    (5) Shock (hypoperfusion)

    (6) Severe burns

    b. Second priority patients are those with:

    (1) Burns without airway problems

Table 33-2. Triage Priorities

Highest Priority (P-1)	Second Priority (P-2)	Lowest Priority (P-3)
Airway and breathing difficulties	Burns without airway problems	Minor painful, swollen, deformed extremities
Uncontrolled or severe bleeding	Major or multiple bone or joint injuries	
Decreased mental status	Back injuries with or without spinal cord damage	Minor soft tissue injuries
Patients with severe medical problems		Death
Signs and symptoms of shock (hypoperfusion)		
Severe burns		

    (2)   Major or multiple bone or joint injuries

    (3)   Back injuries with or without spinal cord damage

  c. Lowest priority patients are those:

    (1)   With minor painful, swollen, deformed extremities

    (2)   With minor soft tissue injuries

    (3)   Who are without vital signs or are obviously dead

GENERAL PROCEDURES

1. The most knowledgeable EMS provider arriving on the scene first becomes the triage officer or IC.

2. Call for additional resources.

3. Perform initial assessment on all patients first.

4. Assign available personnel and equipment to priority one patients.

5. Patient transport decisions are based on a variety of factors:

  a. Prioritization

  b. Destination facilities

  c. Transportation resources

6. Triage officer remains at the scene to assign and coordinate personnel, supplies, and vehicles.

REVIEW QUESTIONS

Directions: Each of the numbered items or incomplete statements in this section is followed by answers or by completions of the statement. Select the ONE lettered answer or completion that is BEST in each case.

1. The Environmental Protection Agency (EPA) has defined four levels of chemical-protective clothing and respiratory protection for entry into hazardous scenes. Personnel should not put on this equipment unless they are specifically trained to do so. The highest level of protection is

  (A)   a level "A" entry suit

  (B)   a level "D" entry suit

  (C)   latex medical gloves, face and eye protection, and a disposable gown

  (D)   firefighter protective clothing with self-contained breathing apparatus (SCBA)

2. When approaching a suspected hazardous materials incident, every effort should be made to approach

  (A)   from upwind and uphill

  (B)   from upwind and downhill

  (C)   from downwind and uphill

  (D)   from downwind and downhill

3. Hazardous materials scenes are divided into zones according to safety. Staging for personnel and equipment at a hazardous materials scene is in which zone?

  (A)   Hot zone

  (B)   End zone

  (C)   Cold zone

  (D)   Warm zone

4. When dealing with multiple-casualty incidents (MCIs), who should be assigned as "triage officer"?

    (A) The highest ranking official
    (B) The first paramedic to arrive at the scene
    (C) The first person to recognize the need for such a person
    (D) The most knowledgeable EMS provider arriving at the scene first

5. According to triage priorities, which of the following patients would be considered the highest priority?

    (A) A 56-year-old male with partial-thickness burns on his left leg
    (B) A 41-year-old female with a red, swollen neck and difficulty breathing
    (C) A 43-year-old female complaining of neck pain who cannot feel or move her legs or arms
    (D) A 23-year-old male who is apneic (not breathing) and pulseless and who has a penetrating injury to the chest

Directions: Each of the numbered questions or incomplete statements in this section refers to

information that precedes them. The numbered questions or incomplete statements are followed by answers or by completions of the statement. Select the answer or completion of the statement that is BEST in each case.

The National Fire Protection Association's (NFPA) Standard 704 designates a hazardous materials classification. Using a diamond-shaped diagram divided into four different colored sections, the NFPA 704 diagram lists hazards in three different categories on a scale of 0 to 4, with 4 being the most hazardous.

Questions 6–7

6. A rating of "4" in the blue portion of the diagram indicates

    (A) extreme frost hazard
    (B) extreme health hazard
    (C) extreme reactivity hazard
    (D) extreme flammability hazard

7. The white portion of the diagram is used to indicate

    (A) antidotes for the contained hazard
    (B) evacuating distance in case of spill or leak
    (C) phone number of the shipping or transport company
    (D) specific hazards (water reactivity, radioactivity, need for specialized equipment)

To assist with the control, direction, and coordination of a complex emergency scene, an incident management system (IMS) has been developed. This system facilitates coordination and interactions between sectors (e.g., extrication sector, transportation sector) and agencies (e.g., emergency departments, dispatch/alarm room, off-site resources). Typically, the emergency response personnel are divided into sectors according to their responsibility at the scene.

Questions 8–10

8. Which sector at a complex emergency scene is responsible for care of patients as they are received from the immediate action area and the movement of these patients to the transportation area?

   (A) Triage sector
   (B) Staging sector
   (C) Extrication sector
   (D) Treatment sector

9. Which sector at a complex emergency scene is responsible for the removal of patients from the immediate action area?

   (A) Triage sector
   (B) Staging sector
   (C) Extrication sector
   (D) Transportation sector

10. At a complex emergency scene, who is responsible for overseeing incident needs, establishing priorities, and developing an action plan?

   (A) The medical director
   (B) The incident commander
   (C) The highest ranking official
   (D) The health care provider with the highest level of certification or licensure

Directions: Each of the numbered questions or incomplete statements in this section refers to a scenario that precedes them. The numbered questions or incomplete statements are followed by answers or by completions of the statement. Select the answer or completion of the statement that is BEST in each case.

Your rescue crew is called to the scene of a "worker down" at a construction site. Upon arrival, you find a male patient unconscious in a 4-foot-deep trench. A 55-gallon container of an unknown substance overturned and leaked into the trench near the patient. On the container is a label with a four-digit number printed on it.

Questions 11–12

11. This placard is a(n)

   (A) MSDS sheet
   (B) UN/DOT placard
   (C) NFPA 704 diamond
   (D) evacuation distance chart

12. To better understand the meaning of this four-digit number and its implications, you should reference this number in

   (A) NFPA 472
   (B) SARA Title III
   (C) OSHA Regulation 1910.120
   (D) the *Emergency Response Guidebook*

ANSWERS AND RATIONALES

1-A. A Level "A" entry suit is a fully encapsulated suit that covers everything including the self-contained breathing apparatus (SCBA). An example of a Level "D" entry suit would be firefighter turnout clothing without the use of an SCBA. Firefighter protective clothing with an SCBA provides little or no protection against absorbed toxins. The use of latex medical gloves, face and eye protection, and a disposable gown provides protection for patient encounters but not for hazardous materials encounters.

2-A. To maximize safety, approach and park uphill and upwind of hazardous materials scenes. If the hazardous material becomes airborne or a large spill occurs, you are less likely to become exposed if you take this stance. Remember, EMS personnel should stage a minimum of 2000 feet from suspected hazardous materials incidents.

3-C. The cold zone is an area safe from exposure or the threat of exposure at hazardous materials scenes. The warm zone is a controlled area for entry into the hot zone and decontamination after exiting the hot zone. All personnel in the warm zone must wear appropriate protective equipment. The hot zone is the danger zone. The size of the hot zone depends on many factors, including the characteristics of the chemical, the amount released (spilled, escaped), the local weather conditions, the local terrain, and other chemicals in the area. The end zone is not an EMS term.

4-D. The task of triaging a multiple-casualty incident (MCI) should occur immediately after scene size-up. The person given the responsibility of triage should be the most knowledgeable EMS provider (EMT-Basic, EMT-Paramedic, nurse, etc.) to arrive at the scene first. Triage should not be delayed until a person of specific rank or certification arrives at the scene.

5-B. High-priority patients are those with airway or breathing problems, uncontrolled or severe bleeding, decreased mental status, severe medical problems (e.g., diabetic and cardiac emergencies), severe burns, or signs of shock (hypoperfusion). The next priority of patients are those with burns without airway or breathing compromise, major or multiple bone or joint injuries, and back injuries with or without spinal cord damage. Relative to high priority patients, care for these patients can be delayed. Finally, the lowest priority patients are those with minor soft tissue or musculoskeletal injuries or those without vital signs or are obviously deceased.

6-B. The blue portion of the diagram deals with health hazards. The red area addresses flammability hazard, and the yellow area addresses reactivity hazard. There is no portion of the diagram that deals specifically with "frost" hazard, although one area of the diagram addresses special hazards.

7-D. The white portion of the diagram lists any special hazards present with the material. For example, if the material reacts violently when exposed to water, a "W̶" (W with a line through it) indicates water reactivity.

8-D. The treatment sector is responsible for the care of patients from time of extrication until time of delivery to the transportation area. If extrication is going to take considerable time, treatment personnel should be involved with patient care during extrication. The triage sector is responsible for assigning patient priorities according to injury. This information should be given to the extrication sector so that the highest priority patients are extricated first. The staging sector is responsible for the movement of equipment and personnel to the scene and the close coordination with the incident commander to ensure that adequate resources are available.

9-C. The extrication sector is responsible for removing trapped patients from the immediate action area. The priority of patients extricated should be coordinated with the incident commander and triage sector. The transportation sector establishes a transportation area (landing zones if necessary). The transportation sector also determines the hospital resources and tracks patients leaving the scene (patient name, unit/agency transporting, and destination facility).

10-B. The incident commander (IC) can be anyone regardless of rank or certification. It is a position that should be determined by coordination and communication competency rather than rank or certification. Certainly, however, the IC must understand the factors involved in the emergency scene and the capabilities and limitations of the operating crews. The IC is ultimately responsible for everything that happens on the emergency scene. Experienced ICs commonly will assign one individual as the scene's safety officer. This person's sole responsibility is to monitor the safety of on-scene working conditions with regard to personal protective equipment, rescue techniques, and overall scene security/safety.

11-B. The UN/DOT placard is required on shipping containers and transport vessels (railroad cars, trucks, ships) if bulk hazardous materials are being transported. The four-digit number corresponds to a specific chemical name or class. MSDS (Material Safety Data Sheets) are required by the Occupational Safety and Health Administration (OSHA) to be kept on site wherever chemicals are used.

12-D. The *Emergency Response Guidebook* is published by the Department of Transportation (DOT) as a quick-reference guide for hazardous materials incidents. Chemicals are listed in the book alphabetically and by their four-digit DOT number. Each chemical is given a reference number that corresponds to a set of instructions and precautions (listed in the back of the book) for dealing with that class of chemical. NFPA 472 is the National Fire Protection Association's Standard for "Professional Competence of Responders to Hazardous Materials Incidents." OSHA Regulation 1910.120 also requires specific training for all EMS personnel who might respond to hazardous materials incidents. SARA (Superfund Amendments and Reauthorization Act of 1989) Title III established hazardous chemical requirements for all government agencies.

BIBLIOGRAPHY

Crosby LA, Lewallen DG (eds): *Emergency Care and Transportation of the Sick and Injured*, 6th ed. Rosemont, IL, American Academy of Orthopaedic Surgeons, 1995.

Grant HD, Murray RH Jr, Bergeron JD: *Emergency Care*, 7th ed. Englewood Cliffs, NJ, Prentice-Hall, 1995.

Hafen BQ, Karren KJ, Mistovich JJ: *Prehospital Emergency Care*, 5th ed. Upper Saddle River, NJ, Prentice-Hall, 1996.

Henry MC, Stapleton ER, Judd RL: *EMT: Prehospital Care*. Philadelphia, WB Saunders, 1992.

Limmer D, Elling B, O'Keefe MF: *Essentials of Emergency Care: A Referesher for the Practicing EMT-Basic*. Upper Saddle River, NJ, Prentice-Hall, 1996.

McSwain NE, White RD, Paturas JL, et al (eds): *The Basic EMT: Comprehensive Prehospital Patient Care*. St. Louis, Mosby-Year Book, 1996.

Stoy WA: *Mosby's EMT-Basic Textbook*. St. Louis, Mosby-Year Book, 1996.

United States Department of Transportation, National Highway Traffic Safety Administration: *Emergency Medical Technician: Basic. National Standard Curriculum*, 1994.

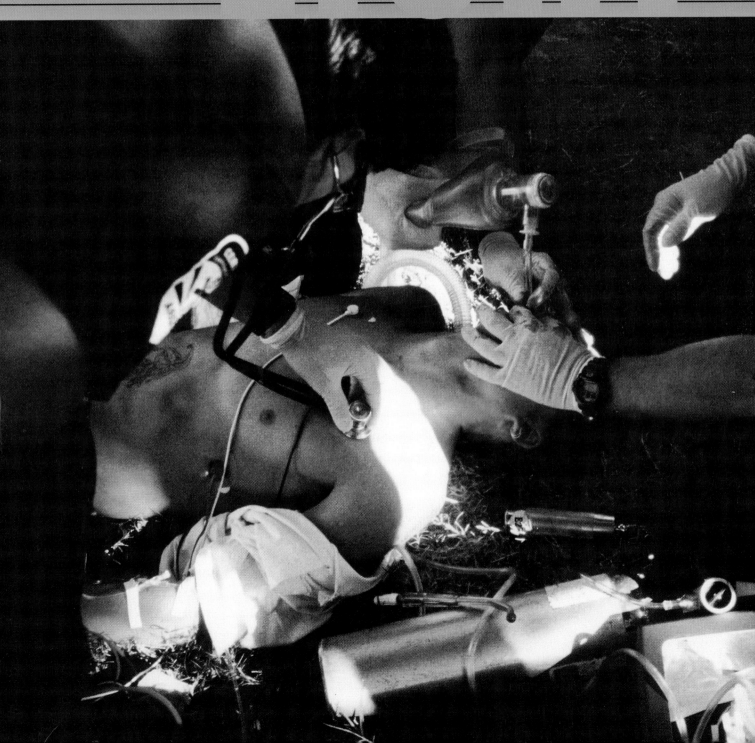

ADVANCED AIRWAY

EIGHT

34 ADVANCED AIRWAY MANAGEMENT

OBJECTIVES

34-1 Identify and describe the airway anatomy in the infant, child, and adult.

34-2 Explain the pathophysiology of airway compromise.

34-3 Differentiate between the airway anatomy in the infant, child, and adult.

34-4 Describe the proper use of airway adjuncts.

*34-5 Describe the purpose of suctioning.

*34-6 List the indications for orotracheal suctioning.

*34-7 List the possible complications of orotracheal suctioning.

*34-8 Describe the technique of orotracheal suctioning.

34-9 Describe the indications, contraindications, and technique for insertion of nasogastric tubes.

*34-10 List the equipment required for nasogastric tube insertion.

*34-11 Describe how to perform the Sellick maneuver (cricoid pressure).

*34-12 Describe the indications for advanced airway management.

*34-13 List the equipment required for orotracheal intubation.

*34-14 Describe the proper use of the straight blade for orotracheal intubation.

*34-15 Describe the proper use of the curved blade for orotracheal intubation.

*34-16 Describe the methods of choosing the appropriate size endotracheal tube in an adult patient.

*34-17 State the reasons for and proper use of the stylet in orotracheal intubation.

*34-18 Describe the skill of orotracheal intubation in the adult patient.

MOTIVATION FOR LEARNING

Advanced airway management by the EMT-Basic is an elective module that may be included in the EMT-Basic course if approved by the state Emergency Medical Services office. If the module is approved, the EMT-Basic will learn how to insert a nasogastric tube for decompression of the stomach of an infant or child patient and how to perform orotracheal intubation of adults, children, and infants.

*34-19 Describe the skill of confirming endotracheal tube placement in the adult, infant, and child patient.

*34-20 Describe the skill of securing the endotracheal tube in the adult, infant, and child patient.

*34-21 State the consequence of and the need to recognize unintentional esophageal intubation.

*34-22 List complications associated with advanced airway management.

*34-23 State the formula for sizing an infant or child endotracheal tube.

*34-24 Define the various alternative methods for sizing the infant and child endotracheal tube.

*34-25 Describe the skill of orotracheal intubation in the infant and child patient.

AIRWAY ANATOMY AND PHYSIOLOGY REVIEW

RESPIRATORY SYSTEM

Components of the respiratory system include:
1. **Nose and mouth**
2. **Pharynx**
   a. Oropharynx
   b. Nasopharynx
3. **Epiglottis,** the leaf-shaped structure that prevents food and liquid from entering the trachea during swallowing
4. **Trachea** (windpipe)
5. **Vallecula,** the area between the base of the tongue and the epiglottis
6. **Cricoid cartilage,** the firm cartilage ring forming the lower portion of the larynx
7. **Larynx** (voice box), which contains the vocal cords
8. **Bronchi,** the two major branches of the trachea to the lungs; each bronchus subdivides into smaller air passages ending at the **alveoli**
9. **Lungs**
10. **Diaphragm**
    a. **Inhalation (active)**
        (1)   The diaphragm and intercostal muscles contract, increasing the size of the thoracic cavity.
            (a) The diaphragm moves slightly downward and flares the lower portion of rib cage.
            (b) Ribs move upward/outward.
        (2)   Air flows into the lungs.
    b. **Exhalation (passive)**
        (1)   The diaphragm and intercostal muscles relax, decreasing the size of the thoracic cavity.
            (a) The diaphragm moves upward.
            (b) Ribs move downward/inward.
        (2)   Air flows out of the lungs.
11. **Respiratory physiology**
    a. **Alveolar/capillary exchange**
        (1)   Oxygen-rich air enters the alveoli during each inspiration.
        (2)   Oxygen-poor blood in the capillaries passes into the alveoli.
        (3)   Oxygen enters the capillaries as carbon dioxide enters the alveoli.
    b. **Capillary/cellular exchange**
        (1)   Cells give up carbon dioxide to the capillaries.
        (2)   Capillaries give up oxygen to the cells.

   c. **Adequate breathing**
     (1)   Normal rates are:
       (a) Adult:12–20 breaths per minute
       (b) Child:15–30 breaths per minute
       (c) Infant: 25–50 breaths per minute
     (2)   Rhythm is regular.
     (3)   Quality is adequate as shown by the following:
       (a) Breath sounds are present and equal bilaterally.
       (b) Chest expansion is adequate and equal.
       (c) Effort of breathing is adequate without use of accessory muscles.
       (d) Depth (tidal volume) is adequate.

 d. **Inadequate breathing**
   (1)   Rate is outside of normal range.
   (2)   Rhythm is irregular.
   (3)   Quality is diminished.
     (a) Breath sounds are diminished or absent.
     (b) Chest expansion is unequal or inadequate.
     (c) Breathing effort is increased. Accessory muscles may be used, especially in infants and children.
   (4)   Depth (tidal volume) is inadequate/shallow.
   (5)   The skin may be pale or cyanotic (blue) and cool and clammy.
   (6)   Retractions may be present above the clavicles, between the ribs, and below the rib cage, especially in children.
   (7)   Nasal flaring may be present, especially in children.
   (8)   Infants may exhibit "seesaw" breathing, in which the abdomen and chest move in opposite directions.
   (9)   **Agonal breathing** (occasional gasping breaths) may be seen just before death.
   (10) Slower than normal heart rate and absent/weak peripheral pulses may be noted in pediatric patients.

INFANT AND CHILD ANATOMY CONSIDERATIONS

1. **Mouth and nose.** In general, all structures are smaller and more easily obstructed than in adults.
2. **Pharynx.** Infants' and children's tongues take up proportionally more space in the mouth than adults'.
3. **Trachea (windpipe)**
   a. Infants and children have narrower tracheas that are obstructed more easily by swelling.
   b. The trachea is softer and more flexible in infants and children.
4. **Cricoid cartilage**
   a. The narrowest area in infants and children is the cricoid cartilage.
   b. Like other cartilage in the infant and child, the cricoid cartilage is less developed and less rigid.
5. **Diaphragm.** The chest wall is softer; infants and children tend to depend more heavily on the diaphragm for breathing.

AIRWAY AND SUCTIONING TECHNIQUES

OPENING THE AIRWAY

1. Use the head-tilt, chin-lift maneuver when there is no suspicion of neck injury.
2. Use the jaw-thrust maneuver when the EMT-Basic suspects spinal injury.
3. Assess need for suction.

TECHNIQUES OF SUCTIONING

1. **Purpose**
   a. Suctioning removes blood, other liquids, and food particles from the airway.
   b. Some suction units are inadequate for removing solid objects like teeth and foreign bodies or food.
   c. A patient needs to be suctioned immediately when a gurgling sound is heard with artificial ventilation.

2. **Types of units**
   a. Suction devices include:
   - (1) Mounted
   - (2) Portable, either electric or hand-operated
   b. Suction catheters include:
   - (1) Hard or rigid catheters
     - (a) Hard or rigid catheters are used to suction the mouth and oropharynx of an unresponsive patient.
     - (b) They should be inserted only as far as you can see.
   - (2) Soft (French) catheters
     - (a) Soft catheters are useful for suctioning the nasopharynx and in other situations where a rigid catheter cannot be used.
     - (b) The catheter should be measured so that it is inserted only as far as the base of the tongue.

3. **Orotracheal suctioning**
   a. Indications include:
   - (1) Obvious secretions
   - (2) Poor compliance with the bag-valve mask
   b. Complications include:
   - (1) Dysrhythmias
   - (2) Hypoxia
   - (3) Coughing
   - (4) Damage to the mucosa
   - (5) Bronchospasm
   c. **Technique**
   - (1) Preoxygenate the patient.
   - (2) Hyperventilate the patient.
   - (3) Check equipment.
   - (4) Use sterile technique.
   - (5) Insert catheter without applying suction.
   - (6) Advance catheter to desired location, typically the carina.
   - (7) Apply suction and withdraw the catheter in a twisting motion.

NASOGASTRIC TUBES

USES

1. Nasogastric tubes decompress the stomach and proximal bowel in response to obstruction or trauma.
2. They may be used to drain the stomach of blood or other substances.
3. They may be used for administration of medications and nutrition.

INDICATIONS

Indications for a nasogastric tube include:
1. Inability to artificially ventilate the infant or child patient because of gastric distension
2. Unresponsive patient

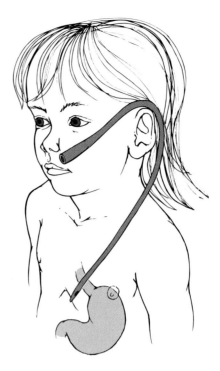

Fig. 34-1. Measure the nasogastric tube from the tip of the nose, around the ear, to below the xiphoid process.

CONTRAINDICATIONS

1. Contraindications include the presence of major facial, head, or spinal trauma.
2. Orogastric technique is preferred in these situations.

COMPLICATIONS

Complications of nasogastric tubes include:
1. Tracheal intubation
2. Nasal trauma
3. Emesis
4. Passage into the cranium in cases of basilar skull fractures

EQUIPMENT

Equipment includes:
1. Nasogastric tube, assorted sizes
    a. Newborn/infant: 8.0 French
    b. Toddler/preschooler: 10.0 French
    c. School-age children: 12.0 French
    d. Adolescent: 14.0–16.0 French
2. 20-milliliter (mL) syringe
3. Water-soluble lubricant
4. Emesis basin
5. Tape
6. Stethoscope
7. Suction unit and suction catheters

INSERTION PROCEDURE—INFANTS AND CHILDREN

1. Prepare and assemble all equipment.
2. Measure tube from the tip of the nose, around the ear, to below the xiphoid process (*Figure 34-1*).

3. Lubricate the distal end of the tube.
4. If trauma is not suspected, place the patient supine, with the head turned to left side.
5. Pass the tube along the nasal floor.
6. Check placement of tube by:
   a. Aspirating stomach contents
   b. Auscultating over the epigastrium while injecting 10–20 mL of air into the tube
7. Aspirate stomach contents.
8. Secure tube in place with tape.

SELLICK MANEUVER (CRICOID PRESSURE)

PURPOSE

1. The Sellick maneuver was developed for use during intubation of patients in the operating room to prevent passive regurgitation related to medication-induced paralysis.
2. It should be used in an unresponsive patient without a cough or gag reflex to help prevent passive regurgitation and aspiration during endotracheal intubation.

ANATOMICAL LOCATION

1. The cricoid cartilage connects the larynx and trachea.
2. It is located below the thyroid cartilage and is attached to the trachea's first ring of cartilage. The cricoid cartilage forms a complete ring and is the narrowest part of the airway in children.
3. The cricothyroid membrane connects the lower border of the thyroid cartilage with the upper portion of the cricoid cartilage. The cricothyroid membrane can be located by palpating the patient's neck, starting at the top. The first structure felt is the thyroid cartilage (more prominent in males than females), and the second prominence is the cricoid cartilage. The depression between these prominences is the cricothyroid membrane.

TECHNIQUE

1. A third provider should find the cricoid cartilage.
2. The rescuer then applies firm posterior pressure just lateral to the midline with the thumb and index finger (*Figure 34-2*).

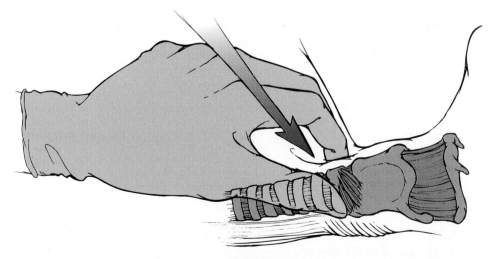

Fig. 34-2. Cricoid pressure (Sellick maneuver) is performed by applying firm posterior pressure to the cricoid cartilage, just lateral to the midline, with the thumb and index finger.

3. Cricoid pressure should be maintained during positive-pressure ventilation until the patient is intubated and the endotracheal cuff is inflated after confirmation of proper tube placement.

SPECIAL CONSIDERATIONS

1. Verify correct anatomy to avoid damage to other structures.
2. The cricoid cartilage is difficult to locate in the child and small adult. Excessive pressure in infants and children may cause tracheal obstruction.
3. Make sure enough personnel are available to perform this maneuver.

ADVANCED AIRWAY MANAGEMENT—OROTRACHEAL INTUBATION

ADULT OROTRACHEAL INTUBATION

1. **Purpose**
   a. Orotracheal intubation is the most effective means of controlling a patient's airway.
   b. Use in apneic patients:
      (1) Provides complete control of the airway
      (2) Reduces risk of aspiration
      (3) Allows for better oxygen delivery
      (4) Allows for deeper suctioning
2. **Indications.** Orotracheal intubation is indicated when:
   a. Prolonged artificial ventilation is required
   b. Adequate artificial ventilation cannot be achieved by other methods
   c. The patient is unresponsive and has no cough or gag reflex
   d. The patient is unable to protect his or her own airway (e.g., cardiac arrest, unresponsive)
3. **Equipment.** Equipment for orotracheal intubation includes:
   a. Gloves, mask, and goggles for body substance isolation (BSI) precautions
   b. Laryngoscope handle with locking bar and, if battery powered, spare batteries
   c. Laryngoscope blades
      (1) **Straight blades**
         (a) Straight blades come in assorted sizes, 0–4.
         (b) The straight blade lifts the epiglottis to allow visualization of the glottic opening and vocal cords.
         (c) The straight blade is preferred in children and infants.
      (2) **Curved blades**
         (a) Curved blades come in assorted sizes, 0–4.
         (b) The curved blade is inserted into the vallecula to allow visualization of the glottic opening and vocal cords.
      (3) Assembly of laryngoscope blade and handle
         (a) The notch on the blade locks onto the locking bar of the laryngoscope handle.
         (b) Lifting the blade up locks it into place and illuminates the light.
         (c) Check light.
            (i) It should be "bright, white, steady, and tight."
            (ii) Spare bulbs should be available; bulbs come in assorted sizes for each blade.
   d. Endotracheal tubes
      (1) Assorted sizes of endotracheal tubes should be available.
         (a) Average sizes are:
            (i) Adult male: 8.0 to 8.5-millimeter (mm) internal diameter (i.d.)
            (ii) Adult female: 7.0–8.0-mm i.d.

        (iii) Emergency rule: 7.5-mm i.d. fits an adult in an emergency
    (b) It is helpful to have one tube larger and one tube smaller than estimated size available.
  (2) Components of the endotracheal tube include:
    (a) 15-mm adapter, which allows attachment of bag-valve mask
    (b) Pilot balloon, which verifies that cuff is inflated
      (i) The cuff holds approximately 10 mL of air.
      (ii) It should be inflated until there is no leak of air around the endotracheal tube.
      (iii) Infant and child endotracheal tubes are uncuffed and should be used in patients younger than 8 years of age.
    (d) Murphy eye, the small hole on the left side across from the bevel that decreases chance of obstruction
    (e) Length of tube for adult: 33 centimeters (cm)
    (f) Helpful hints: average adult
      (i) 15 cm to the cords
      (ii) 20 cm teeth to sternal notch
      (iii) 25 cm teeth to carina
      (iv) "Teeth and tube at 22"

e. Stylet
  (1) The stylet is made of malleable metal and is inserted into the endotracheal tube to provide stiffness and shape of the tube.
    (b) Consider lubrication to allow for easy removal.
    (c) Once inserted, the stylet should be used to form a "hockey stick" shape for the endotracheal tube.
    (d) It should not be inserted beyond the Murphy eye; best if kept 1/4″ from the cuff, or proximal end of Murphy eye.

f. Water-soluble lubricant, which is applied to the endotracheal tube for ease of insertion and the stylet for ease of removal

g. 10-mL syringe
  (1) The syringe is used to test the cuff before insertion of the endotracheal tube.
  (2) Following the verification of integrity of the pilot balloon, the syringe should remain attached.
  (3) It is used to inflate the cuff once tube has been placed.

h. Securing device
  (1) Many securing devices are available, including tape and commercial devices.
  (2) Medical direction should approve taping technique or use of a commercial device.
  (3) The securing device should have an oropharyngeal airway (OPA) or similar device as a bite block.

i. Suction unit
  (1) The suction unit should be readily available to clear any fluid or particulate debris.
  (2) A large-bore catheter is needed to suction during intubation.
  (3) Later, a soft catheter can be used for endotracheal suctioning.

j. Towels, which can be used to raise the patient's shoulders or occiput to align the patient's airway

4. Insertion technique
  a. Take BSI precautions.
  b. Ensure that adequate artificial ventilation by bag-valve mask and oxygen is being performed.
  c. Hyperventilate the patient at a rate of 24 breaths per minute before any intubation attempt.
  d. Assemble and test all intubation equipment.

  e. Position the patient's head to assure ease of visualization.
- **(1)** If trauma is not suspected, tilt the head, lift the chin, and attempt to visualize the cords.
  - **(a)** If unable to visualize the cords, raise the patient's shoulders approximately 1 inch (may be more based on age) by placing a towel beneath them.
  - **(b)** Attempt visualization again.
- **(2)** If trauma is suspected, the patient must be intubated with the head and neck in a neutral position while a second rescuer maintains in-line stabilization.

  f. Holding the laryngoscope handle in the left hand, insert the laryngoscope blade into the right corner of the patient's mouth.

  g. With a sweeping motion, lift the tongue up and to the left, out of the way.

  h. Insert the blade into the proper anatomical landmark.
- **(1)** Curved blade is inserted into the vallecula.
- **(2)** Straight blade lifts the epiglottis.

  i. Lift the laryngoscope up and away from the patient.

  j. Use great care to avoid using the teeth as a fulcrum.

  k. Application of cricoid pressure (Sellick maneuver) during attempts at visualization may be beneficial.
- **(1)** Cricoid pressure should be used if you suspect the patient may vomit.
- **(2)** Thyroid pressure should be used to assist in visualizing the cords.

  l. Visualize the glottic opening and the vocal cords; do not lose sight of the vocal cords.

  m. With the right hand, gently insert the endotracheal tube until the cuff just passes the vocal cords. Note the markings on the tube at the upper teeth or gum line and record.

  n. Remove the laryngoscope blade and extinguish the lamp.

  o. Remove the stylet, if used.

  p. Inflate the cuff with 5 to 10 mL of air and remove the syringe.

  q. Continue to hold the endotracheal tube until the tube is secured in place.

  r. Have a partner attach the bag-valve mask and deliver positive-pressure ventilations.

  s. Confirm tube placement.
- **(1)** Visualization of the tube passing through the cords is the only true way of confirming placement.
- **(2)** All other methods are for verification, including:
  - **(a)** Rise and fall of the patient's chest
  - **(b)** Carbon dioxide detectors
  - **(c)** Auscultation of breath sounds
    - **(i)** Begin over epigastrium. No sounds should be heard during artificial ventilation.
    - **(ii)** Listen to the left apex. Compare with the right apex. Breath sounds should be equal bilaterally.
    - **(iii)** Listen to the left base. Compare to the right base. Breath sounds should be equal bilaterally.
  - **(d)** Other methods
    - **(i)** Pulse oximetry
    - **(ii)** Patient becomes more combative, indicating incorrect tube placement

  t. If breath sounds are bilaterally equal, and no sounds are heard in the epigastrium, the endotracheal tube should be secured in place using tape or a commercial device approved by medical direction.
- **(1)** The patient should then be artificially ventilated at an age-appropriate rate.
- **(2)** Remember to note the distance that the tube has been inserted.

(3) An OPA may be inserted to act as a bite block.

u. If breath sounds are diminished or absent on the left, most likely a right mainstem bronchus intubation has occurred.

(1) Deflate the cuff and gently withdraw the tube while artificially ventilating and auscultating over the left chest.

(2) Take care not to completely remove the endotracheal tube.

(3) Compare the right and left breath sounds.

(4) If bilaterally equal, follow the previous directions regarding inflation of the cuff, securing the tube, and artificially ventilating the patient.

v. If sounds are only present in the epigastrium, an esophageal intubation has occurred.

(1) An unrecognized esophageal intubation is fatal.

(2) Deflate the cuff, remove the tube, and hyperventilate the patient for an additional 2–5 minutes before your second and final intubation attempt.

w. Be sure to reassess breath sounds following every major move (e.g., from the scene to the ambulance, from the ambulance to the receiving facility).

5. Complications

a. Stimulation of the airway may cause the heart rate to decrease. The heart rate should be continuously monitored.

b. Soft tissue trauma to lips, teeth, tongue, gums, and airway structures may occur.

c. Prolonged attempts may lead to inadequate oxygenation.

d. The right mainstem bronchus or esophagus may be inadvertently intubated instead of the trachea.

d. Vomiting may occur.

g. Self extubation may occur. Be sure to reassess chest wall motion, breath sounds following every major move (e.g., from the scene to the ambulance, from the ambulance to the receiving facility) because moving the patient is a primary cause of extubation in infants and children.

INFANT AND CHILD OROTRACHEAL INTUBATION

1. Special considerations for intubation

a. It is difficult to create a single, clear visual plane from the mouth through the pharynx to the glottis for orotracheal intubation in infants and children.

b. Because the cricoid ring is the narrowest part of the child's airway, sizing of the endotracheal tube must be selected based on the size of the cricoid ring rather than the glottic opening.

2. Purpose

a. Orotracheal intubation is the most effective means of controlling a patient's airway.

b. Use in apneic patients:

(1) Provides complete control of the airway

(2) Reduces risk of aspiration

(3) Allows for better oxygen delivery

(4) Allows for deeper suctioning

3. Indications. Orotracheal intubation is indicated when:

a. Prolonged artificial ventilation is required

b. Adequate artificial ventilation cannot be achieved by other methods

c. The patient is clearly apneic

d. The patient is unresponsive with no cough or gag reflex

4. Advantages. Orotracheal intubation:

a. Prevents gastric distention

b. Reduces risk of aspiration

c. Permits suctioning of airway secretions

5. Equipment. Equipment for orotracheal intubation includes:

a. Gloves, mask, and goggles for BSI precautions

b. Bag-valve mask with correct size mask (it is very important to ventilate the patient before and after intubation)

c. Laryngoscope handle with locking bar and, if battery powered, spare batteries

d. Laryngoscope blades

  (1) Straight blades

    (a) The straight blade is preferred in children and infants.

      (i) It provides greater displacement of the tongue.

      (ii) It provides for better visualization of the glottis.

    (b) Straight blades come in assorted sizes, 0–4.

    (c) The straight blade lifts the epiglottis to allow visualization of the glottic opening and vocal cords.

  (2) Curved blades

    (a) The curved blade is preferred in older children; broader base and flange provide displacement of the tongue.

    (b) Curved blades come in assorted sizes, 0–4.

    (c) The curved blade is inserted into the vallecula to allow visualization of the glottic opening and vocal cords.

  (3) Assembly of laryngoscope blade and handle

    (a) The notch on the blade locks onto the locking bar of the laryngoscope handle.

    (b) Lifting the blade up locks it into place and illuminates the light.

    (c) Check light.

      (i) It should be "bright, white, steady, and tight."

      (ii) Spare bulbs should be available; bulbs come in assorted sizes for each blade.

e. Endotracheal tubes

  (1) Assorted sizes of endotracheal tubes should be available.

    (a) Average sizes

      (i) Newborns and small infants: 3.0–3.5 mm i.d.

      (ii) Up to 1 year old: 4.0 mm i.d.

    (b) Formula

      (i) 16 + patient's age in years divided by 4 = tube size, or

      (ii) Patient's age in years divided by 4, + 4 = tube size

    (c) Alternate sizing

      (i) Diameter of patient's little finger

      (ii) Diameter of patient's nasal opening

    (d) It is helpful to have one tube ½ cm size larger and one tube ½ cm size smaller than estimated size available.

  (2) Choice of sizes and type of infant and child endotracheal tubes used is age-dependent.

    (a) Uncuffed tubes are used in patients younger than 8 years old. The circular narrowing at the level of the cricoid cartilage serves as a functional cuff.

    (b) Cuffed tubes should be used for children older than 8 years old.

    (c) A vocal cord marker should be used to assure that the tip of the tube is placed in a midtracheal position.

    (d) Measurement of the endotracheal tube at the teeth (*Box 34-1*):

      (i) 6 months to 1 year of age: 12 cm midtrachea to teeth

      (ii) 2 years of age: 14 cm midtrachea to teeth

      (iii) 4–6 years of age: 16 cm midtrachea to teeth

      (iv) 6–10 years: 18 cm midtrachea to teeth

      (v) 10–12 years: 20 cm midtrachea to teeth

f. Stylet

  (1) The stylet is made of malleable metal and is inserted into the endotracheal tube to provide stiffness and shape of the tube.

  (2) It should be lubricated to allow for easy removal.

> **Box 34-1.** **Measurement of the Endotracheal Tube at the Teeth**
>
> 6 months to 1 year of age: 12 centimeters (cm) midtrachea to teeth
> 2 years of age: 14 cm midtrachea to teeth
> 4–6 years of age: 16 cm midtrachea to teeth
> 6–10 years of age: 18 cm midtrachea to teeth
> 10–12 years of age: 20 cm midtrachea to teeth

    (3) Once inserted, the stylet should be used to form a "hockey stick" shape for the endotracheal tube.

    (4) It should not be inserted beyond the Murphy eye; in pediatric patients, the stylet should be kept just above the Murphy eye.

g. Water-soluble lubricant, which is applied to the endotracheal tube for ease of insertion and the stylet for ease of removal. Types include:

    (1) KY® gel

    (2) Surgi-lube®

h. 10-mL syringe

    (1) The syringe is used to test the cuff before insertion of the endotracheal tube.

    (2) It is used to inflate the cuff once tube has been placed.

i. Securing device

    (1) Many securing devices are available, including tape and commercial devices.

    (2) Medical direction should approve taping technique or use of a commercial device.

    (3) The securing device should have an OPA or similar device as a bite block.

j. Suction unit

    (1) The suction unit should be readily available in case of emesis.

    (2) A large-bore catheter is needed to suction during intubation.

    (3) Later, a soft catheter can be used for endotracheal suctioning.

k. Towels, which can be used to raise the patient's shoulders or occiput to align the patient's airway

6. Insertion technique

a. Ensure adequate artificial ventilation by bag-valve mask and oxygen is being performed.

b. Patient must be hyperventilated at an age appropriate rate before any intubation attempt.

c. Assemble and test all equipment.

d. Take BSI precautions.

e. Heart rate should be continuously monitored during intubation attempts.

    (1) Mechanical stimulation of the airway may cause the heart rate to decrease.

    (2) If a slow heart rate is noted, the intubation attempt should be interrupted to reventilate the infant or child.

f. Position the patient's head to assure ease of visualization.

    (1) If trauma is not suspected, tilt the head, lift the chin, and attempt to visualize the cords.

        (a) If unable to visualize the cords, raise the patient's shoulders approximately 1 inch (may be more based on age).

        (b) Attempt visualization again.

    (2) If trauma is suspected, the patient must be intubated with the head and neck in a neutral position using in-line stabilization.

g. Very little force is necessary for intubation, technique is critical.

h. Holding the laryngoscope handle in the left hand, insert the laryngoscope blade into the right corner of the mouth, following the natural contour of the pharynx.

(1) Once the blade is at the back of the tongue, with a sweeping motion control the tongue and lift it out of the way.

(2) Insert the blade into the proper anatomical landmark.

    (a) Curved blade is inserted into the vallecula.

    (b) Straight blade lifts epiglottis.

        (i) The epiglottis of infants and children is made of cartilage that is less developed than an adult's.

        (ii) As a result, the epiglottis is more likely to block the airway and will require more attention to visualize the airway.

(3) Lift up and away from the patient.

(4) Use great care to avoid using the teeth as a fulcrum.

i. Application of cricoid pressure (Sellick maneuver) during attempts at visualization may be beneficial.

j. Visualize the glottic opening and the vocal cords; do not lose sight of the vocal cords.

k. With the right hand, gently insert the endotracheal tube until the glottic marker, if present, is placed at the level of the vocal cords.

l. If a cuffed tube is used, the tube is inserted until the cuff just passes the vocal cords.

m. Continue to hold the endotracheal tube until the tube is secured in place.

n. Remove the stylet, if used.

o. Remove the laryngoscope blade and extinguish the lamp.

p. Have your partner attach the bag-valve mask and deliver positive-pressure ventilations.

q. Confirm tube placement

    (1) In infants and children, assess for symmetrical rise and fall of the chest. This is the best indicator as breath sounds may be misleading.

    (2) Assess for an improvement in heart rate and skin color.

    (3) Auscultate breath sounds.

        (a) Begin over epigastrium. There should be an absence of insufflation or gurgling sounds.

        (b) Listen to the left apex.

            (i) Compare with the right apex.

            (ii) Breath sounds should be equal bilaterally.

        (c) Listen to the left base.

            (i) Compare with the right base.

            (ii) Breath sounds should be equal bilaterally.

        (d) Listen at the sternal notch.

r. If breath sounds are equal bilaterally and no sounds are heard in the epigastrium, the endotracheal tube should be secured in place using tape or an approved commercial device.

    (1) Remember to inflate the cuff if a cuffed tube was used.

    (2) After securing the tube, reconfirm tube placement.

s. The patient should then be artificially ventilated at an age-appropriate rate.

    (1) Remember to note the distance that the tube has been inserted.

    (2) An OPA may be inserted to act as a bite block.

t. If breath sounds are diminished or absent on the left, most likely a right mainstem bronchus intubation has occurred.

    (1) Deflate the cuff (if a cuffed tube was used) and gently withdraw the tube while artificially ventilating and auscultating over the left chest.

    (2) Take care not to completely remove the endotracheal tube.

    (3) Compare the right and left breath sounds. If equal bilaterally, follow the previous directions regarding securing the tube, and artificially ventilating the patient.

u. If breath sounds are only present in the epigastrium, an esophageal intubation has occurred.

      (1) An unrecognized esophageal intubation is fatal.

      (2) Deflate the cuff (if a cuffed tube was used), remove the tube, and hyperventilate the patient for an additional 2–5 minutes before your second and final intubation attempt.

  v. Once the tube is secured, the patient should be secured to an appropriate device to help minimize movement of the head that may dislodge the tube.

  w. Be sure to reassess chest wall motion and breath sounds following every major move, e.g., from the scene to the ambulance, from the ambulance to the receiving facility.

  x. If the tube is properly placed but inadequate lung expansion occurs, search for one of the following possible causes:

      (1) The tube is too small and a large air leak is present at the glottic opening.

         (a) A too-small tube can be assessed by auscultation of the neck.

         (b) The tube should be replaced with a larger tube.

         (c) In children older than 8 years of age, consider a cuffed tube.

      (2) The pop-off valve on the bag-valve mask has not been deactivated.

      (3) There is a leak in the bag-valve device.

      (4) The ventilator is delivering inadequate breaths.

      (5) The tube is blocked with secretions.

         (a) Treat with endotracheal suctioning.

         (b) If suctioning fails, the tube may have to be removed.

7. Complications

  a. Stimulation of the airway may cause the heart rate to decrease. The heart rate should be continuously monitored.

  b. Soft tissue trauma to lips teeth, tongue, gums, and airway structures may occur.

  c. Prolonged attempts may lead to inadequate oxygenation.

  d. The right mainstem bronchus or esophagus may be inadvertently intubated instead of the trachea.

  d. Vomiting may occur.

  g. Self extubation may occur. Be sure to reassess chest wall motion, breath sounds following every major move (e.g., from the scene to the ambulance, from the ambulance to the receiving facility) because moving the patient is a primary cause of extubation in infants and children.

  h. Collapse of a lung may occur.

REVIEW QUESTIONS

Directions: Each of the numbered items or incomplete statements in this section is followed by answers or by completions of the statement. Select the ONE lettered answer or completion that is BEST in each case.

1. The leaf-shaped structure that prevents food and liquid from entering the windpipe during swallowing is the

  (A) pharynx
  (B) trachea
  (C) epiglottis
  (D) esophagus

2. There are several anatomical differences between adults and children/infants. For example, the narrowest aspect of the adult upper airway is the glottic opening at the vocal cords. For children and infants, the narrowest aspect of the upper airway is the

   (A) pharynx
   (B) esophagus
   (C) cricoid cartilage
   (D) thyroid cartilage

3. The correct formula for approximating the appropriate size endotracheal tube for an infant or child is

   (A) the patient's age in months divided by 4
   (B) the patient's age in years multiplied by 2
   (C) the patient's age in months divided by 16
   (D) the patient's age in years plus 16, then divided by 4

4. Due to anatomical differences between adult and pediatric patients, different endotracheal tubes must be used. Cuffed endotracheal tubes should be used for patients

   (A) younger than 1 year of age
   (B) younger than 6 years of age
   (C) older than 1 year of age
   (D) older than 8 years of age

5. You are called to a long-term care facility for a 96-year-old female patient in cardiac arrest. You arrive to find the patient unconscious and pulseless. You note she takes a gasping breath once every 10–15 seconds. This is most likely

   (A) agonal breathing
   (B) Kussmaul respirations
   (C) hyperventilation
   (D) her normal respiratory rate and effort

6. Your rescue crew is called to the scene of a 92-year-old male patient in cardiopulmonary arrest. Upon arrival, you confirm the patient is pulseless and apneic, and cardiopulmonary resuscitation (CPR) is initiated. Which of the following should be done first?

   (A) Insert a nasogastric tube
   (B) Gather a SAMPLE history
   (C) Perform orotracheal intubation
   (D) Apply the automated external defibrillator (AED) and analyze the patient's heart rhythm

> **Directions:** Each of the numbered questions or incomplete statements in this section refers to a scenario that precedes them. The numbered questions or incomplete statements are followed by answers or by completions of the statement. Select the answer or completion of the statement that is BEST in each case.

Your rescue crew is called to the home of a 56-year-old male patient complaining of chest pain. Upon arrival, you find this patient lying in bed. He is not breathing and does not have a palpable pulse. Cardiopulmonary resuscitation (CPR) is initiated. While preparing this patient for transport, you decide to perform orotracheal intubation.

Questions 7–13

7. Before intubating this patient, you should

   (A) provide high-flow oxygen therapy by nonrebreather mask at 15 liters per
       minute (LPM)
   (B) provide high-flow oxygen therapy by nonrebreather mask at 25 LPM
   (C) hyperventilate the patient with a bag-valve mask and supplemental oxygen at
       a rate of 20 to 24 breaths per minute
   (D) hyperventilate the patient with a bag-valve mask and supplemental oxygen at
       a rate of 60 breaths per minute

8. What size endotracheal tube might you initially use on this adult male patient?

   (A) 3.0
   (B) 6.0
   (C) 7.0
   (D) 8.0

9. You decide to use a size 4 curved laryngoscope blade. The laryngoscope handle
   should be held in your _____ hand, and the tip of the blade should be placed
   into the patient's _____.

   (A) Left/vallecula
   (B) Right/vallecula
   (C) Left/glottic opening
   (D) Right/glottic opening

10. While intubating this patient, what can be done to prevent the liklihood of vomit-
    ing and aspiration of stomach contents?

    (A) Cricoid pressure
    (B) Chest compressions
    (C) Subdiaphragmatic abdominal thrusts
    (D) Insertion of an oropharyngeal airway (OPA)

11. The endotracheal tube is placed in the hand opposite the laryngoscope handle, and
    the tube is gently inserted into the patient's airway. What is the only true way of
    confirming correct placement of the endotracheal tube?

    (A) Visualization of the tube passing the carina
    (B) Visualization of the tube passing the esophagus
    (C) Visualization of the tube passing the base of the tongue
    (D) Visualization of the tube passing through the vocal cords

12. Once the endotracheal tube is in position, you must confirm proper placement.
    Confirmation is done by auscultation (listening with a stethoscope). The first place
    you should listen to confirm correct placement is

    (A) over the epigastrium
    (B) the left lateral chest wall
    (C) the left anterior chest wall
    (D) the right anterior chest wall

13. Initially, the endotracheal tube appears to have been placed properly. However,
    after the patient has been moved several times to get him in the ambulance, you
    reassess lung sounds and hear no air movement over the left chest wall. You should

    (A) immediately remove the endotracheal tube
    (B) ventilate at a faster rate (30 ventilations per minute)

    (C)   deflate the balloon and gently withdraw the tube a short distance

    (D)   insert another endotracheal tube on the left side of the original tube

Your rescue crew is called to the home of a 21-year-old female patient who is unresponsive after injecting heroin. Local law enforcement is already at the scene. Your initial assessment reveals that this patient is unresponsive to painful stimuli. She is not breathing but does have a weak, irregular pulse at 120 beats per minute.

Questions 14–17

14. Which of the following should be done first?

    (A)   Insert a nasogastric tube

    (B)   Perform orotracheal intubation

    (C)   Begin cardiopulmonary resuscitation (CPR)

    (D)   Begin assisting ventilations with a bag-valve mask

15. While assessing this patient for life-threatening injuries, you note she has a large, swollen bruise over her left eye. There is a small amount of blood leaking from a cut at the center of the bruise. If this patient is to be intubated, you must

    (A)   intubate by inserting the tube through the nose instead of the mouth

    (B)   intubate with the head and neck in a neutral position

    (C)   intubate without the use of a stylet in the endotracheal tube

    (D)   intubate with the head elevated on a folded towel or small pillow

16. Your initial attempt at intubating this patient was unsuccessful. Between intubation attempts you should

    (A)   perform chest compressions

    (B)   continuously suction the oropharynx

    (C)   hyperventilate the patient for 2 to 5 minutes

    (D)   provide high-flow oxygen by nonrebreather mask at 15 liters per minute (LPM)

17. As an EMT-Basic, you are allowed a maximum of how many attempts at intubating this patient?

    (A)   Two

    (B)   Three

    (C)   Four

    (D)   Unlimited if the patient is apneic (not breathing)

Your rescue crew is called to the home of an 18-month-old female patient found floating in a pool. Upon arrival, a neighbor is performing cardiopulmonary resuscitation (CPR). You perform an initial assessment and confirm the patient is pulseless and apneic (not breathing). CPR is resumed.

Questions 18–20

18. While providing artificial ventilations with the bag-valve mask, you hear a gurgling noise coming from the patient's mouth. You should immediately

    (A)   deliver 5 abdominal thrusts

    (B)   suction the patient's airway

    (C)   perform orotracheal intubation

    (D)   turn the patient over and deliver 5 back blows

19. After the airway is cleared, you observe while ventilating the patient that you are unable to deliver as much air as you anticipated due to lack of expansion of the lungs. Which of the following procedures may help resolve this complication?

(A) Insert a nasogastric tube
(B) Perform orotracheal intubation
(C) Suction the patient's mouth and nose
(D) Hyperextend the patient's head and neck

20. After successfully intubating this patient, you should initially hyperventilate and then deliver artificial ventilations at what rate?

(A) One breath every 1 second
(B) One breath every 3 seconds
(C) One breath every 5 seconds
(D) As fast as possible

ANSWERS AND RATIONALES

1-C. The epiglottis is the leaf-shaped structure that prevents food and liquid from entering the trachea during swallowing. The pharynx is the common passageway for food and air. The trachea (windpipe) is anterior to the esophagus. It extends from the larynx and divides into two main-stem bronchi. The esophagus is the passageway for food into the stomach.

2-C. Because the cricoid cartilage is the narrowest part of the upper airway of an infant and young child, intubation is different from adults. In adults, the endotracheal tube is advanced until the inflatable cuff is just past the glottic opening (vocal cords). The endotracheal tube cuff is then inflated. In infants and young children, endotracheal tubes without inflatable cuffs are used because of the narrow diameter of the trachea. The cricoid cartilage provides a natural cuff for the endotracheal tube. Extreme care should be taken to secure the endotracheal tube in children due to the susceptibility of these tubes to become displaced.

3-D. The formula used to determine the appropriate size endotracheal tube for an infant or child is:

16 + patient's age in years divided by 4 = tube size, or
Patient's age in years divided by 4, + 4 = tube size

For example, a 6-year-old would most likely require a 5.5 endotracheal tube (16 + 6 = 22; 22 divided by 4 = 5.5).

4-D. The narrowest portion of the infant and young child's upper airway is the cricoid cartilage (see question and answer/rationale 2). A cuffed endotracheal tube is generally used in children 8–10 years of age or older because the anatomical proportions of the child's airway more closely resemble those of an adult.

5-A. Agonal breathing (occasional gasping breaths) may be seen just before death. Kussmaul respirations are rapid, sighing respirations associated with disorders such as diabetes. Hyperventilation is the increased inspiration and expiration of air because of an increase in the rate or depth of breathing, or both. A gasping breath taken once every 10–15 seconds is not normal. Treatment for this patient should include scene size-up with body substance isolation (BSI) precautions and calling for advanced-life-support (ALS) care if available. Initial assessment has revealed the need for cardiopulmonary resuscitation (CPR). The automated external defibrillator (AED) should be applied because the patient is pulseless. Prepare for rapid transport to the closest appropriate facility.

6-D. The automated external defibrillator (AED) should be applied after confirming that the patient is unresponsive, apneic (not breathing), and pulseless. Remember the four links in the "Chain of Survival": early access (9-1-1), early cardiopulmonary resuscitation (CPR), early defibrillation, and early advanced-life-support (ALS) care. Although advanced airway management, insertion of a nasogastric tube, and gathering of a SAMPLE history are important, the priority in this situation is early defibrillation.

7-C. Before intubating, hyperventilate the patient at a rate of 20 to 24 breaths per minute. If the patient is not breathing, a nonrebreather mask is not the device of choice to administer supplemental oxygen. An intubation attempt should not take longer than 30 seconds. If approximately 30 seconds has passed during an intubation attempt, stop and reoxygenate the patient before attempting to intubate again.

8-D. For the average-sized adult male, an 8.0- or 8.5-mm internal diameter (i.d.) endotracheal tube is recommended. For the average-sized adult female, a 7.0- to 8.0-mm i.d.endotracheal tube is recommended. Remember the Emergency Rule: a 7.5-mm i.d. endotracheal tube may be used for an adult. When intubating, having one tube larger and one tube smaller than the estimated size available is helpful.

9-A. The laryngoscope should be held in the left hand and the laryngoscope blade inserted in the right side of the patient's mouth. The laryngoscope blade is used to sweep the tongue to the patient's left to move the tongue out of the way. The curved laryngoscope blade is designed to follow the natural curvature of the tongue. The tip of the curved blade fits into the vallecula (the "valley" formed by the base of the tongue and the base of the epiglottis). Upward pressure on the vallecula lifts the epiglottis, exposing the glottic opening. The straight blade is used to lift the epiglottis and expose the glottic opening.

10-A. During intubation, application of cricoid pressure (the Sellick maneuver) may be helpful. Cricoid pressure reduces the likelihood that the patient will aspirate vomitus into his or her lungs. Thyroid pressure should be used to assist in visualizing the vocal cords.

11-D. The one true way of ensuring that an endotracheal tube is properly placed is to visualize its passage into the trachea (through the vocal cords). Other methods for assessing endotracheal tube placement include listening for breath sounds, observing rise and fall of the chest wall, and use of an end-tidal carbon dioxide detector.

12-A. Inadvertent esophageal intubation (without correction) can be fatal. If the endotracheal tube is in the esophagus, gurgling sounds will be heard over the stomach (epigastrium). If gurgling is heard, the endotracheal tube should be removed immediately. Anticipate vomiting as the tube is removed and during successive intubation attempts due to gastric distention (air in the stomach). Insertion of a nasogastric tube will help decrease the air build-up in the stomach. If no gurgling sounds are heard over the epigastrium, assess sounds in all lung fields.

13-C. An endotracheal tube inserted too far will usually go down the right main-stem bronchus. This may occur during the initial intubation attempt or because of excessive patient movement without careful management of the endotracheal tube. If the endotracheal tube is in the right main-stem bronchus, assessment of the patient will reveal breath sounds heard over the right lung and diminished lung sounds over the left. To correct this problem, deflate the cuff and gently pull the tube back slightly (approximately a centimeter at a time) while artificially ventilating and auscultating over the left chest. Stop when breath sounds appear equal on both sides of the chest. Reinflate the cuff and secure the endotracheal tube in place. Note the markings on the tube at the upper teeth or gum line and record.

14-D. Once you have established that the patient is not breathing, immediately begin positive-pressure ventilation with a bag-valve mask. Intubation should occur (according to local protocol) only after you have confirmed that the patient has a patent (open) airway and the patient has been hyperventilated. Insertion of a nasogastric tube may be beneficial, particularly if the patient has a full stomach; however, this procedure is not your first priority. Cardiopulmonary resuscitation (CPR) is not indicated because the patient has a palpable pulse.

15-B. Extreme caution should be exercised when intubating patients with a possible spinal injury. Ask another rescuer to maintain spinal immobilization while you attempt intubation with the head and neck in a neutral position.

16-C. This patient is not breathing and will receive no oxygen during the intubation attempt. Therefore, oxygenation of the patient between intubation attempts is essential to ensure that the patient does not become hypoxic (low oxygen content in the blood). Ventilate the patient for 2 to 5 minutes between intubation attempts. Continuous suction will only worsen hypoxia. Chest compressions are unnecessary if the patient has a palpable pulse. A nonrebreather mask is not the device of choice to deliver supplemental oxygen in a patient who is not breathing.

17-A. The EMT-Basic is permitted two attempts to intubate (check local protocol). If intubation is unsuccessful, ventilate the patient with a bag-valve mask connected to supplemental oxygen. If possible, insert an oropharyngeal (OPA) or nasopharyngeal airway (NPA) and be prepared to suction as necessary.

18-B. The gurgling sound suggests the presence of secretions or vomitus in the patient's airway. Suctioning should be performed for a maximum of 5 seconds per attempt. Back blows and chest thrusts are indicated in cases of complete airway obstruction in infants. Abdominal thrusts are indicated in cases of complete airway obstruction in children older than 1 year of age. Intubation should be delayed until the airway is cleared and the patient is hyperventilated.

19-A. It is very likely that this patient's stomach is full of air or water. When the stomach fills, the diaphragm is unable to expand fully. Inserting a nasogastric tube may help resolve this problem by removing excess air or fluid from the patient's stomach.

20-B. When delivering positive-pressure ventilations to infants and children, the desired rate is 1 breath every 3 seconds, or 20 respirations per minute. Adults should be ventilated at a rate of 1 breath every 5 seconds, or 12 respirations per minute. Ventilating the patient as fast as possible may be harmful to the patient, resulting in excessive removal of carbon dioxide.

BIBLIOGRAPHY

Crosby LA, Lewallen DG (eds): *Emergency Care and Transportation of the Sick and Injured*, 6th ed. Rosemont, IL, American Academy of Orthopaedic Surgeons, 1995.

Grant HD, Murray RH Jr, Bergeron JD: *Emergency Care*, 7th ed. Englewood Cliffs, NJ, Prentice-Hall, 1995.

Hafen BQ, Karren KJ, Mistovich JJ: *Prehospital Emergency Care*, 5th ed. Upper Saddle River, NJ, Prentice-Hall, 1996.

Henry MC, Stapleton ER, Judd RL: *EMT: Prehospital Care*. Philadelphia, WB Saunders, 1992.

McSwain NE, White RD, Paturas JL, et al (eds): *The Basic EMT: Comprehensive Prehospital Patient Care*. St. Louis, Mosby-Year Book, 1996.

Stoy WA: *Mosby's EMT-Basic Textbook*. St. Louis, Mosby-Year Book, 1996.

United States Department of Transportation, National Highway Traffic Safety Administration: *Emergency Medical Technician: Basic. National Standard Curriculum*, 1994.

GLOSSARY

Abandonment termination of care without reasonable notice or turning the patient over to less-qualified personnel when the patient still needs and desires continuing attention.

Abdomen the part of the body trunk below the ribs and above the pelvis.

Abdominal cavity the part of the body trunk below the ribs and above the pelvis; contains the stomach, intestines, liver, gallbladder, pancreas, and spleen.

Abnormal behavior a manner of acting or conducting oneself that is not consistent with society's norms and expectations, interferes with the individual's well-being and ability to function, and may be harmful to the individual or others.

Abortion the termination of pregnancy before the fetus is capable of survival outside the uterus (age of viability).

Abrasion damage to the outermost layer of skin (epidermis) by shearing forces (e.g., rubbing or scraping).

Abruptio placenta a condition that occurs when a normally implanted placenta separates prematurely from the wall of the uterus during the last trimester of pregnancy. The uterus may separate partially or completely.

Absorption the process by which a drug is transferred from its site of administration into the circulation.

Abuse improper or excessive action so as to injure or cause harm.

Acceptance a defense mechanism in which the patient believes that he or she has done all that is possible in preparation to die.

Accessory organs of digestion the teeth and tongue, salivary glands, liver, gallbladder, and pancreas.

Acetabulum socket of the hip bone.

Active rewarming adding heat directly to the surface of the patient's body.

Acute myocardial infarction (AMI; "heart attack") a condition that occurs when the affected portion of the heart muscle is deprived of oxygen long enough so that the area dies (necrosis).

Addiction a psychological and physical dependence on a substance that has gone beyond voluntary control.

Administration the route by which a drug is given (e.g., oral, sublingual, inhalation, intravenous, intramuscular).

Adolescent an individual 12–18 years of age.

Adrenal glands endocrine glands located on top of each kidney; release epinephrine in response to stress.

Advance directive written instructions that specify a person's health care wishes when he or she becomes unable to make decisions for himself or herself.

Adverse effect an unintended and undesirable response to a drug.

Agonal respirations occasional gasping breaths seen just before death.

Agoraphobia a fear of open spaces.

Allergen any substance that causes signs and symptoms of an allergic response.

Allergic reaction an abnormal response by the immune system to a foreign substance.

Alveolar ducts microscopic tubes that are subdivisions of bronchioles.

Alveoli the functional units of the respiratory system; grape-like clusters of alveolar sacs where gases (oxygen and carbon dioxide) are exchanged between the air and blood.

AMA Drug Evaluation a reference published by the American Medical Association (AMA) that provides information on drug groups, dosages, and use.

American Hospital Formulary Service (AHFS) a loose-leaf book published by the American Society of Hospital Pharmacists that contains a comprehensive evaluation of individual drugs and some investigational uses of medications.

Amniotic sac a membranous bag that surrounds the fetus inside the uterus; bag of waters.

Anal canal the end of the large intestine, about $1\frac{1}{2}$ inches long, that remains closed except during defecation.

Anaphylaxis an unusual or exaggerated allergic reaction to a foreign substance.

Anger a defense mechanism related to a patient's inability to control a situation; aggressiveness aroused by a real or supposed wrong.

Angina pectoris literally, "choking in the chest"; a symptom of coronary artery disease that occurs when the heart's need for oxygen exceeds its supply.

Anisocoria unequal pupil size; may be normal or congenital.

Anterior (ventral) toward the front of the body.

Antibody a protein substance produced by the body to defend it against bacteria, viruses, or other antigens.

Antidote an agent that neutralizes or counteracts the effects of a drug or poison.

Antigen any substance that is foreign to an individual and causes antibody production.

Anxiety a state of apprehension and uneasiness, usually triggered by a vague or imagined situation. Anxiety includes a feeling of "losing control" and/or a feeling of not being able to meet another person's expectations.

Anxiety disorder a disorder that is more intense than normal anxiety (e.g., panic attacks), lasts longer (e.g., lasts for months instead of going away after a stressful situation is over), and may lead to phobias that interfere with the individual's life.

Aorta the largest artery of the body.

Aortic valve semilunar valve located at the junction of the left ventricle and aorta.

Apgar score acronym used to evaluate an infant's condition at 1 and 5 minutes after birth; stands for **a**ppearance (color), **p**ulse (heart rate), **g**rimace (irritability), **a**ctivity (muscle tone), and **r**espirations.

Apparent life-threatening events (ALTEs) formerly known as "near-miss SIDS." An ALTE is described as an episode that is frightening to the observer, who feels the child died or would have died without vigorous intervention. The child has some combination of apnea, color change (cyanosis or pallor), marked change in muscle tone, usually extreme limpness, or choking or gagging.

Appendicular skeleton the bones of the upper extremities (shoulder girdles, arms, wrists, and hands) and lower extremities (pelvic girdles, legs, ankles, and feet).

Aqueous humor fluid in the anterior chamber in front of the lens of the eye; nourishes the lens and cornea.

Arachnoid literally, "resembling a spider's web"; middle meningeal layer with delicate fibers resembling a spider's web; it contains few blood vessels.

Arrhythmia a pulse with an irregular rhythm.

Arteries high-pressure vessels that carry blood away from the heart and help maintain blood pressure.

Arterioles the smallest branches of arteries leading to the capillaries.

Ascending colon the part of the large intestine that passes upward from the cecum to the lower edge of the liver where it turns to become the transverse colon.

Assault threatening, attempting, or causing fear of offensive physical contact with a patient or other individual.

Asthma widespread, reversible narrowing of the bronchioles that results in airflow obstruction.

Atria thin-walled, low-pressure chambers of the heart that receive blood from the systemic circulation and lungs.

Aura a peculiar sensation that may precede a seizure. Typical auras include an unusual taste, a dreamy feeling, a visual disturbance (e.g., flashing light, floating light), an unpleasant odor, or a rising or sinking feeling in the stomach.

Auscultation the process of listening for sounds in some of the body cavities with a stethoscope.

Automated external defibrillator (AED) a machine that analyzes a patient's heart rhythm and, if indicated, delivers an electrical shock.

Avulsion soft tissue injury in which a flap of skin or tissue is torn loose or pulled completely off. The tissue is usually pulled away where it separates from different tissue (e.g., skin from subcutaneous tissue or subcutaneous tissue from muscle). Bleeding is usually significant.

Axial skeleton the bones of the skull, spine, and chest and the hyoid bone.

Bacteria one-celled organisms that can live outside the human body and do not depend on other organisms to live and grow.

Bandage material used to secure a dressing in place.

Bargaining a defense mechanism in which a patient attempts to enter into an "agreement" that he or she hopes may postpone or change the inevitable.

Barotrauma injury caused by pressure.

Base of support the foundation on which an object rests.

Base station a transmitter/receiver at a stationary site such as a hospital, mountain top, or public safety agency with a typical power output of 45–275 watts.

Baseline vital signs an initial set of vital sign measurements against which succeeding measurements can be compared.

Basket stretcher also called the Stokes basket. The device is usually made of plastic and shaped like a long basket and can accommodate a scoop stretcher or a long backboard. The basket stretcher is used for moving patients over rough terrain and is often used in water rescues or high-angle rescues.

Battery unlawful touching of another person without consent.

Battle's sign bluish discoloration (ecchymosis) over the mastoid process (behind the ear) that suggests a possible skull fracture.

Behavior the manner in which a person acts or performs. It includes any or all activities of a person, including physical and mental activity.

Behavioral emergency a situation in which the patient exhibits abnormal behavior within a given situation that is unacceptable or intolerable to the patient, family members, or community. A behavioral emergency can be due to extremes of emotion leading to violence or other inappropriate behavior or a psychological or physical condition (e.g., mental illness, lack of oxygen, low blood sugar).

Bent-arm drag emergency move in which the rescuer puts his or her hands under the patient's armpits (from the back), grasps the patient's forearms, and drags the patient.

Bilateral pertaining to both sides.

Binaurals metal pieces of a stethoscope that connect the earpieces to the plastic or rubber tubing.

Bipolar disorder (manic-depressive disorder) a mental disorder in which a patient has alternating episodes of mood elevation (mania) and depression.

Blanket drag emergency move in which the rescuer places the patient on a blanket and drags the blanket.

Blood pressure the force exerted by the blood on the inner walls of the heart and blood vessels.

Bloody show during early labor, the expulsion of the mucus plug, sometimes mixed with blood, from the vagina.

Blow-out fracture fracture of the bones that make up the orbit of the eye.

Body alignment the positioning of the body's parts in relation to one another while in a standing, sitting, or lying position. Proper body alignment is synonymous with good posture.

Body cavity a hollow space in the body that contains organs.

Body mechanics the field of physiology that studies muscular actions and the function of muscles in maintaining the posture of the body. This term is also used to describe the coordinated effort of the musculoskeletal and nervous systems to maintain proper balance, posture, and body alignment during lifting, bending, moving, and other activities of daily living.

Body substance isolation (BSI) self-protection against *all* body fluids and substances (blood, urine, semen, feces, vaginal secretions, tears, saliva, cerebrospinal fluid, etc.).

Body temperature the balance between the heat produced by the body and the heat lost from the body; measured in heat units called degrees (°).

Brachial pulse peripheral pulse located on the medial aspect of the upper arm, midway between the shoulder and elbow.

Bradycardia in an adult, a heart rate of less than 60 beats per minute.

Bradypnea an excessively slow rate of breathing.

Brain stem part of the brain that consists of the midbrain, pons, and medulla oblongata.

Breathing (pulmonary ventilation) the mechanical process of moving air into and out of the lungs.

Breech presentation presentation of the buttocks or feet first instead of the head during childbirth.

Bronchiole division of the primary bronchi; smaller airway passage for air to and from the alveoli.

Bronchus large air passage for air to and from the alveoli.

Buccal pertaining to the cheek.

Bulb syringe suction device used to remove secretions from the mouth or nose in an infant.

Bulbourethral (Cowper's) glands glands embedded in the male urethra that secrete mucus-like fluid to lubricate the urethra.

Bystander a citizen responder, not part of the EMS response team, on the scene of an illness or injury incident irrespective of training.

Capillaries microscopic vessels that are one cell thick that serve as vessels for exchange of wastes, fluids, and nutrients between the blood and tissues; connect arterioles and venules.

Capillary refill assessment tool used in infants and children; performed by pressing on the patient's skin or nailbeds and determining the time for return to initial color. Normal capillary refill in infants and children is less than 2 seconds. Delayed (greater than 2 seconds) capillary refill suggests circulatory compromise.

Capsules liquid, dry, or beaded drug particles enclosed in a gelatin container (e.g., Actifed®).

Cardiac arrest a condition that occurs when the contraction of the heart stops; confirmed by unresponsiveness, absent breathing, and absent pulses.

Cardiogenic shock shock that occurs when the heart muscle fails to pump blood effectively to all parts of the body.

Cardiovascular system the heart, blood vessels, and blood.

Carina internal ridge formed at the point at which the trachea divides into two primary bronchi.

Carotid pulse central pulse located on either side of the neck.

Carpals wrist bones.

Carrier a person or animal who shows no signs or symptoms of illness but has pathogens in or on its body that can be transferred to others.

Caudal toward the tail (lower end of the spine).

Cecum a blind pouch or cul-de-sac that forms the first part of the large intestine.

Cell the smallest living unit in the body.

Center of gravity the point at which the mass of an object is centered.

Centers for Disease Control (CDC) a division of the United States Public Health Service that has developed standards to reduce the risk of infection.

Central line an intravenous (IV) line placed near the heart for long-term use.

Central nervous system (CNS) the brain and spinal cord.

Cerebellum second largest part of the human brain; responsible for precise control of muscle movements and maintenance of posture and equilibrium.

Cerebral contusion bruising of the brain; bleeding and swelling of brain tissue.

Cerebral hematoma bleeding within the brain.

Cerebrospinal fluid fluid that surrounds the brain and spinal cord and acts as a shock-absorber for the central nervous system.

Cerebrovascular accident (stroke) brain injury caused by the blockage or rupture of an artery supplying the brain. Strokes cause brain injury because the blood supply to the brain is reduced or cut off, depriving brain cells of necessary oxygen and nutrients.

Cerebrum the largest part of the human brain.

Cervix the narrow opening at the distal end of the uterus that connects the uterus to the vagina.

Chain of survival the four components of EMS response to out-of-hospital cardiac arrest that are thought to be the most critical to survival of cardiac arrest: early access, early cardiopulmonary resuscitation (CPR), early defibrillation, and early advanced care.

Chemical name the precise description of a drug's chemical composition and molecular structure.

Chickenpox (varicella) an airborne disease spread by droplets.

Chief complaint the reason EMS was called, usually in the patient's own words.

Child maltreatment includes intentional physical abuse or neglect, emotional abuse or neglect, and sexual abuse of children, usually by adults.

Child neglect the failure of a parent or other person legally responsible for the child's welfare to provide for the child's basic needs and an adequate level of care. Child neglect is the most common form of maltreatment.

Chlamydia a sexually transmitted disease.

Chronic bronchitis sputum production for 3 months of a year for at least 2 consecutive years; the primary cause of chronic bronchitis is cigarette smoking.

Circumoral cyanosis blue-gray color around the mouth; suggests inadequate oxygenation or poor perfusion.

Civil law a branch of law that deals with torts (civil wrongs) committed by one individual against another.

Clavicle collar bone.

Clothing drag emergency move in which a rescuer pulls on the patient's clothing in the neck and shoulder area.

Common law "case" or "judge-made" law; laws derived from society's acceptance of customs or norms over time.

Communicable (contagious) disease a disease that can be spread from one person or animal to another, either directly or indirectly.

Compression injury in which the weight of the head or pelvis is driven into stationary neck or torso.

Concussion a temporary loss of function for some or all of the brain.

Conduction the transfer of heat between objects that are in direct contact.

Congestive heart failure (CHF) a condition in which one or both sides of the heart fail to pump efficiently.

Conjunctiva mucous membrane that covers the front surface of the sclera and the inner eyelid.

Continuing education knowledge acquired by means of skill labs, lectures, workshops, conferences, seminars, case reviews, quality improvement reviews, reading professional journals, and/or reviewing videotapes or audiotapes after the EMT-Basic's initial education program. Continuing education helps the EMT-Basic retain skills and knowledge learned during initial training; provides information about advances in medicine, skills, and equipment; and educates the EMT-Basic about changes in local protocols and national guidelines.

Contraindication a condition for which a drug should not be used because it may cause harm to the patient or offer no improvement of the patient's condition or illness.

Contusion bruise.

Convection the transfer of heat by the movement of air currents.

Coordinated body movement one of the basic elements of body mechanics.

Coronary artery disease a term used for diseases that reduce or stop blood flow through the coronary arteries.

Corpus callosum collection of nerve fibers in the brain that connect the left and right cerebral hemispheres.

Crackles (rales) intermittent high-pitched "popping" sounds produced by the passage of air through moisture.

Cranial (cephalic) toward the head.

Cranial cavity cavity that houses the brain.

Cranial nerves 12 pairs of nerves that connect the brain with the neck and structures in the thorax and abdomen.

Cranium the skull.

Crepitation the grating sound heard or sensation felt when broken bone ends rub together.

Cricoid cartilage the most inferior of the cartilages of the larynx.

Cricoid pressure (Sellick maneuver) technique used in an unresponsive patient without a cough or gag reflex to help prevent passive regurgitation and aspiration during endotracheal intubation.

Criminal abortion an illegally performed abortion, usually in undesirable conditions by unqualified medical personnel.

Criminal law the area of law in which the federal, state, or local government prosecutes individuals on behalf of society for violating laws designed to safeguard society.

Critical incident a situation that causes a prehospital care provider to experience unusually strong emotions and may interfere with the provider's ability to function immediately or later.

Critical incident stress debriefing (CISD) a group meeting led by a mental health professional and peer support personnel to allow rescuers to share thoughts, emotions, and other reactions about a critical event.

Crossed-finger technique technique that may be used to open the mouth of an unconscious patient.

Croup a viral infection that causes inflammation and swelling beneath the larynx and glottis.

Crowing a long, high-pitched sound heard on inspiration.

Cyanosis blue-gray color of the skin that suggests inadequate oxygenation or poor perfusion.

Damages patient injury, either physical or psychological, as a result of a breach of duty.

DCAP-BTLS a mnemonic used during evaluation of a patient to determine the presence of injuries; stands for **d**eformities, **c**ontusions (bruises), **a**brasions (scrapes), **p**unctures or **p**enetrating wounds, **b**urns, **t**enderness to palpation, **l**acerations (cuts), and **s**welling.

Decontamination the use of physical or chemical means to remove, inactivate, or destroy bloodborne pathogens on a surface or item to the point where they are no longer capable of transmitting infectious particles, and the surface or item is considered safe for handling, use, or disposal.

Defecation the elimination of undigested waste.

Defibrillator a device that delivers a controlled electrical shock to a patient to stop an abnormal heart rhythm; defibrillation is the technique of administering the electrical shock.

Defusing a shorter, less structured version of a debriefing for rescuers held immediately after a critical event.

Delivery actual birth of the baby at the end of the second stage of labor.

Delusions false beliefs that the patient maintains are true, despite facts to the contrary.

Denial a defense mechanism characterized by an inability or refusal to believe the reality of an event.

Dependent lividity discoloration due to the pooling of blood in the lowest body areas after death.

Depression a mental state characterized by feelings of sadness, worthlessness, and discouragement. Often occurs in response to a loss (e.g., loss of job or independence, death of a loved one, end of a relationship).

Dermis deeper and thicker layer of skin containing sweat and sebaceous glands, hair follicles, blood vessels, and nerve endings.

Descending colon the part of the large intestine descending from the left colic (splenic) flexure to the brim of the pelvis.

Detailed physical examination head-to-toes physical examination that is patient- and injury-specific.

Diaphragm the dome-shaped muscle used in breathing.

Diastolic blood pressure the pressure exerted against the walls of the arteries when the left ventricle is at rest.

Diffusion the movement of gases or particles from an area of higher concentration to an area of lower concentration.

Digestion the chemical breakdown of food into small parts so absorption can occur.

Direct contact physical transfer of a pathogen between an infected person and a susceptible host, e.g., sexual contact with an infected person or contact with excretions from an open sore or ulcer.

Disentanglement the moving or removing of materials that are trapping a victim.

Distal farthest from the point of reference; away from or farthest from the trunk.

Distention the condition of being expanded or swollen; appearing larger than normal.

Distraction pulling apart of the spine.

Distribution the means by which drugs are transported by body fluids to their intended sites of action.

Dorsalis pedis pulse peripheral pulse located on the top surface of the foot.

Dosage the frequency, size, and number of doses.

Dose the amount of a drug that should be administered to a patient at one time.

Dressing any material that covers a wound.

Drowning death that occurs within 24 hours of submersion/suffocation in fluid.

Drug a chemical substance used in the diagnosis, treatment, or prevention of disease.

Dura mater literally, "hard" or "tough mother"; tough, durable, outermost layer of the meninges that adheres to the inner surface of the cranium.

Durable power of attorney for health care a written document that identifies a legal guardian to make decisions for a patient when the patient can no longer make such decisions.

Dyspnea a sensation of shortness of breath; difficulty breathing.

Dysrhythmia a pulse with an irregular rhythm.

Ecchymosis bluish discoloration due to leakage of blood into the skin or mucous membrane.

Eclampsia the convulsive phase of preeclampsia; associated with a significant risk of death of the mother and fetus.

Ectopic pregnancy a condition that occurs when a fertilized egg implants outside the uterus, usually inside the fallopian tube. As the fetus grows, the fallopian tube tears and eventually ruptures.

Elective abortion an abortion performed at the request of the mother.

Elimination the process by which a drug is removed from the body (e.g., urine, feces, saliva, expired air).

Elixirs clear liquids made with alcohol, water, flavors, or sweeteners (e.g., terpin hydrate, Nyquil®).

Emergency doctrine (implied consent) consent assumed from a patient requiring emergency intervention who is mentally, physically, or emotionally unable to provide expressed consent.

Emergency Medical Dispatcher (EMD) a trained public safety telecommunicator with additional training and specific emergency medical knowledge essential for the efficient management of emergency medical communications.

Emergency Medical Radio Service (EMRS) a group of frequencies designated by the Federal Communications Commission exclusively for use by EMS providers.

Emergency Medical Technician (EMT) a member of the emergency medical services team who provides prehospital emergency care.

Emotional abuse the deliberate attempt to destroy or impair an individual's self-esteem or competence.

Emotional neglect failure to meet an individual's needs for attention, affection, and emotional growth.

Emphysema an irreversible enlargement of the air spaces distal to the terminal bronchioles that leads to the destruction of the walls of the alveoli, distention of the alveolar sacs, and a loss of lung elasticity.

Emergency Medical Services (EMS) system a network of emergency medical personnel, supplies, and equipment designed to function in a coordinated manner. The EMS system is part of the health care system and may exist at local, regional, state, or national levels.

EMT-Basic (EMT-B) an emergency medical technician (EMT) who has taken a minimum 110-hour course as required by the United States Department of Transportation (DOT).

EMT-Intermediate (EMT-I) an emergency medical technician who has completed the EMT-Basic course and additional training in skills such as patient assessment, intravenous therapy, advanced airway procedures, defibrillation, and administration of some medications.

EMT-Paramedic (EMT-P) an emergency medical technician who has completed the EMT-Basic course and has additional training in skills such as patient assessment, intravenous therapy, invasive airway procedures, electrocardiogram (ECG) interpretation, manual defibrillation, and administration of additional medications.

Emulsions mixtures of two liquids, one distributed throughout the other in small globules (e.g., cold cream).

Endocrine system a system of ductless glands that secrete chemicals, such as insulin and adrenalin, that regulate and influence body activities and functions.

Enhanced 9-1-1 a computerized 9-1-1 access telephone system that provides additional information to the dispatcher, such as the street or billing address of the caller and the caller's telephone number.

Enteral drugs drugs administered through the gastrointestinal tract.

Epidermis outermost skin layer.

Epiglottis leaf-shaped cartilage that covers the opening to the larynx during swallowing, preventing food and liquids from entering the airway.

Epiglottitis a bacterial infection of the epiglottis most commonly occurring in children between 3 and 7 years of age, although it may also occur in adults.

Epilepsy a condition of recurrent seizures in which the cause is usually irreversible.

Erythrocytes red blood cells, formed elements of blood.

Esophagus the portion of the digestive canal between the pharynx and stomach that transports food from the pharynx to the stomach by peristalsis.

Ethics principles that identify conduct deemed morally desirable, i.e., what a person *ought* to do.

Evaporation a loss of heat by vaporization of moisture on the body surface.

Evisceration organs protruding through an open abdominal wound.

Excessive extension (hyperextension) injury in which there is severe backward movement of the head or neck.

Excessive flexion (hyperflexion) injury in which there is severe forward movement of the head onto the chest.

Expiration (exhalation) the process of breathing out and moving air out of the lungs.

Exposure contact with infected blood, body fluids, tissues, or airborne droplets, either directly or indirectly.

Expressed consent agreement to accept treatment and/or transport; may be given verbally, by written communication, or nonverbally, i.e., expressed by action or allowing care to be rendered.

External nares nostrils.

Extrication freeing from entrapment.

Fallopian tubes (oviducts) in the female, tubes that receive and transport the egg to the uterus after ovulation.

False imprisonment intentional and unjustifiable detention.

False ribs rib pairs 8–10; attach to the cartilage of the seventh ribs.

Falsify to state untruthfully; misrepresent.

Federal Communications Commission (FCC) federal agency that regulates the use of nongovernment radio frequencies including AM, FM, television, aircraft, marine, and land-mobile frequency ranges.

Feeding button a small, silicone device with a one-way valve that accepts a feeding tube. Used in children who require long-term gastrostomy feedings.

Femoral pulse central pulse located in the fold between the thigh and pelvis.

Femur the thigh; the longest, heaviest, and strongest bone of the body.

Fetus unborn infant.

Fibula bone that runs parallel to the tibia along the lateral side of the lower leg.

First responder the first person with emergency care training who arrives at the scene (e.g., schoolteacher, law enforcement personnel, lifeguard).

Flail chest a condition in which three or more adjacent ribs are fractured in two or more places or when the sternum is detached. The section of the chest wall between the fractured ribs becomes free-floating because it is no longer in continuity with the thorax. This free-floating section of the chest wall is called the "flail segment."

Flexible (Reeves) stretcher a device made of canvas or synthetic flexible material with carrying handles. The flexible stretcher is useful when space is limited to access the patient, such as in narrow hallways, stairs, or cramped corners.

Fontanel "soft spot" in the skull of an infant.

Fowler's position lying on the back with the upper body elevated at a 45° to 60° angle.

Fracture a break in the continuity of a bone.

Friction a force that resists the motion of two objects in contact. Friction must be overcome when moving a patient.

Frontal plane the lengthwise field that passes through the body from side to side, dividing the body into anterior (ventral) and posterior (dorsal) parts.

Gallbladder pear-shaped sac on the undersurface of the liver that stores bile until it is needed by the small intestine.

Gastrostomy tube a special catheter placed directly into the stomach for feeding. It is most often used for children in whom passage of a tube through the mouth, pharynx, or esophagus is contraindicated or impossible.

Gel clear or translucent semisolid substance that liquefies when applied to the skin or a mucous membrane (e.g., glucose).

Generic name usually the name given to a drug by the company that first manufactures it; a simplified version of the chemical name.

Glottis space between the vocal cords.

Glucagon pancreatic hormone that increases blood glucose concentration.

Gonorrhea a sexually transmitted disease.

Greater trochanter the large, bony prominence on the lateral shaft of the femur to which the buttock muscles are attached.

Grunting the sound created when the patient forcefully exhales against a closed glottis; traps air and keeps the alveoli open.

Gurgling the sound heard as air passes through moist secretions in the airway.

Hallucinations false perceptions (e.g., the patient sees things others cannot see). Hallucinations can be auditory (hearing voices), visual (worms or snakes crawling on the floor), or tactile (insects crawling on the skin).

Hard palate floor of the nasal cavity.

Hazardous material any substance or material in a quantity or form that poses an unreasonable risk to health, safety, and property when transported in commerce.

Head-tilt, chin-lift maneuver a technique used to open the airway when a patient is unresponsive and cervical spine injury is not suspected.

Health care system a network of people, facilities, and equipment designed to provide for the general health care needs of the population. This system may exist at local, regional, or national levels and consists of speciality facilities such as trauma centers, burn centers, children's hospitals, poison centers, and neurological centers.

Heart primary organ of the cardiovascular system; lies in the thoracic cavity (mediastinum) behind the sternum and between the lungs.

Hematemesis vomiting blood.

Hematuria blood in the urine.

Hematoma a collection of blood beneath the skin; larger amount of tissue damage as compared to contusion.

Hemoglobin an iron-containing protein that chemically bonds with oxygen; the part of the red blood cell that carries oxygen from the lungs to the tissues. Hemoglobin is red and gives blood its red color.

Hemoptysis coughing up blood.

Hemorrhagic shock shock caused by severe bleeding.

Hemorrhagic stroke also called cerebral hemorrhage; a type of stroke (cerebrovascular accident) caused by bleeding into the brain.

Hemothorax a collection of blood in the pleural space that may result from injury to the chest wall, the major blood vessels, or the lung due to penetrating or blunt trauma.

Hepatitis A a foodborne disease spread by improper handling of food or by poor personal hygiene.

Hepatitis B virus (HBV) a bloodborne disease spread by contact with blood or body fluids of an infected person.

Hepatitis C a bloodborne disease spread by contact with blood or body fluids of an infected person.

High-Efficiency Particulate Air (HEPA) respirator a special mask that should be worn by emergency workers when managing patients with known or suspected tuberculosis.

High-level disinfection a method of decontamination that destroys all microorganisms except large numbers of bacterial spores.

Host a plant, person, or animal capable of harboring and providing nourishment for another organism (the parasite).

Human immunodeficiency virus (HIV) a virus spread by contact with blood or body fluids of an infected person; causes acquired immune deficiency syndrome (AIDS).

Humerus largest bone of the upper extremity.

Hydrocephalus a condition in which there is an excess of cerebrospinal fluid within the brain.

Hyperglycemia a higher-than-normal blood sugar level.

Hypersensitivity an exaggerated response to a drug by an individual.

Hyperthermia high core body temperature.

Hyphema hemorrhage into the anterior chamber of the eye

Hypoglycemia a lower-than-normal blood sugar level.

Hypoperfusion (shock) the inadequate circulation of blood through an organ or a part of the body; a state of profound depression of the vital processes of the body.

Hypothermia low body temperature.

Hypovolemic shock shock caused by either a loss of plasma (e.g., excessive sweating, dehydration due to vomiting or diarrhea, burns) or blood.

Idiosyncrasy a reaction to a drug that is peculiar to an individual and not usually seen in the rest of the population.

Iliac crest lateral bones of the hip that form the wings of the pelvis.

Implantable defibrillator a device that is electronically programmed to identify and stop life-threatening heart rhythms in patients at high risk for sudden cardiac death.

Implied consent (emergency doctrine) consent assumed from a patient requiring emergency intervention who is mentally, physically, or emotionally unable to provide expressed consent.

Incomplete abortion an abortion in which part of the products of conception have been passed, but some remain in the uterus.

Indication   a condition for which a specific drug has documented usefulness.

Indirect contact   contact by a susceptible host with contaminated substances or inanimate objects, e.g., intravenous tubing, needles, toys, eating utensils and glasses, towels, sheets, and wound dressings.

Induced abortion   an abortion performed under sterile conditions in an authorized medical setting.

Infant   child from birth to 1 year of age.

Infection   the invasion and growth of microorganisms in a host, with or without detectable signs of illness.

Infectious disease   a communicable disease caused by microorganisms such as bacteria.

Inferior   below, lower, toward the feet.

Ingestion   bringing nutrients, water, and electrolytes into the body.

Inspiration (inhalation)   the process of breathing in and moving air into the lungs.

Insulin   hormone that decreases blood glucose concentration.

Interatrial septum   wall of myocardium that separates the left and right atria.

Intercostal muscles   muscles located between the ribs.

Intermediate-level disinfection   a method of decontamination that destroys tuberculosis bacteria, vegetative bacteria, and most viruses and fungi, but not bacterial spores.

Iris   visible colored part of the eye; consists of muscles that control the diameter of the pupil, thus controlling the amount of light entering the eye.

Ischemia   a reduction in blood flow to an organ or tissue.

Ischemic stroke   a type of stroke (cerebrovascular accident) caused by a blood clot that decreases blood flow to the brain.

Ischium   inferior portion of pelvis; lower, posterior portion on which we sit.

Islets of Langerhans   located in the pancreas; alpha cells secrete glucagon, which increases blood glucose level; beta cells secrete insulin, which decreases blood glucose level.

Jaundice   yellow coloration of the skin that suggests the presence of liver disease or hepatitis.

Jaw-thrust maneuver   a technique used to open the airway when a patient is unresponsive and cervical spine injury is suspected.

Joint   the place where two bones meet; also called an articulation.

Jugular venous distention (JVD)   distention of the neck veins when the patient is placed in a sitting position at a 45° angle.

Kidney   one of two organs located at the back of the abdominal cavity on each side of the spinal column that produce urine, maintain water balance, aid in regulation of blood pressure, and regulate levels of many chemicals in the blood.

Labor   the time and process in which the uterus repeatedly contracts to push the fetus and placenta out of the mother's body. It begins with the first uterine muscle contraction and ends with delivery of the placenta.

Labored breathing   an increase in the effort of breathing.

Laceration   a break in the skin of varying depth that may be linear (regular) or stellate (irregular); caused by forceful impact with a sharp object (e.g., knife, razor blade, glass).

Lacrimal glands   glands that produce tears that act as a lubricant between the eyelid and the cornea and flood foreign material out of the eye.

Large intestine (colon)   the portion of the gastrointestinal system that extends from the ileum of the small intestine to the anus; subdivided into the following sections (listed in the order in which food passes through them): cecum, ascending colon, transverse colon, descending colon, sigmoid colon, rectum, and anal canal.

Laryngectomy   surgical removal of the larynx.

Laryngopharynx   the most inferior portion of the pharynx; serves as a passageway for both food and air.

Larynx   voice box.

Lateral   away from the midline or middle; toward the side.

Lateral bending   injury in which a sudden side impact moves the torso sideways; the head remains in place until moved along by its attachments to the cervical spine.

Lateral recumbent   lying in a horizontal position on either the right or left side.

Lens   transparent structure separating the posterior chamber and vitreous body of the eye; located directly behind the pupil, changes shape to focus images on the retina.

Leukocytes   white blood cells, formed elements of blood.

Libel   injuring a person's character, name, or reputation by false and malicious writings.

Line of gravity   an imaginary vertical line drawn through an object's center of gravity.

Liniments   preparations in an oily, alcoholic, or soapy base that are applied to the skin.

Liver   largest organ of the body responsible for many functions including the production of bile, storage of minerals and fat-soluble vitamins, and storage of blood.

Local effect   an effect of a drug that usually occurs at the site of drug application.

Long backboard   device that is 6–7 feet long and commonly made of wood, metal, or plastic; usually has holes spaced along the head and foot ends and sides for handholds and insertion of straps; used for spinal immobilization of patients.

Lotions   preparations applied to protect the skin or treat a skin disorder (e.g., Calamine® lotion).

Low-level disinfection   a method of decontamination that destroys most bacteria, some viruses and fungi, but not tuberculosis bacteria or bacterial spores.

Lower respiratory tract   consists of parts found almost entirely within the chest cavity, i.e., the trachea and lungs (including the bronchial tree and alveoli); conducts air to the alveoli where gas exchange occurs.

Lungs   spongy, air-filled organs that bring air into contact with blood so oxygen and carbon dioxide can be exchanged in the alveoli.

Lymphatic system   lymph, lymph nodes, lymph vessels, tonsils, spleen, and thymus gland.

Malfeasance   performing a wrongful or unlawful act.

Mammary glands (breasts)   glands in the female that function in milk production after delivery of an infant.

Manubrium   the superior portion of the sternum (breastbone); connects with the clavicle and first rib.

Massive hemothorax   blood loss of more than 1500 milliliters in the chest cavity.

Measles   an airborne disease spread by droplets.

Mechanism of action   how a drug exerts its effect on body cells and tissues.

Mechanism of injury   refers to the manner in which an injury occurs and the forces involved in producing the injury.

Meconium   material that collects in the intestines of a fetus and forms the first stools of a newborn.

Medial toward the midline or middle.

Mediastinum the area between the lungs that extends from the sternum to the vertebral column; includes all of the contents of the thoracic cavity (except the lungs), including the esophagus, trachea, heart, and large blood vessels.

Medical direction the physician responsible for management, supervision, and guidance of all aspects of an EMS system to ensure its quality of care. Every ambulance service and rescue squad must have physician medical direction.

Medical practice act legislation that governs the practice of medicine; this act varies from state to state.

Meninges literally, membranes; three layers of connective tissue coverings that surround the brain and spinal cord.

Meningitis an airborne disease spread by droplets.

Menstruation the periodic discharge of bloody fluid from the nonpregnant uterus through the vagina during the life of a woman from puberty to menopause.

Metacarpals bones that form the support for the palm of the hand.

Metatarsals bones that form the part of the foot to which the toes attach.

Metered dose inhaler aerosol can containing medication that is released in a specific dose with each spray.

Microorganism an organism too small to be seen with the unaided eye; bacteria, some fungi, and protozoa are microorganisms.

Midaxillary line an imaginary line drawn vertically from the middle of the patient's armpits to the ankle that divides the body into anterior and posterior sections.

Midclavicular line an imaginary line drawn vertically in the middle of the clavicle, parallel to the midline.

Midline an imaginary line drawn vertically through the middle of the body from the nose to the umbilicus (navel) that divides the body into right and left halves.

Misfeasance performing a legal act in a harmful or injurious way.

Mitral (bicuspid) valve atrioventricular (AV) valve located between the left atrium and left ventricle.

Mobile two-way radio a vehicular-mounted communication device that usually transmits at a lower power than base stations (typically 20–50 watts). The typical transmission range is 10–15 miles over average terrain.

Motor nerves transmit impulses from the brain.

Mounted suction device also called a fixed suction unit; suction device mounted (built-in) in ambulances and usually powered by the vehicle's battery.

Mucous membrane a thin sheet or layer of pliable tissue that lines a body cavity that opens to the exterior.

Mucus plug during pregnancy, thick fluid that seals the opening to the uterus, keeping bacteria from entering.

Multiple casualty incident (MCI) any event that places a great demand on resources, be it equipment or personnel.

Multiple-casualty situation (MCS) also called a mass-casualty incident (MCI) or multiple-casualty incident; any event that places a great demand on resources, be it equipment or personnel.

Myocardial contusion bruising of the heart due to blunt chest trauma.

Nasal cavity the open area in the nose that warms and moistens inhaled air; contains sense organs of smell and aids in speech; divided into two chambers by the nasal septum.

Nasal flaring excessive widening of the nostrils with respiration.

Nasopharynx portion of the pharynx located directly behind the nasal cavity; serves as a passageway for air only.

National Highway Traffic Safety Administration (NHTSA) part of the United States Department of Transportation (DOT) whose goal is to reduce the number of deaths and disabilities caused by motor vehicle collisions on the nation's highways. NHTSA has developed standards in 10 areas to guarantee high-quality EMS systems (National Highway Traffic Safety Administration Technical Assistance Program).

Nature of the illness the cause, or signs and symptoms, of the patient's problem.

Near-drowning at least a temporary recovery (more than 24 hours) after a submersion injury.

Neglect giving insufficient attention or respect to someone who has a claim to that attention.

Negligence a deviation from the accepted standard of care resulting in further injury to the patient.

Neonate a child in the first 4 weeks of life.

Nervous system controls the voluntary and involuntary activities of the body; divided into the central nervous system (CNS) and the peripheral nervous system (PNS).

Neurogenic shock shock by loss of blood vessel control by the nervous system.

Nonfeasance failure to perform a required act or duty.

Nose warms and moistens inhaled air, contains sense organs of smell, and aids in speech.

Nuchal cord presence of the umbilical cord around an infant's neck during childbirth.

Occupational Safety and Health Administration (OSHA) a division of the United States Department of Labor that is responsible for safety in the workplace.

Official name the name under which a drug is listed in the *United States Pharmacopeia*.

Off-line medical direction (indirect medical direction) medical direction of prehospital personnel through use of protocols, standing orders, training programs, case review, and quality improvement review.

Olecranon elbow.

Ongoing assessment a repeat of the initial assessment in order to identify and treat life-threatening injuries, reassessment of vital signs to note changes or trends in the patient's condition, and a repeat of the focused assessment.

One-person stretcher (roll-in stretcher) a wheeled stretcher with special loading wheels at the head, allowing it to be rolled in and out of the ambulance by one person. Despite its name, many agencies recommend using two rescuers when loading and unloading this stretcher from an ambulance.

On-line medical direction (direct medical direction) medical supervision of EMS personnel by a physician or physician designee by means of a radio, telephone, or the presence of the physician or designee on the scene.

Open pneumothorax "sucking chest wound" caused by penetrating trauma.

OPQRST an acronym used by the EMT-Basic that may help identify the type and location of the patient's complaint. OPQRST stands for **o**nset, **p**rovocation, **q**uality, **r**egion/**r**adiation, **s**everity, and **t**ime.

Optic nerve nerve that transmits visual messages to the brain.

Oral mucosa mucous membranes of the mouth.

Orbit eye socket.

Organ a collection of different types of tissues.

Oropharynx middle portion of the pharynx that opens into the mouth and serves as a passageway for both food and air.

Orthopnea breathlessness when lying flat that is relieved when the patient sits or stands.

Ovary one of two glands in the female that produce the female reproductive cell (the egg) and the hormones estrogen and progesterone.

Overdose exposure to excessive amounts of a substance.

Over-the-counter (OTC) drug a drug that may be purchased without a prescription.

Ovulation the release of an egg from the ovary; occurs approximately 14 days before the next menstrual period.

Palpitations an abnormal awareness of one's heart beat.

Pancreas gland that secretes juices that contain enzymes for protein, carbohydrate, and fat digestion into the small intestine.

Panic attack an intense state of fear that occurs for no apparent reason.

Paradoxical motion (of a segment of the chest wall) part of the chest moves in an opposite direction from the rest during respiration.

Paranoia a mental disorder characterized by excessive suspiciousness or other delusions, often of persecution or grandeur.

Parasite a plant or animal that lives on or within and obtains nourishment from another living organism.

Parathyroid glands endocrine glands located on the back of the thyroid gland; control calcium and phosphorus metabolism and activate vitamin D.

Parenteral administration of a drug by means other than through the gastrointestinal tract; this term is more commonly used to describe medications administered by injection.

Parietal pleura the outer pleural lining that lines the wall of the thoracic cavity (rib cage, diaphragm, and mediastinum).

Paroxysmal nocturnal dyspnea a sudden onset of difficulty breathing that occurs at night; it occurs because of an accumulation of fluid in the alveoli or pooling of secretions during sleep.

Passive rewarming the warming of the patient without the use of additional heat sources beyond the patient's own heat production.

Patella kneecap.

Pathogen a microorganism capable of producing disease.

Pelvic cavity lowest part of the body trunk; contains the urinary bladder, rectum, and reproductive organs.

Pelvis a bony ring formed by three separate bones that fuse to become one in an adult.

Perfusion the circulation of blood through an organ or a part of the body.

Pericardial tamponade condition that occurs when blood enters the pericardial sac because of laceration of a coronary blood vessel, a ruptured coronary artery, laceration of a chamber of the heart, or a significant cardiac contusion. The blood in the pericardial sac compresses the heart, decreasing the amount of blood the heart can pump out with each contraction.

Perineum in a female, the area between the vaginal opening and anus.

Peripheral nervous system (PNS) consists of all nervous tissue found outside the brain and spinal cord.

Peristalsis the involuntary wavelike contraction of smooth muscle that moves material through the digestive tract.

Personal protective equipment (PPE) a barrier between an emergency worker and infectious material. PPE must be worn when an exposure to blood or other potentially infectious material can be reasonably anticipated and includes eye protection, protective gloves, gowns, and masks.

Pertinent negative a finding expected to accompany the patient's chief complaint but not found during the patient assessment.

Phalanges bones of the fingers and toes.

Pharmacology the study of drugs and their actions on the body.

Pharynx a muscular tube that is a passageway for food, liquids, and air that is common to both the respiratory and digestive tracts.

Phobia an irrational and persistent fear of a specific activity, object, or situation.

Physical abuse the deliberate act of causing physical injury to another.

Physical neglect the lack of necessities such as food, clothing, shelter, medical care, education, and supervision.

Physician's Desk Reference (PDR) a publication that is a compilation of package inserts provided by drug manufacturers. Information includes the accepted use, dosages, and side effects for commercially available drugs.

Pia mater literally, "gentle mother"; delicate inner layer of the meninges that clings gently to the brain and spinal cord; it contains many blood vessels that supply the nervous tissue.

Pills powdered drugs mixed with a liquid and formed into round or oval shapes (e.g., iron).

Pituitary gland endocrine gland that is buried deep in the cranial cavity at the base of the brain; "master gland" of the body; regulates growth and controls other endocrine glands.

Placenta a temporary structure in the uterus through which the fetus takes its nourishment; afterbirth.

Placenta previa a condition that occurs when part or all of the placenta covers the opening of the cervix (e.g., the placenta is the presenting part).

Plasma clear, straw-colored liquid component of blood (blood minus its formed elements); carries nutrients to the cells and waste products from the cells.

Platelets thrombocytes, essential for the formation of blood clots; function to stop bleeding and repair ruptured blood vessels.

Pleura the serous (oily) double-walled membrane that encloses each lung.

Pleural space a space between the visceral and parietal pleura filled with a small amount of serous (oily) fluid that allows the lungs to glide easily against each other as the lungs fill and empty during breathing.

Pleurisy inflammation of the pleura.

Pneumonia an infection that often impairs gas exchange in the lung. It may involve the distal airways and alveoli, part of a lobe, or an entire lobe of the lung.

Poison any substance taken into the body that interferes with normal body function.

Poisoning exposure to a substance that is harmful in any dosage.

Portable radio a handheld communication device used for radio communication away from the emergency vehicle. Typical power output is 1–5 watts, which limits its range.

Portable stretcher device that may be used for carrying patients down stairs, downhill, or over rough terrain; removing patients from spaces too confined or narrow for a wheeled stretcher; or in multiple casualty incidents.

Posterior (dorsal) toward the back of the body.

Posterior tibial pulse peripheral pulse located behind the ankle bone.

Postictal phase the period of gradual awakening following a seizure characterized by confusion, disorientation, and fatigue.

Powders drugs ground into fine particles (e.g., calcium carbonate).

Power grip technique used to get maximum force from the hands when lifting. The hands are placed at least 10 inches apart. The palms should face up and palm and fingers should be in complete contact with the stretcher, with all fingers bent at the same angles.

Power (squat) lift recommended technique for lifting; useful for persons with weak knees or thighs.

Preeclampsia a condition of pregnancy characterized by abnormal weight gain; swelling of the face, hands, and lower back; visual disturbances, headaches, irritability, and increased blood pressure (more than 140/90).

Pregnancy-induced hypertension (PIH) a disorder of pregnancy in which the patient has a blood pressure of 140/90 or more during pregnancy but had a normal blood pressure before the pregnancy.

Prehospital care report (PCR) a document used by health care providers to note changes in patient condition; these changes are important to health care personnel assuming care of the patient.

Preschooler child 3–6 years of age.

Prescription a written direction for the preparation and administration of a drug.

Prolapsed cord a serious emergency that endangers the life of the unborn fetus. Prolapsed cord occurs when the umbilical cord falls down below the presenting part of the fetus and presents through the birth canal before delivery of the head.

Prone lying face down and flat.

Prostate gland secretes fluid that enhances sperm motility and neutralizes the acidity of the vagina during intercourse.

Proximal nearest the point of reference; toward or nearest the trunk.

Proximate cause in a negligence case, proximate cause is established (usually by expert testimony) when the action or inaction of the EMT-Basic was the cause of, or contributed to, the patient's injury and the EMT-Basic could reasonably foresee that his or her action or inaction would result in the damage.

Pubis the anterior portion of pelvis.

Public service answering point (PSAP) a facility equipped and staffed to receive and control 9-1-1 access calls.

Pulmonary arteries blood vessels that originate at the right ventricle of the heart; carry oxygen-poor blood from the right ventricle to the lungs.

Pulmonary contusion bruising of the lung.

Pulmonary edema fluid in the lung tissues, most commonly due to failure of the left ventricle of the heart.

Pulmonary embolus a clot that usually originates from the deep veins in the leg that travels through the veins to the heart and then to the pulmonary circulation. The clot becomes trapped in the smaller branches of the pulmonary arteries, causing partial or complete blood flow obstruction. As a result, a portion of the lung is ventilated but not perfused.

Pulmonary veins blood vessels that carry oxygen-rich blood from the lungs to the left atrium.

Pulmonic valve semilunar valve located at the junction of the right ventricle and pulmonary artery.

Pulse the regular expansion and contraction of an artery caused by the movement of blood from the heart as it contracts. A pulse can normally be felt anywhere an artery passes over a bone and lies near the skin.

Pulse pressure the difference between the systolic and diastolic blood pressures.

Pulse rhythm the pattern of heart beats and the interval between the beats.

Pulse strength the force of the pressure wave as blood is pumped through the body.

Puncture piercing of the skin with a pointed object such as a nail, pencil, ice pick, splinter, piece of glass, bullet, or a knife resulting in little or no external bleeding (internal bleeding may be severe).

Pupil rounded opening in the iris through which light enters the interior of the eye.

Quality improvement a system of internal and external reviews and audits of all aspects of an EMS system to identify those aspects needing improvement to assure that the public receives the highest quality of prehospital care.

Raccoon eyes bilateral bluish discoloration (ecchymosis) around the eyes.

Radial pulse peripheral pulse located proximal to the thumb on the wrist.

Radiation the transfer of heat, as infrared heat rays, from the surface of one object to the surface of another without contact between the two objects.

Radius lateral bone of the forearm.

Rapid trauma assessment a head-to-toes physical examination performed to detect the presence of life-threatening injuries.

Record keeping setting down in permanent form.

Recovery position lying on the left or right side.

Rectum the lower part of the large intestine, about 5 inches long, between the sigmoid colon and the anal canal.

Red blood cells erythrocytes; transport oxygen to body cells and carbon dioxide away from body cells; each red blood cell contains hemoglobin.

Repeater a device that receives a transmission from a low-power portable or mobile radio on one frequency and then retransmits it at a higher power on another frequency so it can be received at a distant location.

Rescue removal of a person from a dangerous or potentially dangerous scene.

Respiration the exchange of gases between a living organism and its environment.

Respiratory depth assessed by observing the amount of movement of the chest wall.

Respiratory equality assessed by observing the amount of movement of the chest wall.

Respiratory quality assessment of the depth and equality of respirations that can be evaluated while determining the respiratory rate.

Respiratory system supplies oxygen from inhaled air to body cells and transports carbon dioxide produced by body cells for exhalation from the body.

Retina innermost layer of the eye; converts light into impulses transmitted by the optic nerve to the brain.

Retractions indentations of the skin above the clavicles (supraclavicular), between the ribs (intercostal), and/or below the rib cage (subcostal).

Rhonchi harsh, low-pitched sounds that are usually the result of narrowing of the larger airways (bronchi) due to mucus or fluid.

Ribs 12 pairs of bones that line the wall of the thorax; all of the ribs are attached posteriorly by ligaments to the thoracic vertebrae.

Rotation mechanism of injury in which there is severe rotation of the torso or head and neck, moving one side of the spinal column against the other.

Rubella an airborne disease spread by droplets.

Sagittal plane the lengthwise field that passes through the body from front to back, dividing the body into right and left sections.

Salivary glands glands of the digestive system that dissolve food chemicals and moisten and lubricate food so it can be swallowed.

Salmonella (food poisoning) a foodborne disease spread by improper handling of food.

SAMPLE an acronym that serves to remind the EMT-Basic of the information that should be gathered when obtaining a patient history. SAMPLE stands for **s**igns and **s**ymptoms, **a**llergies, **m**edications, pertinent **p**ast medical history, **l**ast oral intake, and **e**vents leading to the injury or illness.

Scapula shoulder blade.

Schizophrenia a group of mental disorders characterized by confusion; combative behavior; acting reserved and withdrawn; delusions and hallucinations; rambling, disorganized speech; bizarre or disorganized behavior; indifference to the feelings of others; preferring to be alone, with few, if any, close friends; and disorganized and fragmented thoughts, perceptions, and emotional reactions. Schizophrenic individuals are at high risk for suicidal and homicidal behavior.

School-age child child 6–12 years of age.

Sclera the outermost layer of the eye; "white" of the eye.

Scoop (orthopedic) stretcher also called a split litter. The scoop stretcher is made of metal and consists of four sections, two sections support the upper body and two sections support the lower body. In the absence of spinal injury, the scoop stretcher may be used to carry a supine patient up or down stairs or in other confined spaces.

Scope of practice the duties and skills an EMT-Basic is legally allowed and expected to perform when necessary.

Scrotum loose sac of skin that houses the male testes.

Seesaw breathing movement of the chest and abdomen in opposite directions during breathing; most readily observed in infants.

Seizure a sudden period of abnormal electrical activity in the brain that causes distinctive changes in behavior and body function. A seizure is a symptom (not a disease) of an underlying problem within the central nervous system.

Self-Contained Breathing Apparatus (SCBA) a device used to aid breathing that does not require outside air.

Sellick maneuver (cricoid pressure) technique used in an unresponsive patient without a cough or gag reflex to help prevent passive regurgitation and aspiration during endotracheal intubation.

Seminal vesicles accessory glands in the male that secrete fluid that nourishes and protects sperm.

Sensory nerves nerves that transmit impulses to the brain.

Septum a wall (partition) that divides two cavities.

Sexual abuse the "use, persuasion, or coercion of any child to engage in sexually explicit conduct (or any simulation of such

conduct) for producing any visual depiction of such conduct, or rape, molestation, prostitution, or incest with children" (The Child Abuse and Prevention Act, Public Law 100-294).

Shock (hypoperfusion) the inadequate circulation of blood through an organ or a part of the body; a state of profound depression of the vital processes of the body.

Shock position lying on the back with the feet elevated approximately 8–12 inches.

Short (half) backboard device that is 3–4 feet long and made of wood, aluminum, or plastic that serves as an intermediate device for immobilizing noncritical patients found in a sitting position. It must be used in conjunction with a long backboard for full spinal immobilization..

Side effect an expected (and usually unavoidable) effect of a drug that usually has no consequence on a drug's intended use.

Sigmoid colon the lower part of the descending colon between the iliac crest and the rectum, shaped like the letter S.

Sign any medical or trauma condition displayed by the patient and identifiable by the EMT-Basic.

Sinuses spaces or cavities inside some cranial bones that drain into the nose.

Skeletal muscle striated or voluntary muscle; forms the major muscle mass of the body.

Skeletal system gives the body shape, support, and form; protects vital internal organs; works with muscles to provide for body movement; stores minerals (calcium, phosphorus); and produces red blood cells.

Skull bones that house and protect the brain.

Slander injuring a person's character, name, or reputation by false and malicious spoken words.

Small intestine the portion of the gastrointestinal system between the stomach and beginning of the large intestine; consists of three parts: duodenum, jejunum, and ileum; receives food from the stomach and secretions from the pancreas and liver; completes the digestion of food that began in the mouth and stomach.

Smooth muscle visceral or involuntary muscle; handles the work of all internal organs except the heart.

Snoring sound that results from partial obstruction of the upper airway by the tongue.

Soft palate fleshy portion of the nasal cavity that extends behind the hard palate. It marks the boundary between the nasopharynx and the rest of the pharynx.

Solutions liquid preparations of one or more chemical substances, usually dissolved in water (e.g., 5% dextrose in water, 0.9% normal saline).

Sphygmomanometer a blood pressure cuff.

Spinal cavity extends from the bottom of the skull to the lower back; contains the spinal cord and is protected by vertebrae.

Spinal (vertebral) column 33 separate but connected bones (vertebrae) that enclose the spinal cord.

Spinal nerves 31 pairs of nerves connected to the spinal cord; sensory nerves transmit messages to the brain and spinal cord from the body; motor nerves transmit messages from the brain and spinal cord to the body.

Spirits volatile substances dissolved in alcohol (e.g., spirit of ammonia).

Spontaneous abortion a natural termination of pregnancy; a miscarriage.

Stair chair device designed for patients who can assume a sitting position while being carried to the ambulance. The stair chair is useful for moving patients up or down stairs, through narrow corridors and doorways, into small elevators, and in narrow aisles in aircraft or buses.

Standard of care   exercising the degree of care, skill, and judgement that would be expected under similar circumstances by a similarly trained, reasonable EMT-Basic.

Status epilepticus   continuous seizures or recurrent seizures that occur at a frequency that prevents the patient from recovering from one seizure before having another one. Status epilepticus is a medical emergency that, if not treated quickly, may result in respiratory failure and death.

Sterilization   a method of decontamination that destroys all microorganisms including highly resistant bacterial spores.

Sternum   breastbone.

Stoma   an artificial opening.

Stomach   a sac between the esophagus and small intestine that stores food.

Stridor   a harsh, high-pitched sound associated with severe upper airway obstruction; most often heard during inspiration and often characterized by the use of accessory muscles.

Subcutaneous emphysema   air trapped beneath the skin; a crackling sensation under the fingers that suggests laceration of a lung and the leakage of air into the pleural space.

Substance abuse   the deliberate, persistent, and excessive self-administration of a substance in a way that is not medically or socially approved.

Substance misuse   the self-administration of a substance for unintended purposes, or for appropriate purposes but in improper amounts or doses.

Sudden cardiac death   the unexpected loss of life occurring either immediately or within 1 hour of onset of cardiac symptoms.

Sudden Infant Death Syndrome (SIDS)   the sudden and unexpected death of an infant or young child in which a careful autopsy cannot find an adequate cause of death. Also called "crib death" or "cot death."

Suicide   any willful act designed to end one's own life.

Superior   above, upper, toward the head.

Supine   lying flat on the back; face up.

Suppositories   drugs mixed in a firm base such as cocoa butter that, when placed into the rectum or vagina, melt at body temperature (e.g., glycerin).

Surfactant   a thin substance that coats each alveolus and prevents the alveoli from collapsing.

Suspensions   drug particles mixed with, but not dissolved in, a liquid (e.g., activated charcoal).

Symptom   any condition described by the patient, e.g., shortness of breath, nausea, dizziness.

Syphilis   a bloodborne disease spread by contact with blood or body fluids of an infected person.

Syrups   drugs suspended in sugar and water (e.g., cough syrup).

Systemic effect   an effect of a drug on the whole body rather than to a single area or part of the body.

System   different types of organs that work together to carry out a complex function or functions.

Systolic blood pressure   the pressure exerted against the walls of the arteries when the left ventricle contracts.

Tablets   powdered drugs, molded or compressed during manufacture (e.g., nitroglycerin).

Tachycardia   in an adult, a heart rate greater than 100 beats per minute.

Tachypnea   an excessively rapid rate of breathing.

Tarsals   bones of the heel and back part of the foot.

Tendons   strong cords of fibrous connective tissue that stretch across joints; create a pull between bones when muscles contract.

Tension pneumothorax   a life-threatening injury in which air enters the pleura during inspiration and progressively accumulates under pressure.

Testis   one of two male reproductive glands located in the scrotum that produce reproductive cells and secrete testosterone.

Therapeutic abortion   an abortion performed for medical reasons, often because the pregnancy poses a threat to the mother's health.

Thoracic (chest) cavity   located in the trunk between the diaphragm and the neck.

Thorax   chest; the upper two-thirds of the trunk; contains the ribs and sternum.

Threatened abortion   a pregnancy in which the cervix remains closed and the fetus remains in the uterus. The patient often complains of vaginal bleeding and/or pain resembling menstrual cramps. A threatened abortion may progress to a complete abortion or may subside, and the pregnancy may continue to term.

Thrombocytes   platelets, formed elements of blood.

Thyroid cartilage   Adam's apple; the largest cartilage of the larynx.

Thyroid gland   endocrine gland that lies in the neck, just below the larynx; regulates metabolic rate.

Tibia   shinbone; the larger of the two bones of the lower leg.

Tidal volume   the amount of air inhaled and exhaled during normal breathing.

Tinctures   alcohol solutions prepared from an animal or vegetable drug or chemical substance (e.g., tincture of iodine).

Tissue   collection of cells with similar features or functions.

Toddler   a child 1–3 years of age.

Tolerance   requiring progressively larger doses of a drug to achieve the desired effect.

Tonic-clonic seizure   a generalized motor seizure.

Toxin   a poisonous substance of plant or animal origin.

Trachea   an elongated tube approximately 4–5 inches long that serves as a passageway for air to and from the lungs; windpipe.

Tracheal stoma   an opening in the neck that opens the trachea to the atmosphere.

Tracheostomy   the creation of a surgical opening into the trachea through the neck, with insertion of a tube to aid passage of air or removal of secretions.

Trade name   also known as the brand name, proprietary name, and trademark; a trade name has the symbol ® in the upper right-hand corner showing the drug is registered by and restricted to a manufacturer. A drug may have several different trade names if it is marketed by different manufacturers.

Transient ischemic attack (TIA)   "mini-stroke," a temporary interruption of the blood supply to the brain. The patient's signs and symptoms resemble those of a stroke but are transient, lasting from a few minutes to several hours. Signs and symptoms completely resolve within 24 hours with no permanent damage.

Transverse colon   the portion of the large intestine extending across the abdomen from the right (hepatic) and left colic (splenic) flexures.

Transverse (horizontal) plane   the crosswise field that divides the body into superior (upper) and inferior (lower) sections.

Traumatic asphyxia   a severe compression injury to the chest.

Trendelenburg position   lying on the back with the head of the bed lowered and the feet raised in a straight incline.

Triage   the sorting of multiple casualties into priorities for emergency care or transportation to definitive care.

Tricuspid valve   atrioventricular (AV) valve located between the right atrium and right ventricle.

Tripod position   seated upright, leaning forward with the head hyperextended in an effort to inhale adequate air.

True ribs   rib pairs 1–7 attached anteriorly to the sternum by cartilage.

Tuberculosis   an airborne disease spread by droplets.

Turbinates   bones found on each side of the nose that are shaped like two inverted cones.

Two-person stretcher (lift-in stretcher)   wheeled stretcher that requires two rescuers on each side when loading and unloading from the ambulance.

UHF   ultra-high frequency radio band (a band is a group of radio frequencies close together).

Ulna   medial bone of the forearm.

Umbilical cord   the attachment that connects the fetus with the placenta; contains two arteries and one vein.

United States Pharmacopeia (USP)   an official publication that lists approved drugs and provides directions for their general use.

Universal precautions   self-protection against diseases transmitted via blood.

Upper respiratory tract   consists of parts of the respiratory system outside the chest cavity, i.e., the nose, pharynx, and larynx; filters, warms, and humidifies the air, protecting the surfaces of the lower respiratory tract.

Ureter   one of two tubes that carry urine from the kidneys to the urinary bladder.

Urethra   canal that transports urine from the urinary bladder to the outside of the body.

Urinary bladder   temporary storage site for urine.

Urinary system   produces and excretes urine from the body.

Urticaria   hives.

Uterine rupture   tearing (rupture) of the womb (uterus).

Uterus   a hollow, muscular organ in a female in which a fertilized ovum implants and receives nourishment until birth; womb.

Uvula   soft tissue that hangs down from the middle of the lower border of the soft palate.

Vagina (birth canal)   in the female, a muscular tube that serves as a passageway between the uterus and the outside. It receives the penis during intercourse and serves as a passageway for menstrual flow and delivery of an infant.

Vallecula   the area between the base of the tongue and the epiglottis.

Veins   low-pressure blood vessels that collect blood for transport back to the heart; contain valves to prevent backflow of blood.

Ventricular fibrillation (VF)   an abnormal heart rhythm in which the heart muscle quivers instead of contracting normally; effective contraction of the heart and pulse are absent.

Ventricular shunt   a drainage system used to remove excess cerebrospinal fluid (CSF) in the brain.

Ventricular tachycardia (VT)   a fast heart rhythm (rate more than 100 beats per minute) that originates in the ventricles.

Venules   the smallest branches of veins leading to the capillaries.

VHF   very high frequency radio band (a band is a group of radio frequencies close together).

Virus   a type of infectious agent that depends on other organisms to live and grow.

Visceral pleura   the inner pleural layer that covers the surface of the lungs.

Vital organs   organs with functions that are essential to life (e.g., brain, heart, lungs).

Vital signs   assessments of breathing, pulse, skin, pupils, and blood pressure.

Vitreous humor   fluid in the posterior chamber behind the lens of the eye; maintains the shape of the eye.

Vocal cords   thin membranes within the larynx that produce sound; the length and tension of the vocal cords determine voice pitch.

Wheezing   a continuous, high-pitched musical sound heard on inspiration or expiration that suggests a narrowed or partially obstructed airway.

White blood cells   leukocytes; defend the body from microorganisms, such as bacteria and viruses, that have invaded the bloodstream or tissues of the body.

Withdrawal   the condition produced when an individual stops using or abusing a drug to which he or she is physically or psychologically addicted.

Xiphoid process   piece of cartilage that makes up the inferior portion of the sternum (breastbone).

APPENDIX A

TEST-TAKING PREPARATION

BECOMING AN EMT-BASIC

Taking the certification examination to become an EMT-Basic can potentially change your life. It may open up new career opportunities, enhance your position in a current career, and give you a heightened sense of community involvement. Whatever the reason you seek certification, your endeavors to come to the aid of the sick and injured are noble and should be commended.

As trends in health care seek to minimize in-hospital stays, the number of out-of-hospital calls for help will continue to rise. Drug use, gang and domestic violence, motor vehicle collisions, and chemical dependencies will also increase the need for prehospital health care providers. EMT-Basics, both paid and volunteer, play a vital role in the health, safety, and welfare of our society.

PREPARING FOR THE "BIG RACE"

Imagine you are going to run a marathon. You would not wake up the day of the race, put on a pair of sneakers, and run competitively. Instead, you would put yourself through a training schedule in the weeks leading up to the race. Likewise, taking the EMT-Basic certification examination requires preparation. Just as an athlete prepares for a marathon, so too must you prepare for the taking the test. In sports, this preparation is sometimes called "tapering." Athletes taper their training so that they are at their peak performance on "game day." This, too, should be your goal.

There are five key elements to ensure your ultimate success on the EMT-Basic certification examination: (1) excellent training facilities and equipment, (2) a training schedule, (3) knowledge about the upcoming event (in your case, the certification exam), (4) event strategy, and (5) a proper frame of mind. A checklist is included at the end of this chapter to help you organize these elements into a workable game plan.

EXCELLENT TRAINING FACILITIES AND EQUIPMENT: BUILDING THE IDEAL TRAINING CENTER

YOUR TRAINING FACILITY

To get the most out of your preparation, your physical surroundings must be conducive to learning and retention. Identifying and limiting possible distractions are key factors in selecting your primary study location. It may not always be possible to study in the same place, but you should choose one area as your "usual" study place.

To select a suitable study site, identify those factors that inhibit your ability to concentrate. Next, eliminate as many of these distractions as possible. Typical study areas include a room in your home, a library, your place of work (after normal working hours), or a friend's house. Consider the following elements when selecting a study area:

- Convenience of the site (close to home, school, or work)
- Availability of the area (compatible with your schedule)
- Physical atmosphere

- Noise
- Space
- Lighting
- Comfort
- Available facilities (restrooms, refreshments, break area)

EQUIPMENT

Once you have selected your training facility, the next step is to prepare and organize your equipment. The equipment you will need for certification examination preparation includes all the resources that may be used to enhance your ability to succeed. These items may include:

- This book and other EMT-Basic texts
- Class notes and handouts
- Study groups
- Results from previous certification exams [the National Registry of EMTs provides a breakdown of test results by specific topic (e.g., "Airway" or "Patient Assessment")].
- Resources from the agency that provided you with your initial EMT training
- Certified EMTs who have taken the certification examination

TRAINING SCHEDULE

Everything should now be in place for you to begin training. The next thing you need is a training schedule. Remember to start preparing early and anticipate distractions. By defining a study schedule and sticking to it, you lay a foundation on which success may be built. However, be realistic when you set your schedule. Avoid starting off with a bang and ending with a whimper.

When should you begin training? The earlier you begin, the more realistic and attainable your training goals will be. When you establish your time line, identify goals and specific dates (e.g., "Read and highlight all study material by July 21."). To help you set your priorities, here is a sample training schedule.

STARTING POINT

- Gather study materials and establish study area(s).
- Establish time line.
- Begin comprehensive review by reading and highlighting all material.
- Answer all end-of-chapter study questions and record your score. Don't review answers and rationales until each test is complete—make it as realistic as possible. After completing all the questions, look at your wrong answers. Review and make sure you understand why you answered the question wrong.
- Submit any paperwork that needs to be filed prior to the certification examination.

HALFWAY TO THREE-QUARTERS POINT

- Your initial comprehensive review should be complete.
- Take the Comprehensive Posttest (Appendix B) as you would a certification examination. Give yourself the same amount of time per question as allotted for the "real" certification examination. For example, if your certification examination contains 150 questions given over a maximum of 2½ hours (150 minutes), you would have an average of one minute to complete each question. Because Appendix B has 100 questions, you should allow yourself 100 minutes to complete the exam. Do not cheat or treat this chapter like an "open-book" test. Rather, use this chapter as an opportunity to appraise your preparedness. Record your results on an answer sheet, and score

the test when finished. Review the results to identify your weaknesses, and then concentrate your studying efforts on these weak areas.
- Review all notes, highlighted areas, and discovered weaknesses.

TEST WEEK

- Relax. Allow your brain some "down" time in which to organize all the information you have been studying. Review areas that still cause you concern.
- Prepare your body and mind:
  Eat well.
  Sleep well. Begin setting your internal clock to coincide with test time. In the days preceding the exam, you may want to review material at the same time of day that the exam will be given. This strategy may help you train and condition your brain. Exercise to rid yourself of nervous energy.
  Avoid use of stimulants, depressants, and alcohol.
  Avoid drastic changes in lifestyle. This is not a good time to quit smoking, quit drinking coffee, or lose 20 pounds.
- Be positive. Tell yourself aloud: "I can do this." Leave yourself notes on the refrigerator that say, "I WILL pass." Positive reinforcement may help decrease test-day anxiety.
- Call the testing facility to ensure that the test is scheduled as planned. Double check the location, parking, room number, and test time. If you are unfamiliar with the site, visit it. Make sure that all required paperwork is complete. Ask the testing agency about anything you may need to have with you the day of the test (e.g., pencils, paper, certification application, identification, CPR card, training center code number, etc.).

TEST DAY

- Don't cram! Resist the urge unless you need to clarify a specific point.
- Allow plenty of time to arrive at the facility—anticipate a flat tire or a dead battery. Consider having a back-up method of getting to the test site.
- Eat a good meal, but not one that is going to make you drowsy.
- Allow enough time for a nervous stomach to run its course if you are prone to this reaction. Know where the restrooms are!
- Take a deep breath; tell yourself, "I can pass this test"; and then do so!

KNOWLEDGE ABOUT THE UPCOMING EVENT

Before taking the test, you need to know certain information about it. This information will help you plan your testing strategy. As early as possible, you should know:

- The scope of the material covered
- The number of questions on the test
- The format of the questions (multiple choice, true/false, short answer) or breakdown of the test
- The amount of time allowed to complete the test
- If there is a penalty for incorrect responses

EVENT STRATEGY

Your test strategy should be based on two factors: the characteristics of the test and your personal style. The characteristics of the test are all the things you have learned about the upcoming event (see the previous section, "Knowledge about the Upcoming Event").

Testing style varies from individual to individual. You may have tried-and-true methods that have worked for you in the past. If so, use these methods. Now is not the time to invent a new method.

A SAMPLE TEST-TAKING STRATEGY

If you are unsure about your testing style, you may want to try the following techniques (for multiple-choice testing formats).

- First, answer all the questions you feel confident about while skipping over questions that puzzle you or take up too much time. (Note: If you skip questions, make sure your answers are recorded correctly. This may be especially difficult when using bubble-type answer sheets.)
- Read each question completely looking for such words as *except, always, never, not, first, last, list, all,* and *incorrect.* These words may change the direction of the answer you are searching for.
- After reading each question, think of an answer. Then read the possible answers while searching for the most correct response. Even if the first response appears to be the correct answer, read all the responses to ensure that you have selected the best answer.
- As you go through the test, be sure to reference the questions you skipped. If scratch paper is allowed, draw a circle on it and record the number(s) of the questions you skipped. If no scratch paper is allowed, put a mark beside the skipped questions on your answer sheet or on the testing materials. However, be sure to erase your marks completely from the answer sheet so that it is scored correctly. And, before marking the testing materials, make sure that they are not used again for other tests.
- Once you have gone through the test and answered all the "easy" questions, start on the questions you skipped. If there is no penalty for marking an answer incorrectly (other than not getting credit for that answer), you should always turn in a completed answer sheet.
- Watch your time limit closely. If there is no penalty for marking an answer incorrectly, give yourself the last minute or so to "Christmas tree" any remaining blank answers, i.e., "decorate" your answer sheet by filling in responses for those multiple-choice questions that you could not answer. This strategy is ONLY recommended when there is no penalty for a wrong answer. It is based on the theory that you may, in fact, hit the correct response.
- As you go back through the tougher questions, select the best answer by comparing the topic covered in the question with the topics addressed in the responses. Sometimes, a subsequent question (especially in scenario-based questions) will give you a hint what the correct answer may be. With most multiple-choice test questions, one or two responses can be thrown out immediately. Once you have the responses narrowed down, reverse the question–answer process: read each response, then read the question to see if the question correctly addresses the subject of the response. This strategy is similar to playing "Jeopardy." Answer all skipped questions this way. If you are absolutely uncertain about the answer, guess. Once you have selected an answer based on an instinct, stick with your initial response unless you are certain that you were originally wrong.
- If time permits, review your test. Again, do not change a response unless you are certain that your initial response was incorrect.
- Periodically during the test you should put down your pencil, clear your head, and stretch your body. Be as comfortable and relaxed as possible.

STRATEGY AFTER THE TEST

Strategy does not stop when you turn in your test. While the test is still clear in your mind, record the subject(s) or specific question(s) that gave you the most trouble. In the event that you do not successfully pass the examination the first time, your post-test notes will be important as you prepare for subsequent certification testing.

PROPER FRAME OF MIND

Organized preparation for the EMT-Basic certification examination will help put you in the proper frame of mind for test day. With proper preparation, you should not "freeze up" while taking the test. Preparation gives you all the tools necessary to succeed on the examination.

If you are prepared, there should be no mysteries or surprises in the certification exam. If you know and understand the concepts covered in this text and can apply those concepts to a written question, you will pass.

Think of the testing process as a means of certifying EMT's rather than a means of turning people away. Your preparation allows you to be confident and relaxed while taking the test. So roll up your sleeves and let's get started.

PREPARATION CHECKLIST

BUILD YOUR TRAINING CENTER

- Select a primary area for preparation that:
  Is comfortable
  Is convenient
  Has available facilities (restrooms, food, drink)
  Limits distractions (noise, TV, friends, coworkers)
- Gather study materials:
  Text
  Study notes
  Class handouts
  Homework and quizzes from class
  Copies of old tests or results from previous certification testing
  Information from testing facility or agency
  Certified EMT-Basics

SET YOUR TRAINING SCHEDULE

Date of Exam
_____

Date you begin preparation
_____

Halfway point date
_____

Goal (How far do you want to be in your preparation by this date?)
_____

_____

_____

_____

Three quarters point date
_____

Goal (How far do you want to be in your preparation by this date?)
_____

_____

_____

Date to take Chapter 35 Comprehensive Exam _____

Score _____

Weak areas identified _____

_____

_____

_____

BE PREPARED FOR TEST DAY

- Submit all paperwork needed to register for the examination.
- Gather all paperwork needed on the day of the examination:
  Application (double-check to ensure completion)
  CPR card
  Testing fee and form of fee (e.g., money order, personal check)
  Picture identification
  Other (Number 2 pencils, erasers, etc.)
- When is the test?
  Date:
  Time:
- Test location
  Directions:
  Mode of transport (and an alternate?):
  Parking:
  Building location:
  Room number:
  Time to be in seat:
  Testing agency contact person and phone number:

Directions: Each of the numbered items or incomplete statements in this section is followed by answers or by completions of the statement. Select the ONE lettered answer or completion that is BEST in each case.

1. Which of the following regarding ongoing assessments is true?

   (A) Ongoing assessments should not influence your long-term care of a patient
   (B) Ongoing assessments should only be performed on critically injured patients.
   (C) Ongoing assessments assess the effectiveness of emergency care interventions provided
   (D) Ongoing assessments should be performed every 15 minutes for seriously injured patients

2. The "emergency rule" size for an endotracheal tube for an adult, regardless of gender, is

   (A) 3.0-millimeter (mm) internal diameter
   (B) 5.0-mm internal diameter
   (C) 6.5-mm internal diameter
   (D) 7.5-mm internal diameter

3. Supplying the body with oxygen and removing "waste" gases (mainly carbon dioxide) are the major functions of the respiratory system. The absorption of oxygen into the bloodstream and the release of waste gases takes place in the

   (A) liver
   (B) kidneys
   (C) bronchioles
   (D) alveoli

4. The spleen is the primary organ of the lymphatic system. It is an extremely vascular organ located in the

   (A) groin
   (B) mediastinum
   (C) left upper abdominal quadrant
   (D) right upper abdominal quadrant

5. The inspection of an ambulance's fluid levels, braking ability, warning lights, audible warning devices, communication systems, and heating/air-conditioning systems should be performed at least

   (A) daily
   (B) weekly
   (C) monthly
   (D) quarterly or every 3000 miles (whichever comes first)

6. When operating an ambulance, you should stay at least how far behind the vehicle in front of you?

   (A) 50 feet
   (B) 100 feet
   (C) 4 seconds
   (D) 10 seconds

7. When establishing a nighttime landing zone for a medical helicopter, the area should be a minimum of

   (A) 50 × 50 feet
   (B) 60 × 60 feet
   (C) 100 × 100 feet
   (D) 500 × 500 feet

8. An early sign of respiratory distress is

   (A) unconsciousness
   (B) tracheal deviation
   (C) agonal respirations
   (D) increased respiratory rate

9. For which of the following patients would it be appropriate to provide oxygen therapy by a nasal cannula at 4 liters per minute (LPM)?

   (A) An asthma patient in severe distress
   (B) A patient complaining of chest pain without a history of respiratory disease
   (C) A patient complaining of nausea with a history of emphysema
   (D) A motor vehicle collision patient complaining of abdominal pain

10. According to the American Heart Association, application of the automated external defibrillator (AED) may be applied to nonbreathing, pulseless patients of what age?

    (A) Older than 1 year of age
    (B) Older than 8 years of age
    (C) Older than 18 years of age
    (D) Older than 40 years of age

11. Which of the following is a common side effect of nitroglycerin administration?

    (A) Hypotension
    (B) Unconsciousness
    (C) Difficulty breathing
    (D) Absent breath sounds on the left side of the chest

12. While analyzing a patient's cardiac rhythm with the automated external defibrillator (AED), you must ensure that

    (A) cardiopulmonary resuscitation (CPR) is continued
    (B) the patient is not wearing any clothing
    (C) no rescuers stand within 10 feet of the patient
    (D) there is no movement or contact with the patient

13. When intubating a patient with an endotracheal tube, the laryngoscope should be held

    (A) in the left hand
    (B) in the right hand

    (C)   in either hand

    (D)   in the same hand as the endotracheal tube

14. When inserting a stylet into an endotracheal tube, the tip of the stylet should

    (A)   remain in the endotracheal tube approximately 1 inch from the tip

    (B)   remain in the endotracheal tube approximately 4–6 inches from the tip

    (C)   extend approximately 4–6 inches beyond the tip of the endotracheal tube

    (D)   extend approximately 1–2 inches beyond the tip of the endotracheal tube

15. Your ambulance crew is transporting a 23-year-old male patient to the hospital. He was injured in a motorcycle collision and has a severe injury to his right leg. You attempted to control bleeding with direct pressure and elevation plus indirect pressure (arterial pressure point), but he continues to bleed uncontrollably. Which of the following regarding the application of a tourniquet is correct?

    (A)   Tourniquets should never be used

    (B)   Tourniquets should be applied for a maximum of 10 minutes, then released

    (C)   Once a tourniquet is applied, it should not be removed in the prehospital setting

    (D)   Once a tourniquet is applied it should not be released unless the patient begins to feel numbness and tingling distal to the tourniquet

16. Your rescue crew is called to the scene of a motor vehicle collision. A 54-year-old male patient is complaining of neck pain. Which of the following should be done first when immobilizing this patient to a backboard?

    (A)   Apply a cervical collar

    (B)   Inspect the neck for signs of trauma

    (C)   Maintain in-line cervical immobilization

    (D)   Have the patient lie down on the backboard

17. Which of the following is the most common cause of distress for a newborn?

    (A)   Failure to dry and warm the child

    (B)   Failure to recognize an airway obstruction

    (C)   Failure to deliver the placenta soon enough

    (D)   Failure to cut the umbilical cord soon enough

18. Normally, the placenta (afterbirth) will deliver

    (A)   Approximately 5 minutes before the delivery of the infant

    (B)   At the same time as the infant

    (C)   Within 20 minutes of delivery of the infant

    (D)   Within 2 to 3 hours of delivery of the infant

19. The normal respiratory rate for a newborn is

    (A)   8–10 breaths per minute

    (B)   10–15 breaths per minute

    (C)   15–30 breaths per minute

    (D)   25–50 breaths per minute

20. When treating a pregnant patient, if the amniotic fluid appears greenish or black in color, you should anticipate

    (A)   twins

    (B)   fetal (infant) distress

    (C)   seizures by the mother

    (D)   excessive vaginal bleeding after delivery

21. Most states allow emergency vehicles, when driving in the emergency mode, to disregard certain laws or regulations. Which of the following should never be disregarded?

    (A) The use of seat belts
    (B) The posted speed limit
    (C) Specific turning directions
    (D) The direction of movement

22. Your rescue crew is called to the scene of a motor vehicle collision. En route, you are provided with additional information that a truck carrying an unknown chemical has overturned and is leaking. Assuming you have no formal hazardous materials training, which of the following would be an appropriate course of action?

    (A) Do not enter the emergency scene
    (B) Enter the emergency scene and treat injured patients
    (C) Enter the emergency scene, treat injured patients, and attempt to contain the spill
    (D) Enter the emergency scene, treat injured patients, and attempt to identify the product

23. Before applying a splint to a painful, swollen, deformed extremity, you should

    (A) apply a tourniquet to any open wounds
    (B) straighten the extremity with a sudden, forceful pull
    (C) assess distal circulation, sensation, and motor function
    (D) wrap tape around the entire extremity to prevent swelling

24. An impaled object should not be removed from the body unless it penetrates the

    (A) groin
    (B) cheek
    (C) abdomen
    (D) leg or arm

25. Which of the following would be appropriate management of an amputated finger?

    (A) Pack with ice
    (B) Submerge in ice water
    (C) Submerge in sterile water
    (D) Wrap with a sterile dressing

26. Your rescue crew is called to a high school for a 16-year-old female patient who injured her eye in wood shop. The patient states that a small chip of wood flew in her eye while she was using a saw. Her eye is red and inflamed. Appropriate management of this patient is to

    (A) irrigate the eye with normal saline
    (B) rub the patient's closed eyelid with a sterile dressing
    (C) scrape the surface of the eyeball with a clean fingernail
    (D) rub the patient's open eye with a sterile, moistened dressing

Directions: Each of the numbered questions or incomplete statements in this section refers to a scenario that precedes them. The numbered questions or incomplete statements are followed by answers or by completions of the statement. Select the answer or completion of the statement that is BEST in each case.

Your rescue crew is called to the home of a 56-year-old male patient complaining of chest pain. When you arrive on the scene, the patient is conscious and alert. He tells you he thinks he has "indigestion." Although the patient is in severe distress, he seems to resent your presence. His wife tells you she called 9-1-1 because the antacid he took did not relieve his discomfort.

Questions 27–33

27. Which of the following regarding consent to provide treatment is correct?

    (A) You may not treat this patient if he does not give you consent
    (B) You may treat this patient if his wife gives you permission
    (C) You may treat this patient under the rules of implied consent
    (D) You may treat this patient if he believes he is having a heart attack

28. You convince this patient that he needs medical care, and he agrees to let you treat him. Which of the following should immediately follow the initial assessment?

    (A) Scene size-up
    (B) Body substance isolation (BSI) precautions
    (C) Focused history and physical examination
    (D) Rapid trauma assessment to detect if life-threatening injuries are present

29. Which of the following acronyms may help you in questioning this patient about his chest discomfort?

    (A) AVPU
    (B) OSHA
    (C) APGAR
    (D) OPQRST

30. This patient is breathing at a rate of 16 breaths per minute with an adequate tidal volume. Which of the following oxygen therapy interventions would be indicated for this patient?

    (A) Apply a nasal cannula at 4 liters per minute (LPM) supplemental oxygen
    (B) Apply a nasal cannula at 10 LPM supplemental oxygen
    (C) Apply a nonrebreather mask at 15 LPM supplemental oxygen
    (D) Assist ventilations with a bag-valve mask connected to high-flow oxygen at a rate of 20 respirations per minute

31. The patient tells you his chest pain is a "9" on a scale of 1 to 10 with 10 being the most severe. He also informs you he has a history of angina and is prescribed nitroglycerin. The guidelines for EMT-Basics assisting in the administration of nitroglycerin are

    (A) the patient has a history of angina and the EMT-Basic has access to nitroglycerin
    (B) the patient has a history of past heart attacks, has physician-prescribed nitroglycerin, and is complaining of chest pain following a severe blow to the head
    (C) the patient is experiencing chest pain, has physician-prescribed nitroglycerin, and the EMT-Basic receives specific authorization from medical direction
    (D) the patient is experiencing chest pain, his systolic blood pressure is below 100 millimeters of mercury (mm Hg), he has physician-prescribed nitroglycerin, and the EMT-Basic requests authorization from medical direction

32. While preparing this patient for transport, he collapses and loses consciousness. Which of the following should you do first?

(A) Check for a pulse
(B) Check for spontaneous breathing
(C) Check the patient's blood pressure
(D) Administer an additional nitroglycerin tablet

33. This patient is apneic (not breathing) and pulseless. You should immediately

(A) suction the patient's airway with a rigid suction catheter
(B) apply and activate the automated external defibrillator (AED)
(C) intubate the patient with an 8.0-millimeter (mm) internal diameter endotracheal tube
(D) perform cardiopulmonary resuscitation (CPR) for 1 minute, reassess the patient's pulse, then apply and activate the automated external defibrillator (AED)

Your ambulance is called to the scene of a motor vehicle collision. Upon arrival, your crew is assigned to treat a 42-year-old female patient thrown from a motorcycle. As you approach this patient, you observe that she is lying face down in the street and is not moving.

Questions 34–37

34. You should immediately

(A) turn the patient over
(B) begin cardiopulmonary resuscitation (CPR)
(C) immobilize the patient's head and neck
(D) apply the automated external defibrillator (AED)

35. During your initial assessment, you note that the patient is unconscious. She is breathing at a rate of 16 breaths per minute and has a weak radial pulse at 124 beats per minute. Which of the following oxygen therapy interventions would be most appropriate?

(A) Nasal cannula at 4 liters per minute (LPM)
(B) Nonrebreather mask at 6 to 8 LPM
(C) Nonrebreather mask at 15 LPM
(D) Bag-valve mask at 15 LPM and ventilate once every 8 seconds

36. Immediately following the initial assessment of this patient, you should

(A) evaluate her mental status
(B) perform a rapid trauma assessment
(C) take body substance isolation (BSI) precautions
(D) perform a focused history and physical examination

37. Which acronym would assist you in completing a physical examination of this injured patient?

(A) NFPA
(B) NTSB
(C) DCAP-BTLS
(D) CHEMTREC

Your rescue crew is called to the home of a 24-year-old male patient with an altered mental status. At the time of dispatch, there is no additional information available.

Questions 38–41

38. When you arrive, the patient is irritable. He is also confused and does not understand the reason for your presence. He complains of a headache and weakness and asks you to leave him alone. You should

(A) respect the patient's request and leave
(B) have the patient sign a refusal form and leave
(C) restrain the patient and take him to the hospital
(D) attempt to convince the patient to consent to treatment and contact medical direction if the patient continues to refuse

39. While you are talking with the patient, his brother arrives. The brother informs you that the patient is a diabetic and that the patient was fine about 30 minutes ago when he left to go shopping. This history is most commonly associated with

(A) hypoglycemia
(B) hyperglycemia
(C) postictal phase
(D) diabetic ketoacidosis

40. After explaining your intentions, the patient agrees to allow you to treat him. This form of consent is

(A) implied
(B) coerced
(C) expressed
(D) minor's consent

41. Given this patient's signs and symptoms, what medication might you consider assisting this patient in taking?

(A) Insulin
(B) Albuterol
(C) Nitroglycerin
(D) Oral glucose

Your ambulance is called to the scene of a house fire. There are two burn victims: a 32-year-old man and his 10-month-old daughter. When you arrive, the man is holding his child in front of their burning home. You observe that the man's face is covered with soot, and the child is crying.

Questions 42–45

42. Which of the following is your priority in treating these patients?

(A) Assess their airways
(B) Perform an initial assessment
(C) Cover them with burn sheets
(D) Move them away from the house

43. The father tells you that a space heater started the fire in the child's room. The infant has burns on the front of both legs (but not the back of the legs) and one entire arm. The skin is red, painful, and beginning to blister. These burns are mostly likely

(A) first-degree or superficial burns
(B) third-degree or full-thickness burns
(C) first-degree or partial-thickness burns
(D) second-degree or partial-thickness burns

44. The percent of total body surface area burned for the infant is

    (A) approximately 18%
    (B) approximately 23%
    (C) approximately 45%
    (D) approximately 54%

45. The father has burns covering his head, neck, chest, abdomen, and one arm. The percent of total body surface area burned for this patient is

    (A) approximately 18%
    (B) approximately 36%
    (C) approximately 54%
    (D) approximately 63%

Your rescue crew is called to a hardware store for a 34-year-old male patient who was exposed to an unknown chemical. Upon arrival, you find the patient standing in an office area. He has a whitish-gray powder on his face and shoulders.

Questions 46–48

46. Your priority is to

    (A) perform a scene size-up
    (B) perform an initial assessment
    (C) assess the patient's mental status
    (D) remove the power from the patient, then begin irrigation

47. To assist you in better understanding the characteristics of this chemical, the business should have specific information on-site that identifies and describes the chemical's properties (product name, physical properties, fire and explosion information, and emergency first-aid treatment). This source of information is

    (A) CHEMTREC
    (B) the DOT placard
    (C) the NFPA 704 information
    (D) the Material Safety Data Sheet (MSDS)

48. While transporting this patient to an appropriate facility, he begins complaining of a burning sensation in his left eye. You should

    (A) cover both eyes with a dry, sterile dressing
    (B) cover both eyes with a moist, sterile dressing
    (C) position the patient on his left side and irrigate the left eye
    (D) position the patient on his right side and irrigate both eyes

Your ambulance is called to the scene of a motor vehicle collision. Information at time of dispatch says that three cars collided at an intersection, and one vehicle may have occupants trapped inside. Another crew arrives at the scene first. This crew initiates an incident management system.

Questions 49–54

49. Your crew is assigned to the treatment sector. Your responsibilities will include

    (A) removing trapped patients

(B) moving patients to the transportation sector
(C) establishing objectives and priorities for the scene
(D) coordinating the establishment of a landing zone for medical helicopters

50. You are assisting in the treatment of four occupants trapped in one of the vehicles. Which of these patients would be the highest priority for treatment and rapid transport?

(A) A 10-year-old boy complaining of neck, back, and right arm pain
(B) A 25-year-old woman who is not breathing and does not have a pulse
(C) A 34-year-old man with an angulated, deformed lower leg with bone ends protruding through the skin
(D) A 65-year-old woman with a history of cardiac problems who is complaining of difficulty breathing

51. While treating the 10-year-old boy, you notice a large flap of skin hanging down from an open cut. This injury is consistent with which type of soft tissue injury?

(A) Abrasion
(B) Avulsion
(C) Contusion
(D) Hematoma

52. This patient tells you that his arm feels numb. The numbness is a

(A) sign
(B) symptom
(C) vital sign
(D) pertinent negative

53. The patient is bleeding profusely from this injury. Appropriate management for this condition would include

(A) Fold the flap of tissue over the wound, apply direct pressure with a sterile dressing, and elevate the wound above the level of the heart
(B) Remove the flap of tissue, apply indirect pressure to the closest arterial pressure point, and elevate the wound above the level of the heart
(C) Fold the flap of tissue over the wound, apply direct pressure with an occlusive dressing, and elevate the wound above the level of the heart
(D) Apply a tourniquet, release the tourniquet every 10 minutes, and elevate the extremity above the level of the heart

54. While preparing to go back in service after this incident, you notice that a member of your crew is unusually quiet. He is normally a very social person, but now is keeping to himself. You ask him if he is okay, but he seems reluctant to talk. He keeps commenting about the 25-year-old woman who was fatally injured in the crash. Which of the following may help this crew member deal with this tragedy?

(A) Tell him to "shake it off"
(B) Tell him it is all part of the job
(C) Tell him about critical incident stress debriefing (CISD) as a resource
(D) Tell him that no one else is having trouble with the incident

Your rescue crew is called to a video arcade for a 14-year-old male patient complaining of difficulty breathing. When you arrive, this patient is sitting upright on a bench. He is in severe respiratory distress. The patient is with his friends, and both of his parents are at work.

55. Which of the following regarding the assessment and treatment of minor patients is correct?

(A) You may not treat minor patients until a parent arrives at the scene
(B) You may not treat minor patients until a parent is contacted either by phone or in person
(C) You may treat minor patients if a life-threatening condition exists without prior parental consent
(D) You may treat any minor despite the parent's wishes if a serious condition exists

56. Immediately following the scene size-up, you perform an initial assessment that reveals that this patient is conscious with a clear airway. He is breathing 32 times per minute and speaks in one- and two-word sentences. His pulse rate is 124 beats per minute, and no other life-threatening condition exists. Your next step is to

(A) perform a rapid trauma assessment
(B) perform a focused history and physical examination
(C) assist the patient with taking his albuterol inhaler
(D) intubate the patient with a 7.5-millimeter (mm) internal diameter endotracheal tube

57. Upon auscultation of this patient's lungs, you hear a high-pitched whistling sound during exhalation. This sound is most likely

(A) stridor
(B) rhonchi
(C) wheezing
(D) rales/crackles

58. The patient shows you an albuterol inhaler and tells you that he tried "puffing" on it once, but was unable to get any relief. Which of the following regarding the assisted administration of this medication by an EMT-Basic is correct?

(A) This medication is not authorized for use in infants or children
(B) This medication should be shaken vigorously before administration
(C) This medication is effective regardless of the patient's tidal volume
(D) This medication is not indicated for patients in severe respiratory distress

59. Specific authorization from medical direction must be obtained before assisting with the administration of this medication. You prepare to contact medical direction by radio. When the physician speaks with you by the stationary transmitter/receiver at the hospital, she is using what communication system component?

(A) A land line
(B) A base station
(C) A portable radio
(D) A mobile two-way radio

60. Medical direction grants authorization to administer albuterol. Before ending your communication with medical direction, you must

(A) begin administering the albuterol
(B) repeat the physician's orders back to her
(C) inform her about the patient's condition after taking the albuterol
(D) give the hospital the patient's full name, date of birth, parents' names, and home address

61. To receive maximal benefit from the metered-dose inhaler, you should tell the patient to

(A) depress the inhaler while taking rapid, short breaths (panting)

(B) exhale completely, and then depress the inhaler while taking a deep breath in

(C) spray the albuterol under the tongue and do not swallow until the strange taste is gone

(D) exhale completely, then take a deep breath in and depress the inhaler when the lungs are completely full

Your ambulance crew is called to the home of a 24-year-old male patient complaining of a headache. His wife meets you at the door and tells you that she called because her husband has been in pain since a car accident 3 days ago. The patient is found sitting in a dark room with a cool, wet towel on his forehead. He is alert and answers questions appropriately and tells you that he does not want your help.

Questions 62–63

62. Which of the following is correct?

(A) The patient must be physically assessed before allowing him to refuse care

(B) Since the patient suffered a head injury, you may legally treat him against his wishes

(C) You should immediately leave the patient's house without any further attempts to provide care

(D) The patient may refuse care, but he must be informed of the possible consequences of such refusal

63. When documenting the patient's refusal of assessment, treatment, and transportation, you should have the patient sign the prehospital care report. Preferably, it should also be witnessed by

(A) a police officer

(B) your supervisor

(C) the patient's wife

(D) your EMT-Basic partner

Your rescue crew is called to a picnic area for a 31-year-old male patient in respiratory distress. You arrive to find the patient sitting on a bench. His face looks flushed (red) and swollen at the lips and cheeks. He is gasping for air, and his eyes keep rolling back in his head. His friends tell you that he was stung by a bee and is allergic to bee stings.

Questions 64–67

64. You should immediately

(A) look for a stinger

(B) lay the patient down

(C) spray the patient's body with bee repellent

(D) ask about the patient's past medical history and prescribed medication

65. Which of the following signs would be consistent with a severe allergic reaction?

(A) Battle's sign

(B) Raccoon eyes

(C) One-sided facial droop

(D) Decreasing mental status

66. During your focused history and physical examination, you discover that the patient has been prescribed an auto-injector medication to treat a severe allergic reaction. The medication in the auto-injector is

    (A) Atrovent®
    (B) Arenalin®
    (C) Bronkosol®
    (D) Solu-Medrol®

67. After receiving authorization to administer this medication, you inject the patient in the thigh. Soon after, you notice that a white circle has developed at the injection site. This circle is an example of

    (A) a local effect of the drug
    (B) a systemic effect of the drug
    (C) an adverse effect of the drug
    (D) an idiosyncratic effect of the drug

Your ambulance crew is called to a local restaurant for a "man down, unknown medical problem." Upon arrival, you find an approximately 54-year-old male patient lying on the pavement. Bystanders state that the patient collapsed in his current position about 25 minutes ago. It is a hot and humid summer day.

Questions 68–72

68. An initial assessment reveals that the patient is unconscious. He has an open airway and is breathing 24 times per minute. His pulse rate is 120 beats per minute and weak at the radial artery. Following the initial assessment, you should

    (A) intubate this patient
    (B) administer oral glucose
    (C) perform a rapid trauma assessment
    (D) perform a focused history and physical examination

69. The patient is lying on hot pavement. The transfer of heat from the pavement to the patient is

    (A) radiation
    (B) conduction
    (C) convection
    (D) evaporation

70. While physically assessing this patient, you note that his skin is dry and very hot. Which of the following should you do first?

    (A) Pour cool water on the patient's lips to encourage drinking
    (B) Move the patient to the back of your air-conditioned ambulance
    (C) Question bystanders about the patient's condition before your arrival
    (D) Look for signs that alcohol may be involved in this patient's condition (e.g., empty bottles, the smell of alcohol on this breath, etc.)

71. When lifting this patient to move him from the ground to a gurney, you should

    (A) keep your feet as close together as possible
    (B) slightly bend the knees and lift with the lower back
    (C) keep the knees locked straight and lift primarily with the arms
    (D) bend at the knees and flex at the hips to assume a squatting position

72. Once in the back of the ambulance, you assess this patient's temperature to be 103.8° Fahrenheit (F). In addition to high-flow oxygen by nonrebreather mask, appropriate treatment for this patient would include

    (A)   wrapping the patient in dry burn sheets

    (B)   encouraging the patient to take sips of a diluted sports drink

    (C)   cooling the patient with cold packs applied to the groin, armpits, and neck; keeping skin moist; and fanning the skin aggressively

    (D)   elevating the patient's legs approximately 8–10 inches and attempting to slowly cool patient by sponging with tepid water

Your rescue crew is called to the home of a 6-year-old female patient who is reportedly choking. You arrive to find the patient standing in the kitchen clutching her throat. She is purple in the face and is unable to speak or cough.

Questions 73–77

73. You should immediately

    (A)   perform 5 back blows between the shoulder blades followed by 5 chest thrusts

    (B)   sweep your index finger through the patient's mouth toward the throat to free the object

    (C)   deliver subdiaphragmatic abdominal thrusts (Heimlich maneuver)

    (D)   lay the patient down, open the airway with the head-tilt, chin-lift maneuver, and attempt to ventilate mouth-to-mouth

74. Your initial attempt to clear the airway fails, and the patient becomes unconscious. She is now supine on the floor. Which of the following is true regarding your attempt to clear this patient's airway?

    (A)   You should attempt to intubate the patient to bypass the obstruction in the airway

    (B)   You must apply and activate the automated external defibrillator (AED) before any further attempts to clear the airway

    (C)   You should deliver 5 subdiaphragmatic abdominal thrusts, then reevaluate the airway

    (D)   You should continue to deliver back blows and chest thrusts until you see an object come out of the patient's mouth

75. Finally, you clear the patient's airway; however, she is not breathing on her own. Her pulse rate is 132 beats per minute and weak at the radial artery. You should

    (A)   begin cardiopulmonary resuscitation (CPR)

    (B)   begin oxygen therapy with a nonrebreather mask

    (C)   begin artificial ventilations at a rate of 12 breaths per minute

    (D)   begin artificial ventilations at a rate of 20 breaths per minute

76. This patient begins to vomit while still unconscious. Appropriate immediate management of this condition would include

    (A)   opening the airway with the head-tilt, chin-lift maneuver and suctioning until the mouth is clear

    (B)   opening the airway with a jaw thrust and suctioning for no more than 30 seconds

    (C)   log rolling the patient onto her side and applying suction while withdrawing a rigid suction catheter

    (D)   log rolling the patient onto her side and inserting a nasogastric tube to decompress the stomach

77. After clearing this patient's airway, she is semiconscious and breathing at a rate of 24 breaths per minute with adequate tidal volume. Her color has improved, and her capillary refill time is less than 2 seconds. She moves her extremities upon command but is not able to verbally answer questions with anything other than a moan. To further aid in maintaining an open airway, you may consider inserting

    (A) a nasogastric (NG) tube
    (B) an endotracheal (ET) tube
    (C) an oropharyngeal airway (OPA)
    (D) a nasopharyngeal airway (NPA)

Your ambulance crew is called to the home of a 2-year-old child experiencing a seizure. When you arrive, the patient is lying on her side on the floor. Her parents inform you that she had a full-body seizure that lasted about 2–3 minutes. She has a past medical history of an earache for the last 3 days.

Questions 78–82

78. The appropriate method for opening this patient's airway is

    (A) turn the head to the left
    (B) hyperextend the head and neck
    (C) turn the head to the right and down
    (D) place the head in a neutral or sniffing position

79. While you are assessing this patient, she begins to seize again. Appropriate management would include

    (A) restrain the patient by holding her tightly
    (B) secure the patient to a backboard to prevent seizing
    (C) place the patient on a soft, flat surface and protect her from further harm
    (D) insert an oropharyngeal airway (OPA) in the patient's mouth and apply a nonrebreather mask

80. The seizing stops after approximately 1 minute. The patient is very slow to respond after the seizure. You should immediately

    (A) check for a pulse
    (B) check for a clear airway
    (C) look for signs of external trauma due to the seizure
    (D) begin ventilating the patient with a bag-valve mask connected to supplemental oxygen at a rate of 1 breath every 3 seconds

81. While assessing this patient, you note that her skin is hot to the touch. You assess her rectal temperature to be 103.8° Fahrenheit (F). Medical direction instructs you to "cool the patient" during transport. Which of the following methods would be appropriate?

    (A) Sponge the patient with rubbing alcohol
    (B) Sponge the patient with lukewarm water
    (C) Submerge the patient's torso in ice water
    (D) Apply ice packs to the patient's armpits, neck area, and groin

82. While you are treating this patient, a neighbor approaches one of your crew members and tells her that this patient has been abused by her parents. Your

crew member brings this to your attention. While performing a physical examination of this patient, you note bruises on her upper arms, jaw, and abdomen. You should

(A) question the parents about their suspected abusive behavior
(B) tell the neighbor to call the police if they want to file a complaint
(C) disregard the neighbor's comment since the patient's seizure is attributed to a high fever and not abuse
(D) document the physical findings, quote the neighbor's statement, and express your concern to the physician at the receiving facility

Your rescue crew is called to a hotel for a 24-year-old female patient who has threatened suicide. Local law enforcement has already secured the scene. As you enter the room, you observe that the patient is lying down in bed. She appears to be sleeping.

Questions 83–87

83. Which of the following should you address first?

(A) Open the patient's airway
(B) Attempt to wake the patient
(C) Assess the patient's surroundings
(D) Perform a rapid trauma assessment

84. When questioned, the patient opens her eyes and tells you that she wants to die. While interacting with this patient, you should

(A) avoid identifying yourself by name
(B) maintain eye contact with the patient
(C) sit or stand above the patient's level to show your authority
(D) tell the patient to keep her explanations as brief as possible

85. The patient informs you that she took approximately 20 sleeping pills and "a handful of aspirin." Which of the following regarding activated charcoal is correct?

(A) Activated charcoal is contraindicated in patients with an altered mental status
(B) Activated charcoal is administered at 1 gram per pound of patient body weight
(C) Activated charcoal is contraindicated since the patient has ingested multiple medications
(D) Activated charcoal may be given without authorization from medical direction since it is merely charcoal

86. A common side effect associated with activated charcoal administration is

(A) slurred speech
(B) unconsciousness
(C) difficulty breathing
(D) abdominal cramping

Your ambulance crew is called to a local frozen lake for an injured fisherman. Upon arrival, you find a 54-year-old male patient in wet clothing. It is a cold [23° Fahrenheit (F)] and windy day. The patient informs you he fell in the water while pulling a fish out of the water. He was able to get himself out, and the incident happened about 20 minutes ago.

87. You should immediately

(A) perform a rapid physical examination
(B) check to ensure that the patient's airway is clear
(C) move the patient to the back of your warmed ambulance
(D) give the patient something warm to drink (e.g., hot coffee or tea)

88. Which of the following signs would lead you to believe that this patient is severely hypothermic (cold)?

(A) He is shivering
(B) His muscles are stiff
(C) His heart rate is increased
(D) His pupils are slow to respond

89. Treatment for this patient should include

(A) sponging the patient with warm water
(B) massaging the muscles of the arms and legs
(C) encouraging physical exertion to promote blood flow
(D) removing wet clothing and covering the patient with a blanket

90. While performing a physical examination, you note that this patient's feet are white, cold, and hard to palpation. You attempt to remove his socks, but they appear frozen to the patient's skin. You should

(A) leave the socks in place
(B) cut the socks off the patient's feet
(C) rub his feet until the socks thaw and then remove them
(D) apply gentle but firm traction until the socks separate from the skin and come off

Your rescue crew is called to the home of a 32-year-old female patient for a "possible childbirth." You arrive to find your patient supine in bed. She is visibly pregnant and conscious and tells you when you enter the room that she thinks she is about to have the baby.

91. Which of the following should be done first?

(A) Assess baseline vital signs
(B) Check for crowning
(C) Put on gloves, mask, gown, and goggles
(D) Perform a focused history and physical examination

92. The patient informs you that she is being treated for high blood pressure associated with the pregnancy. She says that the doctor informed her that she was "preeclamptic." Treatment of this patient should include a calm environment to avoid what possible effect associated with this patient's condition?

(A) Stroke
(B) Seizures
(C) Diabetes
(D) Heart attack

93. Which of the following may indicate that birth is imminent and transportation should be delayed until the birth of the child?

(A)   The hospital is more than 15 minutes away
(B)   The mother feels that she needs to move her bowels
(C)   The contractions are 5–10 minutes apart and last about 20–30 seconds
(D)   This is the mother's first pregnancy and she has been feeling contractions for about an hour

94. Upon inspection of the birth canal, you observe that the baby's head is emerging. You should

(A)   stay back until the entire body emerges from the birth canal
(B)   grasp the head with two hands and pull while the mother pushes
(C)   apply gentle pressure against the infant's head and support it as it emerges
(D)   insert a gloved hand into the birth canal to create an airway for the infant to breathe

95. The infant's airway should first be suctioned

(A)   immediately after the entire body is delivered
(B)   immediately after the body is wiped dry and put in a warm towel
(C)   only when airway obstruction or breathing difficulties are observed
(D)   immediately after the head is delivered and before the rest of the body is delivered

Your ambulance crew is called to the scene of a motor vehicle collision. A 41-year-old woman was hit by a car while crossing the street. Upon arrival, this patient is found lying in the crosswalk. She is conscious and in severe pain.

Questions 96–97

96. A traction split may be applied to which of the following injuries?

(A)   A painful, swollen, deformed foot
(B)   A painful, swollen, deformed shin
(C)   A painful, swollen, deformed midthigh
(D)   A painful, swollen, deformed knee joint

97. When applying the traction splint, which of the following should be performed first?

(A)   Apply the support straps to the leg
(B)   Apply mechanical traction to the leg
(C)   Apply the distal securing device to the ankle
(D)   Apply the proximal securing strap to the groin area

Your ambulance crew is called to the home of a 32-year-old male patient who cut his finger while cooking. You arrive to find this patient sitting on the floor in the kitchen with a towel wrapped around his left hand. The towel is soaked with blood. The patient is conscious but appears very pale.

Questions 98–100

98. When the towel is removed to inspect the wound, you notice an open cut on the wrist. Blood is spurting from the wound. This suggests what type of bleeding?

(A)   Alveolar
(B)   Arterial
(C)   Venous
(D)   Capillary

99. Direct pressure and elevation successfully stop the bleeding; however, the patient still appears very distressed. Which of the following signs would be consistent with shock?

   (A)   An altered mental status
   (B)   A pulse rate of 60 beats per minute
   (C)   A respiratory rate of 12 breaths per minute
   (D)   A capillary refill time of less than 2 seconds

100. To treat this patient for shock, you apply a nonrebreather mask connected to oxygen at 15 liters per minute (LPM). During transport, the patient should be positioned

   (A)   sitting upright
   (B)   lying flat on his stomach (prone)
   (C)   lying with his legs elevated 8–12 inches
   (D)   lying with his legs dangling over the edge of the gurney

ANSWERS AND RATIONALES

1-C. Ongoing assessments should be performed on all patients. Ongoing assessments should evaluate the effectiveness of emergency care interventions, identify previously missed injuries or conditions, monitor the patient's progress, and alter emergency care interventions as necessary to provide appropriate patient management. These assessments should be performed at least every 5 minutes in unstable patients and at least every 15 minutes in stable patients.

2-D. The typical-size endotracheal tube for an adult female is 7.0- to 8.0-millimeter (mm) internal diameter, and the typical-size tube for an adult male is 8.0- to 8.5-mm internal diameter. The emergency rule is that, when in doubt, a 7.5-mm endotracheal tube can be used in an adult, regardless of gender.

3-D. The absorption of oxygen and the removal of waste gases take place at the alveolar-capillary membrane (the terminal air sacs in the lungs). The liver is responsible for removing some toxins from the bloodstream and producing bile for the digestion of fats. The kidneys are responsible for regulating salt and fluid levels in the body. Finally, the bronchioles are the smaller air passages that lead to the alveolar sacs; however, gases are not absorbed or removed in these air passages.

4-C. The spleen is located just below the diaphragm in the left upper abdominal quadrant. The stomach and pancreas are also located in the left upper abdominal quadrant. The liver and gallbladder are located in the right upper abdominal quadrant. The mediastinum is a term for the central portion of the chest cavity. It houses the heart, trachea, esophagus, and major blood vessels.

5-A. Daily apparatus checks should be completed with strict attention to detail. These daily checks ensure the safety of the crew, the safety of the patient, and the longevity of the vehicle. A log should be kept to record daily checks and any discrepancies noted.

6-C. To provide for adequate reaction and braking time, you should follow no closer than 4 seconds from the vehicle in front of you. At very slow speeds, 50 feet or 100 feet may be appropriate, but at high speeds these distances may be grossly inappropriate.

7-C. Nighttime landing zones should be at least 100 feet × 100 feet. The area should be secure from vehicle or pedestrian traffic and free of hazards, such as overhead power lines or unsecured objects that may become airborne from the helicopter's turbulence. This landing zone may be 60 feet × 60 feet during daylight hours.

8-D. One of the first compensatory mechanisms for patients in respiratory distress is an increase in respiratory rate. Unconsciousness is a late sign associated with severe hypoxia (low oxygen content in the blood). Agonal respirations (slow, gasping breaths) are typically seen shortly before a patient goes into cardiopulmonary arrest. Tracheal deviation is a late sign of respiratory arrest associated with chest trauma (specifically a tension pneumothorax).

9-C. Oxygen should never be withheld from a patient who needs it. However, patients with a history of emphysema or chronic bronchitis should only be given as much oxygen as necessary to treat their complaint. When treating patients with a history of emphysema or chronic bronchitis, closely monitor their respiratory rate and be prepared to assist ventilations if their breathing slows.

10-B. According to the American Heart Association, the automated external defibrillator (AED) may be applied to patients older than 8 years of age.

11-A. Blood pressure is controlled by the constriction and dilation of the blood vessels. Nitroglycerin causes vasodilation (dilation of the blood vessels), thus lowering blood pressure. The benefit of this vasodilation is that by dilating the coronary arteries, more blood is able to get to the heart muscle. Other side effects of nitroglycerin administration include headache, pulse rate changes, and dizziness.

12-D. While the automated external defibrillator (AED) is analyzing a patient's heart rhythm, you must ensure that no one is touching the patient. Cardiopulmonary resuscitation (CPR) may be stopped for as long as 90 seconds to allow for proper operation of the AED. The patient does not need to be completely disrobed for the AED to be operated; however, the entire chest should be exposed. Rescuers do not need to stand 10 feet from the patient, but rescuers should make sure that they are not in contact with any metal or liquid with which the patient is in contact.

13-A. The laryngoscope should be held in the left hand and the endotracheal tube in the right hand. The laryngoscope blade is designed to allow the endotracheal tube to be passed to the right of the blade. When inserting the laryngoscope blade, be extremely cautious not to use the patient's teeth as a fulcrum to open the airway. Practice until proficient on an intubation mannequin.

14-A. To prevent damage to the airway, the stylet should not extend beyond the tip of the endotracheal tube. However, the stylet should be extended far enough into the endotracheal tube to provide adequate support and structure for the tube. By positioning the stylet approximately 1 inch from the distal end, adequate support may be achieved.

15-C. Once a tourniquet is applied, it should not be removed outside a hospital setting. If the tourniquet is released, toxins and blood clots may enter the patient's bloodstream resulting in serious damage or death. All other techniques for controlling bleeding must be attempted before applying a tourniquet. If you are considering applying a tourniquet to a patient, contact medical direction to review your decision.

16-C. In-line cervical immobilization should be initiated as part of the initial assessment whenever the mechanism of injury suggests that head or neck injury may be present. The correct steps to immobilizing a patient to a backboard are as follows: maintain in-line immobilization, assess distal motor and sensory functions and circulation, inspect the neck (DCAP-BTLS), apply a cervical collar, apply the backboard without manipulating the patient's spine, pad any voids between the patient and the backboard, secure the patient's torso to the board, secure the patient's head to the board, secure the patient's extremities to the board, and reassess motor and sensory functions and circulation.

17-A. Infants are incapable of generating sufficient heat to keep themselves from becoming severely hypothermic; therefore, it is imperative that you thoroughly dry and warm the infant. The infant should be completely dried with soft towels; then wrapped in clean, dry towels and protected against drafts. Since approximately half of our heat is lost through the head, particular attention should be paid to carefully wrapping the infant's head while leaving the face visible for airway and breathing assessment.

18-C. Normally the placenta will deliver within about 10 to 20 minutes of the infant. You should not be overly concerned about the placenta: if it delivers, retain it for inspection at the hospital; if it does not deliver, make sure you pass that information on to the receiving facility.

19-D. Infants normally breathe at a rate of 25 to 50 breaths per minute. If your assessment of a newborn reveals slow or shallow respirations, stimulate the infant and administer 100% oxygen. If there is no improvement after 5 to 10 seconds, provide positive-pressure ventilation with 100% oxygen. If respirations are absent or gasping, begin positive-pressure ventilation with 100% oxygen immediately. Ventilate at a rate of 40 to 60 breaths per minute and reassess after 30 seconds. If there is improvement, continue ventilations and reassessments.

20-B. Meconium is a greenish black substance that lines the fetal gastrointestinal tract. If the fetus becomes distressed, he or she may have a bowel movement of this meconium. If meconium is present in the amniotic fluid, you should anticipate a distressed infant, and should take measures to ensure that the infant does not inhale meconium with his or her first breath. If meconium is present, suction the infant's airway until clear once the head has delivered. Also, once the entire body has delivered, suction the mouth and nose until clear before stimulating the infant to cry or breathe. Infants are primarily "nose breathers." The mouth should be suctioned first to be sure there is nothing for the infant to aspirate if he or she should gasp when the nose is suctioned. Suctioning should be limited to 3 to 5 seconds per attempt.

21-A. You should always wear your seat belt no matter what your position in the vehicle. While some states allow emergency vehicles to travel against traffic, make otherwise illegal turns, and drive faster than posted speed limits, you must remember that you do not, by virtue of being the operator of an emergency vehicle, automatically have the right-of-way. Your lights and sirens are a visual and auditory request to other drivers asking them to yield to you.

22-A. Unless you have received specific training in hazardous materials, you should not enter this scene. You should stage a minimum of 2000 feet from the accident scene and make sure that the appropriate agencies have been notified (e.g., fire department hazardous materials response team). If you enter the scene, you may end up becoming part of the problem rather than part of the solution.

23-C. Before splinting or immobilizing any body part, you should assess the patient's distal (on the other side of the injury) circulation, sensation, and motor function. These parameters should be reassessed after application of the splinting device to ensure that you have not caused further compromise to the injury. A tourniquet should be applied only if all other measures at controlling bleeding have failed. If the extremity is angulated at the injury, you may attempt to straighten the extremity with gentle traction (check local protocol); however, if any resistance is met, you should splint the injury in place. Tape should not be wrapped around the entire extremity. If the extremity swells, the tape may become nothing more than a large tourniquet.

24-B. Generally, impaled objects should not be removed from the body. Exceptions to this rule are impaled objects in the cheek or impaled objects that interfere with chest compressions for cardiopulmonary resuscitation (CPR) or the ability to transport the patient.

25-D. All soft tissue injuries resulting in amputation are treated the same way. First, wrap the amputated part in a sterile dressing and place in a waterproof bag. Then place the bag in a container and keep it cool (without freezing). Transport the amputated part with the patient. Submerging the part in any fluid may result in severe damage to the tissues.

26-A. A gentle flow of normal saline fluid across the affected eye may free the foreign object. Rubbing the patient's eye whether closed or open may cause the foreign object to scratch the eye more. Do not scrape the eye with anything. If a saline flush does not remove the object, the eyelid may be rolled back over a cotton-tipped applicator for better inspection and irrigation of the eye.

27-A. Any conscious, mentally competent adult may legally refuse treatment, regardless of the possible developments (e.g., death from a heart attack). You should try to convince the patient that it would be in his best interest to seek medical attention. You must inform the patient of the possible consequences of his refusal of treatment. For example, it would be appropriate to say, "Sir, do you understand that you may be having a heart attack and that by delaying or refusing medical treatment, you may suffer severe damage, possibly even death?" If the patient continues to refuse care, contact medical direction.

28-C. The focused history and physical examination should follow the initial assessment in conscious patients. Question the patient about his condition and then perform a physical examination based on the patient's complaint and presentation. Scene size-up should occur before the initial assessment. Scene size-up includes taking appropriate body substance isolation (BSI) precautions. A rapid trauma assessment would be appropriate if the patient were unconscious and unable to give you information for a focused history.

29-D. The acronym OPQRST is useful when evaluating a patient's complaint of pain or discomfort. **"O"** stands for onset: "What were you doing when the pain/discomfort began?" **"P"** stands for provoke: "Is there anything that makes this pain feel better or worse?" **"Q"** stands for quality: "Describe how the pain feels." **"R"** stands for radiation: "Does the pain stay in one place or does it move to another area?" **"S"** stands for severity: "On a scale of 1 to 10, with 10 being the most severe pain you have experienced, how would you rate this episode?" **"T"** stands for time: "How long has this been going on?" Ask open-ended questions as much as possible. AVPU is an acronym for evaluation of level of consciousness. AVPU stands for **a**lert, responds to a **v**erbal stimulus, responds to a **p**ainful stimulus, and **u**nresponsive. OSHA is the Occupational Safety and Health Administration. APGAR is an acronym used to assess a newborn. It stands for **a**ppearance, **p**ulse, **g**rimace, **a**ctivity, and **r**espiratory rate.

30-C. Because the patient's respiratory rate and tidal volume appear adequate, assisting ventilations with positive-pressure ventilation is not necessary. Your treatment should include oxygen administration by nonrebreather mask at 15 liters per minute (LPM). Do not use a nasal cannula with an oxygen flow rate of more than 6 LPM because it is uncomfortable for the patient and does not significantly increase oxygen delivery.

31-C. Before assisting a patient with nitroglycerin administration, determine the following:
- Is the patient complaining of chest pain?
- Has the patient been prescribed nitroglycerin by a physician?
- Is the prescribed nitroglycerin available?

- Have you received specific authorization from medical direction to assist this patient in taking nitroglycerin?
- Are there any contraindications for the use of nitroglycerin? [For example, systolic blood pressure is less than 100 millimeters of mercury (mm Hg), the patient has a head injury, or the patient has already taken the maximum recommended dose before the arrival of EMS personnel.]

32-B. If the patient's mental status changes, immediately reevaluate the patient's airway, breathing, circulation, and any life-threatening conditions that may have been previously overlooked. The initial assessment and any later reassessments should be done in this order. Nitroglycerin should never be given to an unconscious patient.

33-B. Once you have confirmed that the patient is apneic and pulseless, the automated external defibrillator (AED) should be applied and activated. If there is any delay in applying or activating the AED, begin cardiopulmonary resuscitation (CPR). Early defibrillation is an essential link in the "chain of survival." Intubation should not occur before the initial application and activation of the AED.

34-C. Assessing the adequacy of the patient's airway and breathing may be difficult in the patient's current position. Before moving this patient, you must immobilize her spine. If the initial assessment cannot be performed with the patient on her stomach (prone), your crew should log roll the patient onto a long backboard while maintaining in-line spinal stabilization. Cardiopulmonary resuscitation (CPR) should be initiated only if the patient is apneic (not breathing) and pulseless. If the patient is apneic and pulseless, the AED should be applied and activated.

35-C. If the patient maintains an adequate respiratory effort, a nonrebreather mask should be used. Because the patient is unconscious, it is especially important to pay close attention to the status of her airway and breathing. If the patient's breathing becomes inadequate, begin ventilating with a bag-valve mask connected to 15 liters per minute (LPM) supplemental oxygen at a rate of 1 breath every 5 seconds.

36-B. A rapid trauma assessment should follow the initial assessment for unconscious patients. The rapid trauma assessment is a head-to-toes evaluation of the patient's body regions to identify and treat injuries. Evaluation of the patient's mental status is part of the initial assessment. Taking appropriate body substance isolation (BSI) precautions is part of the scene size-up. If this patient were conscious, a focused history and physical examination would follow the initial assessment.

37-C. DCAP-BTLS is a helpful acronym to use when performing a physical examination on an injured patient. It stands for: **d**eformities, **c**ontusions (bruises), **a**brasions (scrapes), **p**unctures or penetrating wounds, **b**urns, **t**enderness to palpation, **l**acerations (cuts), and **s**welling. NFPA is the National Fire Protection Association. NTSB is the National Transportation Safety Board. CHEMTREC is the Chemical Transportation Emergency Center. CHEMTREC operates a hotline for hazardous materials information (1-800-424-9300).

38-D. Given the patient's altered mental status, more information should be obtained before deciding if the patient is mentally competent to refuse treatment. Conscious, mentally competent adults have the right to refuse care. It is your duty to ensure that the patient can make an informed decision. Tactfully and carefully attempt to allow the patient to accept your medical assessment. For example, say, "Sir, if you will permit us to ask you a few questions and take a quick look at you, we will leave you alone if there are no problems."

39-A. Hypoglycemia is a diabetic emergency that has a rapid onset. Hyperglycemia (also called diabetic ketoacidosis) develops over days or weeks. Hypoglycemia may develop if the diabetic takes too much insulin, does not eat enough after taking insulin, vomits after eating, or exercises excessively. Postictal phase is the sleepy post-seizure presentation for patients who have experienced a grand mal (full-body) seizure.

40-C. Expressed consent is the acceptance of care via verbal, nonverbal, or written communication from the patient or the patient's guardian. Implied consent applies when rescuers provide care based on the assumption that the patient would want care but is unable to express consent due to mental, physical, or emotional compromise.

41-D. The indications for administration of oral glucose include:
- The patient has a medical history of diabetes and is experiencing an altered mental status
- The patient is able to swallow
  EMT-Basics are not authorized to assist diabetic patients with the administration of insulin. Albuterol is used to treat patients with difficulty breathing. Nitroglycerin is used to treat patients with chest pain.

42-D. As part of the scene size-up, you should move the patients to a safe area. Once in the safe area, immediately begin an initial assessment of both patients. Make sure you have adequate resources to care for two potentially critical patients. You may need to request additional rescue personnel, supplies, and ambulances.

43-D. Second-degree burns, also known as partial-thickness burns, are characterized by intense pain, white or red skin with blisters, and damage to the epidermis and dermis. First-degree burns, also known as superficial burns, are characterized by pain and reddening at the site. Third-degree burns, also called full-thickness burns, appear as either white, brown, or charred skin. The burn is not painful since the underlying nerves have been destroyed. All layers of skin and some underlying tissue are destroyed by full-thickness burns.

44-B. To calculate the percent of total body surface area affected, you must use the Rule of Nines adjusted for the patient's age. For infants, each leg is equal to approximately 14% of the total body surface area. Half of each leg was affected, thus equaling 14% of the total body surface area. One arm is equal to 9% of the total body surface area. Therefore, the total percent affected is 23% (14 + 9 = 23).

45-B. The head and neck of an adult accounts for 9% of total body surface area. The chest and abdomen are an additional 18%, and one arm is another 9%. Therefore, this patient has suffered burns to approximately 36% of his total body surface area (9 + 18 + 9 = 36).

46-A. Your priority is a rapid but complete scene size-up. Specific to this incident, you need to address your safety and the safety of your crew, particularly concerning the suspected hazardous material involved. You may require additional resources, such as the fire department, a hazardous materials team, advanced-life-support (ALS) providers, law enforcement for evacuation assistance, and/or local health officials. You also need to confirm that there is only one patient exposed. Only after ensuring that the proper level of personal protective equipment is in place should you approach the patient.

47-D. Material Safety Data Sheets (MSDS) are an excellent source of initial information about specific chemicals. The Occupational Safety and Health Administration (OSHA) requires that employers have copies of the appropriate MSDS paperwork on the site and available to all employees. Information on the MSDS may play an important role in the approach, assessment, and care of this patient. CHEMTREC is the Chemical Transportation Emergency Center that operates a hotline for hazardous materials information (1-800-424-9300). The DOT (Department of Transportation) placard is the sign on shipping vessels and containers that shows the general class of material being shipped (e.g., poisonous gas, explosive agent, or flammable liquid). The NFPA 704 Hazard Classification System is a diamond-shaped diagram that shows a chemical's health dangers, flammability, reactivity, and special hazards or dangers. The NFPA 704 diagram lists the different hazards on a scale of 0 to 4, with 4 being extremely hazardous.

48-C. Treatment for chemical burns to the eyes is prompt and continuous irrigation of the affected eye. If only one eye is affected, caution should be taken to protect the unaffected eye. Acceptable irrigation solutions include normal saline or sterile water. The eye should be irrigated for a minimum of 20 minutes. Continuing irrigation until arrival at the receiving facility is preferable (check local protocol).

49-B. Typically, the responsibilities of the treatment sector are to provide care during prolonged extrication, provide care in the treatment area (if one is established), and move patients to the transportation area. Removing trapped patients is generally the duty of the extrication sector. Establishing on-scene objectives and priorities is the task of the incident commander, and coordinating the establishment of a transportation area (including landing zones) is the responsibility of the transportation sector. As tasks are concluded within a sector, personnel may be reassigned to a different sector or task.

50-D. The highest priority patients are those with airway or breathing difficulties, uncontrolled or severe bleeding, decreased mental status, severe medical problems, severe shock, or severe burns. Because the 65-year-old woman has breathing difficulty and a history of a severe medical problem, she is the highest priority patient. The 25-year-old woman without a pulse or respiratory effort is the lowest priority patient. The 10-year-old boy and the 34-year-old man fall between these two patients. To better understand your position and priorities, discuss specific triage issues with your medical director (before being involved in a similar situation).

51-B. An avulsion is characterized by an open cut with a flap of tissue, while an abrasion is a scrape. Contusions (bruises) and hematomas (a severe contusion) are closed skin injuries.

52-B. A symptom is something a patient tells you to describe a condition. A sign is something you are able to observe by visualization, listening, and/or palpating. The actual injury is a sign, but the complaint of numbness is a symptom. Vital signs are the patient's blood pressure, pulse rate, respiratory rate, skin condition, and pupil reactivity. A pertinent negative is the absence of a particular condition generally associated with the patient's complaint. For example, the ability to speak in complete sentences without difficulty is a pertinent negative for a patient complaining of difficulty breathing.

53-A. When a flap of tissue is present with an open injury to the skin, the flap should be realigned in its original position and direct pressure applied with a sterile dressing to control bleeding. Elevating the injury above the level of the heart may assist in controlling bleeding. If bleeding is still profuse after your initial efforts, the dressing may be removed momentarily to confirm that direct pressure is being applied over the correct area. If direct pressure fails to stop bleeding, the next step is indirect pressure (arterial pressure point). The closest arterial pressure point should be compressed with continued direct pressure. The last measure to take is the application of a tourniquet. A tourniquet should be reserved for exceptional instances when severe, life-threatening bleeding cannot be controlled by any other means, and transportation is delayed or lengthy. When in doubt, contact medical direction.

54-C. Not all patients respond in the same way under similar circumstances. Likewise, not all care providers react in the same way in similar situations. People cope with emotional trauma in different ways, and some need professional help to cope with this trauma. The need for professional help is not a sign of weakness, but another illustration of how different we are as individuals.

55-C. If the parent or guardian of a minor patient is present, you must receive expressed consent to treat the patient. However, in the absence of a parent or guardian, you may assess and treat a minor patient if serious injury or illness exists.

56-B. For conscious patients, the focused history and physical exam should follow the initial assessment. During the focused history and physical examination, information should be sought regarding the patient's present condition, past history, and pertinent physical findings related to the current complaint. A rapid trauma assessment would follow the initial assessment if the patient were unconscious. Certain criteria must be met before you can assist the patient with administering a medication, and intubation does not appear necessary for this patient at this time.

57-C. Wheezes are the whistling sounds created as air moves through narrowed bronchiole passages. Wheezing is generally more noticeable on exhalation than inhalation. Wheezes may be caused by asthma, chronic obstructive pulmonary disease, infection, allergies, cardiac problems, or physical exertion. Stridor is an abnormal breathing sound associated with upper airway obstruction. It is generally more noticeable on inhalation. Rhonchi are harsh, low-pitched sounds of the lower airway created by the accumulation of fluid or mucus in the larger air passages. Rales or crackles are an intermittent high-pitched "popping" sound produced as air moves through fluid in the lower air passages.

58-B. Metered-dose inhaler medications should be shaken before administration to allow atomization of a full dose. These medications are commonly prescribed for children with a history of respiratory distress. These medications are absorbed at the alveolar-capillary membrane; therefore, it is important that the patient be capable of taking a deep breath so the medication reaches this membrane.

59-B. A base station is a stationary transmitter/receiver that can typically transmit 45–275 watts. A land line is another term for traditional telephone communication. A portable radio is also called a hand held radio. These units typically have a power output of 1 to 5 watts. A portable radio is generally mounted in a vehicle (ambulance or fire truck) and puts out about 20–50 watts of transmitting power.

60-B. Get in the habit of repeating any orders given by medical direction. For example, if medical direction says, "Go ahead and assist this patient with administering his metered-dose inhaler for a maximum of three doses," your reply should be, "Copy, we will assist the patient in administering his metered-dose albuterol for a maximum of three doses." You need not begin the albuterol therapy before ending communication with the physician, and reestablishing communication to update the receiving facility about the patient's response to the albuterol is optional. Since this communication is being transmitted over radio frequencies that may be monitored, protect the patient's right to privacy by not transmitting his full name, parents' names, or home address.

61-B. Since this medication is absorbed in the alveoli, it is imperative that this patient inhale the medication as deeply as possible. Coach the patient to exhale completely, then simultaneously inhale deeply and depress the inhaler. Instruct the patient to momentarily hold his breath at maximum inhalation before exhaling.

62-D. If this patient is capable of processing information and making coherent decisions, he may refuse your assistance regardless of whether you agree with his decision. Your job is to ensure that the patient understands your intent and the possible consequences of refusing care. You should, as always, be nonthreatening, patient, and understanding. However, you must be very careful about addressing the possible consequences of refusing care: "Sir, I understand that you have been feeling poorly since your vehicle crash three days ago. There is a possibility that your current condition is related to an injury you sustained because of that crash. I am very concerned that you may have suffered an injury to the brain. By refusing or delaying care, you may suffer permanent damage or even die. Do you understand what I am telling you?"

63-C. Preferably, this form would be witnessed by someone other than your crew or other emergency response personnel. Explain the refusal to both the patient and his wife, allow time for questions, and have both sign the form. Make sure that you inform them that signing the refusal form does not preclude them from calling for assistance later if the patient changes his mind.

64-B. This patient appears to be on the verge of passing out. Your initial concern (after the scene size-up) should be to protect the patient from further harm. Lay the patient down (be careful not to lay the patient down in an area where there may be more bees) and then begin your initial assessment. Never spray a patient with any chemical not specifically authorized by medical direction. Inquiries about medical history and prescribed medications should be conducted during the focused history and physical examination that follows the initial assessment.

65-D. A decreasing mental status may be attributed to the onset of shock and a decrease in the oxygen reaching the brain. A few of the other signs associated with a severe allergic reaction may include swelling of the face, neck, hands, or feet, hives, flushed (red) skin, abnormal breathing sounds, rapid breathing, decreased blood pressure, and a feeling of impending doom. Battle's sign (bruising behind the ears) and raccoon eyes (bilateral black eyes) are associated with head trauma, specifically a skull fracture. A one-sided facial droop is generally attributed to neurological damage such as a cerebrovascular accident (stroke).

66-B. Adrenalin® is a trade name of epinephrine, the medication prescribed in auto-injectors for anaphylaxis (severe allergic reactions). Atrovent® is a trade name for a bronchodilator, as is Bronkosol®. Solu-Medrol® is a trade name for a steroid medication that may be given by advanced-life-support (ALS) personnel or by hospital personnel for patients in anaphylaxis.

67-A. This common effect from the administration of an epinephrine auto-injector is a local effect, since it occurs at the injection site. A systemic effect is an effect that occurs as the result of a medication being absorbed into the bloodstream and distributed throughout the body. An adverse effect is an unintended and undesirable response to a medication. An idiosyncratic effect is a reaction to the drug that is peculiar to an individual and not usually seen in the general population.

68-C. For unconscious patients, a rapid trauma assessment should follow the initial assessment. It would not make sense to attempt a focused history and physical examination if the patient is unable to respond to your questions. Oral glucose should never be given to an unconscious patient due to possible airway compromise. Intubation may be performed later if the patient remains unable to protect his own airway and you are authorized to perform this skill.

69-B. Conduction is the transfer of energy through direct contact. Radiation is the transfer of energy as light waves while convection is the transfer of energy by air or fluid currents. Evaporation is the change in the physical characteristic from a liquid to a gas.

70-B. Your initial action should be to protect this patient from further harm. Here, the oppressive weather is causing the harm. Allowing this patient to remain in the heat may cause his condition to worsen. Nothing should be put in this patient's mouth due to possible airway compromise. Questioning bystanders and looking for clues to help put all the pieces of the puzzle together should be done only after ensuring the safety and appropriate management of this unstable patient.

71-D. Proper lifting technique would include making sure you have adequate personnel available to move this patient, using the leg muscles to do most of the work, and maintaining a wide stance for increased stability.

72-C. This patient needs to be aggressively cooled before permanent neurological damage sets in. Apply cool packs to the groin, armpits, and the back of the neck. Keep the patient's skin moist with cool water, and facilitate evaporation with aggressive fanning. Elevating the legs and slowly cooling with tepid water, while appropriate for moderate heat exposure patients, would not be appropriate due to this patient's level of distress.

73-C. Appropriate management for a conscious child (1–8 years of age) with an airway obstruction is subdiaphragmatic abdominal thrusts. Rather than lifting the patient off the ground, you must kneel to be level with the patient. Never sweep your finger through the mouth of any conscious patient. Back blows and chest thrusts would be appropriate if this patient were an infant (younger than 1 year of age).

74-C. With the patient supine, you should visualize the airway for obstruction, attempt to ventilate, reposition and reattempt to ventilate, then deliver 5 abdominal thrusts with one hand placed between the xiphoid process and navel. Place your other hand on top of the first. Press both hands into the abdomen. With a quick upward thrust, perform a series of 5 thrusts. Intubation would not be appropriate since it would not bypass the obstruction. Application of the automated external defibrillator (AED) is also not appropriate due to the patient's age and the fact that you must first correct airway problems before addressing possible cardiac problems.

75-D. The patient is not breathing but does have a pulse; therefore, you should begin rescue breathing (ventilations) with a bag-valve mask connected to supplemental oxygen. The rate of ventilation for a child is 1 breath every 3 seconds, or 20 breaths per minute.

76-C. This patient should be immediately log rolled onto her side to prevent vomitus from entering the lungs. Suction should be applied with a rigid catheter. Activate suction while withdrawing the catheter. Since this patient is a child, suctioning should not last more than 5 seconds per attempt (10 seconds for adults). A nasogastric (NG) tube may be inserted after suctioning to facilitate the decompression of the stomach, thus decreasing the chances of subsequent vomiting.

77-D. A nasopharyngeal airway (NPA) may be tolerated by semiconscious patients, whereas an oropharyngeal airway (OPA) would not be tolerated. A nasogastric (NG) tube may prevent further vomiting, but it does not aid in maintaining an open airway. While an endotracheal tube provides maximum airway protection, it is not indicated since this patient seems to be regaining consciousness. She would most likely cough and gag while the endotracheal tube was being inserted and pull on or bite the tube as she becomes more alert.

78-D. The appropriate method for opening the airway of an infant (younger than 1 year of age) is to place the airway in a neutral or sniffing position. If the airway is hyperextended, the windpipe (trachea) may kink, creating an even greater airway problem. Turning the head to either side may fail to remove the tongue from the back of the throat, thus resulting in an obstructed airway.

79-C. Do not attempt to restrain a seizing patient. During an active seizure, direct your efforts at preventing further harm to the patient. This can be done by putting a pad between the patient's head and the ground and moving any objects out of the patient's path. Inserting an oropharyngeal airway (OPA) during an active seizure may cause further harm to the patient.

80-B. After the seizure, you should reassess the initial assessment parameters starting with an evaluation of the patient's airway. Patients often have a build-up of saliva in the mouth following a seizure. You may need to suction the airway. If you determine during the assessment of the patient's breathing status that her respiratory effort is inadequate, begin artificial ventilations with a bag-valve mask at a rate of 1 breath every 3 seconds. Assessment of circulatory status should occur after airway and breathing assessment, as would an inspection for injury (external trauma).

81-B. You should attempt to cool the patient gradually. Ice packs or ice water would most likely cause the patient to shiver, thus increasing heat production. Lukewarm water is ideal for gradually bringing a febrile infant's temperature down. Rubbing alcohol should never be used to cool a patient.

82-D. As an EMT-Basic, you are responsible for ensuring that claims of abuse are brought to the attention of the appropriate personnel (physician, law enforcement, or whatever local protocol dictates). Carefully document your physical findings without bias. Your documentation should not include any of your conclusions or assumptions. Include what you were told by the neighbor by quoting the neighbor's exact words. Attempt to get the neighbor's name or address to pass on to the appropriate authorities for investigation.

83-C. Your first actions should be a rapid but thorough scene size-up. In particular, look for any weapons, medication bottles, alcohol, suicide notes, or blood. After the scene size-up, immediately begin your initial assessment. Be extremely cautious, as this patient has the potential for becoming violent.

84-B. Maintaining eye contact with the patient is important in establishing a trusting relationship. Identify yourself. "Hi, my name is Greg" sounds much better than "I am EMT-Basic Jeffries." Attempt to stay at the patient's eye level. Rather than showing authority, you should show competence and compassion. Do not rush this patient. It may take some time to establish rapport.

85-A. Since activated charcoal is given orally, it is contraindicated in patients with an altered mental status due to airway concerns. It is also contraindicated in patients who have ingested acids or alkalis or are unable to swallow for any reason. You must obtain authorization to administer this medication. The correct dose is 1 gram of activated charcoal per kilogram (2.2 pounds) of body weight.

86-D. The side effects associated with activated charcoal administration include abdominal cramping, constipation, and black stools. Some patients may vomit from taking activated charcoal. If a patient exhibits slurred speech, unconsciousness, or difficulty breathing, it is most likely that the ingested poison has caused these effects, not the activated charcoal.

87-C. Consider this part of the scene size-up under the heading of safety. This patient is in danger of becoming more severely injured from staying out in the cold weather. On cold days, you should always preheat your ambulance before arriving at the scene of any injury or illness. Preserving a patient's body temperature is an important part of treating shock. The ambulance should always be brought as close to the patient as feasible for the scene. Once in the back of the ambulance, you should begin the initial assessment. Hypothermic patients should not be encouraged to drink any caffeinated products or other stimulants.

88-D. A very late sign associated with cold exposure compensation is a sluggish response of the pupils. Early signs of cold exposure include increased heart rate, cool skin, shivering, stiffness, and difficulty speaking. Late signs include low or absent blood pressure; muscular rigidity (more severe than stiff); slow or absent breathing; slowly responding pupils; and an irregular, slow, or barely palpable pulse rate.

89-D. The patient's wet clothing will continue to draw heat out of his body and should be removed. A blanket should cover the patient's entire body with only the face showing to allow evaluation of airway and breathing status. Sponging the patient with warm water will cause the patient to cool further due to evaporation. Massage or physical movement should be avoided. The blood in the extremities is most likely colder than the blood at the core. Massage or physical movement may shunt this cold blood to the body core and possibly cause cardiopulmonary arrest.

90-A. If you forcibly attempt to remove the patient's frozen clothing, you may end up tearing the patient's skin and underlying tissues. Leave the socks in place until they thaw on their own, then remove.

91-C. As part of your scene size-up, you should initiate body substance isolation (BSI) precautions. Full-body BSI precautions are a must. Only after fully protecting yourself should you approach and assess this patient. Any rescuer who may potentially assist in treating this patient or the infant should take full-body BSI precautions before entering the scene.

92-B. In addition to high blood pressure, other signs associated with preeclampsia are abnormal weight gain; swelling of the hands, face, and lower back; visual disturbances; headaches; irritability; and right upper abdominal quadrant pain. The real danger with preeclampsia is the possibility that it will progress to seizures (eclampsia). The mortality rate of pregnancy-related seizures is relatively high for both mother and infant. Since seizures may be induced by rough handling, flashing or bright lights, or loud noises, you must manage preeclamptic patients with great care.

93-B. It is common for a woman in labor to have the sensation that she needs to move her bowels immediately before delivery. As the infant enters the birth canal, the nerves of the rectum are stimulated due to the size of the head. This gives the sensation that the bowels need to be moved. Do not allow the mother to leave the room to move her bowels. Other signs of imminent delivery are crowning (observing the infant's head at the vaginal opening) and regular contractions lasting 45–60 seconds that are 1–2 minutes apart.

94-C. Gentle pressure against the infant's head helps reduce the possibility of an "explosive" birth that may cause serious trauma to the mother's perineum (the area between the vagina and the anus). Be very cautious to avoid pressing on the fontanels (soft spots on the head where the skull is not yet fused). Provide support for the head as it emerges.

95-D. When the head has delivered, tell the mother to stop pushing and "breathe through" the contractions. This will allow you time to suction the infant's mouth and nose with a bulb syringe. When using the bulb syringe, make sure to depress the syringe before inserting it in the infant's airway. Suction the mouth and nasal passages until clear. Then help delivery of the top shoulder and finally the bottom shoulder. Once the shoulders have delivered, the rest of the infant will emerge quickly.

96-C. Traction splints may be applied to closed midthigh injuries if no trauma exists to the pelvis, knee, or lower leg. The traction splint helps relieve pain and reduces injury by pulling fractured bone ends back in line with each other.

97-D. The steps for application of the traction splint are as follows: assess distal motor and sensory functions and circulation, manually stabilize the leg, apply manual traction until the patient experiences a relief of pain or both legs are the same length, adjust the splint to proper length and position on injured leg, apply the proximal strap to groin/waist, apply the distal securing device to the ankle, apply mechanical traction, apply support straps to leg, reevaluate all straps, and reevaluate motor and sensory functions and circulation.

98-B. Arterial bleeding is characterized by spurting bright red blood; it is rapid and potentially severe. Venous bleeding is characterized by a continuous flow of dark-red blood, while capillary bleeds appear as an oozing wound with clear or blood-tinged fluid. Alveoli are the air sacs in the lungs.

99-A. Some signs of hypoperfusion (shock) include an altered mental status (from poor perfusion of the brain); a rapid heart rate; rapid, shallow breathing; dilated pupils; and nausea. In children under the age of 6, delayed capillary refill time (greater than 2 seconds) is associated with shock; however, capillary refill is not accurate in patients older than 6 years of age.

100-C. If spinal immobilization is not indicated, patients in shock should be transported with their legs slightly elevated. If the patient were transported sitting upright, gravity would work against blood being pumped to the brain. If the patient were transported prone, it would be more difficult to reassess the patient's airway and breathing. If the patient were transported with his legs dangling over the edge of the gurney, the heart would have to work harder to pump the blood back from the legs due to gravity.

INDEX

Note: Page numbers in *italic* indicate illustrations, those followed by t indicate tables.